EIGHTH EDITION

IMMUNOLOGY

David Male PhD MA
Professor of Biology
Department of Life Sciences
The Open University
Milton Keynes, UK

Jonathan Brostoff MA DM DSc FRCP FRCPath FIBiol
Professor Emeritus of Allergy and Environmental Health
School of Biomedical and Health Sciences
King's College London
London, UK

David B Roth MD PhD
Simon Flexner Professor and Chair of Pathology and Laboratory Medicine
Department of Pathology and Laboratory Medicine
University of Pennsylvania
Philadelphia, Pennsylvania, USA

Ivan M Roitt MA DSc (Oxon) Hon FRCP (Lon) FRCPath FRS
Director, Centre for Investigative and Diagnostic Oncology
Middlesex University
London, UK

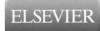
ELSEVIER

ELSEVIER
SAUNDERS

Notice
Knowledge and best practice in this field are constantly changing. As new research and experience broaden our knowledge, changes in practice, treatment and drug therapy may become necessary or appropriate. Readers are advised to check the most current information provided (i) on procedures featured or (ii) by the manufacturer of each product to be administered, to verify the recommended dose or formula, the method and duration of administration, and contraindications. It is the responsibility of the practitioner, relying on their own experience and knowledge of the patient, to make diagnoses, to determine dosages and the best treatment for each individual patient, and to take all appropriate safety precautions. To the fullest extent of the law, neither the Publisher nor the Editors assumes any liability for any injury and/or damage to persons or property arising out of or related to any use of the material contained in this book.

The Publisher

British Library Cataloguing in Publication Data
A catalogue record for this book is available from the British Library.

Library of Congress Cataloging in Publication Data
A catalog record for this book is available from the Library of Congress.

Main edition
ISBN: 978-0-323-08058-3

International edition
ISBN: 978-0-702-04548-6

Printed in China.

your source for books,
journals and multimedia
in the health sciences

www.elsevierhealth.com

Working together to grow
libraries in developing countries

www.elsevier.com | www.bookaid.org | www.sabre.org

ELSEVIER   BOOK AID
              International   Sabre Foundation

The
Publisher's
policy is to use
**paper manufactured
from sustainable forests**

Contents

Contents

Preface

In previous editions of *Immunology*, we have used the preface to outline the major immunological advances that have taken place since the previous edition. Recently, however, advances in the teaching of biomedical science have been just as striking as advances in immunology. Students now learn from a variety of interlinked media, including books, DVDs, and websites. This edition of *Immunology* reflects these changes in science teaching. We have produced this edition as an integrated teaching package, which is presented in two formats. In both cases they can be read as a continuous narrative but they have slightly different content:

- the book contains what we consider to be the core areas and concepts of immunology
- the electronic teaching package includes all the material in the book, plus additional sections within the chapters, which expand on the core material and provide background on immunological methods. It also provides active links to the publisher's website and external websites, and allows more innovative use of video and questions within the text and at the end of the chapters.

Moreover, the availability of much essential information online means that it is now better to provide links to websites that are updated regularly, rather than rely on printed tables of, for example, CD molecules and cytokines.

In the past 5 years, there have also been major advances in immunology, particularly in our understanding of innate immune defenses, and immune recognition systems. These evolutionarily ancient mechanisms for recognizing pathogen, have been retained in mammals and indeed have developed alongside the adaptive immune system. In the eighth edition of *Immunology*, we have expanded on innate immunity throughout the text. This truly reflects the way the immune system operates with the integration of ancient and recently-evolved immune defenses.

Other areas that receive greater coverage are tissue-specific immune defenses, T cell subsets and the use of monoclonal antibodies in disease therapy. It is very exciting to see how advances in antibody technology have now combined with our knowledge of the immune system to provide effective treatments for a number of diseases, including multiple sclerosis and rheumatoid arthritis.

Despite these changes, we have retained the overall organization of the subject material within five sections. The opening section describes the building blocks of the immune system – cells, organs, complement, and the major receptor molecules, including antibodies, T cell receptors, and MHC molecules. The second section deals with the initiation of the immune response starting with innate defenses and mononuclear phagocytes. The unit on antigen presentation, costimulation and cell activation pathways precedes units on the principal effector arms of the immune response, TH2 responses with antibody production, TH1 responses and mononuclear phagocytes, TH17 cells and inflammation and the functions of cytotoxic T cells and NK cells. The final units in this section look into the regulation of the immune response, and there is an expanded unit on the distinctive types of immune response that develop in different tissues of the body. Although it has long been recognized that immune responses in tissues vary, the underlying reasons for the differences are only just being elucidated.

Section three describes the immune responses that develop against different types of infection, and how immunodeficiency leads to increased susceptibility to particular infections. Indeed the diversity and complexity of the immune system can only be understood in relation to the diversity of the pathogens which it protects against. In recent years, the devious strategies employed by pathogens to evade immune responses have provided some quite startling revelations, both on the adaptability of the pathogens and on the flexibility of the immune system. Ultimately the immune system can only be understood in relation to its principal function – defense against pathogens.

Section four describes immune responses against tissues, and section five hypersensitivity. These areas are of great clinical importance. One aim of this book is to provide readers with a sound understanding of the immune responses which underlie clinically important areas including hypersensitivity states and allergy, immunopathology, tumor immunotherapy, and transplantation. In these sections, we have maintained what we believe to be an important feature of the book, namely a clear description of the scientific principles of clinical immunology, integrated with histology, pathology, and clinical examples.

A feature of the text is the inclusion of in-text questions. These are designed to check that the reader understands the implications of the preceding paragraphs or can relate that material to information in earlier units. Another useful learning aid is the critical thinking sections at the end of each unit. Finally, we have put a lot of care into the summaries, ensuring that they really do distil the key aspects, into a manageable overview. The summaries make an excellent revision guide for exams, in addition to setting the framework for each subject area.

The contributors to this volume include many experts in different areas of immunology, including 14 new contributors who have brought new perspectives on their own areas of expertise. We also greatly appreciate the hard work of our publishers and their colleagues, particularly, Andrea Vosburgh, Lucy Boon and Madelene Hyde from Elsevier.

Immunology bridges basic sciences and medicine and encompasses approaches from numerous fields, including biochemistry, genetics, cell biology, structural biology and molecular biology. For the past century, immunology has fascinated and inspired some of the greatest scientific thinkers of our time. We wish our readers well in their study of immunology, a subject which continues to excite and surprise us, and which underpins many other areas of biology and biomedical sciences.

David Male
Jonathan Brostoff
David Roth
Ivan Roitt 2012

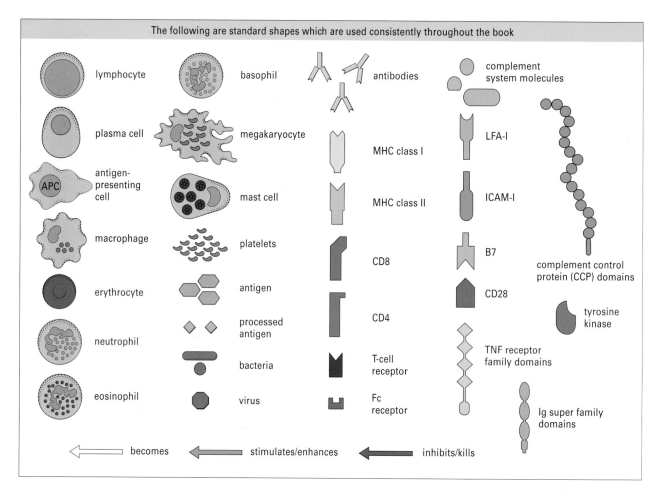

– where this icon is found in the margin, it indicates more material is available on studentconsult.com

List of Contributors

Gregory J Bancroft BSc(Hons) PhD
Reader
Department of Immunology and Infection
London School of Hygiene and Tropical Medicine
London, UK

David Bending MA PhD
Arthritis Research UK Foundation Fellow
UCL, Institute of Child Health
London, UK

Persephone Borrow PhD
Reader
Nuffield Department of Clinical Medicine
University of Oxford
Oxford, UK

Warwick J Britton PhD MB BS BScMed FRACP FRCP FRCPA DTM&H
Bosch Professor of Medicine and Professor
of Immunology
Department of Medicine
Sydney Medical School
University of Sydney;
Head, Mycobacterial Research Program
Centenary Institute
Sydney, NSW, Australia

Jonathan Brostoff MA DM DSc FRCP FRCPath FIBiol
Professor Emeritus of Allergy and Environmental Health
School of Biomedical and Health Sciences
King's College London
London, UK

Colin Casimir BSc PhD
Senior Lecturer
Department of Natural Sciences
Middlesex University
London, UK

David P D'Cruz MD FRCP
Consultant Rheumatologist and Reader
The Louise Coote Lupus Unit
St Thomas' Hospital
London, UK

Andrew J T George MA PhD FRCPath FHEA FRSA
Professor of Molecular Immunology
Department of Immunology, Division of Medicine
Imperial College London
London, UK

Siamon Gordon MBDhB PhD
Glaxo Wellcome Professor of Cellular Pathology
Emeritus
Sir William Dunn School of Pathology
Oxford University
Oxford, UK

David A Isenberg
The Centre for Rheumatology Research
Department of Medicine
University College London
London, UK

Roy Jefferis BSc PhD FRSC CChem MRCP FRCPath DSc
Professor Emeritus
School of Immunity and Infection
University of Birmingham
Birmingham, West Midlands, UK

Thomas Kamradt Dr med
Professor
Institute of Immunology
University of Jena
Jena, Germany

Dean H Kedes BSc PhD MD
Associate Professor
Myles H Thaler Center for AIDS and
Retrovirology Research
Departments of Microbiology and Medicine
University of Virginia
Charlottesville, Virginia, USA

Peter M Lydyard MSc PhD FRCPath
Emeritus Professor
Division of Infection and Immunity
University College London;
Visiting Professor
School of Biosciences
University of Westminster;
Emeritus Professor
Medical and Healthcare Education
St George's University of London
London; UK

David Male PhD MA
Professor of Biology
Department of Life Sciences
The Open University
Milton Keynes, UK

Victoria Male MA PhD
Faculty of Natural Science
Imperial College London
London, UK

Joseph C Marini PhD
Centocor Research and Development, Inc.
Radnor, Pennsylvania, USA

Luisa Martinez-Pomares BSc PhD
Lecturer
Faculty of Medicine and Health Services
School of Molecular Medical Sciences
University of Nottingham
Nottingham, UK

B Paul Morgan BSc MBChB PhD FRCPath MRCP
Dean of Medicine
School of Medicine
Cardiff University
Cardiff, UK

Anthony A Nash PhD FRSE FmedSci
Professor
The Roslin Institute
University of Edinburgh
Edinburgh, UK

Lisa A Nichols PhD
Research Associate
Department of Microbiology
University of Virginia
Charlottesville, Virginia, USA

Luigi D Notarangelo MD
Professor of Pediatrics and Pathology
Department of Medicine
Children's Hospital Boston;
Harvard Medical School
Boston, Massachusetts, USA

James E Peters MBChB MRCP BSc
Dr, Centre for Rheumatology
Department of Medicine
University College London
London, UK

Thomas A E Platts-Mills MD PhD FRS
Head, Asthma and Allergic Disease Center
Department of Medicine
University of Virginia
Charlottesville, Virginia, USA

Richard J Pleass PhD
Professor
Department of Molecular Parasitology
Liverpool School of Tropical Medicine
Liverpool, UK

Nino Porakishvili PhD
Dr, School of Life Sciences
University of Westminster
London, UK;
Emeritus Professor
Department of Immunology and Microbiology
Javakishvili Tbilisi State University
Tbilisi, Georgia

Ivan M Roitt MA DSC (Oxon) Hon FRCP (Lon) FRCPath FRS
Director, Centre for Investigative
and Diagnostic Oncology
Middlesex University
London, UK

David B Roth MD PhD
Simon Flexner Professor and Chair of Pathology
and Laboratory Medicine
Department of Pathology and Laboratory Medicine
University of Pennsylvania
Philadelphia, Pennsylvania, USA

Pramod K Srivastava PhD MD
Professor and Chairman
Department of Immunology
University of Connecticut School of Medicine
Farmington, Connecticut, USA

Kalpit A Vora PhD
Vaccine Basic Research
Merck Research Laboratory
West Point, Pennsylvania, USA

Components of the Immune System

CHAPTER 1

Introduction to the Immune System

SUMMARY

- **The immune system has evolved to protect us from pathogens.** Intracellular pathogens infect individual cells (e.g. viruses), whereas extracellular pathogens divide outside cells in blood, tissues or the body cavities (e.g. many bacteria and parasites). These two kinds of pathogens require fundamentally different immune responses.

- **Phagocytes and lymphocytes are key mediators of immunity.** Phagocytes internalize pathogens and degrade them. Lymphocytes (B and T cells) have receptors that recognize specific molecular components of pathogens and have specialized functions. B cells make antibodies (effective against extracellular pathogens), cytotoxic T lymphocytes (CTLs) kill virally infected cells, and helper T cells coordinate the immune response by direct cell–cell interactions and the release of cytokines.

- **Specificity and memory are two essential features of adaptive immune responses.** As a result, the adaptive arm of the immune system (B and T lymphocytes) mounts a more effective response on second and subsequent encounters with a particular antigen. Non-adaptive (innate) immune responses (mediated, for example, by complement, phagocytes, and natural killer cells) do not alter on repeated exposure to an infectious agent.

- **Antigens are molecules that are recognized by receptors on lymphocytes.** B cells usually recognize intact antigen molecules, whereas T cells recognize antigen fragments displayed on the surface of the body's own cells.

- **An immune response occurs in two phases – antigen recognition and antigen eradication.** In the first phase clonal selection involves recognition of antigen by particular clones of lymphocytes, leading to clonal expansion of specific clones of T and B cells and differentiation to effector and memory cells. In the effector phase, these lymphocytes coordinate an immune response, which eliminates the source of the antigen.

- **Vaccination depends on the specificity and memory of adaptive immunity.** Vaccination is based on the key elements of adaptive immunity, namely specificity and memory. Memory cells allow the immune system to mount a much stronger and more rapid response on a second encounter with antigen.

- **Inflammation is a response to tissue damage.** It allows antibodies, complement system molecules, and leukocytes to enter the tissue at the site of infection, resulting in phagocytosis and destruction of the pathogens. Lymphocytes are also required to recognize and destroy infected cells in the tissues.

- **The immune system may fail (immunopathology).** This can be a result of immunodeficiency, hypersensitivity, or dysregulation leading to autoimmune diseases.

- **Normal immune reactions can be inconvenient in modern medicine**, for example blood transfusion reactions and graft rejection.

The immune system is fundamental to survival, as it protects the body from **pathogens**, viruses, bacteria and parasites that cause disease. To do so, it has evolved a powerful collection of defense mechanisms to recognize and protect against potential invaders that would otherwise take advantage of the rich source of nutrients provided by the vertebrate host. At the same time it must differentiate between the individual's own cells and those of harmful invading organisms while not attacking the beneficial commensal flora that inhabit the gut, skin, and other tissues.

This chapter provides an overview of the complex network of processes that form the immune system of higher vertebrates. It:

- illustrates how the components of the immune system fit together to allow students to grasp the 'big picture' before delving into the material in more depth in subsequent chapters;

- introduces the basic elements of the immune system and of immune responses, which are mediated principally by white blood cells or **leukocytes** (from the Greek for 'white cell') and are detailed in Chapters 2–12.

Over many millions of years, different types of immune defense, appropriate to the infecting pathogens, have evolved in different groups of organisms. In this book, we concentrate on the immune systems of mammals, especially humans. Because mammals are warm-blooded and long-lived, their immune systems have evolved particularly sophisticated systems for recognizing and destroying pathogens.

Q. Why do warm-blooded, long-lived animals require particularly complex immune defenses?
A. Infectious agents such as bacteria can divide rapidly in warm-blooded creatures. Animals have to remain healthy during their reproductive years to raise offspring.

Many of the immune defenses that have evolved in other vertebrates (e.g. reptiles, amphibians) and other phyla (e.g. sponges, worms, insects) are also present in some form in mammals. Consequently the mammalian immune system consists of multi-layered, interlocking defense mechanisms that incorporate both primitive and recently evolved elements.

Cells and soluble mediators of the immune system

Cells of the immune system

Immune responses are mediated by a variety of cells and the soluble molecules that these cells secrete (Fig. 1.1). Although the leukocytes are central to all immune responses, other cells in the tissues also participate, by signaling to the lymphocytes and responding to the cytokines (soluble intercellular signaling molecules) released by T cells and macrophages.

Phagocytes internalize antigens and pathogens, and break them down

The most important long-lived phagocytic cells belong to the **mononuclear phagocyte** lineage. These cells are all derived from bone marrow stem cells, and their function is to engulf particles, including infectious agents, internalize them and destroy them. To do so, mononuclear phagocytes have surface receptors that allow them to recognize and bind to a wide variety of microbial macromolecules. They can then internalize and kill the micro-organism (Fig. 1.2). The process of **phagocytosis** describes the internalization (endocytosis) of large particles or microbes. The primitive responses of phagocytes are highly effective, and people with genetic defects in phagocytic cells often succumb to infections in infancy.

To intercept pathogens, mononuclear phagocytes are strategically placed where they will encounter them. For example, the Kupffer cells of the liver line the sinusoids along which blood flows, while the synovial A cells line the synovial cavity (Fig. 1.3).

Leukocytes of the mononuclear phagocyte lineage are called **monocytes**. These cells migrate from the blood into the tissues, where they develop into tissue **macrophages**.

Polymorphonuclear neutrophils (often just called **neutrophils** or **PMNs**) are another important group of phagocytes. Neutrophils constitute the majority of the blood leukocytes and develop from the same early precursors as monocytes and macrophages. Like monocytes, neutrophils migrate into tissues, particularly at sites of inflammation, However, neutrophils are short-lived cells that phagocytose material, destroy it, and then die within a few days.

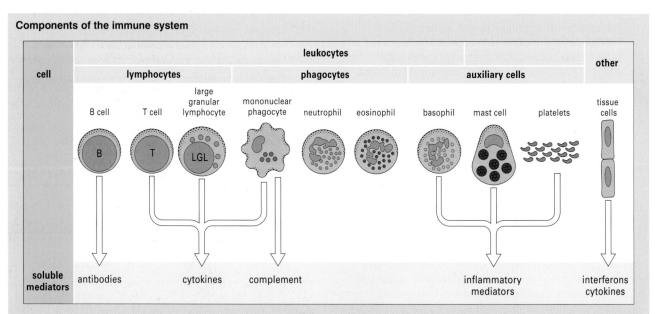

Fig. 1.1 The principal cells of the immune system and the mediators they produce are shown. Neutrophils, eosinophils, and basophils are collectively known as polymorphonuclear granulocytes (see Chapter 2). Cytotoxic cells include cytotoxic T lymphocytes (CTLs), natural killer (NK) cells (large granular lymphocytes [LGLs]), and eosinophils. Complement is made primarily by the liver, though there is some synthesis by mononuclear phagocytes. Note that each cell produces and secretes only a particular set of cytokines or inflammatory mediators.

Phagocytes internalize and kill invading organisms

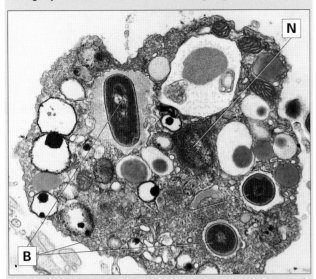

Fig. 1.2 Electron micrograph of a phagocyte from a tunicate (sea squirt) that has endocytosed three bacteria (B). (N, nucleus.) *(Courtesy of Dr AF Rowley.)*

Cells of the mononuclear phagocyte lineage

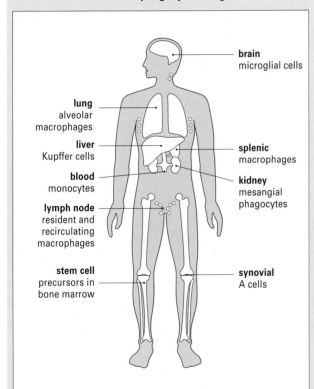

Fig. 1.3 Many organs contain cells belonging to the mononuclear phagocyte lineage. These cells are derived from blood monocytes and ultimately from stem cells in the bone marrow.

B cells and T cells are responsible for the specific recognition of antigens

Adaptive immune responses are mediated by a specialized group of leukocytes, the **lymphocytes**, which include T and B lymphocytes (T cells and B cells) that specifically recognize foreign material or **antigens**. All lymphocytes are derived from bone marrow stem cells, but T cells then develop in the thymus, while B cells develop in the bone marrow (in adult mammals).

These two classes of lymphocytes carry out very different protective functions:

- **B cells** are responsible for the production of antibodies that act against extracellular pathogens
- **T cells** are mainly concerned with cellular immune responses to intracellular pathogens, such as viruses. They also regulate the responses of B cells and the overall immune response.

B cells express specific antigen receptors (**immunoglobulin molecules**) on their cell surface during their development and, when mature, secrete soluble immunoglobulin molecules (also known as antibodies) into the extracellular fluids. Each B cell is genetically programmed to express a surface receptor which is specific for a particular antigen. If a B cell binds to its specific antigen, it will multiply and differentiate into **plasma cells**, which produce large amounts of the antibody, but in a secreted form.

Secreted antibody molecules are large glycoproteins found in the blood and tissue fluids. Because secreted antibody molecules are a soluble version of the original receptor molecule (antibody), they bind to the same antigen that initially activated the B cells. Antibodies are an essential component of an immune response, and, when bound to their cognate antigens, they help phagocytes to take up antigens, a process called **opsonization** (from the Latin, opsono, 'to prepare victuals for').

There are several different types of T cell, and they have a variety of functions (Fig 1.4):

- one group interacts with mononuclear phagocytes and helps them destroy intracellular pathogens – these are called type 1 helper T cells or TH1 cells;
- another group interacts with B cells and helps them to divide, differentiate, and make antibody – these are the type 2 helper T cells or TH2 cells;
- a third group of T cells is responsible for the destruction of host cells that have become infected by viruses or other intracellular pathogens – this kind of action is called cytotoxicity and these T cells are therefore called cytotoxic T lymphocytes (CTLs or TC cells).

A fourth group of T-cells, **regulatory T cells** or **Tregs**, help to control the development of immune responses, and limit reactions against self tissues.

In every case, the T cells recognize antigens present on the surface of other cells using a specific receptor – the **T cell antigen receptor (TCR)** – which is quite distinct from, but related in structure to, the antigen receptor (antibody) on B cells. T cells generate their effects either by releasing soluble proteins, called **cytokines**, which signal to other cells, or by direct cell–cell interactions.

Functions of different types of lymphocyte

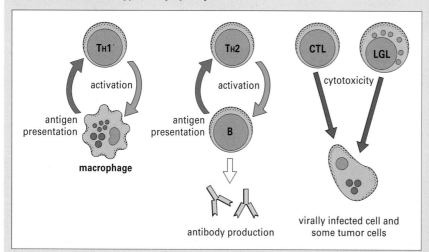

Fig. 1.4 Macrophages present antigen to TH1 cells, which then activate the macrophages to destroy phagocytosed pathogens. B cells present antigen to TH2 cells, which activate the B cells, causing them to divide and differentiate. Cytotoxic T lymphocytes (CTLs) and large granular lymphocytes (LGLs) recognize and destroy virally infected cells.

Cytotoxic cells recognize and destroy other cells that have become infected

Several cell types have the capacity to kill other cells should they become infected. Cytotoxic cells include CTLs, natural killer (NK) cells (large granular lymphocytes), and eosinophils. Of these, the CTL is especially important, but other cell types may be active against particular types of infection.

All of these cell types damage their different targets by releasing the contents of their intracellular granules close to them. Cytokines secreted by the cytotoxic cells, but not stored in granules, contribute to the damage.

Lymphocytes known as **large granular lymphocytes (LGLs)** have the capacity to recognize the surface changes that occur on a variety of tumor cells and virally infected cells. LGLs damage these target cells, but use a different recognition system to CTLs. This action is sometimes called NK cell activity, so these cells are also described as **NK cells**.

Eosinophils are a specialized group of leukocytes that have the ability to engage and damage large extracellular parasites, such as schistosomes.

Auxiliary cells control inflammation

The main purpose of inflammation is to attract leukocytes and the soluble mediators of immunity towards a site of infection. Inflammation is mediated by a variety of other cells including basophils, mast cells and platelets.

Basophils and **mast cells** have granules that contain a variety of mediators, which induce inflammation in surrounding tissues and are released when the cells are triggered. Basophils and mast cells can also synthesize and secrete a number of mediators that control the development of immune reactions. Mast cells lie close to blood vessels in all tissues, and some of their mediators act on cells in the vessel walls. Basophils are functionally similar to mast cells, but are mobile, circulating cells.

Platelets are small cellular fragments which are essential in blood clotting, but they can also be activated during immune responses to release mediators of inflammation.

Soluble mediators of immunity

A wide variety of molecules are involved in the development of immune responses, including antibodies, opsonins and complement system molecules. The serum concentration of a number of these proteins increases rapidly during infection and they are therefore called **acute phase proteins**.

One example of an acute phase protein is **C reactive protein (CRP)**, so-called because of its ability to bind to the C protein of pneumococci; it promotes the uptake of pneumococci by phagocytes. Molecules such as antibody and CRP that promote phagocytosis are said to act as **opsonins**.

Another important group of molecules that can act as opsonins are components of the complement system.

Complement proteins mediate phagocytosis, control inflammation and interact with antibodies in immune defense

The complement system, a key component of innate immunity, is a group of about 20 serum proteins whose overall function is the control of inflammation (Fig. 1.5). The components interact with each other, and with other elements of the immune system. For example:

- a number of microorganisms spontaneously activate the complement system, via the so-called 'alternative pathway', which is an innate immune defense – this results in the microorganism being opsonized (i.e. coated by complement molecules, leading to its uptake by phagocytes);
- the complement system can also be activated by antibodies or by mannose binding lectin bound to the pathogen surface via the 'classical pathway'.

Complement activation is a cascade reaction, where one component acts enzymatically on the next component in the cascade to generate an enzyme, which mediates the following step in the reaction sequence, and so on. (The blood clotting system also works as an enzyme cascade.)

Functions of complement

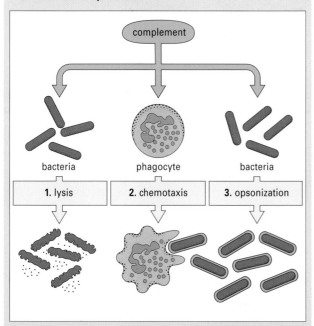

Fig. 1.5 Components of the complement system can lyse many bacterial species (**1**). Complement fragments released in this reaction attract phagocytes to the site of the reaction (**2**). Complement components opsonize the bacteria for phagocytosis (**3**). In addition to the responses shown here, activation of the complement system increases blood flow and vascular permeability at the site of activation. Activated components can also induce the release of inflammatory mediators from mast cells.

Activation of the complement system generates protein molecules or peptide fragments, which have the following effects:

- opsonization of microorganisms for uptake by phagocytes and eventual intracellular killing;
- attraction of phagocytes to sites of infection (chemotaxis);
- increased blood flow to the site of activation and increased permeability of capillaries to plasma molecules;
- damage to plasma membranes on cells, Gram-negative bacteria, enveloped viruses, or other organisms that have caused complement activation. This can result in lysis of the cell or virus and so reduce the infection;
- release of inflammatory mediators from mast cells.

Cytokines signal between lymphocytes, phagocytes and other cells of the body

Cytokine is the general term for a large group of secreted molecules involved in signaling between cells during immune responses. All cytokines are proteins or glycoproteins. The different cytokines fall into a number of categories, and the principal subgroups of cytokines are outlined below.

Interferons (IFNs) are cytokines that are particularly important in limiting the spread of certain viral infections:

Interferons

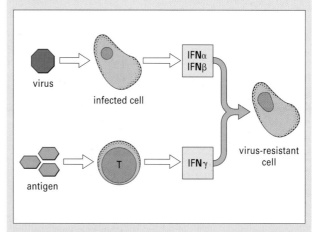

Fig. 1.6 Host cells that have been infected by virus secrete interferon-α (IFNα) and/or interferon-β (IFNβ). TH1 cells secrete interferon-γ (IFNγ) after activation by antigen. IFNs act on other host cells to induce resistance to viral infection. IFNγ has many other effects as well.

- one group of interferons (IFNα and IFNβ or type-1 interferons) is produced by cells that have become infected by a virus;
- another type, IFNγ, is released by activated TH1 cells.

IFNs induce a state of antiviral resistance in uninfected cells (Fig. 1.6). They are produced very early in infection and are important in delaying the spread of a virus until the adaptive immune response has developed.

The **interleukins (ILs)** are a large group of cytokines produced mainly by T cells, though some are also produced by mononuclear phagocytes or by tissue cells. They have a variety of functions. Many interleukins cause other cells to divide and differentiate.

Colony stimulating factors (CSFs) are cytokines primarily involved in directing the division and differentiation of bone marrow stem cells, and the precursors of blood leukocytes. The CSFs partially control how many leukocytes of each type are released from the bone marrow. Some CSFs also promote subsequent differentiation of cells. For example, macrophage CSF (M-CSF) promotes the development of monocytes in bone marrow and macrophages in tissues.

Chemokines are a large group of chemotactic cytokines that direct the movement of leukocytes around the body, from the blood stream into the tissues and to the appropriate location within each tissue. Some chemokines also activate cells to carry out particular functions.

Tumor necrosis factors, TNFα and TNFβ, have a variety of functions, but are particularly important in mediating inflammation and cytotoxic reactions.

Transforming growth factors (e.g. TGFβ) are important in controlling cell division and tissue repair.

Each set of cells releases a particular blend of cytokines, depending on the type of cell and whether, and how, it has been activated. For example:

- TH1 cells release one set of cytokines, which promote TH1 cell interactions with mononuclear phagocytes;
- TH2 cells release a different set of cytokines, which activate B cells.

Some cytokines may be produced by all T cells, and some just by a specific subset.

Equally important is the expression of cytokine receptors. Only a cell that has the appropriate receptors can respond to a particular cytokine. For example the receptors for interferons are present on all nucleated cells in the body whereas other receptors are much more restricted in their distribution. In general, cytokine receptors are specific for their own individual cytokine, but this is not always so. In particular, many chemokine receptors respond to several different chemokines.

Immune responses to pathogens

Effective immune responses vary depending on the pathogen

The primary function of the immune system is to prevent entry of and/or to eliminate infectious agents and minimize the damage they cause, ensuring that most infections in normal individuals are short-lived and leave little permanent damage. Pathogens, however come in many different forms, with various modes of transmission and reproductive cycles, so the immune system has evolved different ways of responding to each of them.

The exterior defenses of the body (Fig. 1.7) present an effective barrier to most organisms. Very few infectious agents can penetrate intact skin. In contrast, many infectious agents gain access to the body across the epithelia of the gastrointestinal or urogenital tracts; others, such as the virus responsible for the common cold, infect the respiratory epithelium of nasopharynx and lung; a small number of infectious agents infect the body only if they enter the blood directly (e.g. malaria and sleeping sickness).

Once inside the body, the site of the infection and the nature of the pathogen largely determine which type of immune response will be induced – most importantly (Fig. 1.8) whether the pathogen is:

- an **intracellular pathogen** (i.e. invades the host cells to divide and reproduce); or
- an **extracellular pathogen** (i.e. does not invade the host cells).

Exterior defenses

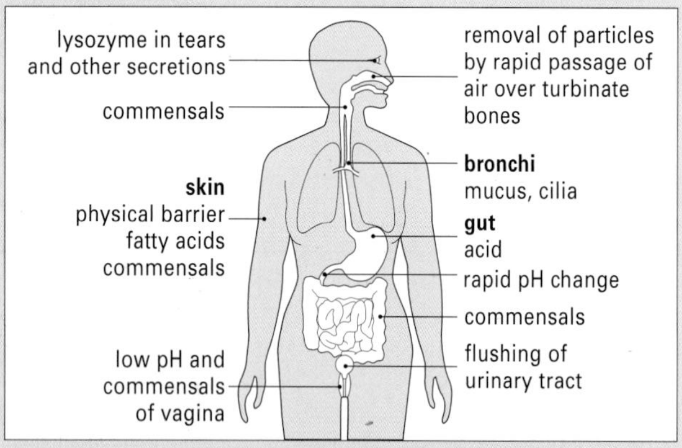

lysozyme in tears and other secretions

commensals

skin
physical barrier
fatty acids
commensals

low pH and commensals of vagina

removal of particles by rapid passage of air over turbinate bones

bronchi
mucus, cilia

gut
acid

rapid pH change

commensals

flushing of urinary tract

Fig. 1.7 Most infectious agents are prevented from entering the body by physical and biochemical barriers. The body tolerates a number of commensal organisms, which compete effectively with many potential pathogens.

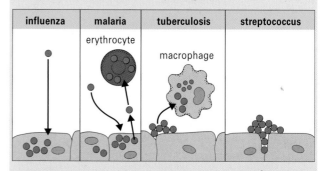

Intracellular and extracellular pathogens

influenza	malaria	tuberculosis	streptococcus
	erythrocyte	macrophage	

Fig. 1.8 All infectious agents spread to infect new cells by passing through the body fluids or tissues. Many are intracellular pathogens and must infect cells of the body to divide and reproduce (e.g. viruses such as influenza viruses and malaria, which has two separate phases of division, either in cells of the liver or in erythrocytes). The mycobacteria that cause tuberculosis can divide outside cells or within macrophages. Some bacteria (e.g. streptococci, which produce sore throats and wound infections) generally divide outside cells and are therefore extracellular pathogens.

Many bacteria and larger parasites live in tissues, body fluids, or other extracellular spaces, and are susceptible to the multitude of immune defenses, such as **antibodies** (see Chapter 3) and **complement** (see Chapter 4), that are present in these areas. Because these components are present in the tissue fluids of the body (the 'humors' of ancient medicine), they have been classically referred to as **humoral immunity**.

Many organisms (e.g. viruses, some bacteria, some parasites) evade these formidable defenses by being intracellular pathogens and replicating within host cells. To clear these infections, the immune system has developed ways to specifically recognize and destroy infected cells. This is largely the job of **cell-mediated immunity**.

Intracellular pathogens cannot, however, wholly evade the extracellular defenses (see Fig. 1.8) because they must reach their host cells by moving through the blood and tissue fluids. As a result they are susceptible to humoral immunity during this portion of their life cycle.

Any immune response involves:

- first, recognition of the pathogen or other foreign material; and
- second, a reaction to eliminate it.

Innate immune responses are the same on each encounter with antigen

Broadly speaking, immune responses fall into two categories – those that become more powerful following repeated encounters with the same antigen (**adaptive immune responses**) and those that do not become more powerful following repeated encounters with the same antigen (**innate immune responses**).

Innate immune responses (see Chapters 6 and 7) can be thought of as simple though remarkably sophisticated systems present in all animals that are the first line of defense against pathogens and allow a rapid response to invasion.

Innate immune response systems range from external barriers (skin, mucous membranes, cilia, secretions, and tissue fluids containing antimicrobial agents; see Fig. 1.7) to sophisticated receptors capable of recognizing broad classes of pathogenic organisms, for example:

- innate immune receptors on certain leukocytes recognize **pathogen-associated molecular patterns (PAMPs)**, which are common to many foreign invaders and are not normally present in the host (e.g. constituents of bacterial cell walls);
- components of the complement system can be specifically activated by bacterial surface molecules.

The innate defenses are closely interlinked with adaptive responses.

Adaptive immune responses display specificity and memory

In contrast to the innate immune response, which recognizes common molecular patterns (PAMPs), the adaptive immune system takes a highly discriminatory approach, with a very large repertoire of specific antigen receptors that can recognize virtually any component of a foreign invader (see Chapters 3 and 5). This use of highly specific antigen receptor molecules provides the following advantages:

- pathogens that lack stereotypical patterns (which might avoid recognition by the innate immune system) can be recognized;
- responses can be highly specific for a given pathogen;
- the **specificity** of the response allows the generation of **immunological memory** – related to its use of highly individual antigen receptors, the adaptive immune system has the capacity to 'remember' a pathogen.

These features underlie the phenomenon of specific immunity (e.g. diseases such as measles and diphtheria induce adaptive immune responses that generate life-long immunity).

Specific immunity can, very often, be induced by artificial means, allowing the development of vaccines (see Chapter 18).

Antigen recognition

Originally the term **antigen** was used for any molecule that induced B cells to produce a specific antibody (*antibody generator*). This term is now more widely used to indicate molecules that are specifically recognized by antigen receptors of either B cells or T cells.

Antigens, defined broadly, are molecules that initiate adaptive immune responses (e.g. components of pathogenic organisms), though purists may prefer the term **immunogen** in this context.

Antigens are not just components of foreign substances, such as pathogens. A large variety of 'self' molecules can serve as antigens as well, provoking autoimmune responses that can be highly damaging, and even lethal (see Chapter 20).

Antigens initiate and direct adaptive immune responses

The immune system has evolved to recognize antigens, destroy them, and eliminate the source of their production – when antigen is eliminated, immune responses switch off.

Both T cell receptors and immunoglobulin molecules (antibodies) bind to their cognate antigens with a high degree of specificity. These two types of receptor molecules have striking structural relationships and are closely related evolutionarily, but bind to very different types of antigens and carry out quite different biological functions.

Antibody specifically binds to antigen

Soluble antibodies are a group of serum molecules closely related to and derived from the antigen receptors on B cells. All antibodies have the same basic Y-shaped structure, with two regions (variable regions) at the tips of the Y that bind to antigen. The stem of the Y is referred to as the constant region and is not involved in antigen binding (see Chapter 3).

The two variable regions contain identical antigen-binding sites that, in general, are specific for only one type of antigen. The amino acid sequences of the variable regions of different antibodies, however, vary greatly between different antibodies. The antibody molecules in the body therefore provide an extremely large repertoire of antigen-binding sites. The way in which this great diversity of antibody variable regions is generated is explained in Chapter 3.

Each antibody binds to a restricted part of the antigen called an epitope

Pathogens typically have many different antigens on their surface. Each antibody binds to an **epitope**, which is a restricted part of the antigen. A particular antigen can have several different epitopes or repeated epitopes (Fig. 1.9). Antibodies are specific for the epitopes rather than the whole antigen molecule.

Q. Many evolutionarily related proteins have conserved amino acid sequences. What consequences might this have in terms of the antigenicity of these proteins?
A. Related proteins (with a high degree of sequence similarity) may contain the same epitopes and therefore be recognized by the same antibodies.

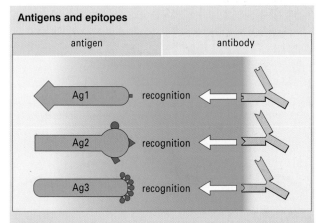

Antigens and epitopes

Fig. 1.9 Antibodies recognize molecular shapes (epitopes) on the surface of antigens. Each antigen (Ag1, Ag2, Ag3) may have several epitopes recognized by different antibodies. Some antigens have repeated epitopes (Ag3).

Fc regions of antibodies act as adapters to link phagocytes to pathogens

The constant region of the antibody (the Fc region) can bind to Fc receptors on phagocytes, so acting as an adapter between the phagocyte and the pathogen (Fig. 1.10). Consequently, if antibody binds to a pathogen, it can link to a phagocyte and promote phagocytosis. The process in which specific binding of an antibody activates an innate immune defense (phagocytosis) is an important example of collaboration between the innate and adaptive immune responses.

Other molecules (such as activated complement proteins) can also enhance phagocytosis when bound to microbial surfaces.

Binding and phagocytosis are most effective when more than one type of adapter molecule (**opsonin**) is present (Fig. 1.11). Note that antibody can act as an adapter in many other circumstances, not just phagocytosis.

Peptides from intracellular pathogens are displayed on the surface of infected cells

Antibodies patrol only extracellular spaces and so only recognize and target extracellular pathogens. Intracellular pathogens (such as viruses) can escape antibody-mediated responses once they are safely ensconced within a host cell. The adaptive immune system has therefore evolved a specific method of displaying portions of virtually all cell proteins on the surface of each nucleated cell in the body so they can be recognized by T cells.

For example, a cell infected with a virus will present fragments of viral proteins (peptides) on its surface that are recognizable by T cells. The antigenic peptides are transported to the cell surface and presented to the T cells by **MHC molecules** (a group of molecules encoded with the Major Histocompatibility Complex, see Chapter 5). T cells use their antigen-specific receptors (T cell receptors – TCRs) to recognize the antigenic peptide–MHC molecule complex (Fig. 1.12).

Opsonization

	phagocyte	opsonin	binding
1		–	±
2		complement C3b	+ +
3		antibody	+ +
4		antibody and complement C3b	+ + + +

Fig. 1.11 Phagocytes have some intrinsic ability to bind to bacteria and other microorganisms (**1**). This is much enhanced if the bacteria have been opsonized by complement C3b (**2**) or antibody (**3**), each of which cross-link the bacteria to receptors on the phagocyte. Antibody can also activate complement, and if antibody and C3b both opsonize the bacteria, binding is greatly enhanced (**4**).

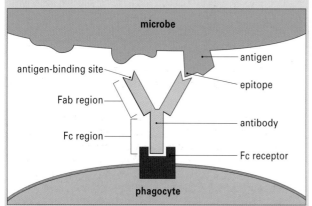

Antibody acts as an adapter that links a microbe to a phagocyte

microbe

antigen-binding site

antigen

epitope

Fab region

antibody

Fc region

Fc receptor

phagocyte

Fig. 1.10 The antibody binds to a region of an antigen (an epitope) on the microbe surface, using one of its antigen-binding sites. These sites are in the Fab regions of the antibody. The stem of the antibody, the Fc region, can attach to receptors on the surface of the phagocytes.

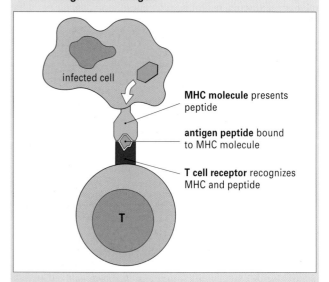

T cell recognition of antigen

infected cell

MHC molecule presents peptide

antigen peptide bound to MHC molecule

T cell receptor recognizes MHC and peptide

T

Fig. 1.12 MHC molecules transport peptides to the surface of an infected cell where they are presented to T cells, which may recognize the MHC–peptide combination. If a cell is infected, MHC molecules present peptides derived from the pathogen, as well as the cell's own proteins.

Q. Why is it necessary to have a mechanism that transports antigen fragments to the host cell surface for cytotoxic T cells to recognize infected cells?
A. The T cell cannot 'see' what is going on inside an infected cell. Its antigen receptor can only interact with and recognize what is present on the surface of cells. Therefore antigen fragments need to be transported to the cell surface for recognition, and this is the key function of MHC molecules.

T cell responses require proper presentation of antigen by MHC molecules (**antigen presentation**). To activate T cell responses this must occur on the surface of specialized **antigen-presenting cells (APCs)**, which internalize antigens by phagocytosis or endocytosis. Several different types of leukocyte can act as APCs, including dendritic cells, macrophages, and B cells.

APCs not only display antigenic peptide–MHC complexes on their surface, but also express co-stimulatory molecules that are essential for initiating immune responses (see Chapter 8). Co-stimulatory signals are upregulated by the presence of pathogens, which can be detected by the engagement of innate immune receptors that recognize PAMPs.

Most immune responses to infectious organisms are made up of a variety of innate and adaptive components:

*   in the earliest stages of infection, innate responses predominate;
*   later the lymphocytes start to generate adaptive immune responses;
*   after recovery, immunological memory remains within the population of lymphocytes, which can then mount a more effective and rapid response if there is a reinfection with the same pathogen at a later date.

The two major phases of any immune response are antigen recognition and a reaction to eradicate the antigen.

Antigen activates specific clones of lymphocytes

In adaptive immune responses, lymphocytes are responsible for immune recognition, and this is achieved by clonal selection. Each lymphocyte is genetically programmed to be capable of recognizing just one particular antigen. However, the immune system as a whole can specifically recognize many thousands of antigens, so the lymphocytes that recognize any particular antigen are only a tiny proportion of the total.

How then is an adequate immune response to an infectious agent generated? The answer is that, when an antigen binds to the few lymphocytes that can recognize it, they are induced to proliferate rapidly. Within a few days there is a sufficient number to mount an adequate immune response. In other words, the antigen selects and activates the specific clones to which it binds (Fig. 1.13), a process called **clonal selection**. This operates for both B cells and T cells.

How can the immune system 'know' which specific antibodies will be needed during an individual's lifetime? It does not know. The immune system generates antibodies (and T cell receptors) that can recognize an enormous range of antigens even before it encounters them. Many of these specificities, which are generated more or less at random (see Chapters 3 and 5), will never be called upon to protect the individual against infection.

B cell clonal selection

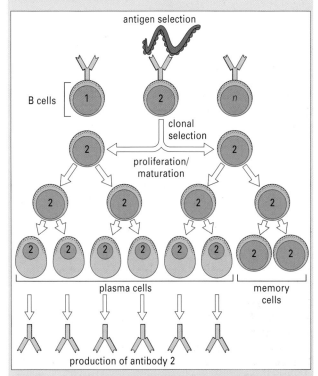

Fig. 1.13 Each B cell expresses just one antibody (i.e. with specificity for a single particular antigen), which it uses as its antigen receptor. Antigen binds only to those B cells with the specific antibody (number 2 in this example), driving these cells to divide and differentiate into plasma cells and memory cells, all having the same specificity as the original B cell. Thus an antigen selects just the clones of B cells that can react against it.

Q. What advantage could there be in having an immune system that generates billions of lymphocytes that do not recognize any known infectious agent?
A. Many pathogens mutate their surface antigens. If the immune system could not recognize new variants of pathogens, it would not be able to make an effective response. By having a wide range of antigen receptors, at least some of the lymphocytes will be able to recognize any pathogen that enters the body.

Lymphocytes that have been stimulated, by binding to their specific antigen, take the first steps towards cell division. They:

*   express new receptors that allow them to respond to cytokines from other cells, which signal proliferation;
*   may start to secrete cytokines themselves;
*   will usually go through a number of cycles of division before differentiating into mature cells, again under the influence of cytokines.

Even when the infection has been overcome, some of the newly produced lymphocytes remain, available for restimulation if the antigen is ever encountered again. These cells are called **memory cells**, because they are generated by past encounters with particular antigens. Memory cells confer lasting immunity to a particular pathogen.

Antigen elimination

Antigen elimination involves effector systems

There are numerous ways in which the immune system can destroy pathogens, each being suited to a given type of infection at a particular stage of its life cycle. These defense mechanisms are often referred to as **effector systems**.

Antibodies can directly neutralise some pathogens

In one of the simplest effector systems, antibodies can combat certain pathogens just by binding to them. For example, antibody to the outer coat proteins of some rhinoviruses (which cause colds) can prevent the viral particles from binding to and infecting host cells.

Phagocytosis is promoted by opsonins

More often antibody activates complement or acts as an opsonin to promote ingestion by phagocytes. Phagocytes that have bound to an opsonized microbe, engulf it by extending pseudopodia around it. These fuse and the microorganism is internalized (endocytosed) in a phagosome. Granules and lysosomes fuse with the phagosome, pouring enzymes into the resulting phagolysosome, to digest the contents (Fig. 1.14).

Phagocytes have several ways of dealing with internalized opsonized microbes in phagosomes. For example:

- macrophages reduce molecular oxygen to form microbicidal reactive oxygen intermediates (ROIs), which are secreted into the phagosome;
- neutrophils contain lactoferrin, which chelates iron and prevents some bacteria from obtaining this vital nutrient.

Cytotoxic cells kill infected target cells

Cytotoxic reactions are effector systems directed against whole cells that are in general too large for phagocytosis.

The target cell may be recognized either by:

- specific antibody bound to the cell surface; or
- T cells using their specific TCRs.

In cytotoxic reactions the attacking cells direct their granules towards the target cell (in contrast to phagocytosis where the contents are directed into the phagosome). As a result granules are discharged into the extracellular space close to the target cell.

The granules of CTLs and NK cells contain molecules called **perforins**, which can punch holes in the outer membrane of the target. (In a similar way, antibody bound to the surface of a target cell can direct complement to make holes in the cell's plasma membrane.) Some cytotoxic cells can signal to the target cell to initiate programmed cell death – a process called **apoptosis**.

Q. What risks are associated with discharging granule contents into the extracellular space?
A. Cells other than the target cell may be damaged. This is minimized by close intercellular contact between the CTL and the target cell.

Termination of immune responses limits damage to host tissues

Although it is important to initiate immune responses quickly, it is also critical to terminate them appropriately once the threat has ended.

To clear the offending pathogen immune responses are often massive, with:

- millions of activated lymphocytes;
- proliferation of large clones of specific T and B cells;
- activation of huge numbers of inflammatory cells.

These responses, if left unchecked, can also damage host tissues.

A number of mechanisms are employed to dampen or terminate immune responses. One is a passive process – that is, simple clearance of antigen should lead to a diminution of immune responses.

Q. Why would removal of antigen lead to the decline in an immune response?
A. Antigen is required to stimulate B cell proliferation and differentiation, with the consequent production of antibody. Antigen combined with antibody activates several effector systems (e.g. complement). Antigen is also required to stimulate T cells with consequent production of cytokines. Therefore removal of antigen takes away the primary stimulus for lymphocyte activation.

Antigen elimination can be a slow process, however, so the immune system also employs a variety of active mechanisms to downregulate responses, as discussed in Chapter 11.

Immune responses to extracellular and intracellular pathogens differ

In dealing with extracellular pathogens, the immune system aims to destroy the pathogen itself and neutralize its products.

In dealing with intracellular pathogens, the immune system has two options:

- T cells can destroy the infected cell (i.e. cytotoxicity); or
- T cells can activate the infected cell to deal with the pathogen itself (e.g. helper T cells release cytokines, which activate macrophages to destroy the organisms they have internalized).

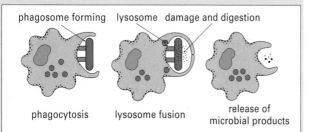

Phagocytosis

phagosome forming   lysosome   damage and digestion

phagocytosis   lysosome fusion   release of microbial products

Fig. 1.14 Phagocytes attach to microorganisms using cell surface receptors for microbial products or via antibody or complement C3b. Pseudopods extend around the microorganism and fuse to form a phagosome. Killing mechanisms are activated and lysosomes fuse with the phagosomes, releasing digestive enzymes that break down the microbe. Undigested microbial products may be released to the outside.

Reaction to extracellular and intracellular pathogens

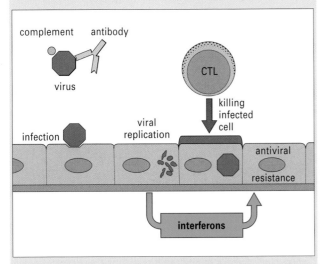

Fig. 1.15 Different immunological systems are effective against different types of infection, here illustrated as a virus infection. Antibodies and complement can block the extracellular phase of the life cycle and promote phagocytosis of the virus. Interferons produced by infected cells signal to uninfected cells to induce a state of antiviral resistance. Viruses can multiply only within living cells; cytotoxic T lymphocytes (CTLs) recognize and destroy the infected cells.

Principle of vaccination

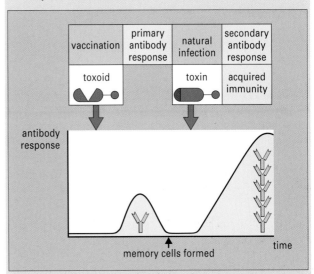

Fig. 1.16 Chemical modification of tetanus toxin produces a toxoid, which has lost its toxicity but retains many of its epitopes. A primary antibody response to these epitopes is produced following vaccination with the toxoid. If a natural infection occurs, the toxin restimulates memory B cells, which produce a faster and more intense secondary response against that epitope, so neutralizing the toxin.

Because many pathogens have both intracellular and extracellular phases of infection, different mechanisms are usually effective at different times. For example, the polio virus travels from the gut, through the blood stream to infect nerve cells in the spinal cord. Antibody is particularly effective at blocking the early phase of infection while the virus is in the blood stream, but to clear an established infection CTLs must kill any cell that has become infected.

Consequently, antibody is important in limiting the spread of infection and preventing reinfection with the same virus, while CTLs are essential to deal with infected cells (Fig. 1.15). These factors play an important part in the development of effective vaccines.

Vaccination

The study of immunology has had its most successful application in vaccination (see Chapter 18), which is based on the key elements of adaptive immunity, namely specificity and memory. Memory cells allow the immune system to mount a much stronger response on a second encounter with antigen. Compared with the primary response, the secondary response is:

- faster to appear;
- more effective.

The aim in vaccine development is to alter a pathogen or its toxins in such a way that they become innocuous without losing antigenicity. This is possible because antibodies and T cells recognize particular parts of antigens (the epitopes), and not the whole organism or toxin.

Take, for example, vaccination against tetanus. The tetanus bacterium produces a toxin that acts on receptors to cause tetanic contractions of muscle. The toxin can be modified by formalin treatment so that it retains its epitopes, but loses its toxicity. The resulting molecule (known as a toxoid) is used as a vaccine (Fig. 1.16).

Whole infectious agents, such as the poliovirus, can be attenuated so they retain their antigenicity, but lose their pathogenicity.

Inflammation

Tissue damage caused by physical agents (e.g. trauma or radiation) or by pathogens results in the tissue response of **inflammation**, which has three principal components:

- increased blood supply to the infected area;
- increased capillary permeability due to retraction of the endothelial cells lining the vessels, permitting larger molecules than usual to escape from the capillaries;
- migration of leukocytes out of the venules into the surrounding tissues – in the earliest stages of inflammation, neutrophils are particularly prevalent, but in later stages monocytes and lymphocytes also migrate towards the site of infection or damage.

Q. What advantage could the inflammatory responses have in the defense against infection?
A. The inflammatory responses allow leukocytes, antibodies, and complement system molecules (all of which are required for the phagocytosis and destruction of pathogens) to enter the tissues at the site of infection. Lymphocytes are also required for the recognition and destruction of infected cells in the tissues.

Three phases in neutrophil migration across endothelium

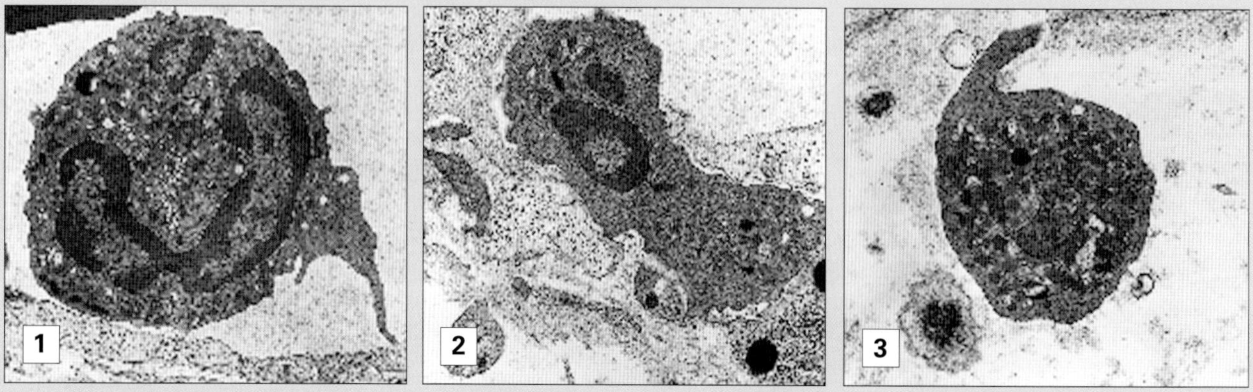

Fig. 1.17   A neutrophil adheres to the endothelium in a venule (**1**). It extends its pseudopodium between the endothelial cells and migrates towards the basement membrane (**2**). After the neutrophil has crossed into the tissue, the endothelium reseals behind (**3**). The entire process is referred to as diapedesis. *(Courtesy of Dr I Jovis.)*

Leukocytes enter inflamed tissue by crossing venular endothelium

The process of leukocyte migration is controlled by **chemokines** (a particular class of cytokines) on the surface of venular endothelium in inflamed tissues. Chemokines activate the circulating leukocytes causing them to bind to the endothelium and initiate migration across the endothelium (Fig. 1.17).

Once in the tissues, the leukocytes migrate towards the site of infection by a process of chemical attraction known as **chemotaxis**. For example, phagocytes will actively migrate up concentration gradients of certain (chemotactic) molecules.

A particularly active chemotactic molecule is **C5a**, which is a fragment of one of the complement components (Fig. 1.18) that attracts both neutrophils and monocytes. When purified C5a is applied to the base of a blister in vivo, neutrophils can be seen sticking to the endothelium of nearby venules shortly afterwards. The cells then squeeze between the endothelial cells and move through the basement membrane of the microvessels to reach the tissues. This process is described more fully in Chapter 6.

Immunopathology

Strong evolutionary pressure from infectious microbes has led to the development of the immune system in its present form. Deficiencies in any part of the system leave the individual exposed to a greater risk of infection, but other parts of the system may partly compensate for such deficiencies. However, there are occasions when the immune system is itself a cause of disease or other undesirable consequences.

In essence the immune system can fail in one of three ways (Fig. 1.19), resulting in autoimmunity, immunodeficiency, or hypersensitivity.

Inappropriate reaction to self antigens – autoimmunity

Normally the immune system recognizes all foreign antigens and reacts against them, while recognizing the body's own tissues as 'self' and making no reaction against them.

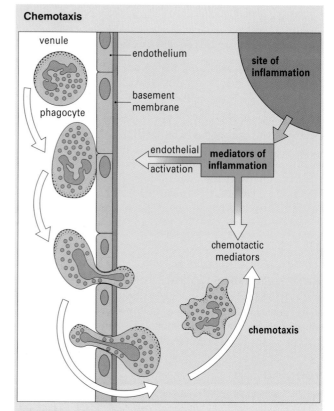

Chemotaxis

Fig. 1.18   At a site of inflammation, tissue damage and complement activation cause the release of chemotactic peptides (e.g. chemokines and C5a), which diffuse to the adjoining venules and signal to circulating phagocytes. Activated cells migrate across the vessel wall and move up a concentration gradient of chemotactic molecules towards the site of inflammation.

The mechanisms by which this discrimination between 'self' and 'non-self' is established are described in Chapter 19.

When the immune system reacts against 'self' components, the result is an **autoimmune disease** (see Chapter 20), for example rheumatoid arthritis or pernicious anemia.

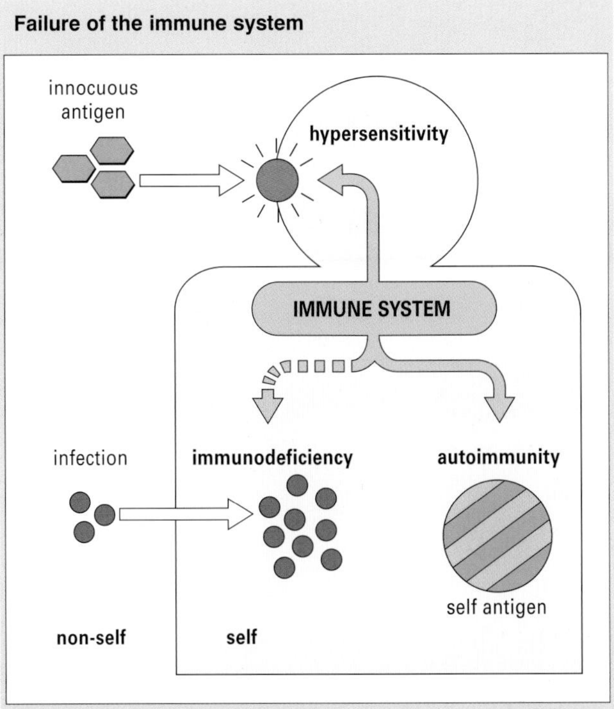

Failure of the immune system

Fig. 1.19 The three principal ways in which the immune system can fail result in hypersensitivity (an overactive immune response to an antigen), immunodeficiency (an ineffective immune response to an infection), and autoimmunity (the immune system reacts against the body's own tissues).

Ineffective immune response – immunodeficiency

If any elements of the immune system are defective, the individual may not be able to fight infections adequately, resulting in **immunodeficiency**. Some immunodeficiency conditions:

- are hereditary and start to manifest shortly after birth; they are primary immundeficiencies (see Chapter 16);
- develop later in life, for example the acquired immune deficiency syndrome (AIDS) and are referred to as secondary immunodeficiencies (see Chapter 17).

Overactive immune response – hypersensitivity

Sometimes immune reactions are out of all proportion to the damage that may be caused by a pathogen. The immune system may also mount a reaction to a harmless antigen, such as a food molecule. Such immune reactions (**hypersensitivity**) may cause more damage than the pathogen or antigen (see Chapters 23–26). For example, molecules on the surface of pollen grains are recognized as antigens by particular individuals, leading to the symptoms of hay fever or asthma.

Normal but inconvenient immune reactions

Q. Can you think of an instance where an individual is treated to suppress an immune reaction that does not fall into one of the three categories of immunopathology described above?
A. Immunosuppression to prevent graft rejection.

The most important examples of normal immune reactions that are inconvenient in the context of modern medicine are:

- blood transfusion reactions (see Chapter 24);
- graft rejection (see Chapter 21).

In these cases it is necessary to carefully match the donor and recipient tissues so that the immune system of the recipient does not attack the donated blood or graft tissue.

CRITICAL THINKING: SPECIFICITY AND MEMORY IN VACCINATION (SEE P. 433 FOR EXPLANATIONS)

The recommended schedules for vaccination against different diseases are strikingly different. Two examples are given in the table. For tetanus, the vaccine is a modified form of the toxin released by the tetanus bacterium. The vaccine for influenza is either an attenuated non-pathogenic variant of the virus, given intranasally, or a killed preparation of virus, given intradermally. Both vaccines induce antibodies that are specific for the inducing antigen.

Schedules for vaccination against tetanus and influenza A

Pathogen	Type of vaccine	Recommended for	Vaccination	Effectiveness (%)
Tetanus	Toxoid	Everyone	Every 10 years	100
Influenza A	Attenuated virus	Health workers and older people	Annually	Variable, 0–90

1 Why is it necessary to vaccinate against tetanus only every 10 years, though antibodies against the toxoid disappear from the circulation within a year?

2 Why is the vaccine against tetanus always effective, whereas the vaccine against influenza protects on some occasions but not others?

3 Why is tetanus recommended for everyone and influenza for only a restricted group of 'at-risk' individuals, even though influenza is a much more common disease than tetanus?

CHAPTER 2

Cells, Tissues, and Organs of the Immune System

SUMMARY

- **Most cells of the immune system** derive from hemopoietic stem cells. The primary lymphoid organs in mammals are the thymus and bone marrow, where lymphocyte differentiation occurs.

- **Phagocytic cells** are found in the circulation as monocytes and granulocytes. Monocytes differentiate into macrophages that reside in tissues (e.g. Kupffer cells in the liver). Neutrophils are short-lived phagocytes present in high numbers in the blood and at sites of acute inflammation.

- **Eosinophils, basophils, mast cells, and platelets, together with cytokines and complement, take part in the inflammatory response**.

- **NK cells recognize and kill virus-infected cells and certain tumor cells** by inducing apoptosis.

- **Antigen-presenting cells** link the innate and adaptive immune systems and are required by T cells to enable them to respond to antigens.

- **Lymphocytes** are heterogeneous phenotypically, functionally, and morphologically.

- **B lymphocytes and T lymphocytes express specific antigen receptors** called the B cell receptor (BCR) and T cell receptor (TCR) respectively.

- **There are three major subpopulations of T cells which have helper, cytotoxic and regulatory activities** (T_H, T_C and Treg).

- **B cells can differentiate into antibody-secreting plasma cells and memory cells.**

- **T cells developing in the thymus** are subject to positive and negative selection processes.

- **Mammalian B cells develop mainly in the fetal liver and from birth onwards in the bone marrow**. This process continues throughout life. B cells also undergo a negative selection process at the site of B cell generation.

- **Lymphocytes** migrate to, and function in, the secondary lymphoid organs and tissues.

- **Secondary lymphoid organs and tissue protect different body sites** – the spleen responds to blood borne organisms; the lymph nodes respond to lymph-borne antigens; and the mucosa-associated lymphoid tissue (**MALT**) protects the mucosal surfaces.

- **Most lymphocytes recirculate around the body**; there is continuous lymphocyte traffic from the blood stream into lymphoid tissues and back again into the blood via the thoracic duct and right lymphatic duct.

Cells of the immune system

There is great heterogeneity in the cells of the immune system, most of which originate from hematopoietic stem cells in the fetal liver and in the postnatal bone marrow – mainly in the vertebrae, sternum, ribs, femur and tibia (Fig. 2.1). This morphological heterogeneity reflects the fact that cells of the immune system are called on to provide a wide variety of functions including:

- phagocytosis;
- antigen presentation;
- lysis of virus-infected cells; and
- secretion of specific antibodies.

In general, cells of the immune system can be divided into two broad functional categories, which work together to provide innate immunity and the adaptive immune response. Innate immunity represents an ancient defense system which has evolved to recognize conserved patterns characteristic of a variety of pathogens, and often serves as the first line of defense. Adaptive immunity, a more recent evolutionary innovation, recognizes novel molecules produced by pathogens by virtue of a large repertoire of specific antigen receptors.

Cells of the innate immune system include monocytes/macrophages, polymorphonuclear granulocytes, NK cells, mast cells, and platelets

Phagocytic cells of the innate immune system belong to the myeloid lineage and include:

- the monocytes: circulating blood cells;
- the macrophages: differentiated from monocytes and residing in various tissues;

Origin of cells of the immune system

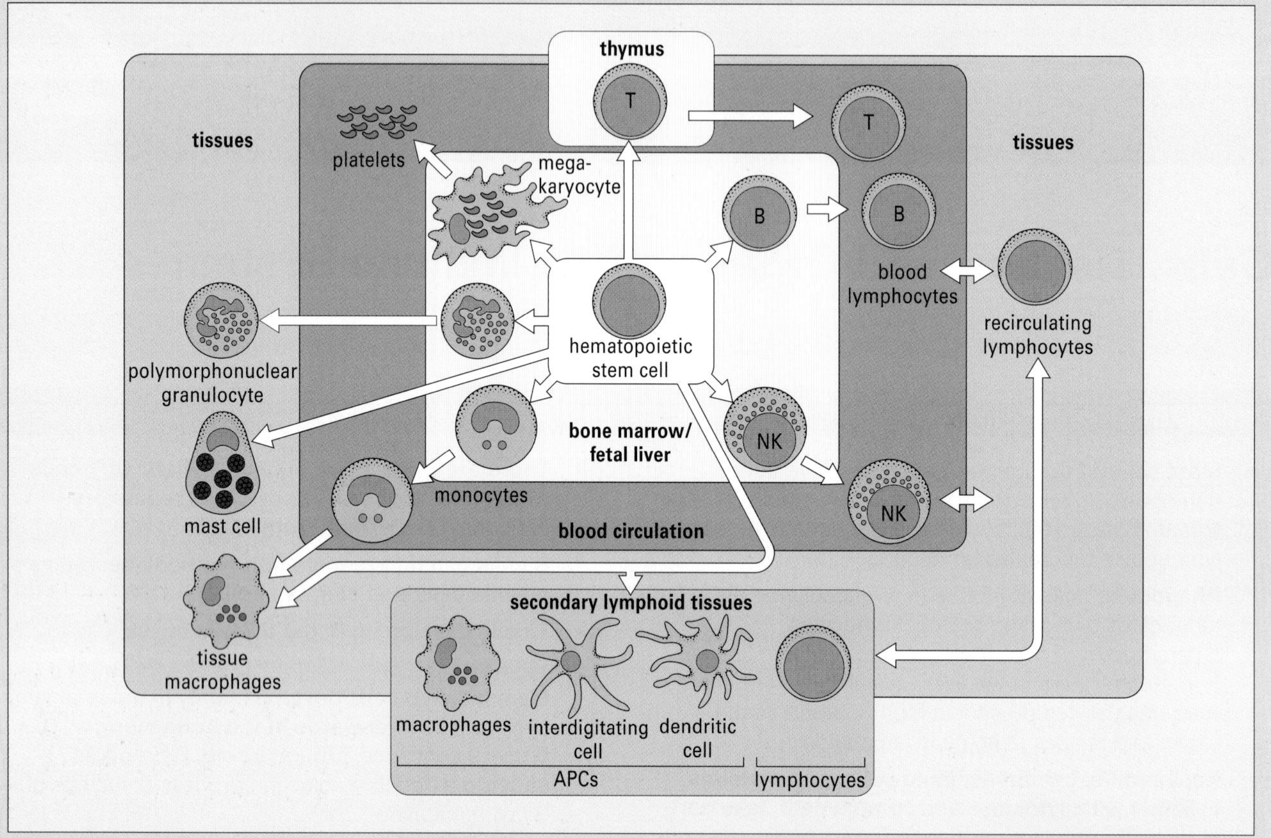

Fig. 2.1 All cells shown here arise from the hematopoietic stem cell. Platelets – cellular fragments produced by megakaryocytes – are released into the circulation. Polymorphonuclear granulocytes and monocytes pass from the circulation into the tissues. Mast cells are identifiable in all tissues. B cells mature in the fetal liver and bone marrow in mammals, whereas T cells mature in the thymus. The origin of the large granular lymphocytes with natural killer (NK) activity is probably the bone marrow. Lymphocytes recirculate through secondary lymphoid tissues. Interdigitating cells and dendritic cells act as antigen-presenting cells (APCs) in secondary lymphoid tissues.

- • the **polymorphonuclear granulocytes** (polymorphonuclear neutrophils [PMNs], basophils, and eosinophils): circulating blood cells.

All phagocytic cells are mainly involved in defense from extracellular microbes.

Natural killer (NK) cells are mainly involved in the defense against intracellular microbes and are responsible for killing virus-infected cells.

Mast cells and platelets are pivotal in inducing and maintaining inflammation.

Microbes express various cell surface and intracellular molecules called pathogen-associated molecular patterns (PAMPs). Cells of the innate system recognize microbes through their receptors to PAMPs called pattern recognition receptors (PRR). PRR have broad specificity and a non-clonal distribution, features which distinguish them from the specific antigen receptors of the adaptive immune system (see Chapter 6).

Antigen-presenting cells (APCs) link the innate and adaptive immune systems

A specialized group of cells termed antigen-presenting cells (APCs) link the innate and adaptive immune systems by taking up and processing antigens so they can be recognized

by T cells, and by producing cytokines. APCs enhance innate immune cell function and they are essential for activation of T cells (Fig. 2.2).

Adaptive immune system cells are lymphocytes

Lymphocytes (T and B cells) recognize antigens through clonally expressed, highly specific antigen receptors (see Chapters 3 and Chapter 5). T cells are produced in the thymus (see Fig. 2.1) and require antigen to be processed and presented to them by specialized APCs.

Whereas the cells of the innate immune system are found in the blood stream and in most organs of the body, lymphocytes are localized to specialized organs and tissues.

The lymphoid organs where the lymphocytes differentiate and mature from stem cells are termed the **primary lymphoid organs** and include:

- • the thymus – the site of T cell development;
- • the fetal liver and postnatal bone marrow – the sites of B cell development.

It is in the primary lymphoid organs that the lymphocytes undergo the antigen independent portion of their differentiation program. Cells of the T and B cell lineages migrate

Antigen-presenting cells (APCs) in the immune system

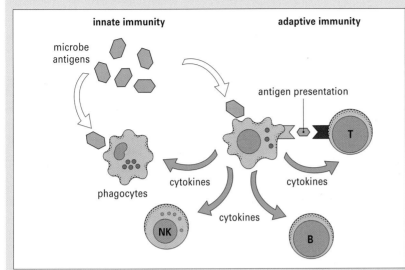

Fig. 2.2 Specialized APCs are involved in both innate and adaptive immunity to bacteria and viruses by the production of cytokines and by presentation of processed antigens to T cells.

from the primary lymphoid organs to function in the **secondary lymphoid organs**. These can be subdivided into:

- encapsulated organs – the spleen and lymph nodes;
- non-encapsulated tissues, e.g. mucosa-associated lymphoid tissues (MALT).

In the secondary lymphoid organs and tissues, lymphocytes undergo their final differentiation steps, which occur in the presence of antigen. Effector B and T cells generated in the secondary lymphoid tissues account for the two major cell types participating in adaptive immune responses of humoral and cellular immunity, respectively.

As the cells of the immune system develop, they acquire molecules that are important for their function. These specific functional molecules are referred to as 'lineage markers' because they identify the cell lineage for example:

- myeloid cells – polymorphs and monocytes;
- lymphoid cells – T and B cells.

Other marker molecules include those involved in regulating cell differentiation (maturation, development), proliferation and function and those involved in regulating the number of cells participating in the immune response. Some of these are called 'death receptors' and mediate the programmed cell death (apoptosis) that occurs as the cells reach the end of their lifespan.

Myeloid cells

Mononuclear phagocytes and polymorphonuclear granulocytes are the two major phagocyte lineages

Phagocytic cells are found both in the circulation and in tissues. Phagocytes belong to two major lineages that differentiate from myeloid precursors:

- mononuclear phagocytes – monocytes/macrophages; and
- polymorphonuclear granulocytes.

The mononuclear phagocytes consist of circulating cells (the monocytes) and macrophages, that differentiate from

monocytes and reside in a variety of organs (e.g. spleen, liver, lungs, kidneys) where they display distinctive morphological features and perform diverse functions.

The other family of phagocytes, polymorphonuclear granulocytes, have a lobed, irregularly shaped (polymorphic) nucleus. On the basis of how their cytoplasmic granules stain with acidic and basic dyes, they are classified into neutrophils, basophils and eosinophils, and have distinct effector functions:

- the neutrophils, also called polymorphonuclear neutrophils (PMNs), are most numerous and constitute the majority of leukocytes (white blood cells) in the blood stream (around 60–70% in adults);
- the primary actions of eosinophils and basophils, which can both function as phagocytes, involve granule release (exocytosis).

The mononuclear phagocytes and polymorphonuclear granulocytes develop from a common precursor.

Mononuclear phagocytes are widely distributed throughout the body

Cells of the mononuclear phagocytic system are found in virtually all organs of the body where the local microenvironment determines their morphology and functional characteristics, e.g. in the lung as alveolar macrophages, in kidney as glomerular mesangial cells, and in the liver as Kupffer cells (Fig. 2.3 and see Fig. 1.2).

The main role of the mononuclear phagocytes is to remove particulate matter of 'foreign' origin (e.g. microbes) or self origin (e.g. aged erythrocytes).

Myeloid progenitors in the bone marrow differentiate into pro-monocytes and then into circulating monocytes, which migrate through the blood vessel walls into organs to become macrophages.

The human blood monocyte:

- is large (10–18 μm in diameter) relative to the lymphocyte;
- has a horseshoe-shaped nucleus;

Kupffer cells

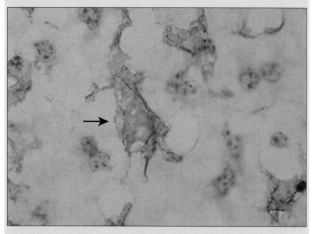

Fig. 2.3 Kupffer cells in the normal mouse liver stain strongly positive with antibody to F4/80 (arrow). Sinusoidal endothelial cells and hepatocytes are F4/80-negative. *(Courtesy of Professor S Gordon and Dr DA Hume.)*

Morphology of the monocyte

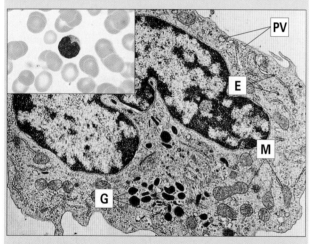

Fig. 2.4 Ultrastructure of a monocyte showing the horseshoe-shaped nucleus, pinocytotic vesicles (PV), lysosomal granules (G), mitochondria (M), and isolated rough endoplasmic reticulum cisternae (E). × 8000. Inset: Light microscope image of a monocyte from the blood. × 1200. *(Courtesy of Dr B Nichols.)*

- contains primary azurophilic (blue-staining) granules; and
- possesses ruffled membranes, a well-developed Golgi complex, and many intracytoplasmic lysosomes (Fig. 2.4).

The lysosomes contain peroxidase and several acid hydrolases, which are important for killing phagocytosed microorganisms. Monocytes/macrophages actively phagocytose microorganisms (mostly bacteria and fungi) and the body's own aged and dead cells, or even tumor cells.

Microbial adherence occurs through pattern recognition receptors (see Chapters 6 and 7), followed by phagocytosis. Coating microbes with complement components and/or antibodies (opsonization) enhances phagocytosis by monocytes/macrophages and is mediated by specialized complement receptors and antibody receptors expressed by the phagocytic cells (see Chapters 3 and 4).

Q. How do macrophages recognize microbes that have been coated with antibody?
A. Macrophages have Fc receptors that recognize the constant domains of the heavy chains of an antibody molecule (see Figs 1.10 and 1.11).

There are three different types of polymorphonuclear granulocyte

The polymorphonuclear granulocytes (often referred to as **polymorphs** or **granulocytes**) consist mainly of neutrophils (PMNs). They:

- are released from the bone marrow at a rate of around 7 million per minute;
- are short-lived (2–3 days) relative to monocytes/macrophages, which may live for months or years.

Like monocytes, PMNs marginate (adhere to endothelial cells lining the blood vessels) and extravasate by squeezing between the endothelial cells to leave the circulation (see Fig. 1.17) to reach the site of infection in tissues. This process is known as **diapedesis**. Adhesion is mediated by receptors on the granulocytes and ligands on the endothelial cells, and is promoted by chemo-attractants (**chemokines**) such as **interleukin-8 (IL-8)** (see Chapter 6).

Like monocytes/macrophages, granulocytes also have pattern recognition receptors, and PMNs play an important role in acute inflammation (usually synergizing with antibodies and complement) in providing protection against microorganisms. Their predominant role is phagocytosis and destruction of pathogens.

The importance of granulocytes is evident from the observation of individuals who have a reduced number of white cells or who have rare genetic defects that prevent polymorph extravasation in response to chemotactic stimuli (see Chapter 16). These individuals have a markedly increased susceptibility to bacterial and fungal infection.

Neutrophils comprise over 95% of the circulating granulocytes

Neutrophils have a characteristic multilobed nucleus and are 10–20 μm in diameter (Fig. 2.5). Chemotactic agents attracting neutrophils to the site of infection include:

- protein fragments released when complement is activated (e.g. C5a);
- factors derived from the fibrinolytic and kinin systems;
- the products of other leukocytes and platelets; and
- the products of certain bacteria (see Chapter 6).

Neutrophils have a large arsenal of enzymes and antimicrobial proteins stored in two main types of granule:

- the primary (azurophilic) granules are lysosomes containing acid hydrolases, myeloperoxidase, and muramidase (lysozyme); they also contain the antimicrobial proteins including defensins, seprocidins, cathelicidins, and bacterial permeability inducing (BPI) protein; and

Morphology of the neutrophil

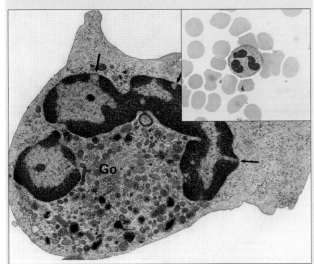

Fig. 2.5 Morphology of the neutrophil. At the ultrastructural level, the azurophilic (primary) granules are larger than the secondary (specific) granules with a strongly electron-dense matrix; the majority of granules are specific granules and contain a variety of toxic materials to kill microbes. A pseudopod (to the right) is devoid of granules. Arrows indicate nuclear pores. Go: Golgi region. Inset: A mature neutrophil in a blood smear showing a multilobed nucleus. × 1500. *(From Zucker-Franklin D, Grossi CE, eds. Atlas of blood cells: function and pathology, 3rd edn. Milan: Edi Ermes; 2003.)*

- the secondary granules (specific to neutrophils) contain lactoferrin and lysozyme (see Fig. 2.5).

During phagocytosis the lysosomes containing the antimicrobial proteins fuse with vacuoles containing ingested microbes (termed **phagosomes**) to become **phagolysosomes** where the killing takes place.

Neutrophils can also release granules and cytotoxic substances extracellularly when they are activated by immune complexes (antibodies bound to their specific antigen molecules) through their Fc receptors. This is an important example of collaboration between the innate and adaptive immune systems, and may be an important pathogenetic mechanism in immune complex diseases (type III hypersensitivity, see Chapter 25).

Granulocytes and mononuclear phagocytes develop from a common precursor

Studies in which colonies have been grown *in vitro* from individual stems cells have shown that the progenitor of the myeloid lineage (CFU-GEMM) can give rise to granulocytes, monocytes and megakaryocytes (Fig. 2.6). Monocytes and neutrophils develop from a common precursor cell, the CFU-granulocyte macrophage cells (CFU-GMs) (see Fig. 2.6). **Myelopoiesis** (the development of myeloid cells) commences in the liver of the human fetus at about 6 weeks of gestation.

CFU-GEMMs mature under the influence of colony-stimulating factors (CSFs) and several interleukins (see Fig. 2.6). These factors, which are relevant for the positive regulation of hemopoiesis, are:

Development of granulocytes and monocytes

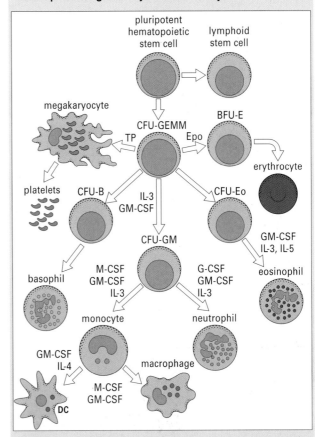

Fig. 2.6 Pluripotent hematopoietic stem cells generate colony-forming units (CFUs) that can give rise to granulocytes, erythrocytes, monocytes, and megakaryocytes (CFU-GEMMs). CFU-GEMMs therefore have the potential to give rise to all blood cells except lymphocytes. IL-3 and granulocyte–macrophage colony-stimulating factor (GM-CSF) are required to induce the CFU-GEMM stem cell to enter one of five pathways (i.e. to give rise to megakaryocytes, erythrocytes via burst-forming units, basophils, neutrophils, or eosinophils). IL-3 and GM-CSF are also required during further differentiation of the granulocytes and monocytes. Eosinophil (Eo) differentiation from CFU-Eo is promoted by IL-5. Neutrophils and monocytes are derived from the CFU-GM through the effects of G-CSF and M-CSF, respectively. Both GM-CSF and M-CSF, and other cytokines (including IL-1, IL-4, and IL-6), promote the differentiation of monocytes into macrophages. Thrombopoietin (TP) promotes the growth of megakaryocytes. (B, basophil; BFU-E, erythrocytic burst-forming unit; DC, dendritic cell; Epo, erythropoietin; G, granulocyte; M, monocyte)

- derived mainly from stromal cells (connective tissue cells) in the bone marrow;
- also produced by mature forms of differentiated myeloid and lymphoid cells.

Bone marrow stromal cells, stromal cell matrix, and cytokines form the microenvironment to support stem cell differentiation into individual cell lineages. Stromal cells produce an extracellular matrix which is very important in establishing cell–cell interactions and enhancing stem cell differentiation. The major components of the matrix are proteoglycans, fibronectin, collagen, laminin, haemonectin and thrombospondin.

Other cytokines, such as transforming growth factor-β (TGFβ) may downregulate hemopoiesis. CFU-GMs taking the monocyte pathway give rise initially to proliferating monoblasts. Proliferating monoblasts differentiate into pro-monocytes and finally into mature circulating monocytes which serve as a replacement pool for the tissue-resident macrophages (e.g. lung macrophages).

Monocytes express CD14 and significant levels of MHC class II molecules

The non-differentiated hemopoietic stem cell marker CD34, like other early markers in this lineage, is lost in mature neutrophils and mononuclear phagocytes. Other markers may be lost as differentiation occurs along one pathway, but retained in the other. For example, the common precursor of monocytes and neutrophils, the CFU-GM cell, expresses **major histocompatibility complex (MHC) class II molecules**, but only monocytes continue to express significant levels of this marker.

> **Q. What is the functional significance of the expression of MHC molecules on monocytes?**
> A. Monocytes can present antigens to helper T cells, but neutrophils generally cannot.

Mononuclear phagocytes and granulocytes display different functional molecules. Mononuclear phagocytes express CD14 which is part of the receptor complex for the lipopolysaccharide of Gram-negative bacteria). In addition, they acquire many of the same surface molecules as mature or activated neutrophils (e.g. the adhesion molecules CD11a and b and Fc receptors which recognize the constant regions of antibodies e.g. CD64 and CD32 – FcγRI and FcγRII respectively).

Neutrophils express adhesion molecules and receptors involved in phagocytosis

CFU-GMs go through several differentiation stages to become neutrophils. As the CFU-GM cell differentiates along the neutrophil pathway, several distinct morphological stages are distinguished. Myeloblasts develop into promyelocytes and myelocytes, which mature and are released into the circulation as neutrophils.

The one-way differentiation of the CFU-GM into mature neutrophils is the result of acquiring specific receptors for growth and differentiation factors at progressive stages of development. Surface differentiation markers disappear or are expressed on the cells as they develop into granulocytes. For example, MHC class II molecules are expressed on the CFU-GM, but not on mature neutrophils.

Other surface molecules acquired during the differentiation process include:

- adhesion molecules (e.g. the leukocyte integrins CD11a, b, and c, associated with CD18 β_2 chains); and
- receptors involved in phagocytosis including complement and antibody Fc receptors.

Neutrophils constitutively express FcγRIII and FcγRII, and FcγRI is induced on activation.

It is difficult to assess the functional activity of different developmental stages of granulocytes, but it seems likely that the full functional potential is realized only when the cells are mature.

There is some evidence that neutrophil activity, as measured by phagocytosis or chemotaxis, is lower in fetal than in adult life. However, this may be due, in part, to the lower levels of opsonins (e.g. complement components and antibodies) in the fetal serum, rather than to a characteristic of the cells themselves.

To become active in the presence of opsonins, neutrophils must interact directly with microorganisms and/or with cytokines generated by a response to antigen. This limitation could reduce neutrophil activity in early life.

Activation of neutrophils by cytokines and chemokines is also a prerequisite for their migration into tissues (see Chapter 9).

Eosinophils, basophils, mast cells and platelets in inflammation

Eosinophils are thought to play a role in immunity to parasitic worms

Eosinophils comprise 2–5% of blood leukocytes in healthy, non-allergic individuals. Human blood eosinophils usually have a bilobed nucleus and many cytoplasmic granules, which stain with acidic dyes such as eosin (Fig. 2.7). Although not their primary function, eosinophils appear to be capable of phagocytosing and killing ingested microorganisms.

The granules in mature eosinophils are membrane-bound organelles with crystalloid cores that differ in electron

Morphology of the eosinophil

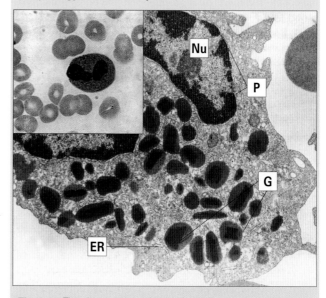

Fig. 2.7 The ultrastructure of a mature eosinophil shows granules (G) with central crystalloids. × 17 500. (ER, endoplasmic reticulum; Nu, nucleus; P, nuclear pores) Inset: A mature eosinophil in a blood smear is shown with a bilobed nucleus and eosinophilic granules. × 1000. (*From Zucker-Franklin D, Grossi CE, eds. Atlas of blood cells: function and pathology, 3rd edn. Milan: Edi Ermes; 2003.*)

density from the surrounding matrix (see Fig. 2.7). The crystalloid core contains the **major basic protein (MBP)**, which:

- is a potent toxin for helminth worms;
- induces histamine release from mast cells;
- activates neutrophils and platelets; and
- of relevance to allergy, provokes bronchospasm.

Other proteins with similar effects are found in the granule matrix, for example:

- eosinophil cationic protein (ECP); and
- eosinophil-derived neurotoxin (EDN).

Release of the granules on eosinophil activation is the only way in which eosinophils can kill large pathogens (e.g. schistosomula), which cannot be phagocytosed. Eosinophils are therefore thought to play a specialized role in immunity to parasitic worms using this mechanism (see Fig. 15.13).

Basophils and mast cells play a role in immunity against parasites

Basophils are found in very small numbers in the circulation and account for less than 0.2% of leukocytes (Fig. 2.8).

The mast cell (Fig. 2.9), which is present in tissues and not in the circulation, is indistinguishable from the basophil in a number of its characteristics, but displays some distinctive morphological features (Fig. 2.10). Their shared functions may indicate a convergent differentiation pathway.

The stimulus for mast cell or basophil degranulation is often an **allergen** (i.e. an antigen causing an allergic reaction). To be effective, an allergen must cross-link IgE molecules bound to the surface of the mast cell or basophil via its high-affinity Fc receptors for IgE (FcεRI). Degranulation of a basophil or mast cell results in all contents of the

Morphology of the basophil

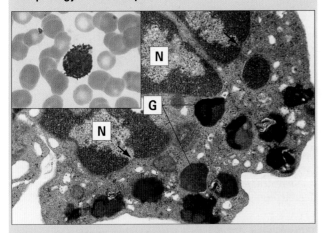

Fig. 2.8 Morphology of the basophil: ultrastructural analysis shows a segmented nucleus (N) and the large cytoplasmic granules (G). Arrows indicate nuclear pores. × 11 000. Inset: This blood smear shows a typical basophil with its deep violet-blue granules. × 1000. *(Adapted from Zucker-Franklin D, Grossi CE, eds. Atlas of blood cells: function and pathology, 3rd edn. Milan: Edi Ermes; 2003.)*

Histological appearance of human connective tissue in mast cells

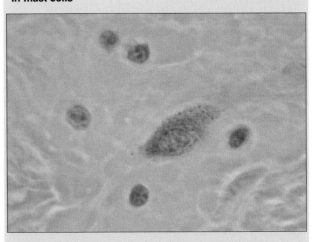

Fig. 2.9 This micrograph of a mast cell shows dark blue cytoplasm with purple granules. Alcian blue and safranin stain. × 600. *(Courtesy of Dr TS Orr.)*

granules being released very rapidly. This occurs by intracytoplasmic fusion of the granules, followed by discharge of their contents (Fig. 2.11).

Mediators such as histamine, released by degranulation, cause the adverse symptoms of allergy, but, on the positive side, also play a role in immunity against parasites by enhancing acute inflammation.

Platelets have a role in clotting and inflammation

Blood platelets (Fig. 2.12) are not cells, but cell fragments derived from megakaryocytes in the bone marrow. They contain granules, microtubules, and actin/myosin filaments, which are involved in clot contraction. Platelets also participate in immune responses, especially in inflammation.

The adult human produces 10^{11} platelets each day. About 30% of platelets are stored in the spleen, but may be released if required.

Q. What circumstance might require the release of additional platelets into the circulation?
A. Severe blood loss.

Platelets express class I MHC products and receptors for IgG (CD32; FcγRII), which are important in platelet activation via IgG immune complexes. In addition, megakaryocytes and platelets carry:

- receptors for clotting factors (e.g. factor VIII); and
- other molecules important for their function, such as the GpIIb/IIIa complex (CD41) responsible for binding to fibrinogen, fibronectin, vitronectin (tissue matrix), and von Willebrand factor (another clotting factor).

Both receptors and adhesion molecules are important in the activation of platelets.

Following injury to endothelial cells, platelets adhere to and aggregate at the damaged endothelial surface. Release

Some distinctive and common characteristics of basophils and mast cells

	basophils	mast cells
origin	bone marrow	bone marrow
site of maturation	bone marrow	connective tissues
presence in the circulation	yes	no
proliferative capacity	no	yes
life span	days	weeks to months
surface expression of FcεR1	yes	yes
granule content		
histamine	yes	yes
heparin	?	yes
cytokine production		
IL-4	yes	yes
IL-13	yes	yes

Fig. 2.10 Some distinctive and common characteristics of basophils and mast cells.

Electron micrograph study of rat mast cells

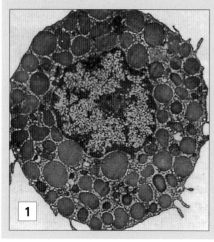 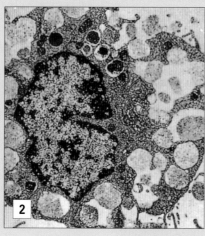

Fig. 2.11 Rat peritoneal mast cells show electron-dense granules (**1**). Vacuolation with exocytosis of the granule contents has occurred after incubation with anti-IgE (**2**). Transmission electron micrographs. × 2700. *(Courtesy of Dr D Lawson.)*

of platelet granule contents, which include *de novo* synthesized serotonin and endocytosed fibrinogen, results in:

- increased capillary permeability, a feature of inflammation;
- activation of complement (and hence attraction of leukocytes); and
- clotting.

NK cells

NK cells account for up to 15% of blood lymphocytes and express neither T cell nor B cell antigen receptors. They are derived from the bone marrow and morphologically have the appearance of large granular lymphocytes (see Fig. 2.19).

Functional NK cells are found in the spleen, and cells found in lymph nodes that express CD56 but not CD16 (see below) might represent immature NK cells.

Nevertheless many surface markers are shared with T cells, monocytes/macrophages or neutrophils.

CD16 and CD56 are important markers of NK cells

The presence of CD16 (FcγRIII) is commonly used to identify NK cells in purified lymphocyte populations. CD16 is involved in one of the activation pathways of NK cells and is also expressed by neutrophils, some macrophages and γδ T cells (see below). However on neutrophils, CD16 is

Ultrastructure of a platelet

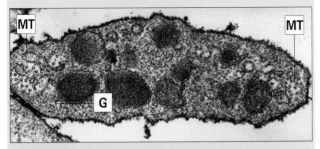

Fig. 2.12   Cross-section of a platelet showing two types of granule (G) and bundles of microtubules (MT) at either end. × 42 000. *(Adapted from Zucker-Franklin D, Grossi CE, eds. Atlas of blood cells: function and pathology, 3rd edn. Milan: Edi Ermes; 2003.)*

linked to the surface membrane by a glycoinositol phospholipid (GPI) linkage, whereas NK cells and γδ T cells express the transmembrane form of the molecule. The CD56 molecule, a homophilic adhesion molecule of the immunoglobulin superfamily (NCAM), is another important marker of NK cells. Combined with the absence of the T cell receptor (CD3), CD56 and CD16 are currently the most reliable markers for NK cells in humans.

Resting NK cells also express the β chain of the IL-2 receptor, and the signal transducing common γ chain of IL-2 and other cytokine receptors (see Fig. 8.18). Therefore, direct stimulation with IL-2 activates NK cells.

The function of NK cells is to recognize and kill virus-infected cells (Fig. 2.13) and certain tumor cells by mechanisms described in chapter 10.

Classical and non-classical MHC class I molecules (see Fig. 5.15) are ligands for inhibitory receptors on the NK cells which prevent killing and this explains why normal body cells (all of which normally express MHC class I molecules) are not targeted by NK cells.

An NK cell attached to a target cell

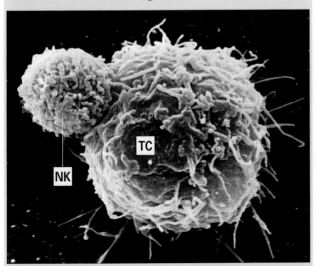

Fig. 2.13   An NK cell (NK) attached to a target cell (TC). × 4500. *(Courtesy of Dr G Arancia and W Malorni, Rome.)*

Downregulation or modification of MHC molecules in virus-infected cells and some tumors makes them susceptible to NK cell-mediated killing.

> **Q. What advantage is there for a virus in causing the loss of MHC class I molecules in the cell it has infected?**
> A. The infected cell can no longer be recognized by cytotoxic T cells (see Fig. 1.12).

NK cells are also able to kill targets coated with IgG antibodies via their receptor for IgG (FcγRIII, CD16). This property is referred to as **antibody-dependent cellular cytotoxicity (ADCC)**.

NK cells release interferon-γ (IFNγ) and other cytokines (e.g. IL-1 and GM-CSF) when activated, which might be important in the regulation of hemopoiesis and immune responses.

Antigen presenting cells

APCs are a heterogeneous population of leukocytes that are important in innate immunity (see Fig. 2.2) and play a pivotal role in the induction of functional activity of T helper (TH) cells.

In this regard, APCs are seen as a critical interface between the innate and adaptive immune systems. There are **professional APCs** (dendritic cells, macrophages and B cells) constitutively expressing MHC class II and co-stimulatory molecules, and **non-professional APCs** which express MHC class II and co-stimulatory molecules for short periods of time throughout sustained inflammatory responses. This group is comprised of fibroblasts, glial cells, pancreatic β cells, thymic epithelial cells, thyroid epithelial cells and vascular endothelial cells.

Both macrophages and B cells are rich in membrane MHC class II molecules, especially after activation, and are thus able to process and present specific antigens to (activated) T cells (see Chapter 8).

Somatic cells other than immune cells do not normally express class II MHC molecules, but cytokines such as IFNγ and tumor necrosis factor-α (TNFα) can induce the expression of class II molecules on some cell types, and thus allow them to present antigen (non-professional APCs). This induction of 'inappropriate' class II expression might contribute to the pathogenesis of autoimmune diseases and to prolonged inflammation (see Chapter 20).

Dendritic cells are derived from several different lineages

Functionally, dendritic cells (DC) are divided into those that both process and present foreign protein antigens to T cells – **'classical' dendritic cells (DCs)** – and a separate type that passively presents foreign antigen in the form of immune complexes to B cells in lymphoid follicles – **follicular dendritic cells (FDCs**; Fig. 2.14).

Most DCs derive from one of two precursors:

- a myeloid progenitor (DC1) that gives rise to myeloid DCs, otherwise called bone-marrow derived or **bm-DCs**; and
- a lymphoid progenitor (DC2) that develops into plasmacytoid DCs (**pDCs**).

Different kinds of antigen-presenting cells (APCs)

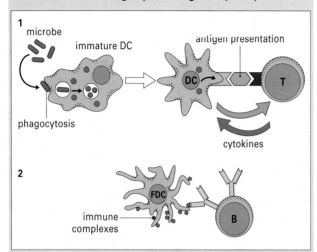

Fig. 2.14 There are two main types of dendritic cells – classical DC and follicular dendritic cells (FDCs). (1) Immature DCs are derived from bone marrow and interact mainly with T cells. They are highly phagocytic, take up microbes, process the foreign microbial antigens into small peptides, and become mature APCs carrying the processed antigen (a peptide) on their surface with specialized MHC molecules. Specific T cells recognize the displayed peptide in a complex with MHC and, in the presence of cytokines produced by the mature DC, proliferate and also produce cytokines. (2) FDCs are not bone marrow derived and interact with B cells. In the B cell follicles of lymphoid organs and tissues they bind small immune complexes (IC, called iccosomes). Antigen contained within the IC is presented to specific B cells in the lymphoid follicles. This protects the B cell from cell death. The B cell then proliferates and with T cell help can leave the follicle and become a plasma cell or a memory cell (see Fig. 2.48).

A summary of the main properties of myeloid and plasmacytoid dendritic cells is shown in Figure 2.15.

Myeloid DCs can also be divided into at least three types: Langerhans' cells (LCs), dermal or interstitial DCs (DDC-IDCs) and blood monocyte-derived DCs (moDCs).

Different populations of DCs can be identified by their surface markers. Myeloid DCs, but not pDCs express CD1a and CD208, whilst DDC-IDC and moDC express also CD11b. Langerhans' cells have so called Birbeck granules containing Langerin. It appears that various populations of myeloid DCs may represent different stages in their maturation and migration in the body (see below).

BM-DCs express various receptors that are involved in antigen uptake:

- C-type lectin receptors – for glycosyl groups, e.g. macrophage mannose receptor (MMR) family;
- Fc receptors for IgG, IgE;
- receptors for heat shock protein–peptide complexes;
- receptors for apoptotic corpses;
- 'scavenger' receptors – for sugars, lipid etc;
- toll-like receptors (TLRs).

Before DCs take up antigen (become loaded) they are called immature DCs and express various markers characteristic for this, resting, stage, the most important being chemokine receptors CCR1, CCR5 and CCR6. DCs are attracted to the infection site by chemokines through these receptors (see Chapter 6).

Mature DCs loaded with antigen down-regulate expression of CCR1, 5, 6 and up-regulate CCR7. This encourages their migration from various tissues into peripheral lymphatics, where CCR7 interacts with secondary lymphoid tissue chemokine SLC (CCL21) expressed on vascular endothelium (see Fig. 6.15).

DCs are found primarily in the skin, lymph nodes, and spleen, and within or underneath most mucosal epithelia. They are also present in the thymus, where they present self antigens to developing T cells.

Langerhans' cells and interdigitating dendritic cells are rich in MHC class II molecules

Langerhans' cells in the epidermis and in other squamous epithelia migrate via the afferent lymphatics into the paracortex of the draining lymph nodes (Fig. 2.16). Here, they interact with T cells and are termed interdigitating cells (IDCs, Fig. 2.17). These DCs are rich in class II MHC molecules, which are important for presenting antigen to helper T cells.

Myeloid and plasmacytoid dendritic cells (DCs)

	myeloid DCs	plasmacytoid DCs
origin of precursor	myeloid (DC1)	lymphoid (DC2)
localization	diffuse – epidermis, mucosae, thymus, and T cell areas of secondary lymphoid organs and tissues	restricted to T cell areas of secondary lymphoid organs and tissues
myeloid markers	many	none
characteristic cytokines produced	mainly IL-8, IL-12	mainly type I interferons (on challenge with enveloped viruses)

Fig. 2.15 There are two main types of dendritic cells defined by their origin. They have differences in their localization markers and cytokine.

Migration of antigen-presenting cells (APCs) into lymphoid tissues

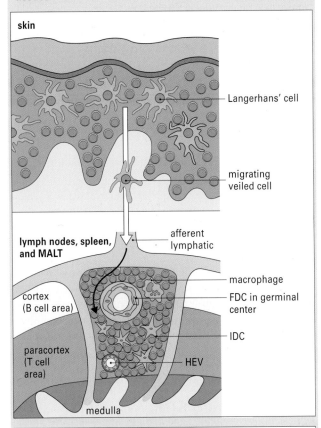

Ultrastructure of an interdigitating dendritic cell (IDC) in the T cell area of a rat lymph node

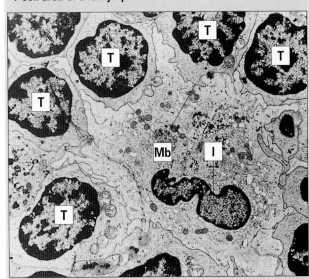

Fig. 2.17   Intimate contacts are made by APCs with the membranes of the surrounding T cells. The cytoplasm contains a well-developed endosomal system and does not show the Birbeck granules characteristic of skin Langerhans' cells. × 2000. (I, IDC nucleus; Mb, IDC membrane; T, T cell nucleus) *(Courtesy of Dr BH Balfour.)*

Q. What function could the migration of Langerhans' cells to the lymph nodes from the mucosa or skin serve?
A. The migration of Langerhans' cells provides an efficient mechanism for carrying antigen from the skin and mucosa to the Tн cells in the lymph nodes, and are rich in class II MHC molecules, which are important for presenting antigen to Tн cells. Lymph nodes provide the appropriate environment for lymphocyte proliferation.

BM-DCs are also present within the germinal centers (GCs) of secondary lymphoid follicles (i.e. they are the MHC class II molecule-positive germinal center DCs [GCDCs]). In contrast to FDCs, they are migrating cells, which on arrival in the GC interact with germinal center T cells and are probably involved in antibody class switching (see Chapter 9).

The thymus is of crucial importance in the development and maturation of T cells. In thymus there are cortical DCs and IDCs which are especially abundant in the medulla (see Fig. 2.16). They participate in two important stages in T cell maturation/differentiation in thymus positive and negative selection respectively (see below).

FDCs lack class II MHC molecules and are found in B cell areas

Unlike the APCs that actively process and present protein antigens to T cells, FDCs have a passive role in presenting antigen in the form of immune complexes to B cells. They are therefore found in the primary and secondary follicles of the B cell areas of the lymph nodes, spleen, and MALT (see Fig. 2.16). They are a non-migratory population of cells and

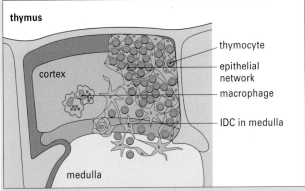

Fig. 2.16   Bone marrow-derived dendritic cells (DCs) are found especially in lymphoid tissues, in the skin, and in mucosa. DCs in the form of Langerhans' cells are found in the epidermis and in mucosa and are characterized by special granules (the tennis racquet-shaped Birbeck granules; not shown here). Langerhans' cells are rich in MHC class II molecules, and carry processed antigens. They migrate via the afferent lymphatics (where they appear as 'veiled' cells) into the paracortex of the draining lymph nodes. Here they make contact with T cells. These 'interdigitating dendritic cells (IDCs)', localized in the T cell areas of the lymph node, present antigen to T helper cells. Antigen is exposed to B cells on the follicular dendritic cells (FDCs) in the germinal centers of B cell follicles. Some macrophages located in the outer cortex and marginal sinus may also act as APCs. In the thymus, APCs occur as IDCs in the medulla. (HEV, high endothelial venule)

Follicular dendritic cell

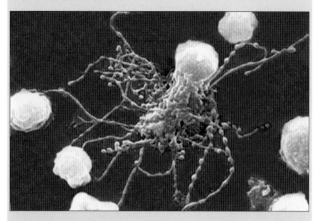

Fig. 2.18 An isolated follicular dendritic cell (FDC) from the lymph node of an immunized mouse 24 hours after injection of antigen. The FDC is of intermediate maturity with smooth filiform dendrites typical of young FDCs, and beaded dendrites, which participate in the formation of iccosomes (immune complexes) in mature FDCs. The adjacent small white cells are lymphocytes. *(Electron micrograph kindly provided by Dr Andras Szakal; reproduced by permission of the Journal of Immunology.)*

form a stable network (a kind of web) by establishing strong intercellular connections via desmosomes.

FDCs lack class II MHC molecules, but bind antigen via complement receptors (CD21 and CD35), which attach to complement associated with immune complexes (iccosomes; Fig. 2.18). They also express Fc receptors. The FDCs produce chemokines that are important in homing of B cells to the follicular areas in lymphoid tissues. They are not bone marrow derived, but are of mesenchymal origin.

Lymphocytes

Lymphocytes are phenotypically and functionally heterogeneous

Large numbers of lymphocytes are produced daily in the primary or central lymphoid organs (i.e. thymus and postnatal bone marrow). Some migrate via the circulation into the secondary lymphoid tissues (i.e. spleen, lymph nodes, and MALT).

The average human adult has about 2×10^{12} lymphoid cells and lymphoid tissue as a whole represents about 2% of total body weight. Lymphoid cells account for about 20% of the leukocytes in the adult circulation.

Many mature lymphoid cells are long-lived, and persist as memory cells for many years.

> **Q. Given that there are roughly 10^9 lymphocytes/liter of blood and an average of 5 liters of blood in an individual, and that roughly 2×10^9 new cells are produced each day, what can you infer about the location and life span of lymphocytes within an individual?**
>
> A. This implies that less than 1% of an individual's lymphocytes are in the circulation. This highly selective population of lymphocytes is mostly en route between tissues. The data also imply that many lymphocytes must die each day to maintain the overall balance of the lymphoid system, and

that the average life span of a lymphocyte will be months to years. The actual values are, however, enormously variable, depending on the type of lymphocyte.

Lymphocytes are morphologically heterogeneous

In a conventional blood smear, lymphocytes vary in both size (from 6–10 μm in diameter) and morphology.

Differences are seen in:

- nuclear to cytoplasmic (N:C) ratio;
- nuclear shape; and
- the presence or absence of azurophilic granules.

Two distinct morphological types of lymphocyte are seen in the circulation as determined by light microscopy and a hematological stain such as Giemsa (Fig. 2.19):

- the first type is relatively small, is typically agranular and has a high nuclear to cytoplasmic (N:C) ratio (Fig. 2.19[1]);
- the second type is larger, has a lower N:C ratio, contains cytoplasmic azurophilic granules, and is known as the large granular lymphocyte (LGL).

LGLs should not be confused with granulocytes, monocytes, or their precursors, which also contain azurophilic granules.

Most T cells express the αβ T cell receptor (see below) and, when resting, can show either of the above morphological patterns.

Most T helper (TH) cells (approximately 95%) and a proportion (approximately 50%) of cytotoxic T cells (TC or CTL) have the morphology shown in Figure 2.19(1).

The LGL morphological pattern displayed in Figure 2.19 (2) is shown by less than 5% of TH cells and by about 30–50% of TC cells. These cells display LGL morphology with primary lysosomes dispersed in the cytoplasm and a well-developed Golgi apparatus, as shown in Figure 2.19(3).

Most B cells, when resting, have a morphology similar to that seen in Figure 2.19(1) under light microscopy.

Lymphocytes express characteristic surface and cytoplasmic markers

Lymphocytes (and other leukocytes) express a large number of different functionally important molecules mostly on their surfaces but also in their cytoplasm, which can be used to distinguish ('mark') cell subsets. Many of these cell markers can be identified by specific monoclonal antibodies (mAb) and can be used to distinguish T cells from B cells (Fig. 2.20).

Lymphocytes express a variety of cell surface molecules that belong to different families, which have probably evolved from a few ancestral genes. These families of molecules are shared with other leukocytes and are distinguished by their structure. The major families include:

- the immunoglobulin superfamily;
- the integrin family;
- selectins;
- proteoglycans.

The **immunoglobulin superfamily** comprises molecules with structural characteristics similar to those of the

Morphological heterogeneity of lymphocytes

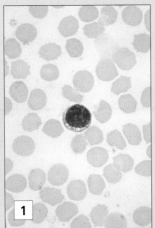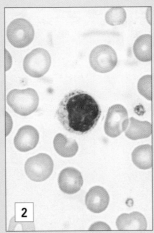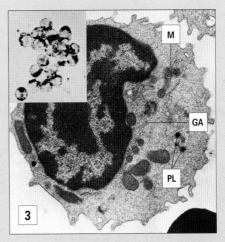

Fig. 2.19 Lymphocyte morphology. (**1**) The small lymphocyte has no granules, a round nucleus, and a high N:C ratio. (**2**) The large granular lymphocyte (LGL) has a lower N:C ratio, indented nucleus, and azurophilic granules in the cytoplasm. Giemsa stain. (**3**) Ultrastructure of the LGL shows characteristic electron-dense peroxidase-negative granules (primary lysosomes, PL), scattered throughout the cytoplasm, with some close to the Golgi apparatus (GA) and many mitochondria (M). × 10 000. ((1) Adapted from Zucker-Franklin D, Grossi CE, eds. Atlas of blood cells: function and pathology, 3rd edn. Milan: Edi Ermes; 2003. (2) Courtesy of Dr A Stevens and Professor J Lowe.)

Main distinguishing markers of T and B cells

CD number	T cells	B cells
antigen receptor	TCR – (αβ or γδ)	immunoglobulin (Ig)
CD1	–	+
CD3	+ (part of the TCR complex)	–
CD4	+ (subset)	–
CD8	+ (subset)	–
CD19	–	+
CD20	–	+
CD23	+ (subset)	+
CD40	–	+
CD79a	–	+ (part of the BCR complex)
CD79b	–	+ (part of the BCR complex)
BCR, B cell receptor; TCR, T cell receptor		

Fig. 2.20 Main distinguishing markers of T and B cells.

immunoglobulins and includes CD2, CD3, CD4, CD8, CD28, MHC class I and II molecules, and many more.

The **integrin** family consists of heterodimeric molecules with α and β chains. There are several integrin subfamilies and all members of a particular subfamily share a common β chain, but each has a unique α chain:

- one integrin subfamily (**the β₂-integrins**) uses CD18 as the β chain, which can be associated with CD11a, CD11b, CD11c, or αd – these combinations make up the lymphocyte function antigens LFA-1, Mac-1 (CR3), p150, 95, and αdβ₂ surface molecules respectively – and are commonly found on leukocytes;
- a second subfamily (**the β₁-integrins**) has CD29 as the β chain, which again is associated with various other peptides and includes the VLA (very late activation) markers.

The **selectins** (CD62, E, L, and P) are expressed on leukocytes (L) or activated endothelial cells and platelets

(E and P). They have lectin-like specificity for a variety of sugars expressed on heavily glycosylated membrane glyco-proteins (e.g. CD43).

The **proteoglycans**, typically CD44, have a number of glycosaminoglycan (GAG) binding sites (e.g. for chondroi-tin sulfate), and bind to extracellular matrix components (typically, hyaluronic acid).

Other families include:

- the tumor necrosis factor (TNF) and nerve growth factor (NGF) receptor superfamily;
- the C-type lectin superfamily;
- the family of receptors with seven transmembrane segments (tm7); and
- the tetraspanins, a superfamily with four membrane-spanning segments (tm4), for example CD20.

Marker molecules allow lymphocytes to communicate with their environment

The major function of the families of marker molecules de-scribed above is to allow lymphocytes to communicate with their environment. They are extremely important in cell trafficking, adhesion, and activation.

Markers expressed by lymphocytes can often be detected on cells of other lineages (e.g. CD44 is commonly expressed by epithelial cells).

T cells can be distinguished by their different antigen receptors

The definitive T cell lineage marker is the T cell antigen receptor (TCR). The two defined types of TCR are:

- a heterodimer of two disulfide-linked polypeptides (α and β);
- a structurally similar heterodimer consisting of γ and δ polypeptides.

Both receptors are associated with a set of five polypeptides (the CD3 complex) and together form the TCR complex (TCR–CD3 complex; see Chapter 5).

Approximately 90–95% of blood T cells in humans are αβ T cells and the remaining 5–10% are γδ T cells.

There are three major subpopulations of αβ T cells

- Helper T cells (TH) that express the **CD4 marker (CD4$^+$ T cells), and mainly** 'helps' or 'induces' immune responses, divided into two main subsets (TH1 and TH2).
- Regulatory T cells (Tregs) that express the **CD4 marker (CD4$^+$T cells)** and regulate immune responses.
- Cytotoxic T cells (Tc) that express the **CD8 marker (CD8$^+$ T cells)** – also called cytotoxic T lymphocytes (CTLs).

CD4$^+$ T cells recognize their specific antigens in association with MHC class II molecules, whereas CD8$^+$ T cells recog-nize antigens in association with MHC class I molecules (see Chapter 7). Thus, the presence of CD4 or CD8 limits (restricts) the type of cell with which the T cell can interact (Fig. 2.21).

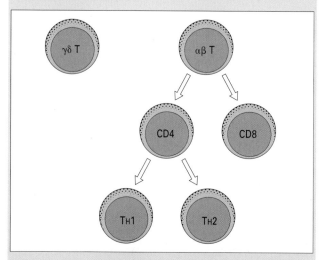

Functional T cell subsets

Fig. 2.21 T cells express either γδ or αβ T cell receptors (TCR). T cells are divided into CD4$^+$ and CD8$^+$ subsets and these subsets determine whether they see antigen (peptides) with MHC class II or I molecules, respectively. CD4$^+$ T cells can be further subdivided into TH1 and TH2 on the basis of their cytokine profiles.

A small proportion of αβ T cells express neither CD4 nor CD8; these 'double negative' T cells might have a regulatory function.

In contrast, while most circulating γδ cells are 'double negative', most γδ T cells in the tissues express CD8.

T helper subsets are distinguished by their cytokine profiles

CD4$^+$ T helper cells can be further divided into functional subsets on the basis of the spectrum of the cytokines they produce:

- TH1 cells secrete IL-2 and IFNγ;
- TH2 cells produce IL-4, IL-5, IL-6, and IL-10 (see Fig. 11.4).

TH1 cells mediate several functions associated with cytotox-icity and local inflammatory reactions. They help cytotoxic T cell precursors develop into effector cells to kill virally-infected target cells and activate macrophages infected with intracellular pathogens (e.g. *Mycobacterium, Chlamydia*) enhancing intracellular killing of the pathogens by the pro-duction of IFNγ. Consequently, they are important for combating intracellular pathogens including viruses, bacte-ria, and parasites. Some TH1 cells also help B cells to pro-duce different classes of antibodies.

Recently a TH17 cell has been described that is similar to the TH1 subset but its induction from TH0 cells is depen-dent on TGFβ and IL-21 and not IL-12 and IFNα. Their in-duction by TGFβ suggests that they are related to the regulatory T cell subsets. They produce both IL-17 and IL-22 and appear to play an important role in maintaining the integrity of mucosal surfaces and thus in protection against microbial entry into the body.

Q. Which cell type do TH1 cells interact with to help combat intracellular pathogens?
A. Mononuclear phagocytes.

TH2 cells are effective at stimulating B cells to proliferate and produce antibodies of some IgG subclasses and especially IgE and therefore function primarily to protect against free-living, extracellular, microorganisms (humoral immunity).

The number of cells producing a given cytokine can be measured using flow cytometry and antibodies that are allowed to penetrate the cells following permeabilization (see Method box 2.1). The same technique can be used to determine the number of B cells producing a particular antibody.

The measurement of single cells secreting a particular cytokine or antibody can be achieved using an enzyme-linked method, namely ELISPOT (see Method box 2.1).

Several CD4$^+$ regulatory T cell populations have been described as being capable of suppressing T cell responses (see below).

Other T cell subsets include γδ T cells and NKT cells

γδ T cells may protect the mucosal surfaces of the body

γδ T cells are relatively frequent in mucosal epithelia, but form only a minor subpopulation of circulating T cells (around 5%). Most intraepithelial lymphocytes (IELs) are γδ T cells and express CD8, a marker not found on most circulating γδ T cells.

γδ T cells have a specific repertoire of TCRs biased towards certain bacterial/viral antigens (**superantigens**, see Fig. 14.16). Human blood γδ T cells have specificity for low molecular mass mycobacterial products (e.g. ethylamine and isopentenyl pyrophosphate).

Current opinion is that γδ T cells may play an important role in protecting the mucosal surfaces of the body. Some γδ T cells may recognize antigens directly (i.e. with no need for MHC molecule-mediated presentation).

γδ T cells display LGL characteristics (see Fig. 2.19) and some have a dendritic morphology in lymphoid tissues (Fig. 2.22). They appear to have a broader specificity for

Dendritic morphology of γδ T cells in the tonsil

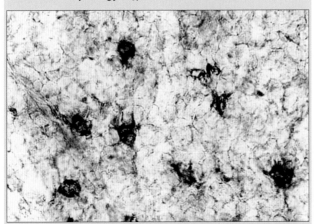

Fig. 2.22 The γδ T cell population is predominantly localized in the interfollicular T cell-dependent zones. Note the dendritic morphology of the cells. Anti-γδ T cell monoclonal antibody and immunoperoxidase. × 900. *(Courtesy of Dr A Favre, from Eur J Immunol 1991;21:173, with permission.)*

recognition of unconventional antigens such as heat shock proteins, phospholipids and phosphoproteins. Unlike αβ T cells, they do not generally recognize antigens in association with classical MHC class I and II molecules. There is evidence that γδ T cells show cytotoxicity and regulatory functions and subsets of them appear to have specific tissue locations.

NKT cells may initiate T cell responses

NKT cells have T markers and also some NK cell markers: they express CD3 and have a unique αβ TCR (expressing an invariant Vα and Vβ11, see Chapter 5).

Q. What markers would one normally use to distinguish T cells from NK cells?
A. CD16 and CD56 are used to distinguish NK cells. CD3 is characteristic of T cells.

NKT cells are thought to recognize glycolipid antigens presented by CD1d molecules (see Chapter 5), but not conventional MHC molecules. In response to antigen they are capable of producing large amounts of IFNγ and IL-4.

NKT cells are therefore thought to act as an interface between the innate and adaptive systems by initiating T cell responses to non-peptide antigens.

NKT cells are also thought to regulate immune responses (especially dendritic cell function) through the production of cytokines (e.g. IL-10).

B cells recognize antigen using the B cell receptor complex

About 5–15% of the circulating lymphoid pool are B cells, which are defined by the presence of **surface immunoglobulin**, transmembrane molecules, which are constitutively produced and inserted into the B cell membrane, where they act as specific antigen receptors.

Most human B cells in peripheral blood express two immunoglobulin isotypes on their surface:

- IgM; and
- IgD (see Chapter 3).

On any B cell, the antigen-binding sites of these IgM and IgD isotypes are identical.

Fewer than 10% of the B cells in the circulation express IgG, IgA, or IgE, but B cells expressing IgG, IgA, or IgE are present in larger numbers in specific locations of the body (e.g. IgA-bearing cells in the intestinal mucosa).

Immunoglobulin associated with other 'accessory' molecules on the B cell surface forms the '**B cell antigen receptor complex' (BCR)**. These 'accessory' molecules consist of disulfide-bonded heterodimers of:

- Igα (CD79a); and
- Igβ (CD79b).

The heterodimers interact with the transmembrane segments of the immunoglobulin receptor (see Fig. 3.1), and, like the separate molecular components of the TCR/CD3 complex (see Fig. 5.2), are involved in cellular activation. Intracellular domains of CD79a/b have immunoreceptor tyrosine-based activation motifs (ITAMs). BCR interaction with specific antigen triggers ITAM phosphorylation and this initiates a downstream cascade of intracellular events leading to the activation-related changes in gene expression.

Other B cell markers include MHC class II antigens and complement and Fc receptors

Most B cells carry MHC class II antigens, which are important for cooperative (cognate) interactions with T cells (see Fig. 5.18).

Complement receptors for C3b (CD35) and C3d (CD21) are commonly found on B cells and are associated with activation and, together with chemokine receptors, possibly 'homing' of the cells in the peripheral lymphoid organs and tissues. CD19/CD21 interactions with complement, associated with antigen, play a role in antigen-induced B cell activation via the antigen-binding antibody receptor.

Fc receptors for exogenous IgG (FcγRII, CD32) are also present on B cells and play a role in negative signaling to the B cell (see Chapter 11).

CD19 and CD20 are the main markers currently used to identify human B cells. Other human B cell markers are CD22 and CD72 to CD78.

Murine B cells also express CD72 (Lyb-2) together with B220, a high molecular weight (220 kDa) isoform of CD45 (Lyb-5).

CD40 is an important molecule on B cells and is involved in cognate interactions between T and B cells (see Fig. 9.6) with T cells expressing CD40 ligand (CD40L).

Activated B cells upregulate expression of B7.1 (CD80) and B7.2 (CD86) molecules that interact with their CD28 expressed by T cells. This provides a co-stimulatory signal for T/B cognate interactions.

CD5+ B-1 cells and marginal zone B cells produce natural antibodies

CD5+ B-1 cells have a variety of roles

Many of the first B cells that appear during ontogeny express CD5, a marker originally found on T cells. These cells (termed B-1 cells) are found predominantly in the peritoneal cavity in mice, and there is some evidence for a separate differentiation pathway from 'conventional' B cells (termed **B-2 cells**).

CD5+ B-1 cells express their immunoglobulins from unmutated or minimally mutated germline genes (see Chapter 3) and produce mostly IgM, but also some IgG and IgA. These so-called natural antibodies are of low avidity, but, unusually, they are polyreactive and are found at high concentration in the adult serum. CD5+ B-1 cells:

- respond well to TI (T-independent) antigens (i.e. antigens that can directly stimulate B cells without T cell help);
- may be involved in antigen processing and antigen presentation to T cells; and
- probably play a role in both tolerance and antibody responses.

Functions proposed for natural antibodies include:

- the first line of defense against microorganisms;
- clearance of damaged self components; and
- regulatory 'idiotype network' interactions within the immune system.

Characteristically, natural antibodies react against autoantigens including:

- DNA;
- Fc of IgG;
- phospholipids; and
- cytoskeletal components.

CD5 has been shown to be expressed by B-2 cells when they are activated appropriately, so there is some controversy about whether CD5 represents an activation antigen on B cells. Current theories therefore support the notion for two different kinds of CD5+ B cells.

Although the function of CD5 on human B cells is unknown, it is associated with the BCR and may be involved in the regulation of B cell activation.

Marginal zone B cells are thought to protect against polysaccharide antigens

Much has been learned about **marginal zone B cells** over the past few years. These cells accumulate slowly in the marginal zone of the spleen – a process that takes between 1 and 2 years in humans.

Like B-1 cells, marginal zone B cells respond to thymus-independent antigens, and they are thought to be our main protection against polysaccharide antigens. They also produce natural antibodies, and together with B-1 cells have recently been termed 'innate-like B cells'.

B cells can differentiate into antibody-secreting plasma cells

Following B cell activation, many B cell blasts mature into **antibody-forming cells** (AFCs), which progress *in vivo* to terminally differentiated **plasma cells**, whilst a subset of B cells remains in the periphery as long-lived memory B cells.

Some B cell blasts do not develop rough endoplasmic reticulum cisternae. These cells are found in germinal centers and are named **follicle center cells** or **centrocytes**.

Under light microscopy, the cytoplasm of the plasma cells is basophilic due to the large amount of RNA being used for antibody synthesis in the rough endoplasmic reticulum. At the ultrastructural level, the rough endoplasmic reticulum can often be seen in parallel arrays (Fig. 2.23).

Plasma cells are infrequent in the blood, comprising less than 0.1% of circulating lymphocytes. They are normally restricted to the secondary lymphoid organs and tissues, but are also abundant in the bone marrow. Since their sole function is to produce immunoglobulins, plasma cells have few surface receptors and do not respond to antigens. Unlike resting B cells or memory B cells, plasma cells do not express surface BCR or MHC class II.

Antibodies produced by a single plasma cell are of one specificity (idiotype) and immunoglobulin class (isotype and allotype; see Chapter 3).

Immunoglobulins can be visualized in the plasma cell cytoplasm by staining with fluorochrome-labeled specific antibodies (Fig. 2.24).

Many plasma cells have a short life span, surviving for a few days and dying by apoptosis (Fig. 2.25). However, a subset of plasma cells with a long life span (months) has recently been described in the bone marrow that might be important in giving rise to sustained antibody responses.

Lymphocyte development

Lymphocytes, the effector cells of the adaptive immune response, are the major component of organs and tissues that collectively form the lymphoid system.

Ultrastructure of the plasma cell

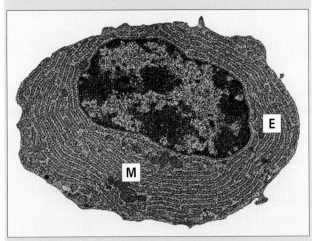

Fig. 2.23 The plasma cell is characterized by parallel arrays of rough endoplasmic reticulum (E). In mature cells, these cisternae become dilated with immunoglobulins. Mitochondria (M) are also seen. × 5000. *(Adapted from Zucker-Franklin D, Grossi CE, eds. Atlas of blood cells: function and pathology, 3rd edn. Milan: Edi Ermes; 2003.)*

Plasma cell death by apoptosis

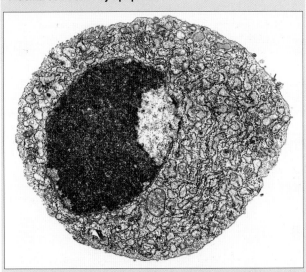

Fig. 2.25 Plasma cells are short-lived and die by apoptosis (cell suicide). Note the nuclear chromatin changes, which are characteristic of apoptosis. × 5000.

Immunofluorescent staining of intracytoplasmic immunoglobulin in plasma cells

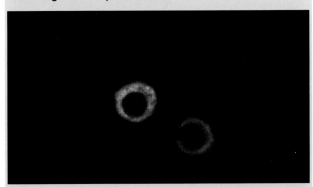

Fig. 2.24 Fixed human plasma cells, treated with fluoresceinated anti-human-IgM (green) antibody and rhodaminated anti-human-IgG (red) antibody, show extensive intracytoplasmic staining. As the distinct staining of the two cells shows, plasma cells normally produce only one class or subclass (isotype) of antibody. × 1500. *(Adapted from Zucker-Franklin D, Grossi CE, eds. Atlas of blood cells: function and pathology, 3rd edn. Milan: Edi Ermes; 2003.)*

Within the lymphoid organs, lymphocytes interact with other cell types of both hematopoietic and non-hematopoietic origin that are important for lymphocyte maturation, selection, function and disposal of terminally differentiated cells.

These other cell types are termed accessory cells and include:

- antigen presenting cells;
- macrophages;
- reticular cells; and
- epithelial cells.

The lymphoid system is arranged into either discrete encapsulated organs or accumulations of diffuse lymphoid tissue, which are classified into primary (central) and secondary (peripheral) organs or tissues (Fig. 2.26).

In essence, lymphocytes:

- are produced, mature, and are selected in primary lymphoid organs; and
- exert their effector functions in the secondary lymphoid organs and tissues.

Tertiary lymphoid tissues are anatomical sites that under normal conditions contain sparse lymphocytes, if any, but may be selectively populated by these cells in pathological conditions (e.g. skin, synovium, lungs).

Lymphoid stem cells develop and mature within primary lymphoid organs

In the primary lymphoid organs, lymphocytes (B and T cells):

- differentiate from lymphoid stem cells;
- proliferate;
- are selected; and
- mature into functional cells.

In mammals, T cells mature in the thymus and B cells mature in the fetal liver and postnatal bone marrow (see Chapter 9). Birds have a specialized site of B cell generation, the bursa of Fabricius.

In the primary lymphoid organs:

- lymphocytes acquire their repertoire of specific antigen receptors to cope with the antigenic challenges that individuals encounter during their lifetime;
- cells with receptors for **autoantigens** are mostly eliminated; and
- in the thymus, T cells also 'learn' to recognize appropriate **self MHC molecules**.

Major lymphoid organs and tissues

primary lymphoid organs	secondary lymphoid organs and tissues

Waldeyer's ring (tonsils and adenoids)

bronchus-associated lymphoid tissue

lymph nodes

bone marrow

spleen

lymphoid nodules

mesenteric lymph nodes

Peyer's patch

urogenital lymphoid tissue

lymph nodes

thymus

bone marrow

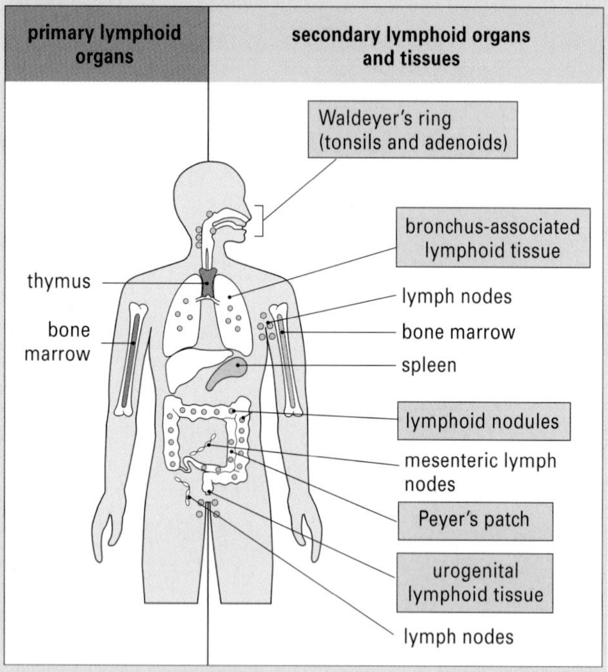

Fig. 2.26 Thymus and bone marrow are the primary (central) lymphoid organs. They are the sites of maturation for T and B cells, respectively. Cellular and humoral immune responses occur in the secondary (peripheral) lymphoid organs and tissues. Secondary lymphoid organs can be classified according to the body regions they defend. The spleen responds predominantly to blood-borne antigens. Lymph nodes mount immune responses to antigens circulating in the lymph, entering through the skin (subcutaneous lymph nodes) or through mucosal surfaces (visceral lymph nodes). Tonsils, Peyer's patches, and other mucosa-associated lymphoid tissues (MALT) (blue boxes) react to antigens that have entered via the surface mucosal barriers. Note that the bone marrow is both a primary and a secondary lymphoid organ because it gives rise to B and NK cells, but is also the site of B cell terminal differentiation (long-lived plasma cells).

There is evidence that some lymphocyte development might occur outside primary lymphoid organs.

Q. Why do lymphocytes need to 'learn' what constitutes self MHC and self antigens?

A. Each individual is different and has a particular set of MHC molecules and particular variants of the many other molecules present in the body. The process of what constitutes immunological 'self' is different in each individual and therefore learning to recognize 'self' is a dialogue between T cells and APCs that takes place in each individual.

T cells develop in the thymus

The thymus in mammals is a bilobed organ in the thoracic cavity overlying the heart and major blood vessels. Each lobe is organized into lobules separated from each other by connective tissue trabeculae.

Thymus section showing the lobular organization

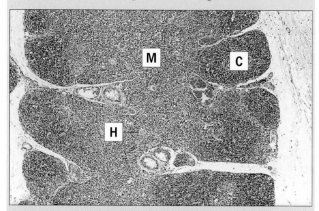

Fig. 2.27 This section shows the two main areas of the thymus lobule – an outer cortex of immature cells (C) and an inner medulla of more mature cells (M). Hassall's corpuscles (H) are found in the medulla. H&E stain. × 25. *(Courtesy of Dr A Stevens and Professor J Lowe.)*

Within each lobule, the lymphoid cells (thymocytes) are arranged into:

- an outer tightly packed cortex, which contains the majority of relatively immature proliferating thymocytes; and
- an inner medulla containing more mature cells, implying a differentiation gradient from cortex to medulla (Fig. 2.27).

The main blood vessels that regulate cell traffic in the thymus are high endothelial venules (HEVs; see Fig. 2.29) at the corticomedullary junction of thymic lobules. It is through these veins that T cell progenitors formed in the fetal liver and bone marrow enter the **epithelial anlage** and migrate towards the cortex.

In the cortex of the thymus the T cell progenitors undergo proliferation and differentiation processes that lead to the generation of mature T cells through a corticomedullary gradient of migration.

A network of epithelial cells throughout the lobules plays a role in the differentiation and selection processes from fetal liver and bone marrow-derived prethymic cells to mature T cells.

The mature T cells probably leave the thymus through the same PCVs, at the corticomedullary junction from which the T cell progenitors entered (Fig. 2.28).

Three types of thymic epithelial cell have important roles in T cell production

At least three types of epithelial cell can be distinguished in the thymic lobules according to distribution, structure, function, and phenotype:

- the epithelial nurse cells are in the outer cortex;
- the cortical thymic epithelial cells (TECs) form an epithelial network; and
- the medullary TECs are mostly organized into clusters (Fig. 2.29).

Cell migration to and within the thymus

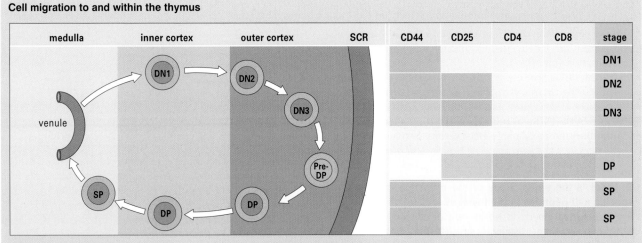

medulla	inner cortex	outer cortex	SCR	CD44	CD25	CD4	CD8	stage
								DN1
								DN2
								DN3
								DP
								SP
								SP

Fig. 2.28 T cell progenitors enter the thymic lobule through postcapillary venules (PCVs) at the corticomedullary junction. These cells are double negative 1 (DN1) for CD4 and CD8 expression but are also CD25$^-$, but CD44$^+$. They move progressively towards the outer cortex and differentiate into DN2 (CD25$^+$, CD44$^+$) and DN3 cells (CD25$^+$, CD44^{lo}). Thymocytes accumulate in the subcapsular region where they actively proliferate and differentiate into double positive (DP; CD4$^+$, CD8$^+$) cells. DP thymocytes reverse their polarity and move towards the medulla. In the course of this migration, thymocytes are selected and as single positive (SP; CD4$^+$ or CD8$^+$) cells ultimately leave the thymus, presumably via HEVs at the corticomedullary junction.

Schematic structure of the thymus

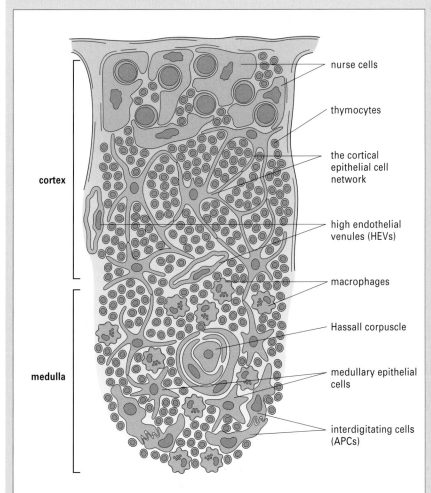

nurse cells

thymocytes

the cortical epithelial cell network

high endothelial venules (HEVs)

macrophages

Hassall corpuscle

medullary epithelial cells

interdigitating cells (APCs)

cortex

medulla

Fig. 2.29 A schematic representation of the cell types found in a fully developed thymic lobule. Subcapsular epithelial cells that produce IL-7 (nurse cells) sustain T lymphoblast proliferation in the outer cortex. Developing T cells interact with the cortical epithelial network where they are positively selected. Apoptotic cells are phagocytosed by macrophages present in the deep cortex and in the medulla. TCR$^+$ thymocytes co-expressing CD4 and CD8 undergo the process of negative selection by interacting with a variety of antigen-presenting cells (APCs), such as dendritic cells, interdigitating cells, macrophages, and epithelial cells. T cells that have survived the selection processes are exported from the thymus via high endothelial venules (HEVs) and lymphatic vessels. *(From Zucker-Franklin D, Grossi CE, eds. Atlas of blood cells: function and pathology, 3rd edn. Milan: Edi Ermes; 2003.)*

These three types of epithelial cell have different roles for thymocyte proliferation, maturation, and selection:

- **nurse cells** in the outer cortex sustain the proliferation of progenitor T cells, mainly through cytokine production (e.g. IL-7);
- **cortical TECs** are responsible for the positive selection of maturing thymocytes, allowing survival of cells that recognize MHC class I and II molecules with associated peptides via TCRs of intermediate affinity; and
- **medullary TECs** display a large variety of organ-specific self peptides through transcription factors such as AIRE (autoimmune regulator).

Q. What is the significance of the presence of organ-specific self peptides in the thymus?

A. An individual needs to be tolerant of antigens that are expressed in other tissues, not just the thymus. By presenting a library of self molecules, the thymus can delete or tolerize lymphocytes that might otherwise react against self molecules once they had migrated into other tissues. Thus TECs, together with other APCs (interdigitating cells and macrophages), play a role in negative selection (i.e. the deletion of self-reactive T cells).

Hassall's corpuscles (see Fig. 2.27) are found in the thymic medulla. Their function is unknown, but they appear to contain degenerating epithelial cells rich in high molecular weight cytokeratins.

The mammalian thymus involutes with age (Fig. 2.30). In humans, atrophy begins at puberty and continues throughout life. Thymic involution begins within the cortex and this region may disappear completely, whereas medullary remnants persist.

Cortical atrophy is related to a sensitivity of the cortical thymocytes to corticosteroid, and all conditions associated with an acute increase in corticosteroids (e.g. pregnancy and stress) promote thymic atrophy.

It is conceivable that T cell generation within the thymus continues into adult life, albeit at a low rate. Evidence for

de novo T cell production in the thymus (recent thymic emigrants) has been shown in humans over the age of 76 years.

Stem cell migration to the thymus initiates T cell development

The thymus develops from the endoderm of the third pharyngeal pouch as an epithelial rudiment that becomes seeded with blood-borne stem cells. Relatively few stem cells appear to be needed to give rise to the enormous repertoire of mature T cells with diverse antigen receptor specificities.

From experimental studies, migration of stem cells into the thymus is not a random process, but results from chemotactic signals periodically emitted from the thymic rudiment. β_2-microglobulin, a component of the MHC class I molecule, is one such putative chemoattractant.

In birds, stem cells enter the thymus in two or possibly three waves, but it is not clear that there are such waves in mammals.

Once in the thymus, the stem cells begin to differentiate into thymic lymphocytes (called thymocytes), under the influence of the epithelial microenvironment.

Whether or not the stem cells are 'pre-T cells' (i.e. are committed to becoming T cells before they arrive in the thymus) is controversial. Although the stem cells express CD7, substantial evidence exists that they are in fact multipotent. Granulocytes, APCs, NK cells, B cells, and myeloid cells have all been generated *in vitro* from hematopoietic precursors isolated from the thymus. This suggests that the prethymic bone marrow-derived cell entering the thymic rudiment is multipotent.

Notch1 receptor has proved to be essential for T cell development, and is involved in T versus B cell fate determination through interaction with thymic epithelial cells expressing Notch ligands. At this particular level Notch1 acts as a lineage specifier. Notch1 deficient bone marrow progenitors migrate from the bone marrow to the thymus but can no longer develop towards the T cell lineage. Since these progenitors are still at least bi-potential they develop into B cells instead.

Epithelial cells, macrophages, and bone marrow-derived IDCs, molecules rich in MHC class II, are important for the differentiation of T cells from this multipotent stem cell. For example, specialized epithelial cells in the peripheral areas of the cortex (the thymic nurse cells, see above) contain thymocytes within pockets in their cytoplasm. The nurse cells support lymphocyte proliferation by producing the cytokine IL-7.

The subcapsular region of the thymus is the only site where thymocyte proliferation occurs. Thymocytes develop into large, actively proliferating, self-renewing lymphoblasts, which generate the thymocyte population.

There are many more developing lymphocytes (85–90%) in the thymic cortex than in the medulla, and studies of function and cell surface markers have indicated that cortical thymocytes are less mature than medullary thymocytes. This reflects the fact that cortical cells migrate to, and mature in, the medulla.

Most mature T cells leave the thymus via HEVs at the corticomedullary junction, though other routes of exit may exist, including lymphatic vessels.

Atrophic adult thymus

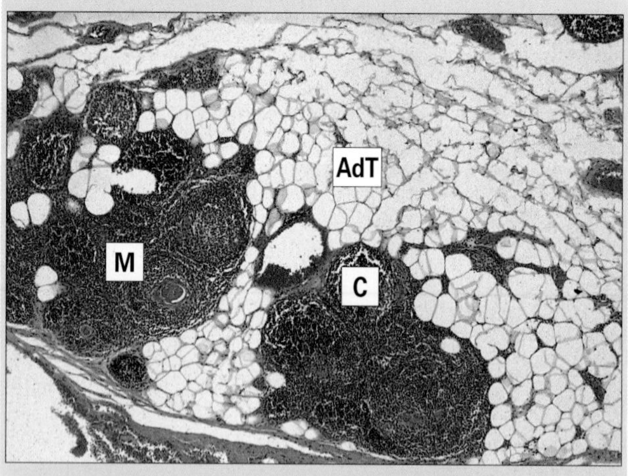

Fig. 2.30 There is an involution of the thymus with replacement by adipose tissue (AdT). The cortex (C) is largely reduced and the less cellular medulla (M) is still apparent. *(Courtesy of Dr A Stevens and Professor J Lowe.)*

The T cell receptor is generated during development in the thymus

TCR gene recombination takes place within the subcapsular and outer cortex of the thymus, where there is active cell proliferation. Through a random assortment of different gene segments, a large number of different TCRs are made and thymocytes that fail to make a functional receptor die. The TCRs associate with peptides of the CD3 complex, which transduces activating signals to the cell (see Chapter 5).

Positive and negative selection of developing T cells takes place in the thymus

The processes involved in the education of T cells are shown in Figure 2.31, and self tolerance is discussed fully in Chapter 11. Positive selection ensures only TCRs with an intermediate affinity for self MHC develop further.

T cells:

- recognize antigenic peptides only when presented by self MHC molecules on APCs; and
- show 'dual recognition' of both the antigenic peptides and the polymorphic part of the MHC molecules.

Positive selection (the first stage of **thymic education**) ensures that only those TCRs with an intermediate affinity for self MHC are allowed to develop further. There is evidence that positive selection is mediated by TECs acting as APCs.

T cells displaying very high or very low receptor affinities for self MHC undergo apoptosis and die in the cortex. Apoptosis is a pre-programmed 'suicide', achieved by activating endogenous nucleases that cause DNA fragmentation.

T cells with TCRs that have intermediate affinities are rescued from apoptosis, survive, and continue along their pathway of maturation. A possible exception is provided by some T cells equipped with $\gamma\delta$ receptors, which (like B cells) recognize native antigenic conformations with no need for APCs.

Negative selection ensures that only T cells that fail to recognize self antigen proceed in their development. Some of the positively selected T cells may have TCRs that recognize self components other than self MHC. These cells are deleted by a 'negative selection' process, which occurs:

- in the deeper cortex;
- at the corticomedullary junction; and
- in the medulla.

T cells interact with antigen presented by interdigitating cells, macrophages, and medullary TECs. The role of medullary TECs for negative selection has been emphasized recently by the finding that these cells express genes for virtually all tissue antigens in the body, and that these genes are activated by certain transcription factors (TF) to express these antigens (e.g. AIRE).

Only T cells that fail to recognize self antigen are allowed to proceed in their development. The rest undergo apoptosis and are destroyed. These, and all the other apoptotic cells generated in the thymus, are phagocytosed by (tingible body) macrophages (see Fig. 2.45) in the deep cortex.

T cells at this stage of maturation (CD4$^+$ CD8$^+$ TCR^{lo}) go on to express TCR at high density and lose either CD4 or CD8 to become 'single positive' mature T cells.

The separate subsets of CD4$^+$ and CD8$^+$ cells possess specialized homing receptors (e.g. CD44), and exit to the

---

T cell differentiation within the thymus

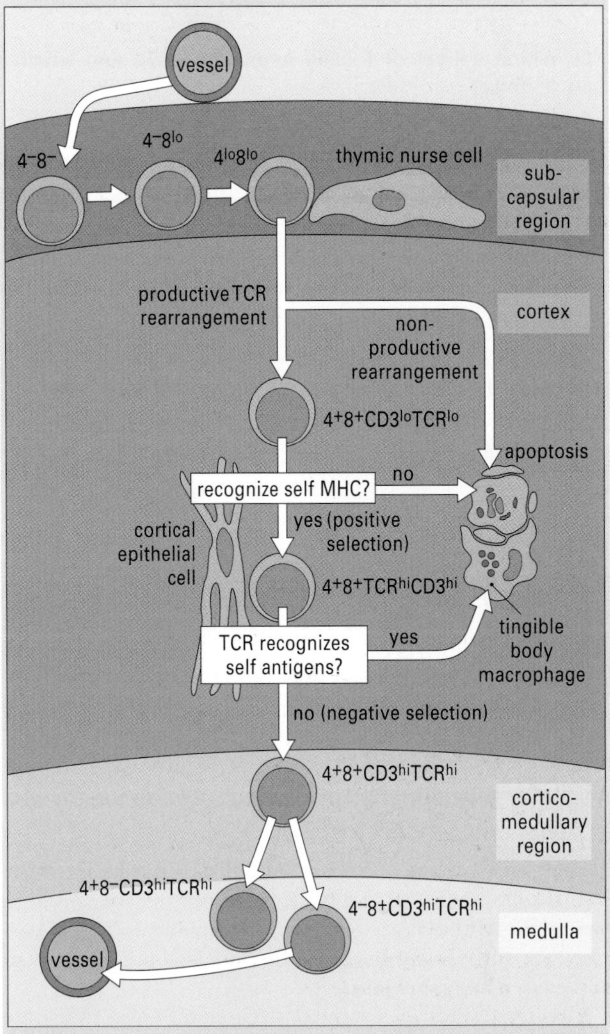

Fig. 2.31 In this model, pre-thymic T cells are attracted to and enter the thymic rudiment at the corticomedullary junction. They reach the subcapsular region where they proliferate as large lymphoblasts, which give rise to a pool of cells entering the differentiation pathway. Many of these cells are associated with epithelial thymic nurse cells. Cells in this region first acquire CD8 and then CD4 at low density. They also rearrange their T cell receptor (TCR) genes and may express the products of these genes at low density on the cell surface. Maturing cells move deeper into the cortex and adhere to cortical epithelial cells. These epithelial cells are elongated and branched, and thus provide a large surface area for contact with thymocytes. The TCRs on the thymocytes are exposed to epithelial MHC molecules through these contacts. This leads to positive selection. Those cells that are not selected undergo apoptosis and are phagocytosed by macrophages. There is an increased expression of CD3, TCR, CD4, and CD8 during thymocyte migration from the subcapsular region to the deeper cortex. Those TCRs with self reactivity are now deleted through contact with autoantigens presented by medullary thymic epithelial cells, interdigitating cells, and macrophages at the corticomedullary junction – a process called negative selection. Following this stage, cells expressing either CD4 or CD8 appear and exit to the periphery via specialized vessels at the corticomedullary junction. *(Adapted from D Zucker-Franklin, CE Grossi, eds. Atlas of blood cells: function and pathology, 3rd edn. Milan: Edi Ermes; 2003.)*

T cell areas of the peripheral (secondary) lymphoid tissues where they function as mature 'helper' and 'cytotoxic' T cells, respectively.

Q. Which subset of T cells functions as TH and which as Tc cells?
A. CD4$^+$ T cells function mainly as TH cells whereas CD8$^+$ T cells are predominantly Tc cells.

Less than 5% of thymocytes leave the thymus as mature T cells. The rest die as the result of:

- selection processes; or
- failure to undergo productive rearrangements of antigen receptor genes.

Adhesion of maturing thymocytes to epithelial and accessory cells is crucial for T cell development

Adhesion of maturing thymocytes to epithelial and other accessory cells is mediated by the interaction of complementary adhesion molecules, such as:

- CD2 with LFA-3 (CD58); and
- LFA-1 (CD11a, CD18) with ICAM-1 (CD54).

These interactions induce the production of the cytokines IL-1, IL-3, IL-6, IL-7, and GM-CSF, which are required for T cell proliferation and maturation in the thymus.

Early thymocytes also express receptors for IL-2, which together with IL-7 sustains cell proliferation.

Negative selection may also occur outside the thymus in peripheral lymphoid tissues

Not all self-reactive T cells are eliminated during intrathymic development, probably because not all self antigens can be presented in the thymus. The thymic epithelial barrier that surrounds blood vessels may also limit access of some circulating antigens.

Given the survival of some self-reacting T cells, a separate mechanism is required to prevent them attacking the body. Experiments with transgenic mice have suggested that peripheral inactivation of self-reactive T cells (**peripheral tolerance**, see Chapter 19) could occur via several mechanisms as follows:

- downregulation of the TCR and CD8 (in cytotoxic cells) so that the cells are unable to interact with target autoantigens;
- **anergy**, due to the lack of crucial co-stimulatory signals provided by the target cells, followed by induction of apoptosis after interaction with autoantigen;
- regulatory T cells (Tregs).

Regulatory T cells are involved in peripheral tolerance

Tregs have been the subject of intensive research over the past few years, especially in the areas of autoimmunity and vaccine development.

In addition to NKT cells and γδ T cells regulating immune responses, there is now substantial evidence that separate CD4$^+$ subsets also have this function. The general consensus is that there are two main types of Treg – naturally occurring, and inducible following activation by specific antigen.

Naturally occurring Tregs:

- constitutively express CD25 (the α chain of the receptor for IL-2);
- constitute about 5–10% of the peripheral CD4$^+$ T cells;
- express the unique transcription factor FoxP3;
- constitutively express the marker CTLA4;
- do not proliferate in response to antigenic challenge;
- are thought to produce their suppressive effects through cell contact (e.g. with APCs, TH1 or TH2 cells).

Antigen-induced Tregs:

- also express CD25;
- can develop from CD25$^-$, CD4$^+$ T cells;
- are believed to exert their suppressive effects through IL-10.

There is some evidence for extrathymic development of T cells

The vast majority of T cells require a functioning thymus for differentiation, but small numbers of cells carrying T cell markers that are often oligoclonal in nature have been found in athymic ('nude') mice. Although the possibility that these mice possess thymic remnants cannot be ruled out, there is accumulating evidence to suggest that bone marrow precursors can home to mucosal epithelia and mature without the need for a thymus to form functional T cells with γδ TCRs and probably also T cells with αβ TCRs.

The importance of extrathymic development in animals that are euthymic (i.e. that have a normal thymus) is at present unclear.

B cells develop mainly in the fetal liver and bone marrow

Unlike birds, which have a discrete organ for the generation of B cells (the bursa of Fabricius), in mammals B cells develop directly from lymphoid stem cells in the hematopoietic tissue of the fetal liver (Fig. 2.32). This occurs at 8–9 weeks of gestation in humans, and by about 14 days in the mouse. Later, the site of B cell production moves from

Hemopoiesis in fetal liver

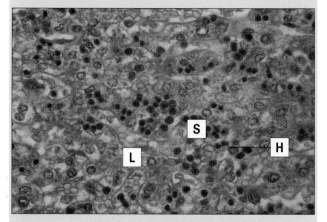

Fig. 2.32 Section of human fetal liver showing islands of hemopoiesis (H). Hematopoietic stem cells are found in the sinusoidal spaces (S) between plates of liver cells (L). *(Courtesy of Dr A Stevens and Professor J Lowe.)*

the liver to the bone marrow, where it continues through adult life. This fetal liver-bone marrow migration of stem cells is also true for cells of other hematopoietic lineages such as erythrocytes, granulocytes, monocytes, and platelets. The B cell lineage specifier is the transcription factor PAX5 which is expressed initially in B cell precursors but then at all stages of B cell development

B cell progenitors are also present in the omental tissue of murine and human fetuses and are the precursors of a self-replicating B cell subset, the B-1 cells (see above).

B cell production in the bone marrow does not occur in distinct domains

B cell progenitors in the bone marrow are seen adjacent to the endosteum of the bone lamellae (Fig. 2.33). Each B cell progenitor, at the stage of immunoglobulin gene rearrangement may produce up to 64 progeny. The progeny migrate towards the center of each cavity of the spongy bone and reach the lumen of a venous sinusoid (Fig. 2.34).

In the bone marrow, B cells mature in close association with **stromal reticular cells**, which are found both adjacent to the endosteum and in close association with the central sinus, where they are termed **adventitial reticular cells**.

Where the B cells differentiate, the reticular cells have mixed phenotypic features with some similarities to fibroblasts, endothelial cells, and myofibroblasts. The reticular cells produce type IV collagen, laminin and the smooth muscle form of actin. Experiments in vitro have shown that reticular cells sustain B cell differentiation, possibly by producing the cytokine IL-7.

Adventitial reticular cells may be important for the release of mature B cells into the central sinus.

B cells are subject to selection processes

Most B cells (>75%) maturing in the bone marrow do not reach the circulation, but (like thymocytes) undergo a process of programmed cell death (apoptosis) and are phagocytosed by bone marrow macrophages.

Bone marrow

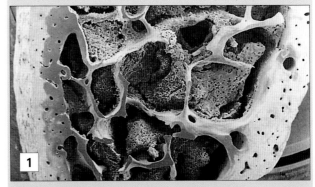
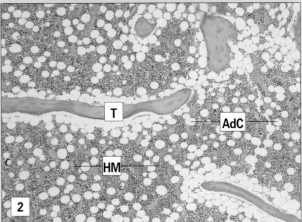

Fig. 2.34 (**1**) Low-power scanning electron micrograph showing the architecture of bone and its relationship to bone marrow. Within the cavities of spongy bone between the bony trabeculae, B cell lymphopoiesis takes place, with maturation occurring in a radial direction towards the center (from the endosteum to the central venous sinus). (**2**) The biopsy below shows hematopoietic bone marrow (HM) in the spaces between the bony trabeculae (lamellae) (T). Some of the space is also occupied by adipocytes (AdC). *(Courtesy of Dr A Stevens and Professor J Lowe.)*

Schematic organization of B cell development in the bone marrow

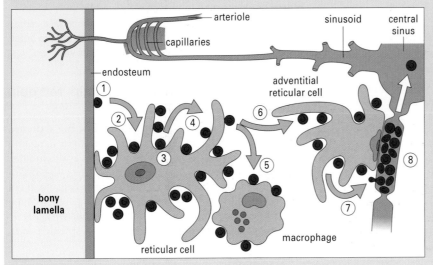

Fig. 2.33 The earliest B cell progenitors are found close to the endosteum (**1**) where they interact with stromal reticular cells (**2**). The stromal reticular cells prompt precursor B cell proliferation and maturation (**3** and **4**). During these processes, selection occurs, which implies B cell apoptosis and phagocytosis of apoptotic cells by macrophages (**5**). B cells that have survived selection mature further and interact with adventitial reticular cells (**6**), which may facilitate their ingress (**7**) into bone marrow sinusoids (**8**) and finally the central venous sinuses, from which they enter the general circulation. In this model, maturation and selection events follow a gradient from the periphery of the bone marrow tissue contained in the bony spaces towards the center.

Q. By analogy with T cell development, infer what determines whether a B cell will die during development in the bone marrow.

A. B cells with a non-productive rearrangement of the immunoglobulin genes do not survive and many self-reactive B cells are also eliminated through negative selection.

B cell–stromal cell interactions enhance the survival of developing B cells and mediate a form of selection that rescues a minority of B cells with productive rearrangements of their immunoglobulin genes from programmed cell death.

Many self-reactive B cells are also eliminated through negative selection in the bone marrow.

From kinetic data, it is estimated that about 5×10^7 murine B cells are produced each day. As the mouse spleen contains approximately 7.5×10^7 B cells, a large proportion of B cells must die, probably at the pre-B cell stage, because of non-productive rearrangements of receptor genes or if they express self-reactive antibodies and are not rescued.

Immunoglobulins are the definitive B cell lineage markers

Lymphoid stem cells expressing terminal deoxynucleotidyl transferase (TdT) proliferate, differentiate, and undergo immunoglobulin gene rearrangements to emerge as pre-B cells (see Chapters 3 and 9). A sequence of immunoglobulin gene rearrangements and phenotypic changes takes place during B cell ontogeny (see Chapter 8), similar to that described above for T cells.

Heavy-chain gene rearrangements occur in B cell progenitors and represent the earliest indication of B lineage commitment. This is followed by light-chain gene rearrangements, which occur at later pre-B cell stages.

Once a B cell has synthesized light chains, it becomes committed to the antigen-binding specificity of its surface IgM (sIgM) antigen receptor.

One B cell can therefore make only one specific antibody – a central tenet of the **clonal selection theory** for antibody production.

Surface immunoglobulin-associated molecules Igα and Igβ (CD79a and b) are present by the pre-B cell stage of development.

B cells migrate to and function in the secondary lymphoid tissues

Early B cell immigrants into fetal lymph nodes (17 weeks in humans) are surface IgM$^+$ and are B-1 cells. CD5$^+$ B cell precursors are found in the fetal omentum.

Some CD5$^+$ B cells are also found in the marginal zone of the spleen and mantle zone of secondary follicles in adult lymph nodes (see Fig. 2.42).

Following antigenic stimulation, mature B cells can develop into memory cells or antibody-forming cells (AFCs).

Surface immunoglobulins (sIg) are usually lost from plasma cells (the terminally differentiated form of an AFC) because their function as a receptor is no longer required. Like any other terminally differentiated hematopoietic cell, the plasma cell has a limited life span, and eventually undergoes apoptosis.

Lymphoid organs

The generation of lymphocytes in primary lymphoid organs is followed by their migration into peripheral secondary tissues, which comprise:

- well-organized encapsulated organs, the spleen and lymph nodes (systemic lymphoid organs); and
- non-encapsulated accumulations of lymphoid tissue.

Lymphoid tissue found in association with mucosal surfaces is called mucosa-associated lymphoid tissue (MALT).

Lymphoid organs and tissues protect different body sites

The systemic lymphoid organs and the mucosal system have different functions in immunity:

- the spleen is responsive to blood-borne antigens, and patients who have had their spleen removed are much more susceptible to pathogens that reach the blood stream;
- the lymph nodes protect the body from antigens that come from skin or from internal surfaces and are transported via the lymphatic vessels;
- the MALT protects mucosal surfaces.

Responses to antigens encountered via the spleen and lymph nodes result in the secretion of antibodies into the circulation and local cell-mediated responses.

Being the major port of entry into the body for pathogens, the mucosa-associated lymphoid tissue is the site of first encounter (priming) of immune cells with antigens entering via mucosal surfaces, and lymphoid tissues are associated with surfaces lining:

- the intestinal tract – gut-associated lymphoid tissue (GALT);
- the respiratory tract – bronchus-associated lymphoid tissue (BALT); and
- the genitourinary tract.

The major effector mechanism at mucosal surfaces is secretory IgA antibody (sIgA), which is actively transported via the mucosal epithelial cells to the lumen of the tracts.

Q. More than 50% of the body's lymphoid tissue is in the MALT and IgA is the most abundant immunoglobulin in the body. What reason could explain this preponderance of immune defenses in mucosal tissues?

A. The mucosal surfaces present a large surface area, vulnerable to infectious agents. Most infectious agents enter the body by infecting and/or crossing mucosal surfaces.

The spleen is made up of white pulp, red pulp, and a marginal zone

The spleen lies at the upper left quadrant of the abdomen, behind the stomach and close to the diaphragm. The adult spleen is around 13×8 cm in size and weighs approximately 180–250 g.

The outer layer of the spleen consists of a capsule of collagenous bundles of fibers, which enter the parenchyma of the organ as short trabeculae. These, together with a reticular framework, support two main types of splenic tissue:

- the white pulp; and
- the red pulp.

A third compartment, the **marginal zone**, is located at the outer limit of the white pulp.

The white pulp consists of lymphoid tissue

The white pulp of the spleen consists of lymphoid tissue, the bulk of which is arranged around a central arteriole to form the periarteriolar lymphoid sheaths (PALS; Fig. 2.35). PALS are composed of T and B cell areas:

* the T cells are found around the central arteriole;
* the B cells may be organized into either primary 'unstimulated' follicles (aggregates of virgin B cells) or secondary 'stimulated' follicles (which possess a germinal center with memory cells).

The germinal centers also contain follicular dendritic cells (FDCs) and phagocytic macrophages. Macrophages and the FDCs present antigen to B cells in the spleen.

B cells and other lymphocytes are free to leave and enter the PALS via branches of the central arterioles, which enter a system of blood vessels in the marginal zone (see below). Some lymphocytes, especially maturing plasmablasts, can pass across the marginal zone via bridges into the red pulp.

The red pulp consists of venous sinuses and cellular cords

The venous sinuses and cellular cords of the red pulp contain:

* resident macrophages;
* erythrocytes;
* platelets;
* granulocytes;
* lymphocytes; and
* numerous plasma cells.

White pulp of the spleen

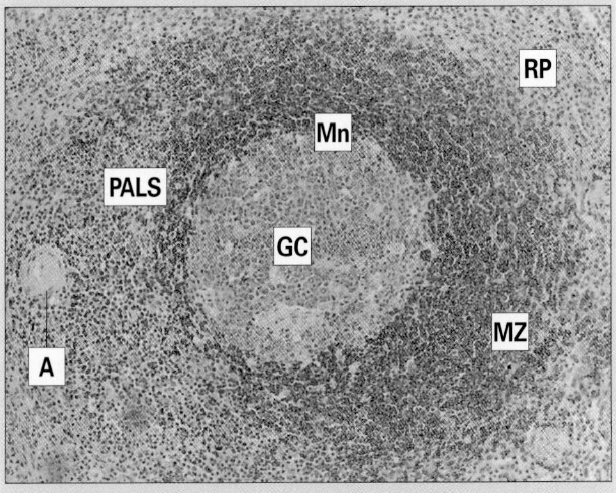

Fig. 2.35 Spleen section showing a white pulp lymphoid aggregate. A secondary lymphoid follicle, with germinal center (GC) and mantle (Mn), is surrounded by the marginal zone (MZ) and red pulp (RP). Adjacent to the follicle, an arteriole (A) is surrounded by the periarteriolar lymphoid sheath (PALS) consisting mainly of T cells. Note that the marginal zone is present only at one side of the secondary follicle. *(Courtesy of Professor I Maclennan.)*

In addition to immunological functions, the spleen serves as a reservoir for platelets, erythrocytes, and granulocytes. Aged platelets and erythrocytes are destroyed in the red pulp in a process referred to as 'hemocatheresis'.

The functions of the spleen are made possible by its vascular organization (Fig. 2.36). Central arteries surrounded by PALS end with arterial capillaries, which open freely into the red pulp cords. Circulating cells can therefore reach these cords and become trapped. Aged platelets and erythrocytes are recognized and phagocytosed by macrophages.

Blood cells that are not ingested and destroyed can re-enter the blood circulation by squeezing through holes in the discontinuous endothelial wall of the venous sinuses, through which plasma flows freely.

The marginal zone contains B cells, macrophages, and dendritic cells

The marginal zone surrounds the white pulp and exhibits two major features, namely:

* a characteristic vascular organization; and
* unique subsets of resident cells (B cells, macrophages, and dendritic cells).

The blood vessels of the marginal zone form a system of communicating sinuses, which receive blood from branches of the central artery (see Fig. 2.36).

Most of the blood from the marginal sinuses enters the red pulp cords and then drains into the venous sinuses, but a small proportion passes directly into the venous sinuses to form a closed circulation.

Cells residing in the marginal zone comprise:

* various types of APC – metallophilic macrophages, marginal zone macrophages, dendritic cells;
* a subset of B cells with distinctive phenotype and function – they express high levels of IgM and low or absent IgD and in humans are long-lived recirculating cells;
* some B-1 cells.

Q. In humans, the marginal zone does not develop fully until 2 years of age. What is the functional consequence of this delay in development of the marginal zone?
A. Marginal zone B cells and B-1 cells respond strongly to thymus-independent antigens, including capsular polysaccharides of bacteria, and the main function of the marginal zone is to mount immune responses to bacteria that have reached the circulation (e.g. streptococci). Infants therefore have a reduced ability to respond to blood-borne infections with certain (encapsulated) bacteria.

Lymph nodes filter antigens from the interstitial tissue fluid and lymph

The lymph nodes form part of a network that filters antigens from the interstitial tissue fluid and lymph during its passage from the periphery to the thoracic duct and the other major collecting ducts (Fig. 2.37).

Lymph nodes frequently occur at the branches of the lymphatic vessels. Clusters of lymph nodes are strategically placed in areas that drain various superficial and deep regions of the body, such as the:

* neck;
* axillae;

Vascular organization of the spleen

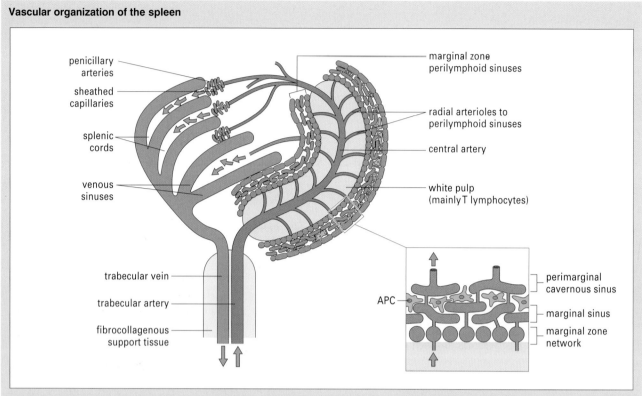

Fig. 2.36 The splenic artery branches to form trabecular arteries, which give rise to central arteries surrounded by periarteriolar lymphoid sheaths (PALS), which are the T cell areas of the white pulp. Leaving the PALS, the central arteries continue as penicillary arteries and sheathed capillaries, which open in the splenic cords of the red pulp. From the red pulp (where hemocatheresis takes place) the blood percolates through the wall of the venous sinuses. The central arterioles surrounded by PALS give collateral branches that reach a series of sinuses in the marginal zone. Most of the blood from the marginal sinuses enters the red pulp cords and then drains into the venous sinuses, but a proportion passes directly into the sinuses to form a closed circulation. *(Courtesy of Dr A Stevens and Professor J Lowe.)*

- groin;
- mediastinum; and
- abdominal cavity.

Lymph nodes protect the skin (superficial subcutaneous nodes) and mucosal surfaces of the respiratory, digestive, and genitourinary tracts (visceral or deep nodes).

Human lymph nodes are 2–10 mm in diameter, are round or kidney shaped, and have an indentation called the hilus where blood vessels enter and leave the node.

Lymph arrives at the lymph node via several afferent lymphatic vessels, and leaves the node through a single efferent lymphatic vessel at the hilus.

Lymph nodes consist of B and T cell areas and a medulla

A typical lymph node is surrounded by a collagenous capsule. Radial trabeculae, together with reticular fibers, support the various cellular components. The lymph node consists of:

- a B cell area (cortex);
- a **T cell area (paracortex)**; and
- a central **medulla**, consisting of cellular cords containing T cells, B cells, abundant plasma cells, and macrophages (Figs 2.38–2.40).

The paracortex contains many APCs (interdigitating cells), which express high levels of MHC class II surface molecules.

These are cells migrating from the skin (Langerhans' cells) or from mucosae (dendritic cells), which transport processed antigens into the lymph nodes from the external and internal surfaces of the body (Fig. 2.41). The bulk of the lymphoid tissue is found in the cortex and paracortex.

The paracortex contains specialized postcapillary vessels – **high endothelial venules (HEVs)** – which allow the traffic of lymphocytes out of the circulation into the lymph node (see 'Lymphocyte traffic' below).

The medulla is organized into cords separated by lymph (medullary) sinuses, which drain into a terminal sinus – the origin of the efferent lymphatic vessel (see Fig. 2.40).

Scavenger phagocytic cells are arranged along the lymph sinuses, especially in the medulla. As the lymph passes across the nodes from the afferent to the efferent lymphatic vessels, particulate antigens are removed by the phagocytic cells and transported into the lymphoid tissue of the lymph node.

The cortex contains aggregates of B cells in the form of primary or secondary follicles.

B cells are also found in the subcapsular region, adjacent to the marginal sinus. It is possible that these cells are similar to the splenic marginal zone B cells that intercept incoming pathogens primarily by mounting a rapid, IgM-based, T-independent response.

T cells are found mainly in the paracortex. Therefore, if an area of skin or mucosa is challenged by a T-dependent

The lymphatic system

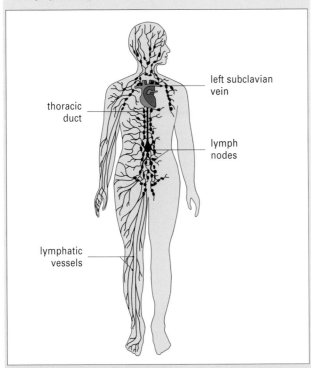

Fig. 2.37 Lymph nodes are found at junctions of lymphatic vessels and form a network that drains and filters interstitial fluid from the tissue spaces. They are either subcutaneous or visceral, the latter draining the deep tissues and internal organs of the body. The lymph eventually reaches the thoracic duct, which opens into the left subclavian vein and thus back into the circulation.

Lymph node section

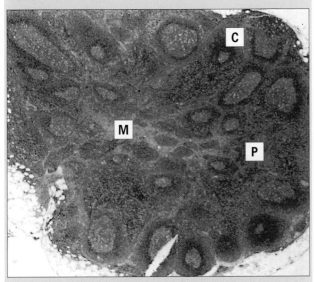

Fig. 2.38 The lymph node is surrounded by a connective tissue capsule and is organized into three main areas: the cortex (C), which is the B cell area; the paracortex (P), which is the T cell area; and the medulla (M), which contains cords of lymphoid tissue (T and B cell areas rich in plasma cells and macrophages). H&E stain. × 10. *(Adapted from Zucker-Franklin D, Grossi CE, eds. Atlas of blood cells: function and pathology, 3rd edn. Milan: Edi Ermes; 2003.)*

Histological structure of the lymph node

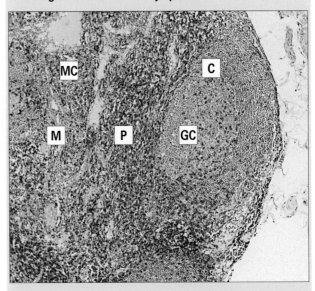

Fig. 2.39 Cortex (C), paracortex (P), and medulla (M) are shown. The section has been stained to show the localization of T cells. They are most abundant in the paracortex, but a few are found in the germinal center (GC) of the secondary lymphoid follicle, in the cortex, and in the medullary cords (MC). *(Courtesy of Dr A Stevens and Professor J Lowe.)*

Schematic structure of the lymph node

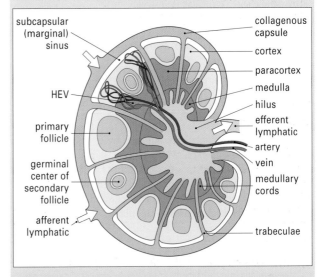

Fig. 2.40 Beneath the collagenous capsule is the subcapsular sinus, which is lined by endothelial and phagocytic cells. Lymphocytes and antigens from surrounding tissue spaces or adjacent nodes pass into the sinus via the afferent lymphatics. The cortex is mainly a B cell area. B cells are organized into primary or, more commonly, secondary follicles – that is, with a germinal center. The paracortex contains mainly T cells. Each lymph node has its own arterial and venous supply. Lymphocytes enter the node from the circulation through the highly specialized high endothelial venules (HEVs) in the paracortex. The medulla contains both T and B cells in addition to most of the lymph node plasma cells organized into cords of lymphoid tissue. Lymphocytes leave the node through the efferent lymphatic vessel.

Intedigitating cells in the lymph node paracortex

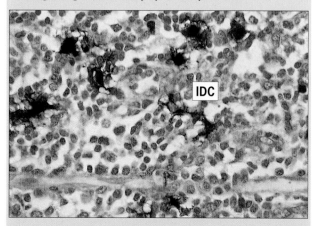

Fig. 2.41 Interdigitating dendritic cells (IDC; stained dark brown) form contacts with each other and with paracortical T cells (see also Fig. 2.16). *(Courtesy of Dr A Stevens and Professor J Lowe.)*

Structure of the secondary follicle

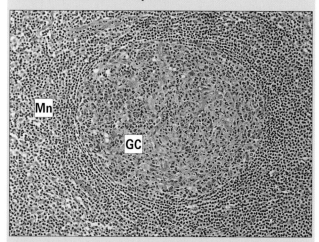

Fig. 2.42 A large germinal center (GC) is surrounded by the mantle zone (Mn).

Distribution of B cells in the lymph node cortex

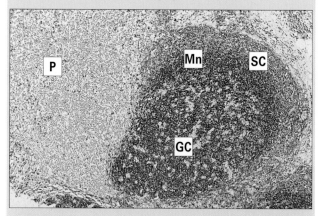

Fig. 2.43 Immunohistochemical staining of B cells for surface immunoglobulin shows that they are concentrated largely in the secondary follicle, germinal centre (GC), mantle zone (Mn), and between the capsule and the follicle – the subcapsular zone (SC). A few B cells are seen in the paracortex (P), which contains mainly T cells (see also Fig. 2.41).

antigen, the lymph nodes draining that particular area show active T cell proliferation in the paracortex.

Q. How is antigen transported from the skin to the para-cortex of the regional lymph nodes?
A. On Langerhans' cells/veiled cells via the afferent lymph.

Further evidence for this localization of T cells in the paracortex comes from patients with congenital thymic aplasia (DiGeorge syndrome), who have fewer T cells in the paracortex than normal. A similar feature is found in neonatally thymectomized or congenitally athymic ('nude') mice or rats.

Secondary follicles are made up of a germinal center and a mantle zone

Germinal centers in secondary follicles are seen in antigen-stimulated lymph nodes. These are similar to the germinal centers seen in the B cell areas of the splenic white pulp and of MALT.

Germinal centers are surrounded by a mantle zone of lymphocytes (Fig. 2.42). Mantle zone B cells (Fig. 2.43) co-express surface IgM, IgD, and CD44. This is taken as evidence that they are naive, actively recirculating B cells.

In most secondary follicles, the thickened mantle zone or corona is oriented towards the capsule of the node. Secondary follicles contain:

- FDCs (Fig. 2.44);
- some macrophages (Fig. 2.45); and
- a few follicular TH cells.

All the cells in the secondary follicle together with specialized marginal sinus macrophages, appear to play a role in generating B cell responses and, in particular, in the development of B cell memory.

In the germinal centers B cells proliferate, are selected, and differentiate into memory cells plasma cell precursors

The germinal center consists of a dark zone and a light zone:

- the dark zone is the site where one or a few B cells enter the primary lymphoid follicle and undergo active

proliferation leading to clonal expansion – these B cells are termed **centroblasts**. Their immunoglobulin genes undergo a process of **somatic hypermutation**, which leads to the generation of cells with a wide range of affinities for antigen;
- in the light zone, B cells (**centrocytes**) encounter the antigen on the surface of FDCs (see Fig. 2.14) and only those cells with higher affinity for antigen survive.

Cells with mutated antibody receptors of lower affinity die by apoptosis and are phagocytosed by germinal center macrophages.

Selected centrocytes interact with germinal center CD4$^+$ TH cells, and their BCRs undergo **class switching** (i.e. replacement of their originally expressed immunoglobulin heavy chain constant region genes by another class – for instance IgM to IgG or IgA, see Chapter 9).

Follicular dendritic cells in a secondary lymphoid follicle

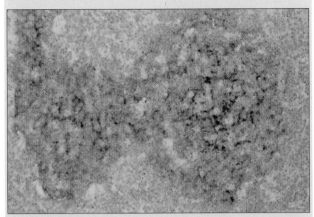

Fig. 2.44 This lymph node follicle is stained with enzyme-labeled monoclonal antibody to demonstrate follicular dendritic cells.

Germinal center macrophages

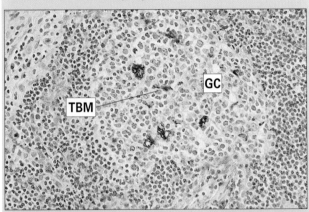

Fig. 2.45 Immunostaining for cathepsin D shows several macrophages localized in the germinal center (GC) of a secondary follicle. These macrophages, which phagocytose apoptotic B cells, are called tingible body macrophages (TBM). *(Courtesy of Dr A Stevens and Professor J Lowe.)*

The selected germinal center B cells differentiate into **memory B cells** or **plasma cell** precursors and leave the germinal center (Fig. 2.46).

MALT includes all lymphoid tissues associated with mucosa

Aggregates of encapsulated and non-encapsulated lymphoid tissue are found especially in the lamina propria and submucosal areas of the gastrointestinal, respiratory, and genitourinary tracts (see Fig. 2.26).

The tonsils contain a considerable amount of lymphoid tissue, often with large secondary follicles and intervening T cell zones with HEVs. The three main kinds of tonsil that constitute Waldeyer's ring are:

- palatine tonsil;
- pharyngeal tonsil (called adenoids when diseased); and
- lingual tonsil (Fig. 2.47).

Aggregates of lymphoid tissue are also seen lining the bronchi and along the genitourinary tract.

The digestive, respiratory, and genitourinary mucosae contain dendritic cells for the uptake, processing, and transport of antigens to the draining lymph nodes.

Lymphoid tissues seen in the lamina propria of the gastrointestinal wall often extend into the submucosa and are found as either:

- solitary nodules (Fig. 2.48); or
- aggregated nodules such as in the appendix (Fig. 2.49).

Follicle-associated epithelium is specialized to transport pathogens into the lymphoid tissue

Peyer's patches are found in the lower ileum. The intestinal epithelium overlying Peyer's patches (follicle-associated epithelium – FAE) and other mucosa-associated lymphoid aggregates (e.g. the tonsils) is specialized to allow the transport of antigens into the lymphoid tissue. This particular function is carried out by epithelial cells termed **M cells**, which are scattered among other epithelial cells and so called because they have numerous microfolds on their luminal surface.

M cells contain deep invaginations in their basolateral plasma membrane, which form pockets containing B and T lymphocytes, dendritic cells, and macrophages (Fig. 2.50). Antigens and microorganisms are transcytosed into the pocket and to the organized mucosal lymphoid tissue under the epithelium (Fig. 2.51) and taken up by the dendritic cells.

M cells are not exclusive to Peyer's patches, but are also found in epithelia associated with lymphoid cell accumulations at 'antigen sampling' areas in other mucosal sites.

The dome area of Peyer's patches and the subepithelial regions of tonsils harbor B cells that display a phenotype and function similar to that seen for the splenic marginal zone B cells (see above).

Q. The major defense at mucosal surfaces is antibody of the IgA isotype. What characteristics of this antibody would be critical in this respect?

A. The IgA isotype antibody produced at the mucosal level is a specific secretory form that can traverse epithelial membranes and helps prevent the entry of infectious microorganisms. Resistance to digestion by enzymes in the gut would also be an important feature of secretory IgA in GALT. Transport of IgA across mucosal epithelium is described in detail in Chapter 3 (see Fig. 3.8).

Lamina propria and intraepithelial lymphocytes are found in mucosa

In addition to organized lymphoid tissue forming the MALT system, a large number of lymphocytes and plasma cells are found in the mucosa of the:

- stomach;
- small and large intestine;
- upper and lower respiratory airways; and
- several other organs.

Lymphocytes are found both in the connective tissue of the lamina propria and within the epithelial layer:

- lamina propria lymphocytes (LPLs) are predominantly activated T cells, but numerous activated B cells and

Structure and function of the germinal center

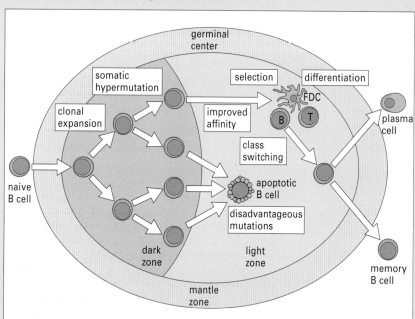

Fig. 2.46 One or a few B cells (founder cells) in the dark zone proliferate actively. This proliferation leads to clonal expansion and is accompanied by somatic hypermutation of the immunoglobulin V region genes. B cells with the same specificity, but different affinity, are therefore generated. In the light zone, B cells with disadvantageous mutations or with low affinity undergo apoptosis and are phagocytosed by macrophages. This process is also called 'affinity maturation'. Cells with appropriate affinity encounter the antigen on the surface of the follicular dendritic cells (FDCs) and, with the help of CD4$^+$ T cells, undergo class switching, leaving the follicle as memory B cells or plasma cells precursors.

Structure of the lingual tonsil

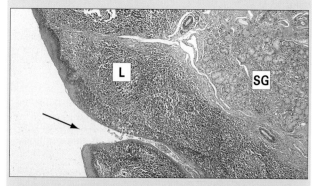

Fig. 2.47 The lingual tonsil, situated in the posterior one-third of the tongue, consists of accumulations of lymphoid tissue (L) with large secondary follicles associated with a mucosa that forms deep cleft-like invaginations (arrow). Mucus-containing salivary glands (SG) are seen around the tonsil. These are common features of all types of tonsil. *(Courtesy of Dr A Stevens and Professor J Lowe.)*

A solitary lymphoid nodule in the large intestine

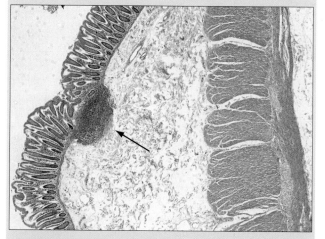

Fig. 2.48 This nodule is localized in the mucosa and submucosa of the intestinal wall (arrow). *(Courtesy of Dr A Stevens and Professor J Lowe.)*

plasma cells are also detected – these plasma cells secrete mainly IgA, which is transported across the epithelial cells and released into the lumen;
- intraepithelial lymphocytes (IELs) are mostly T cells – the population is different from the LPLs because it includes a high proportion of γδ T cells (10–40%) and CD8$^+$ cells (70%).

Most LPL and IEL T cells belong to the CD45RO$^+$ subset of memory cells. They respond poorly to stimulation with antibodies to the TCR (CD3), but may be triggered via other activation pathways (e.g. via CD2 or CD28).

The integrin αE chain HML-1 (CD103) is not present on resting circulating T cells, but is expressed following phytohemagglutinin (PHA) stimulation. Antibodies to CD103 are mitogenic and induce expression of the low-affinity IL-2 receptor α chain (CD25) on peripheral blood T cells. αE is coupled with a β$_7$ chain to form an αE/β$_7$ heterodimer, which is an integrin expressed by IELs and other activated leukocytes. E-cadherin on epithelial cells is the ligand for αE/β$_7$. Binding of αE/β$_7$ to E-cadherin may be important in the homing and retention of αE/β$_7$-expressing lymphocytes in the intestinal epithelium.

Lymphoid nodules in the human appendix

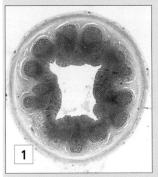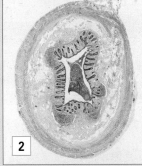

Fig. 2.49 (**1**) Appendix of a 10-year-old child showing large lymphoid nodules extending into the submucosa. (**2**) Appendix from a 36-year-old man. Note the dramatic reduction of lymphoid tissue, with the virtual disappearance of lymphoid follicles. This illustrates the atrophy of lymphoid tissues during aging, which is not limited to the appendix. (*Courtesy of Dr A Stevens and Professor J Lowe.*)

Location of M cells

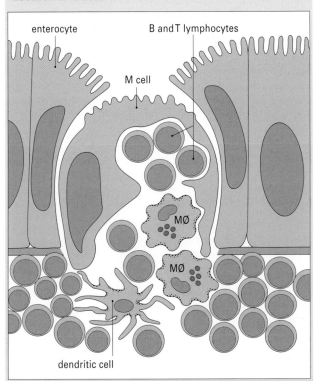

Fig. 2.50 The intestinal follicle-associated epithelium contains M cells. Note the lymphocytes and occasional macrophages (MØ) in the pocket formed by invagination of the basolateral membrane of the M cell. Antigens endocytosed by the M cell are passed via this pocket into the subepithelial tissues (not shown).

IELs are known to release cytokines, including IFNγ and IL-5. One function suggested for IELs is immune surveillance against mutated or virus-infected host cells.

Lymphocyte recirculation

Once in the secondary tissues the lymphocytes do not simply remain there; many move from one lymphoid organ to another via the blood and lymph (Fig. 2.52).

Lymphocytes leave the blood via high endothelial venules

Although some lymphocytes leave the blood through non-specialized venules, the main exit route in mammals is through a specialized section known as high endothelial venules (HEVs; Figs 2.53 and 2.54). In the lymph nodes these are mainly in the paracortex, with fewer in the cortex and none in the medulla.

Some lymphocytes, primarily T cells, arrive from the drainage area of the node through the afferent lymphatics, not via HEVs – this is the main route by which antigen enters the nodes.

Besides lymph nodes, HEVs are also found in MALT and in the thymus (see Fig. 2.29).

> **Q. What types of molecule required for the movement of lymphocytes would you expect to be expressed on HEVs?**
> A. HEVs express a distinctive set of chemokines that signal lymphocytes to migrate into the lymphoid tissue. They also have a specialized set of adhesion molecules that allow the cells to attach to the endothelial cells, as they migrate.

HEVs are permanent features of secondary lymphoid tissues, but can also develop from normal endothelium at sites of chronic inflammatory reactions (e.g. in the skin and in the synovium). This, in turn, may direct specific T cell subsets to the area where HEVs have formed.

The movement of lymphocytes across endothelium is controlled by adhesion molecules and chemokines (see Chapters 6 and 12). For example:

- the adhesion molecule MadCAM-1 is expressed on endothelial cells in intestinal tissues;
- VCAM-1 is present on endothelial cells in the lung and skin.

Homing molecules on lymphocytes selectively direct lymphocytes to particular organs by interaction with these adhesion molecules (see Chapter 6). In the case of the intestine, a critical role is played by $\alpha_4\beta_7$-integrins, which mediate adherence of lymphocytes to HEVs of Peyer's patches that express MadCAM-1.

Lymphocyte trafficking exposes antigen to a large number of lymphocytes

Lymphoid cells within lymph nodes return to the circulation by way of the efferent lymphatics, which pass via the thoracic duct into the left subclavian vein. About 1–2% of the lymphocyte pool recirculates each hour.

Mucosal lymphoid tissue

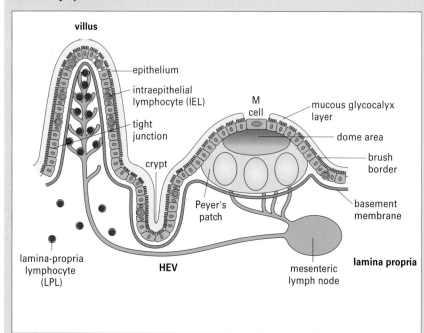

Fig. 2.51 Peyer's patches, as well as tonsils and other lymphoid areas of MALT, are sites of lymphocyte priming by antigens, which are internalized by M cells in the follicle-associated epithelium (FAE). The subepithelial region, the dome, is rich in APCs and also contains a subset of B cells similar to those found in the splenic marginal zone. Lymphoid follicles and intervening T-dependent zones are localized under the dome region. Lymphocytes primed by antigens in these initiation sites of the gut mucosa migrate to the mesenteric lymph nodes and then to the effector sites (the intestinal villi), where they are found both in the lamina propria (LPLs) and within the surface epithelium (IELs)

Overall, this process allows a large number of antigen-specific lymphocytes to come into contact with their specific antigen in the microenvironment of the peripheral lymphoid organs.

Q. Why is it important that antigen can contact many lymphocytes?

A. Lymphoid cells are monospecific and only a limited number of lymphocytes are capable of recognizing any particular antigen. Lymphocyte recirculation and the movement of an antigen and APCs increase the opportunity for lymphocytes to encounter their specific antigen soon after infection.

Under normal conditions there is continuous lymphocyte traffic through the lymph nodes, but when antigen enters the lymph nodes of an animal already sensitized to that antigen there is a temporary shutdown in the traffic, which lasts for approximately 24 hours. Thus, antigen-specific lymphocytes are preferentially retained in the lymph nodes draining the source of antigen. In particular, blast cells do not recirculate but appear to remain in one site.

Patterns of lymphocyte traffic

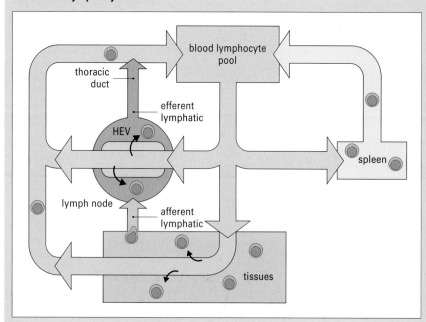

Fig 2.52 Lymphocytes move through the circulation and enter the lymph nodes and MALT via the specialized endothelial cells of the postcapillary venules (i.e. high endothelial venules [HEVs]). They leave the lymph nodes and MALT through the efferent lymphatic vessels and pass through other nodes, finally entering the thoracic duct, which empties into the circulation at the left subclavian vein (in humans). Lymphocytes enter the white pulp areas of the spleen in the marginal zones, pass into the sinusoids of the red pulp, and leave via the splenic vein.

Lymph node paracortex showing high endothelial venules (HEVs)

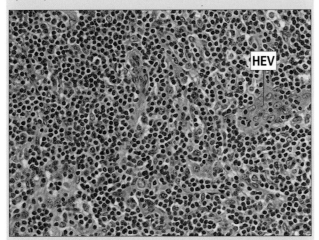

Fig. 2.53 Lymphocytes leave the circulation through HEVs and enter the node. H&E. × 200. *(Courtesy of Dr A Stevens and Professor J Lowe.)*

Electron micrograph showing a high endothelial venule (HEV) in the paracortex of a lymph node

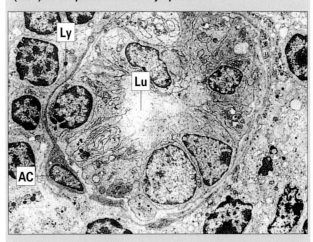

Fig. 2.54 A lymphocyte (Ly) in transit from the lumen (Lu) of the HEV can be seen close to the basal lamina. The HEV is partly surrounded by an adventitial cell (AC). × 1600.

Antigen stimulation at one mucosal area elicits an antibody response largely restricted to MALT

One reason for considering MALT as a system distinct from the systemic lymphoid organs is that mucosa-associated lymphoid cells mainly recirculate within the mucosal lymphoid system. Thus, lymphoid cells stimulated in Peyer's patches pass via regional lymph nodes to the blood stream and then 'home' back into the intestinal lamina propria (Fig. 2.55 and see Fig. 2.51).

Specific recirculation is made possible because the lymphoid cells expressing homing molecules attach to adhesion

Lymphocyte circulation within the mucosal lymphoid system

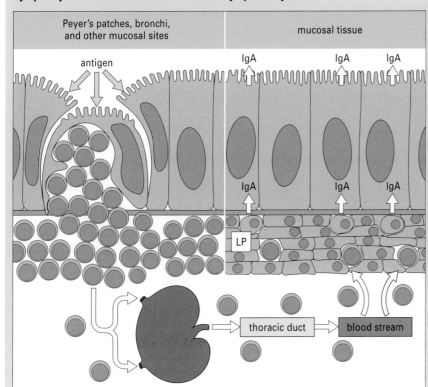

Fig. 2.55 Lymphoid cells that are stimulated by antigen in Peyer's patches (or the bronchi or another mucosal site) migrate via the regional lymph nodes and thoracic duct into the blood stream and hence to the lamina propria (LP) of the gut or other mucosal surfaces, which might be close to or distant from the site of priming. Thus lymphocytes stimulated at one mucosal surface may become distributed selectively throughout the MALT system. This is mediated through specific adhesion molecules on the lymphocytes and mucosal HEV.

molecules that are specifically expressed on endothelial cells of the mucosal venules, but are absent from lymph node HEVs (see above).

Thus, antigen stimulation at one mucosal area elicits an antibody response largely, but not exclusively, restricted to mucosal tissues.

CRITICAL THINKING: DEVELOPMENT OF THE IMMUNE SYSTEM (SEE P. 433 FOR EXPLANATIONS)

Immunodeficiencies can tell us a lot about the way the immune system functions normally. Mice that congenitally lack a thymus (and have an associated gene defect that produces hairlessness), termed 'nude mice', are often used in research.

1 What effect would you expect this defect to have on numbers and types of lymphocytes in the blood? How would this affect the structure of the lymph nodes? What effect would this have on the ability of the mice to fight infections?

   Occasionally adult patients develop a tumor in the thymus (thymoma) and it is necessary to completely remove the thymus gland.

2 What effect would you expect adult thymectomy to have on the ability of such patients to fight infections?

With the development of modern techniques in molecular biology, it is possible to produce animals that completely lack individual genes. Such animals are called 'gene knockouts'. Sometimes these knockouts can have quite surprising effects on development, and sometimes only minor effects. Others, like the immunodeficiencies, are very informative. Based on the information provided in Chapter 2, what effects would you expect the following 'knockouts' to have on the development of leukocytes and/or lymphoid organs?

3 RAG-1? (*RAG-1* and *RAG-2* genes are involved in the recombination processes that generate antigen receptors on B and T cells.)

4 Interleukin-7?

5 The β_7-integrin chain?

Further reading

Kindt TJ, Osborne BA, Goldsby RA. Kuby Immunology, 6th edn. Oxford: WH Freeman; 2006.

Lamm ME, Strober W, McGhee JR, Mayer L, eds. Mestecky J, Bienenstock J. Mucosal Immunology. San Diego: Academic Press; 2005.

Steinman RM, Odoyaga J. Features of the dendritic cell lineage. Immunol Rev 2010;234:5–17.

Lydyard PM, Whelan A, Fanger MW. Instant Notes in Immunology, 2nd edn. London: Garland Science/Bios Scientific Publishing; 2004.

Playfair JHL, Chain BM. Immunology at a Glance, 9th edn Wiley-Blackwell; 2009.

Reddy KV, Yedery RD, Aranha C. Antimicrobial peptides: premises and promises. Int J Antimicrob Agents 2004;24:536–547.

Roitt IM, Delves P. Essential Immunology, 10th edn. Oxford: Blackwell Scientific Publications; 2001.

Shevach E. Regulatory/suppressor T cells in health and disease. Arthritis Rheum 2004;50:2721–2724.

Von Andrian UH, Mempel TR. Homing and cellular traffic in lymph nodes. Nat Rev Immunol 2003;3:867–878.

CHAPTER 3

Antibodies

SUMMARY

- **Circulating antibodies (also called immunoglobulins) are soluble glycoproteins that recognize and bind antigens, specifically.** They are present in serum, tissue fluids or on cell membranes. Their purpose is to help eliminate microorganisms bearing those antigens. Antibodies also function as membrane-bound antigen receptors on B cells, and play key roles in B cell differentiation.

- **There are five classes of antibody in mammals** – IgG, IgA, IgM, IgD, and IgE. In humans, four subclasses of IgG and two of IgA are also defined. Thus, collectively, there are nine **isotypes**: IgM, IgA1, IgA2, IgG1, IgG2, IgG3, IgG4, IgD, and IgE.

- **Antibodies have a basic structure of four polypeptide chains** – two identical light chains and two identical heavy chains. The N- terminal ~110 amino acid residues of the light and heavy chains are highly variable in sequence; referred to as the variable regions V_L and V_H, respectively. The unique sequence of a VL/VH pair forms the specific antigen-binding site or **paratope**. The C-terminal regions of the light and heavy chains form the constant regions (C_L and C_H, respectively), which determine the effector functions of an antibody.

- **Antigen-binding sites of antibodies are specific for the three-dimensional shape (conformation) of their target** — the antigenic determinant or **epitope**.

- **Antibody affinity** is a measure of the strength of the interaction between an antibody combining site (paratope) and its epitope. The avidity (or functional affinity) of an antibody depends on its number of binding sites (two for IgG) and its ability to engage multiple epitopes on the antigen – the more epitopes it binds, the greater the avidity.

- **Receptors for antibody heavy chain constant regions (Fc receptors)** are expressed by mononuclear cells, neutrophils, natural killer cells, eosinophils, basophils and mast cells. They interact with the Fc regions of different isotypes of antibody and promote activities such as phagocytosis, tumor cell killing and mast cell degranulation.

- **A vast repertoire of antigen-binding sites is achieved by random selection and recombination** of a limited number of V, D and J gene segments that encode the variable (V) regions (domains). This process is known as V(D)J recombination and generates the primary antibody repertoire.

- **Repeated rounds of somatic hypermutation and selection** act on the primary repertoire to generate a secondary repertoire of antibodies with higher specificity and affinity for the stimulating antigen.

- **Class switching** combines rearranged VDJ genes with different heavy chain constant region genes so that the same antigen receptor can activate a variety of effector functions.

Antibodies recognize and bind antigens

Highly specific recognition of antigen is the hallmark of the adaptive immune response. Two principal molecules are involved in this process:

- antibodies (immunoglobulins); and
- T-cell antigen receptors (TCRs).

Structural and functional diversity are characteristic features of these molecules.

Antibody genes have diversified in different species by multiple gene duplications and subsequent divergence. In many species, including man, diversity is further amplified by extensive gene rearrangement and somatic mutation during the lifetime of an individual.

Antibodies function as membrane-bound antigen receptors on B cells and soluble circulating antibodies

Antibodies are glycoproteins expressed as:

- membrane-bound receptors on the surface of B cells; or
- soluble molecules (secreted from plasma cells) present in serum and tissue fluids.

Contact between the B cell receptor on a particular B cell and the antigen it recognizes results in B cell activation and differentiation to generate a clone of **plasma cells**, which secrete large amounts of antibody. Each clone secretes only one type of antibody, with a unique specificity. The secreted antibody has the same binding specificity as the original B cell receptor (Fig. 3.1).

Surface and secreted antibodies

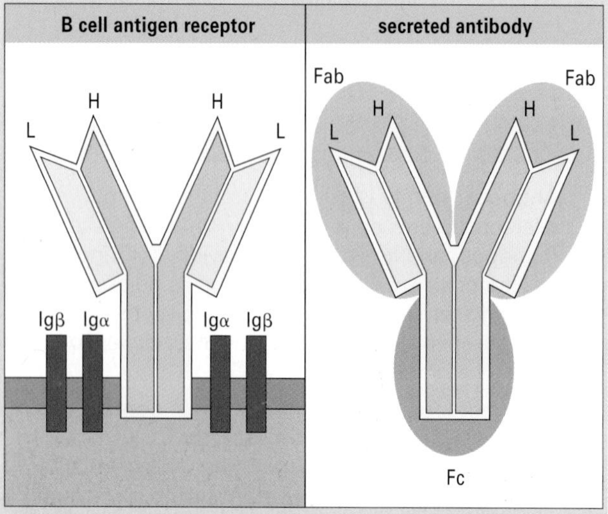

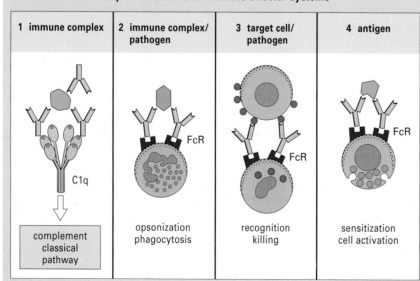

Fig. 3.1 The B cell antigen receptor (left) consists of two identical heavy (H) chains and two identical light (L) chains. In addition, secondary components (Igα and Igβ) are closely associated with the primary receptor and are thought to couple it to intracellular signaling pathways. Circulating antibodies (right) are structurally identical to the primary B cell antigen receptors except they lack the transmembrane and intracytoplasmic sections. Many proteolytic enzymes cleave antibody molecules into three fragments – two identical Fab (antigen binding) fragments and one Fc (crystallizable) fragment.

Antibodies are a family of glycoproteins

Five distinct **classes of antibody** molecule are recognized in most mammals, namely IgG, IgA, IgM, IgD, and IgE. They differ in:

- size, e.g. the number of polypeptide chains;
- charge;
- amino acid sequence; and
- carbohydrate content.

In humans, four subclasses of IgG and two of IgA are defined. Collectively there are nine antibody isotypes: IgM, IgA1, IgA2, IgG1, IgG2, IgG3, IgG4, IgD, and IgE. Each isotype is defined by the amino acid sequence of the heavy chain constant region and encoded by a unique gene. Antibodies present in blood (serum) are polyclonal, i.e. structurally heterogeneous reflecting their ability to recognize and bind different antigens; they are products of different plasma cell clones.

All antibody isotypes except IgD are bifunctional

Antibodies are bifunctional molecules. They:

- recognize and bind antigen; and
- promote the killing and/or removal of the immune complex formed through the activation of effector mechanisms.

One part of the antibody molecule determines its antigen specificity while another determines which effector functions will be activated. Effector functions include binding of the heavy chain constant regions (Fc) to:

- receptors expressed on host tissues (e.g. FcγRI on phagocytic cells); and
- the first component (C1q) of the complement system to initiate the classical pathway complement cascade (Fig. 3.2).

Antibodies act as adapter molecules for immune effector systems

1 immune complex	2 immune complex/ pathogen	3 target cell/ pathogen	4 antigen
C1q	FcR	FcR	FcR
complement classical pathway	opsonization phagocytosis	recognition killing	sensitization cell activation

Fig. 3.2 Antibodies act as adapter molecules for different immune effector systems, linking antigens to receptor molecules (C1q and FcR) of the immune system. (**1**) Immune complexes can activate the complement classical pathway. (**2**) Antibodies bound to the surface of pathogens opsonize them for phagocytosis. (**3**) Antibodies bound to cells can promote their recognition and killing by NK cells. (Similarly recognition of some parasitic worms by eosinophils, mediated by antibodies, targets them for killing.) (**4**) Antibody bound to Fc receptors sensitizes cells so that they can recognize antigen, and the cell becomes activated if antigen binds to the surface antibody.

Antibody class and subclass is determined by the structure of the heavy chain

The basic structure of each antibody molecule is a unit consisting of:

- two light polypeptide chains (~25 kDa); and
- two heavy polypeptide chains (~55 kDa).

In an individual antibody molecule the amino acid sequences of the two light chains are identical, as are the sequences of the two heavy chains. Both light and both heavy chains are folded into a series of discrete domains. The sequence of the constant region of the heavy chain determines the class and subclass, or isotype, of the antibody. The heavy chains are designated:

- μ (IgM);
- γ1, γ2, γ3, and γ4 (IgG1, IgG2, IgG3, IgG4);
- α1 and α2 (IgA1, IgA2);
- δ (IgD);
- ε (IgE).

There are no subclasses of IgM, IgD, or IgE (Fig. 3.3).

Different antibody isotypes activate different effector systems

The human IgG subclasses (IgG1–IgG4), which are are present in serum in the approximate proportions of 66, 23, 7, and 4%, respectively, have arisen after the divergence of evolutionary lines leading to humans and the mouse. Consequently, despite their similar nomenclature there is no direct structural or functional correlation between the four human and mouse IgG molecules identified by the same nomenclature (IgG1, IgG2, etc.).

The relative proportions of IgA1 and IgA2 vary between serum and external secretion, where IgA is present in a secretory form (see Fig. 3.3).

Q. What advantage might there be in having such a variety of different antibody classes?
A. Each antibody isotype acts as an adapter molecule forming a bridge between the antigen and effector molecules. The immune system can respond individually to each pathogen with the generation of antibody isotypes most effective in its immobilization and elimination.

IgG is the predominant antibody isotype in normal human serum

IgG accounts for 70–75% of the total serum antibody pool and consists of a monomeric four-chain molecule. Normal concentration range: 6.0–16 g/L.

IgM accounts for about 10% of the serum antibody pool

IgM accounts for approximately 10% of the serum antibody pool. It is a pentamer of a basic four-chain structure with a mass of ~970 kDa; polymerization to the pentamer is aided by the presence of the J (joining) polypeptide chain of mass ~15 kDa. Normal concentration range: 0.5–2.0 g/L. A transmembrane monomeric form (mIgM) is present as an antigen-specific receptor on mature B cells.

IgA is the predominant antibody isotype present in seromucous secretions

IgA accounts for approximately 15–20% of the serum antibody pool. In humans over 80% of serum IgA has a four chain monomer. Normal concentration range: 0.8–4.0 g/L. In the serum of most mammals IgA is polymeric, mostly as a dimer.

IgA is the predominant antibody isotype present in seromucous secretions such as saliva, colostrum, milk, and tracheobronchial and genitourinary secretions.

IgD is an antigen-specific receptor (mIgD) on mature B cells

IgD, a four chain monomer, accounts for less than 1% of the serum antibody pool. Normal concentration range: 2.0–100 mg/L.

Physicochemical properties of human immunoglobulin classes

property	immunoglobulin type									
	IgG1	IgG2	IgG3	IgG4	IgM	IgA1	IgA2	sIgA	IgD	IgE
heavy chain	γ_1	γ_2	γ_3	γ_4	μ	α_1	α_2	α_1/α_2	δ	ε
mean serum conc. (mg/ml)	9	3	1	0.5	1.5	3.0	0.5	0.05	0.03	0.00005
sedimentation constant	7s	7s	7s	7s	19s	7s	7s	11s	7s	8s
mol. wt (kDa)	146	146	170	146	970	160	160	385	184	188
half-life (days)	21	20	7	21	10	6	6	?	3	2
% intravascular distribution	45	45	45	45	80	42	42	trace	75	50
carbohydrate (%)	2–3	2–3	2–3	2–3	12	7–11	7–11	7–11	9–14	12

Fig. 3.3 Each immunoglobulin class has a characteristic type of heavy chain. Thus IgG possesses γ chains; IgM, μ chains; IgA, α chains; IgD, δ chains; and IgE, ε chains. Variation in heavy chain structure within a class gives rise to immunoglobulin subclasses. For example, the human IgG pool consists of four subclasses reflecting four distinct types of heavy chain. The properties of the immunoglobulins vary between the different classes. In secretions, IgA occurs in a dimeric form (sIgA) in association with a protein chain termed the secretory component. The serum concentration of sIgA is very low, whereas the level in intestinal secretions can be very high.

Basophils and mast cells are continuously saturated with IgE

Serum IgE levels are very low (0–90 IU/mL) relative to the other antibody isotypes. However, basophils and mast cells express an IgE-specific receptor of very high affinity with the result that they are continuously saturated with IgE.

Antibodies have a basic four chain structure

The basic four chain structure and folding of antibody molecules is illustrated for IgG1 (Fig. 3.4).

The **light chains** (25 kDa) are bound to the heavy chains (55 kDa) by interchain disulfide bridges and multiple non-covalent interactions.

The **heavy chains** are similarly bound to each other by interchain disulfide bridges and multiple non-covalent interactions.

Each segment of ~110 amino acids folds to form a compact domain, which is stabilized through a multiple non-covalent interaction and a covalent intrachain disulfide bond. Thus:

- the light chain has two domains and an intrachain disulfide bond in each of the V_L and C_L domains;
- the heavy chain has four domains and an intrachain disulfide in each of the VH, CH1, CH2, and CH3 domains.

Each disulfide bond encloses a peptide loop of 60–70 amino acid residues.

The basic structure of IgG1

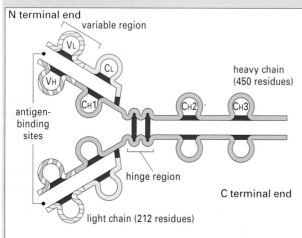

N terminal end

variable region

VL

CL

VH

CH1

CH2

CH3

heavy chain (450 residues)

antigen-binding sites

hinge region

C terminal end

light chain (212 residues)

Fig. 3.4 The N terminal end of IgG1 is characterized by sequence variability (V) in both the heavy and light chains, referred to as the VH and VL regions, respectively. The rest of the molecule has a relatively constant (C) structure. The constant portion of the light chain is termed the CL region. The constant portion of the heavy chain is further divided into three structurally discrete regions: CH1, CH2, and CH3. These globular regions, which are stabilized by intrachain disulfide bonds, are referred to as 'domains'. The sites at which the antibody binds antigen are located in the variable domains. The hinge region is a segment of heavy chain between the CH1 and CH2 domains. Flexibility in this area permits the two antigen-binding sites to operate independently. There is close pairing of the domains except in the CH2 region (see Fig. 3.8). Carbohydrate moieties are attached to the CH2 domains.

There is significant amino acid sequence homology between antibody domains which is reflected in a common conformational motif, referred to as the **immunoglobulin fold**. This characteristic fold defines the immunoglobulin superfamily members.

Antibodies are prototypes of the immunoglobulin superfamily

The three dimensional structure of each ~110 amino acid homology region (domain) of an antibody is designated as the immunoglobulin fold. It is also present in many proteins and provides for both stability and a multiplicity of structural and functional variants, which may or may not have an overt immune function. Examples include:

- the adhesion molecules ICAM-1 and VCAM-1 (see Chapter 6);
- the TCR (see Chapter 5);
- MHC molecules (see Chapter 5);
- cellular receptors for antibodies.

Such molecules are said to belong to the **immunoglobulin supergene family (IgSF)**.

The principal elements of the domain are two opposed β-pleated sheets, stabilized by one or more disulfide bonds between the β-pleated sheets. This structure is sometimes referred to as a **β barrel**.

The overall structure of an antibody depends on its class and subclass

X-ray crystallography has provided structural data on complete IgG molecules (Fig. 3.5). Mobility around the hinge region of IgG allows for the generation of the Y- and T-shaped structures visualized by electron microscopy.

For all antibody isotypes there is pairing between VH/VL and CH1/CL domains through extensive non-covalent interactions to form the antigen binding (Fab) region.

Antigen binding is a common feature for IgG-Fab regions of each of the four human IgG subclasses; however, although there is >95% sequence homology between the IgG-Fc regions each IgG subclass exhibits a unique profile of effector activities.

The hinge regions are structurally distinct and determine the relative mobilities of the IgG-Fab and IgG-Fc moieties within the intact molecule. The equivalent of the IgG hinge region is present in all isotypes, except IgM.

In addition to the pairing of the VL/VH and CL/CH1 domains the CH3 domains of the IgG-Fc are also paired through non-covalent interactions.

The CH2 domains are not paired and, potentially, present a hydrophobic surface to solvent. This unfavorable property is avoided by interactions with a hydrophilic N-linked oligosaccharide moiety.

The N-linked oligosaccharide of the CH2 domain, although accounting for only 2–3% of the mass of the IgG molecule, is crucial to the expression of effector functions. The conformation of the CH2 domain protein moiety, and ultimately the IgG-Fc, results from reciprocal interactions between the CH2 protein and the oligosaccharide. The oligosaccharide exhibits structural heterogeneity and effector functions may be modulated depending on the particular oligosaccharide structure (glycoform) attached.

Model of an IgG molecule

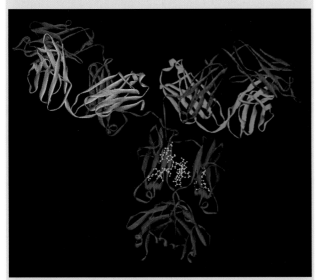

Fig. 3.5 A model of an IgG molecule showing the polypeptide backbones of the four chains as a ribbon. Heavy chains are shown in dark blue and dark green. The antigen-binding sites are at the tips of the arms of the Y-shaped molecule and are formed by domains from both the heavy and light chains. The extended, unfolded hinge region lies at the center of the molecule. Carbohydrate units are shown as ball and stick structures, covalently linked to the Fc region.

Electron micrographs of IgM molecules

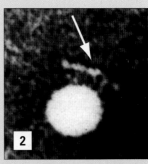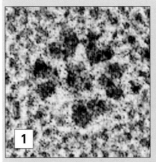

Fig. 3.6 (**1**) In free solution, deer IgM adopts the characteristic star-shaped configuration. ×195 000. (**2**) Rabbit IgM antibody (arrow) in 'crab-like' configuration with partly visible central ring structure bound to a poliovirus virion. × 190 000. *((1) Courtesy of Drs E Holm Nielson, P Storgaard, and Professor S-E Svehag. (2) Courtesy of Dr B Chesebro and Professor S-E Svehag.)*

Assembled IgM molecules have a 'star' conformation

IgM is present in human serum as a pentamer of the basic four-chain structure (see Fig. 3.w3). Each heavy chain is comprised of a VH and four CH domains. One advantage of this pentameric structure is that it provides 10 identical binding sites, which can dramatically increase the avidity with which IgM binds its cognate antigen. Given that serum IgM commonly functions to eliminate bacteria containing low affinity, polysaccharide antigens, the increased avidity provided by the pentameric structure provides an important functional advantage.

Covalent disulfide bonds between adjacent CH2 and CH3 domains, the C terminal 18-residue peptide sequence, referred to as the 'tailpiece', and J chain link the subunits of the pentamer.

J chain is synthesized within plasma cells, has a mass of ~15 kDa and folds to form an immunoglobulin domain. Each heavy chain bears four N-linked oligosaccharide moieties, however, the oligosaccharides are not integral to the protein structure in the same way as in IgG-Fc. Oligosaccharides present on IgM activate the complement cascade via binding to the mannose binding lectin (see Chapter 4).

In electron micrographs the assembled IgM molecule is seen to have a 'star' conformation with a densely packed central region and radiating arms (Fig. 3.6); however, electron micrographs of IgM antibodies binding to poliovirus show molecules adopting a 'staple' or 'crab-like' configuration (see Fig. 3.6), which suggests that flexion readily occurs between the CH2 and CH3 domains, though this region is

not structurally homologous to the IgG hinge. Distortion of this region, referred to as **dislocation**, results in the 'staple' configuration of IgM required to activate complement.

Secretory IgA is a complex of IgA, J chain and secretory component

IgA present in serum is produced by bone marrow plasma cells and secreted as a monomer with the basic four-chain structure. Each heavy chain is comprised of a VH and three CH domains.

The IgA1 and IgA2 subclasses differ substantially in the structure of their hinge regions:

- the hinge of IgA1 is extended and bears O-linked oligosaccharides;
- the hinge of IgA2 is truncated, relative to IgA1.

A deficit in the addition of O-linked sugars within the hinge region of IgA1 protein has been linked with the disease IgA nephropathy.

IgA is the predominant antibody isotype in external secretions but is present as a complex secretory form. IgA is secreted by gut localized plasma cells as a dimer in which the heavy chain 'tailpiece' is covalently bound to a J chain, through a disulphide bond (see Fig. 3.w3).

Electron micrographs of IgA dimers show double Y-shaped structures, suggesting that the monomeric subunits are linked end-to-end through the C terminal Cα3 regions (Fig. 3.7).

The dimeric form of IgA binds a **poly-Ig receptor** (Fig. 3.8) expressed on the basolateral surface of epithelial cells. The complex is internalized, transported to the apical surface where the poly-Ig receptor is cleaved to yield the secretory component (SC) that is released still bound to the IgA dimer. The released secretory form of IgA is relatively resistant to cleavage by enzymes in the gut and is comprised of:

- two units of IgA;
- J chain; and
- a secretory component (mass 70 kDa) (see Figs. 3.w3 and 3.8).

Electron micrographs of human dimeric IgA molecules

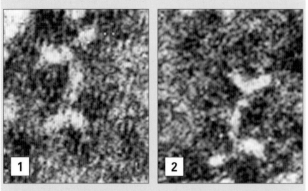

Fig. 3.7   The double Y-shaped appearance suggests that the monomeric subunits are linked end to end through the C terminal Cα3 domain. × 250 000. *(Courtesy of Professor S-E Svehag.)*

Transport of IgA across the mucosal epithelium

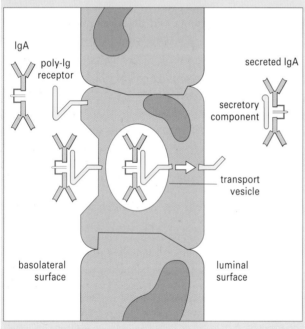

Fig. 3.8   IgA dimers secreted into the intestinal lamina propria by plasma cells bind to poly-Ig receptors on the internal (basolateral) surface of the epithelial cells. The sIgA–receptor complex is then endocytosed and transported across the cell while still bound to the membrane of transport vesicles. These vesicles fuse with the plasma membrane at the luminal surface, releasing IgA dimers with bound secretory component derived from cleavage of the receptor. The dimeric IgA is protected from proteolytic enzymes in the lumen by the presence of this secretory component.

Serum IgD has antigen specificity but not effector functions

Serum IgD accounts for less than 1% of the total serum immunoglobulin. Although serum IgD has been shown to have specific antigen binding activity no effector functions have been identified. Each heavy chain is comprised of a VH domain and three CH domains with an extended hinge region (see Figs. 3.w3). IgD also functions as an antigen specific receptor on B cells, together with IgM, and as such exhibits the same diversity of antigen specificity.

The heavy chain of IgE is comprised of four constant region domains

It is estimated that ∼50% of total body IgE is present in the blood, with the remainder being bound to mast cells and basophils through their high-affinity IgE Fcε receptor (FcεRI). IgE also binds the low affinity receptor (FcεRII) expressed on B cells and cells of the myeloid lineage.

Each heavy chain is comprised of a VH and four CH domains and bears six N-linked oligosaccharides (see Figs. 3.w3). An N-linked oligosaccharide, present in the CH3 domain, and equivalent to CH2 in IgG, influences binding to FcεRII but not FcεRI.

Antigen–antibody interactions

The conformations of the epitope and the paratope are complementary

Protein molecules are not rigid structures, but exist in a dynamic equilibrium between structures that differ in their ability to form a **primary interaction** with specific **ligands**.

Following a primary interaction, each 'partner' may influence the final **conformation** within the complex. This concept approximates to the 'induced fit' model of protein–protein interactions.

An examination of the interaction between the Fab fragment of the mouse D1.3 monoclonal antibody and hen egg white lysozyme (HEL) reveals the complementary surfaces of the epitope and the antibody's combining site (paratope); comprised of 17 amino acid residues of the antibody and 16 residues of the lysozyme molecule (Fig. 3.9). All hypervariable regions of the heavy and light chains contribute, though the third hypervariable region in the heavy chain appears to be most important.

The paratope of the D1.3 monoclonal antibody may be regarded as 'classical'. The structures of other lysozyme–antibody complexes have been solved and show differing involvement of hypervariable and framework residues.

Such structural studies are essential when engineering antibody molecules (e.g. when 'humanizing' a mouse antibody to generate an antibody therapeutic, see Method box 3.1).

Antibody affinity is a measure of the strength of interaction between a paratope and its epitope

The affinity of a protein–protein interaction is a thermodynamically defined measure of the strength of interaction between reciprocal binding sites, i.e as for the paratope of a Fab fragment and the epitope of an antigen. Since an antibody has two Fab moieties it can form multiple or three dimensional complexes; thus the apparent affinity is enhanced and is referred to as the avidity.

Antibodies form multiple non-covalent bonds with antigen

The antigen–antibody interaction results from the formation of multiple non-covalent bonds. These attractive forces consist of:

- hydrogen bonds;
- electrostatic bonds;
- van der Waals forces; and
- hydrophobic forces.

Each bond is relatively weak in comparison with covalent bonds, but together they can generate a high-affinity interaction.

The Fab–lysozyme complex

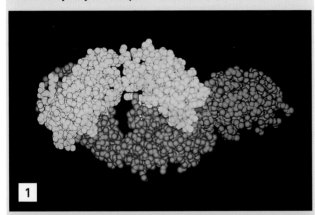

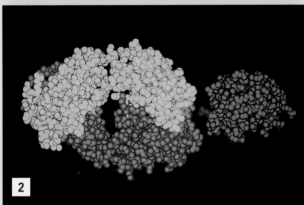

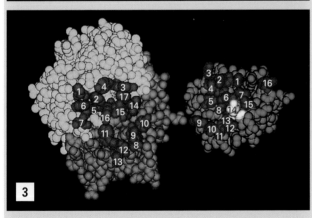

Fig. 3.9 (**1**) Lysozyme (green) binds to the hypervariable regions of the heavy (blue) and light (yellow) chains of the Fab fragment of antibody D1.3. (**2**) The separated complex with Glu121 visible (red). This residue fits into the center of the cleft between the heavy and light chains. (**3**) The same molecules rotated 90° to show the contact residues that contribute to the antigen–antibody bond. *(Reprinted with permission from Poljak RJ, Science 1986;233: 747–753. Copyright 1986 AAAS and reprinted with permission from Garcia KC et al, Science 1996;274:209–219. Copyright 1996 AAAS.)*

The strength of a non-covalent bond is critically dependent on the distance (d) between the interacting groups, being proportional to $1/d^2$ for electrostatic forces, and to $1/d^7$ for van der Waals forces.

Thus interacting groups must be in intimate contact before these attractive forces come into play.

For a paratope to combine with its epitope (see Fig. 3.9) the interacting sites must be complementary in shape, charge distribution, and hydrophobicity, and in terms of donor and acceptor groups, capable of forming hydrogen bonds.

Close proximity of two protein surfaces can also generate repulsive forces (proportional to $1/d^{12}$) if electron clouds overlap.

In combination, the attractive and repulsive forces have a vital role in determining the specificity of the antibody molecule and its ability to discriminate between structurally similar molecules.

The great specificity of the antigen–antibody interaction is exploited in a number of widely used assays (see Method box 3.2).

Antigen–antibody interactions are reversible

The affinity of an antibody is the sum of the attractive and repulsive forces resulting from binding between the paratope of a monovalent Fab fragment and its epitope. This interaction will be reversible, so at equilibrium the Law of Mass Action can be applied and an equilibrium constant, K (the association constant), can be determined (Fig. 3.10). In practice, due to the divalency of antibody and multiple epitopes expressed on an antigen, large three dimensional complexes may be formed that do not readily dissociate; when a paratope–epitope interaction is broken both the antibody and antigen remain in proximity due to other paratope–epitope interactions, thus reassociation is favored.

Avidity is likely to be more relevant than affinity

Because each antibody unit of four polypeptide chains has two antigen-binding sites, antibodies are potentially multivalent in their reaction with antigen.

Calculation of antibody affinity

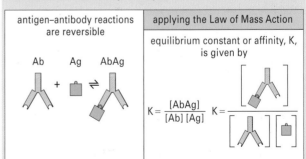

antigen–antibody reactions are reversible	applying the Law of Mass Action

$$K = \frac{[AbAg]}{[Ab][Ag]}$$

Fig. 3.10 All antigen–antibody reactions are reversible. The Law of Mass Action can therefore be applied, and the antibody affinity (given by the equilibrium constant, K) can be calculated. (Square brackets refer to the concentrations of the reactants)

Affinity and avidity

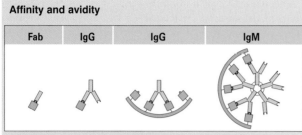

antibody	Fab	IgG	IgG	IgM
effective antibody valence	1	1	2	up to 10
antigen valence	1	1	n	n
equilibrium constant (L/mol)	10^4	10^4	10^7	10^{11}
advantage of multivalence	–	–	10^3-fold	10^7-fold
definition of binding	affinity	affinity	avidity	avidity
		intrinsic affinity		functional affinity

Fig. 3.11 Multivalent binding between antibody and antigen (avidity or functional affinity) results in a considerable increase in stability as measured by the equilibrium constant, compared with simple monovalent binding (affinity or intrinsic affinity, here arbitrarily assigned a value of 10^4 L/mol). This is sometimes referred to as the 'bonus effect' of multivalency. Thus there may be a 10^3-fold increase in the binding energy of IgG when both valencies (combining sites) are used and a 10^7-fold increase when IgM binds antigen in a multivalent manner.

In addition, antigen can be:

- monovalent (e.g. small chemical groups, haptens); or
- multivalent (e.g. microorganisms).

The strength with which a multivalent antibody binds a multivalent antigen is termed **avidity** to differentiate it from the **affinity**, which is determined for a univalent antibody fragment binding to a single antigenic determinant.

The avidity of an antibody for its antigen is dependent on the affinities of the individual antigen-combining sites for the epitopes on the antigen. Avidity will be greater than the sum of these affinities if both antibody-binding sites bind to the antigen because all antigen–antibody bonds would have to be broken simultaneously for the complex to dissociate (Fig. 3.11).

In physiological situations, avidity is likely to be more relevant than affinity because antibodies are at least divalent and most naturally occurring antigens are multivalent.

In practice we determine the association constant at equilibrium when the rate of formation of complex (ka) is equal to the spontaneous rate of dissociation (kd). The association or equilibrium constant is defined as K = ka/kd.

It has been suggested that B cell selection and stimulation during a maturing antibody response depend upon selection for the ability of antibodies to bind to antigens both:

- rapidly (kinetic selection); and
- tightly (thermodynamic selection).

Cross-reactive antibodies recognize more than one antigen

Antigen–antibody reactions can show a high level of specificity, but can also be **cross-reactive**, binding to a structurally related but different antigen (Fig. 3.12). Thus,

Specificity, cross-reactivity, and non-reactivity

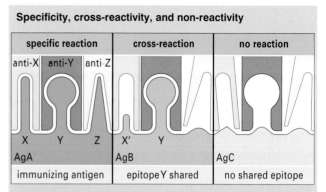

specific reaction	cross-reaction	no reaction
anti-X anti-Y anti-Z		
X Y Z	X' Y	
AgA	AgB	AgC
immunizing antigen	epitope Y shared	no shared epitope

Fig. 3.12 Antiserum specificity results from the action of a population of individual antibody molecules (anti-X, anti-Y, anti-Z) directed against different epitopes (X, Y, Z) on the same or different antigen molecules. Antigen A (AgA) and antigen B (AgB) have epitope Y in common. Antiserum raised against AgA (anti-XYZ) not only reacts specifically with AgA, but cross-reacts with AgB (through recognition of epitopes Y and X'). The antiserum gives no reaction with AgC because there are no shared epitopes.

monoclonal antibodies to hen egg lysozyme (HEL) may also bind structurally homologous duck egg lysozyme (DEL). A polyclonal antiserum to HEL will contain populations of antibodies specific for HEL and others that cross-react with DEL.

Antibodies recognize the conformation of antigenic determinants

Analysis of antibodies to protein antigens reveals that specificity may be for epitopes:

- consisting of a single contiguous stretch of amino acids (**a continuous epitope**);
- dependent on the native conformation of the antigen and formed from two or more stretches of sequence separated in the primary structure (**discontinuous or conformational epitopes**).

Continuous epitopes are unique three dimensional structures whilst discontinuous epitopes may be formed of a flexible peptide that assumes a unique conformation when bound to a paratope. i.e., the paratope may influence the conformation of the epitope by an induced fit mechanism.

Q. How might these differing characteristics of antigen be relevant when producing antibodies for immunological assays?

A. Antibodies specific for discontinuous epitopes may not bind denatured antigen, for example on immunoblots (see Method box 3.3), whereas antibodies to continuous epitopes may bind denatured antigen.

Antibodies are capable of expressing remarkable specificity and are able to distinguish small differences in the shape and chemical properties (e.g. charge, hydrophobicity) of epitopes. Small changes in the epitope, such as the position of a single chemical group, can therefore abolish binding (Figs. 3.13 and 3.14).

Specificity and cross-reacitivity

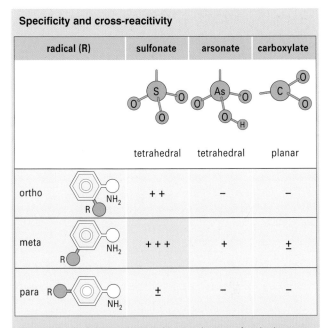

radical (R)	sulfonate	arsonate	carboxylate
	tetrahedral	tetrahedral	planar
ortho	+ +	–	–
meta	+ + +	+	±
para	±	–	–

Fig. 3.13 Antiserum raised to the meta isomer of aminobenzene sulfonate (the immunizing hapten) is mixed with ortho and para isomers of aminobenzene sulfonate, and also with the three isomers (ortho, meta, para) of two different, but related, antigens: aminobenzene arsonate and aminobenzene carboxylate. The antiserum reacts specifically with the sulfonate group in the meta position, but will cross-react (although more weakly) with sulfonate in the ortho position. Further, weaker cross-reactions are possible when the antiserum is reacted with either the arsonate group or the carboxylate group in the meta, but not in the ortho or para, position. Arsonate is larger than sulfonate and has an extra hydrogen atom, while carboxylate is the smallest of the three groups. These data suggest that an antigen's configuration is as important as the individual chemical groupings that it contains.

Configurational specificity

antiserum	antigen		
	lysozyme	isolated 'loop' peptide	reduced 'loop'
anti-lysozyme	+ +	+	–
anti-'loop' peptide	+	+ +	–

Fig. 3.14 The lysozyme molecule possesses an intrachain bond (red), which produces a loop in the peptide chain. Antisera raised against whole lysozyme (anti-lysozyme) and the isolated loop (anti-'loop' peptide) are able to distinguish between the two. Neither antiserum reacts with the isolated loop in its linear reduced form. This demonstrates the importance of tertiary structure in determining antibody specificity.

Q. Consider an antibody that recognizes an antigen on the outer envelope of a virus. If the antigen mutated, what would be the effect on its ability to bind antibody?
A. It depends on the nature of the mutation. Only mutations that affect the structure of the epitope could affect binding. However, if the mutation caused a radical change in the epitope structure (e.g. charge change or the insertion of a bulky amino acid residue), then the ability to bind might be lost or the affinity of binding drastically reduced.

Q. What effect would it have on the virus if a mutation of the epitope prevented it from being recognized by the antibody?
A. Viruses that mutate to avoid recognition by antibody will be at a selective advantage because they will not be destroyed by the immune system or prevented from attaching to host cells. Many viruses, including influenza and HIV, mutate their surface molecules and so evade recognition by antibodies.

Antibody effector functions

Antibodies are bifunctional because they both:

- specifically bind antigen to form large complexes thus limiting the spread of pathogens in vivo; and
- the immune complexes formed elicit host responses to facilitate their removal and destruction.

The nature of the constant region determines the effector function of the antibody and the host responses elicited, e.g. complement activation, phagocytosis.

In antibody–antigen complexes the antibody molecules are essentially aggregated such that the multiple Fc regions are able to engage, cross link and activate ligands or receptors (e.g. FcγR and C1q) (Fig. 3.15). Antibody is said to be an **opsonin**; it **opsonizes** the antigen (bacterium, virus); to opsonise means to make the antigen more 'tasty' or 'attractive' targets for phagocytic cells, i.e. they ingest or eat the complexes.

IgM predominates in the primary immune response

IgM is the first antibody produced in the primary immune response and is largely confined to the intravascular pool. It is frequently associated with the immune response to antigenically complex, blood-borne infectious organisms.

Once bound to its target, IgM is a potent activator of the classical pathway of complement.

Although the pentameric IgM antibody molecule consists of five Fcμ regions, it does not activate the classical pathway of complement in its uncomplexed form. However, when bound to an antigen with repeating identical epitopes, it forms a 'staple' structure (see Fig. 3.6), undergoing a conformational change referred to as **dislocation**, and the multiple Fcμ presented in this form are able to initiate the classical complement cascade.

IgG is the predominant isotype of secondary immune responses

The four IgG subclasses are highly homologous in structure, but each exhibits a unique profile of effector functions; thus, in activating the classical pathway of complement, complexes formed with:

- IgG1 and IgG3 antibodies are efficient;
- IgG2 antibodies are less effective;
- IgG4 antibodies are inactive.

Biological properties of human immunoglobulins

isotype	IgG1	IgG2	IgG3	IgG4	IgA1	IgA2	IgM	IgD	IgE
complement activation									
classical pathway	++	+	+++	–	–	–	+++	–	–
alternative pathway	varies with epitope density and antibody/antigen ratio								
lectin pathway	varies with glycosylation status								
Fc receptor binding									
FcγRI (monocytes)	+++	–	+++	++	–	–	–	–	–
FcγRIIa (monocytes, neutrophils, eosinophils, platelets)	+	±*	+	–	–	–	–	–	–
FcγRIIb (lymphocytes)	+	?	+	–					
FcγRIII (neutrophils, eosinophils, macrophages, LGLs, NK cells, T cells)	+	–	+	±	–	–	–	–	–
FcεRI (mast cells, basophils)	–	–	–	–	–	–	–	–	+++
FcεRII (monocytes, platelets, neutrophils, B and T cells, eosinophils)	–	–	–	–	–	–	–	–	++
FcαR (monocytes, neutrophils, eosinophils, T and B lymphocytes)	–	–	–	–	+	+	–	–	–
FcμR (T cells, macrophages)	–	–	–	–	–	–	+	–	–
FcδR (T and B cells)	–	–	–	–	+	–	–	+	–
pIgR, poly-Ig receptor; mucosal transport	–	–	–	–	+	+	+	–	–
FcRn, placental transport and catabolism	+	+	+	+	–	–	–	–	–
products of microorganisms									
SpA, staphylococcal protein A	+	+	–	+					
SpG, streptococcal protein G	+	+	+	+	–	–	–	–	–

*dependent on the allotype of FcγRIIa; LGLs, large granular lymphocytes; NK cells, natural killer cells

Fig. 3.15 The biological functions of different antibody classes and subclasses depend on which receptors they bind to and the cellular distribution of those receptors mediated by acting as adapters that bind via their Fc region to Fc receptors on different cell types.

The IgG subclasses also interact with a complex array of cellular Fc receptors (FcλR) expressed on various cell types (see Fig. 3.15 and below). IgG equilibrates between the intravascular and extravascular pools, so providing comprehensive systemic protection.

In humans, the newborn infant is not immunologically competent and the fetus is protected by passive IgG antibody selectively transported across the placenta (Fig. 3.16). Transport is mediated by the neonatal Fc receptor (FcRn) – all IgG subclasses are transported but the cord/maternal blood ratios differ, being approximately 1.2 for IgG1 and approximately 0.8 for IgG2.

Q. How do you interpret these ratios with respect to IgG transport across the placenta?

A. IgG1 is transported more efficiently than IgG2. Also, because the ratio for IgG1 is >1, the antibody is moving up a concentration gradient; therefore it must be active transport.

In some species (e.g. the rat), maternal immunoglobulin, present in colostrum or milk, is transferred to the offspring in the postnatal period through selective transport of IgG across the gastrointestinal tract via a homologous FcRn receptor.

Serum IgA is produced during a secondary immune response

Serum IgA is a product of a secondary immune response. Immune complexes of IgA opsonize antigens and activate phagocytosis through cellular Fc receptors (FcαR).

A predominant role for IgA antibody is in its secretory form, affording protection of the respiratory, gastrointestinal, and reproductive tracts.

The IgA1 subclass predominates in:

- human serum (approximately 90% of total IgA); and
- secretions such as nasal mucus, tears, saliva, and milk (70–95% of total IgA).

Immunoglobulins in the serum of the fetus and newborn child

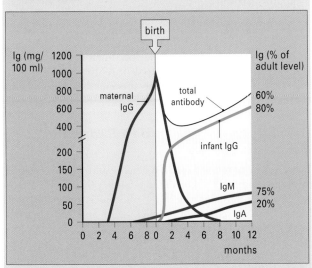

Fig. 3.16 IgG in the fetus and newborn infant is derived solely from the mother. This maternal IgG has disappeared by the age of 9 months, by which time the infant is synthesizing its own IgG. The neonate produces its own IgM and IgA; these classes cannot cross the placenta. By the age of 12 months, the infant produces 80% of its adult level of IgG, 75% of its adult IgM level, and 20% of its adult IgA level.

In the colon, IgA2 predominates (approximately 60% of the total IgA). Many microorganisms that can infect the upper respiratory and gastrointestinal tracts have adapted to their environment by releasing proteases that cleave IgA1 within the extended hinge region, whereas the short hinge region of IgA2 is not vulnerable to these enzymes.

IgD is a transmembrane antigen receptor on B cells

IgD has no known effector functions as a serum protein. It functions as a transmembrane antigen receptor on mature B lymphocytes.

IgE may have evolved to protect against helminth parasites infecting the gut

Despite its low serum concentration, the IgE class:

- is characterized by its ability to bind avidly to circulating basophils and tissue mast cells through the high-affinity FcεRI receptor (see below);
- sensitizes cells on mucosal surfaces such as the conjunctival, nasal, and bronchial mucosae.

IgE may have evolved to provide immunity against helminth parasites, but in developed countries it is now more commonly associated with allergic diseases such as asthma and sensitivity to peanuts, eggs, fish, etc.

Fc receptors

Antibodies sometimes protect just by binding to a pathogen, so preventing the pathogen from attaching to cells of the body and infecting them. More often, the biological and protective functions of antibodies are mediated by acting as adapters that bind antigen, via the paratope, and via their Fc region to Fc receptors (FcR) expressed on the above cell types. Three classes of FcR are defined that recognize the Fc regions of IgG (FcγR), IgA (FcαR) and IgE (FcεR); within each class of FcR there are several different types, e.g. FcγRI, FcγRII and FcγRIII.

The three types of Fc receptor for IgG are FcγRI, FcγRII, and FcγRIII

Three types of cell surface receptor for IgG (FcγR) are defined in humans:

- FcγRI (CD64);
- FcγRII (CD32); and
- FcγRIII (CD16).

Each receptor is characterized by a glycoprotein **α** chain that has an extracellular domain, homologous with immunoglobulin domains, that binds to antibody (Fig. 3.17) – that is, they belong to the immunoglobulin superfamily, as do receptors for IgA (FcαR) and IgE (FcεRI).

FcγRs are expressed constitutively but differentially on a variety of cell types but may be upregulated or induced by environmental factors (e.g. cytokines).

Biological activation results from aggregation (cross-linking) of the FcγR on the cell surface with consequent signal transduction and subsequent activation of **immunoreceptor tyrosine-based activation (ITAM)** or **immunoreceptor tyrosine-based inhibitory (ITIM)** motifs in the cytoplasmic sequences.

Fcγ receptors

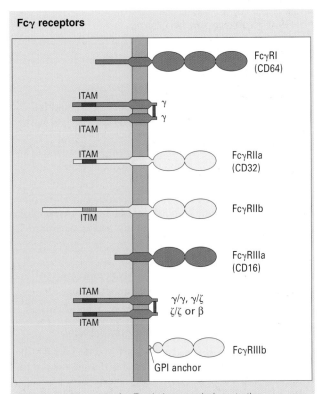

Fig. 3.17 Receptors for Fcγ in humans belong to the immunoglobulin superfamily, and have either two or three extracellular immunoglobulin domains. Motifs (ITAM, ITIM) on the intracellular segments or on associated polypeptides are targets for tyrosine kinases involved in initiating intracellular signaling pathways.

Phosphorylation of the ITAM motif triggers activities such as:

- phagocytosis;
- antibody-dependent cell-mediated cytotoxicity (ADCC);
- apoptosis;
- mediator release;
- enhancement of antigen presentation.

In contrast, phosphorylation of ITIM blocks cellular activation.

FcγRI is involved in phagocytosis of immune complexes and mediator release

It is common practice to refer to FcR as being of high, medium or low affinity. However, these descriptions are imprecise and relative; the affinity values vary considerably depending on the methods of determination.

FcγRI (CD64) binds:

- monomeric IgG1 and IgG3 with high affinity; relative to
- IgG4, low affinity;
- IgG2 does not have detectable binding affinity.

FcγRI has a restricted cellular distribution but is expressed on all cells of the mononuclear phagocyte lineage, and is involved in the phagocytosis of immune complexes, mediator release, etc.

The extra-cellular region of the α chain is comprised of three immunoglobulin domains; the cytoplasmic domain is associated with a γ chain that bears an ITAM motif.

FcγRII is expressed in two forms

FcγRII (CD32a; CD32b) is expressed as structurally and functionally distinct FcγRIIa and FcγRIIb forms with wide but differing cellular distribution.

The α chain of FcγRIIa:

- has moderate affinity for monomeric IgG1 and IgG3;
- binds complexed (multivalent, aggregated) IgG with high avidity;
- expresses an ITAM motif within its cytoplasmic tail; and
- may be produced as a polymorphic form which can bind monomeric IgG2.

Polymorphism in the FcγRIIA gene results in the presence of histidine or arginine at position 131 in the extracellular domains – the His[131] allotype binds and is activated by immune complexes of IgG2.

The FcγRIIb molecule:

- expresses an ITIM motif within its cytoplasmic tail; and
- when cross-linked inhibits cellular activation, particularly on B cells (see Fig. 11.13).

FcγRIII is expressed as FcγRIIIa and FcγRIIIb

FcγRIIIa (CD16a) is structurally and functionally distinct from FcγRIII (CD16b) and they have different cellular distributions. Both are extensively glycosylated.

FcγRIIIa is a transmembrane protein (like FcγRI, FcγRIIa, and FcγRIIb), whereas FcγRIIIb is GPI (glycosyl phosphatidyl inositol) anchored (see Fig. 3.17).

The α chains of FcγRIIIa:

- have a moderate affinity for monomeric IgG; and
- may be associated with γ/ξ and/or β chains bearing ITAM motifs.

FcγRIIIa is expressed on monocytes, macrophages, NK cells, and a fraction of T cells.

The FcγRIIIb form:

- is selectively expressed on neutrophils and basophils; and
- has a low affinity for monomeric IgG.

Engagement and cross-linking of FcγRIIIb can result cellular activation due to lipid raft formation by association with other membrane proteins bearing signaling motifs.

Polymorphism in FcγRIIIa and FcγRIIIb may affect disease susceptibility

Polymorphism in the FcγRIIIA gene results in the presence of phenylalanine (Phe) or valine (Val) at position 158 in the extracellular domains; the Val[158] allotype is associated with higher binding affinity for IgG1/IgG3 and consequently more efficient NK cell activation.

Polymorphism in the FcγRIIIB gene results in multiple amino acid sequence differences, including the generation of an N-linked glycosylation motif in the FcγRIIIb-NA2 and consequently the extent of glycosylation.

The relative expression of the FcγRIIIb-NA1 and FcγRIIIb-NA2 forms are reported to be associated with differing susceptibility to infection.

Q. What factors determine whether a particular IgG subclass will have a particular biological function (e.g. the ability to opsonize a bacterium for phagocytosis by a macrophage)?

A., The ability of each subclass of antibody to bind to Fc receptors, the affinity of binding and the distribution of Fc receptors between different effector cells.

IgG Fc interaction sites for several ligands have been identified

Application of site-directed mutagenesis, X-ray crystallography and nuclear magnetic resonance spectroscopy has allowed elucidation of the molecular topography of IgG Fc interaction sites for several ligands that bind overlapping non-identical sites at the CH2/CH3 interface, for example:

- staphylococcal protein A;
- streptococcal protein G;
- FcRn; and
- FcγRIIIB.

The interactions between maternal IgG and the MHC class I molecule-like FcRn expressed on the intestinal epithelium of the neonatal rat have now been studied at high resolution (Fig. 3.18) and are believed to mimic closely the binding of the human placental counterpart, hFcRn, with maternal IgG. Titration of IgG histidine residues in the binding site for FcRn may explain its:

- pH sensitivity;
- ability to bind at pH 6.5 (the pH within vacuoles); and
- dissociation at pH 7.4 (the pH of blood).

Given the symmetry of the Fc region, the fragments used in the experiments above are functionally divalent and may form multimeric complexes.

If monomeric IgG were divalent for FcγR and C1q, however, it would not function properly because circulating

Neonatal rat intestinal Fc receptor FcRn

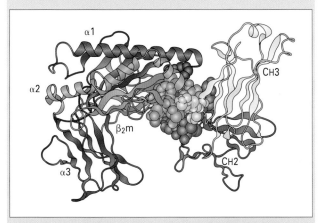

Fig. 3.18 Principal interactions between neonatal rat intestinal FcRn and the Fc of maternal IgG (derived from milk) are illustrated by ribbon diagrams of FcRn (domains α1, α2, α3, and β₂m are shown in red, light green, purple, and gray, respectively) and of Fc (CH2 and CH3 domains are shown in blue and yellow). The main contact residues of the FcRn (α1 domain, 90; α2, 113–119 and 131–135; β₂m, 1–4 and 86) are depicted as space-filling structures. *(Reproduced from Ravetch JV, Margulies DH. New tricks for old molecules. Nature 1994;372:323–324.)*

monomeric IgG could form activating multimers. The interaction sites for these ligands (e.g. FcγR and C1q) have been 'mapped' to the CH2 domain next to the hinge. The crystal structure of an IgG Fc/FcγRIIIb complex reveals an asymmetric interaction site embracing the CH2 domains of both heavy chains, thereby ensuring monovalency.

IgM–antigen complexes are very efficient activators of the classical complement system, but the mechanism by which IgM binds C1q appears different from that of IgG. The conformational change from a 'star' to a 'staple' conformation upon binding to multivalent antigen is thought to un-veil a ring of occult C1q-binding sites that are not accessible in the star-shaped configuration (see Fig. 3.6).

Glycosylation is important for receptor binding to IgG

N-linked glycosylation of the IgG Cγ2 domain is essential for the binding and activation of FcγRI, FcγRII, FcγRIII, and C1q. The oligosaccharide is of the complex type and is heterogeneous, generating multiple glycoforms. In addition to the covalent link to asparagine 297 it forms multiple non-covalent interactions with the CH2 domain such that it appears to be sequestered within the protein structure and inaccessible for direct interactions with the FcγRI, FcγRII, FcγRIII, and C1q ligands.

Fidelity of glycosylation has become an important issue in the production of monoclonal antibodies for therapy because glycosylation is a species- and tissue-specific post-translational modification (see Method box 3.1).

The FcR for IgA is FcαRI

The receptor for IgA is FcαRI (CD89):
- it is comprised of two Ig superfamily domains;
- it is associated with a γ chain;
- it is expressed on myeloid cells;
- can trigger phagocytosis, cell lysis and the release of inflammatory mediators; and
- can bind both IgA1 and IgA2.

The two types of Fc receptor for IgE are FcεRI and FcεRII

Two types of Fc receptor for IgE (FcεR) are defined in humans (Fig. 3.19):
- the high-affinity FcεRI which is expressed on mast cells and basophils and is the 'classical' IgE receptor; and
- the low-affinity FcεRII (CD23), which is expressed on leukocytes and lymphocytes.

The α chain of FcεRI is a glycoprotein and has two extracellular domains homologous to immunoglobulin domains and is a member of the immunoglobulin superfamily.

The low-affinity FcεRII is not a member of the immunoglobulin superfamily, but has substantial structural homology with several animal C-type lectins (e.g. mannose-binding lectin [MBL]).

Cross-linking of IgE bound to FcεRI results in histamine release

The high-affinity receptor (FcεRI) is present on the surface of mast cells and basophils as a complex with a β (33 kDa) and two γ (99 kDa) chains to form the αβγ₂ receptor unit (see Fig. 3.19).

FcεRI binds IgE with an affinity of approximately 10^{10} L/mol such that, although the serum concentration of IgE is very low, the receptors are permanently saturated.

Models for FcεRI and FcεRII

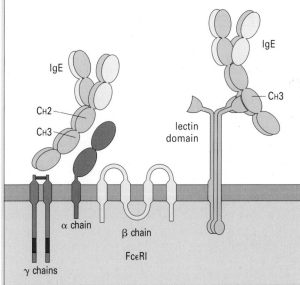

Fig. 3.19 Models for the high-affinity IgE receptor (FcεRI), which binds to IgE via its α chain, and the low-affinity receptor (FcεRII), which binds using its lectin domains. Both receptors are shown with IgE bound in the activation and release of histamine and other vasoactive and inflammatory mediators.

Cross-linking of the IgE bound to these receptors results in the activation and release of histamine and other vasoactive mediators.

FcεRII is a type 2 transmembrane molecule

FcεRII is the low-affinity (CD23) receptor and is a type 2 transmembrane molecule (i.e. one in which the C termini of the polypeptides are extracellular, see Fig. 3.19). The two forms of human CD23 are:

- **CD23a**, which is expressed in antigen-activated B cells and influences IgE production;
- **CD23b**, expression of which is induced in a wide range of cells by IL-4.

CD23a and CD23b differ by six or seven amino acids in their cytoplasmic N termini and contain different signaling motifs that modify their functions.

IgE receptors bind to IgE by different mechanisms

Decades of research and controversy surround the identification of the interaction site on IgE for the high-affinity FcεRI receptor.

Recent crystal structures of a Cε2Cε3Cε4 fragment and Cε3Cε4–FcεRI complex seem to have resolved the issue, and there is a striking structural homology between this site and the site on IgG Fc that binds FcγRIII. One distinctive feature is that, unlike IgG binding to FcγR, binding of IgE to its FcεRI receptor does not appear to depend on glycosylation of the immunoglobulin; however, binding to FcεRII does because it is a lectin. These studies should be interpreted with caution because the antibody fragments were not produced in mammalian cells.

Possible models for the interaction of IgE with the FcεRI and FcεRII receptors are illustrated in Figure 3.19. The low-affinity IgE Fc receptor, FcεRII (CD23), is a C-type lectin and is therefore sensitive to glycosylation status.

Development of the antibody repertoire by gene recombination

How can a finite genome provide the information required for the vast repertoire of antibody molecules that an individual can synthesize? This question posed an intellectual and practical challenge for decades.

Ehrlich's side-chain hypothesis, put forward at the beginning of the 20th century (Fig. 3.20), proposed antigen-induced selection. His model is close to our present view of clonal selection, except that he placed receptors of several different specificities on the same cell and did not address the question of how the diverse receptors were generated.

Later it was shown that light chains were comprised of a variable N-terminal half and a constant C-terminal region. This led Dreyer and Bennett to propose the 'two genes one polypeptide chain' hypothesis, i.e. the light chain sequence is encoded by at least two different genes, contrary to a central dogma of molecular biology at the time ('one gene, one protein').

Shortly thereafter, Tonegawa proved the Dreyer and Bennett hypothesis by demonstrating that the DNA encoding the variable and constant region were located at distant sites, on the same chromosome. Subsequently it was shown

Ehrlich's side-chain theory

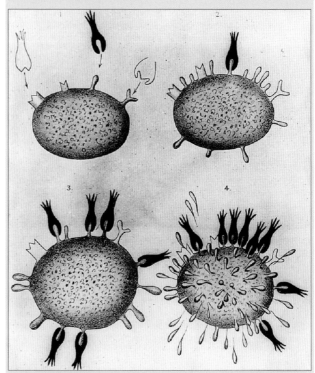

Fig. 3.20 Ehrlich proposed that the combination of antigen with a preformed B cell receptor (now known to be antibody) triggered the cell to produce and secrete more of those receptors. Although the diagram indicates that he thought a single cell could produce antibodies to bind more than one type of antigen, it is evident that he anticipated both the clonal selection theory and the idea that the immune system could generate receptors before contact with antigen.

that light and heavy variable regions were comprised of the product of two (VL, JL) or three (VH, DH, and JH) separate gene libraries of DNA sequences, respectively, which are rearranged into a complete antigen receptor gene via recombination events (termed 'V(D)J recombination') that occur at specific times during B cell differentiation. Combinatorial assembly of antigen receptor genes from these libraries of gene segments, described in more detail below, allows a limited amount of genetic material to generate the vast antigen receptor repertoire required for humoral immune protection. A similar process is used to assemble the genes encoding the antigen binding domains of T cell receptors.

Q. Given that one human can produce more heavy chains and more light chains than there are genes in the entire human genome, what mechanism(s) could lead to the presence of the great diversity of immunoglobulin genes seen in different B cells, each encoding a specific antibody?

A. The antibody genes could be produced by splicing together different gene segments, with a different combination of segments used in different B cells. Another mechanism could involve mutation of the original gene(s) with different mutations occurring in different B cells. In fact, both of these mechanisms take place in human B cells.

The two mechanisms occurring within individual B cells – gene segment recombination and gene mutation – described above, are termed **somatic recombination** and **somatic mutation** to distinguish them from the related processes that occur in germ cells.

In addition to the diversity generated by somatic recombination and somatic mutation, the pairing of a unique V_L domain with a unique V_H domain generates a unique antigen-binding site. This is referred to as **combinatorial pairing**.

An exception to this rule is present in the Camelidae family in which a high proportion of circulating antibody is comprised of a functional heavy chain only. This suggests possibilities for using just V_H domains as therapeutics that may have advantages for penetrating solid tumors.

Heavy chain gene recombination precedes light chain recombination

The revealed organization of mammalian genomes invalidated the earlier dogma of 'one gene, one polypeptide chain' and replaced it with 'genes in pieces' as coding (exons) and non-coding (introns) DNA sequences were identified. Generally:

- an open reading frame is transcribed to nuclear RNA;
- the introns are 'spliced' out of nuclear RNA to yield a continuous messenger RNA (mRNA);
- protein is translated from continuous mRNA.

Germline DNA encoding immunoglobulin polypeptide chains shows a further level of complexity. Information for the variable domains is present in two or three libraries containing multiple alternative versions of **V, D, and J gene segments.** These families of gene segments are widely separated from exons encoding the constant regions. Recombination events during B cell differentiation choose a particular V, D, and J gene segment from each library and assemble them into a continuous DNA sequence encoding the V domain. However, in the initial nuclear RNA transcript the information for the V and C domains is still widely separated.

The DNA encoding the leader peptide to the end of the C gene, including introns, is transcribed into heterogeneous nuclear RNA (hnRNA). The hnRNA is processed with the 'splicing out' of introns to yield the mRNA encoding the polypeptide V and C domains within a continuous RNA sequence that is translated into protein.

The primary antibody repertoire is:

- generated through recombination of germline gene segments, with selection to eliminate B cells producing anti-self antibodies;
- present in the B cell population and expressed as membrane-bound IgM and IgD acting as antigen receptors.

Antibody genes undergo rearrangement during B cell development

Antibody gene rearrangement is initiated at the heavy chain locus. If a 'productive' rearrangement occurs (i.e. generating a functional gene product), then rearrangement at the κ locus is initiated:

- if the κ rearrangement is productive, the assembled antibody is expressed as a membrane receptor;
- if recombination at the κ locus is not productive, rearrangement at the λ locus proceeds.

A number of **pseudogenes** (non-functional genes with high homology to the heavy chain genes) and **orphan genes** (putative genes with no known homology to known functional genes) have been identified as related to functional heavy and light chain genes. For example, the heavy chain locus includes approximately 78 related pseudogenes, and orphan genes occur on chromosomes other than 14.

Rearrangement at the heavy chain V_H locus precedes rearrangement at light chain loci

The germline human heavy chain locus, on chromosome 14 (Fig. 3.21), contains a library of 38 to 46 functional V_H gene segments that encode the N-terminal 95 residues of the V_H region.

The C terminal residues of the V_H region are encoded within 23 D_H and six J_H gene segments (see Fig. 3.21).

Productive rearrangement at the V_H locus is an obligatory and early event in the generation of B cells that precedes rearrangement at light chain loci.

The first event is recombination between a J_H gene segment and D_H segments, followed by recombination with a V_H gene segment

D_H segments:

- are highly variable, both in the number of codons and in the nucleotide sequence;
- may be read in three possible reading frames without generating stop codons; and
- can be used singly or in combinations.

Heavy chain VDJ recombination in humans

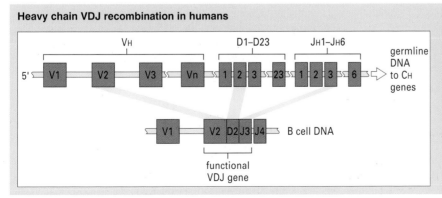

Fig. 3.21 The heavy chain gene loci recombine three segments to produce a VDJ gene, which encodes the V_H domain. Of some 80 V genes, about 50 are functional and the others are pseudogenes. The V gene segment recombines with one of 23 D_H segments and one of six J_H segments to produce a functional VDJ gene in the B cell.

Productive recombination between DH and JH gene segments signals recombination of this DJ sequence to a VH gene segment, forming a contiguous DNA sequence encoding the entire VH protein sequence (see Fig. 3.21).

The recombined VH, DH, and JH gene segments generate widely diverse hypervariable Hv3 (CDR3) sequences, which contribute greatly to the diversity of the primary antibody repertoire.

Rearrangement results in a Vκ gene segment becoming contiguous with a Jκ gene segment

The germline human κ light chain locus on chromosome 2 (Fig. 3.22) contains a library of 31–35 functional Vκ gene segments that encode the N terminal 95 residues of the Vκ region.

The C terminal residues of the Vκ region are encoded within five Jκ gene segments (see Fig. 3.22).

During B cell development, rearrangement of the DNA occurs such that one of the Vκ genes becomes contiguous with one of five Jκ genes.

Q. If there are 31 Vκ segments and five Jκ segments, what is the theoretical maximum number of rearrangements that could occur at this locus?
A. 155 (i.e. 31 × 5), but imprecise joining introduces additional diversity (see below).

The κ locus also includes over 30 related pseudogenes, and orphan genes are present on other chromosomes.

A leader or signal sequence (a short hydrophobic segment responsible for targeting the chain to the endoplasmic reticulum) precedes each Vκ segment. The leader sequence is cleaved in the endoplasmic reticulum, and the antibody molecule is then processed through the intracellular secretory pathway.

Recombination results in a Vλ gene segment becoming contiguous with a functional Jλ gene segment

The germline human λ light chain locus (Fig. 3.23) on chromosome 22 contains a library of 29–33 functional Vλ gene segments that encode the N terminal 95 residues of the Vλ region.

κ chain production in humans

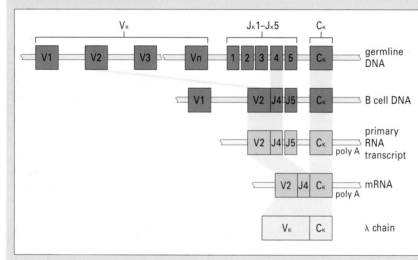

Fig. 3.22 During differentiation of the pre-B cell, one of several Vκ genes on the germline DNA (V1–Vn) is recombined and apposed to a Jκ segment (Jκ1–Jκ5). The B cell transcribes a segment of DNA into a primary RNA transcript that contains a long intervening sequence of additional J segments and introns. This transcript is processed into mRNA by splicing the exons together, and is translated by ribosomes into κ chains. The rearrangement illustrated is only one of the many possible recombinations. (B cell DNA is colored light brown; RNA is colored green; and immunoglobulin peptides are colored yellow.)

λ chain production in humans

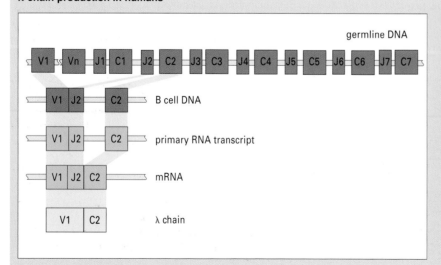

Fig. 3.23 During B cell differentiation, one of the germline Vλ genes recombines with a J segment to form a VJ combination. The rearranged gene is transcribed into a primary RNA transcript complete with introns (non-coding segments occurring between the genes), exons (which code for protein), and a poly A tail. This is spliced to form mRNA with loss of the introns, and then translated into protein.

There are 7–11 Jλ gene segments with each linked to a Cλ gene sequence (see Fig. 3.23) – the number of JλCλ sequences depends on the haplotype.

During the generation of B cells, unproductive rearrangement at the κ locus leads to recombination at the λ locus such that one of the Vλ genes becomes contiguous with one of four or five functional Jλ genes.

The number of possible λ chain variable regions that could be produced in this way is approximately 120–160. Imprecise joining introduces additional diversity (see below).

The λ locus also includes over 35 related pseudogenes, and orphan genes are present on other chromosomes.

Following recombination between Vλ and Jλ genes, there is still an intron (a non-coding intervening sequence) between the recombined VλJλ gene and the exon encoding the C region.

Recombination involves recognition of signal sequences by the V(D)J recombinase

Recombination of germline gene segments is a key feature in the generation of the primary antibody repertoire. How is the recombination effected?

Each V, D, and J segment is flanked by **recombination signal sequences (RSS)**:

- a signal sequence found downstream (3′) of VH,VL, and DH gene segments consists of a heptamer CACAGTG or its analog, followed by a spacer of non-conserved sequence (12 or 23 bases), and then a nonamer ACAAAAACC or its analog (Fig. 3.24);
- immediately upstream (5′) of a germline JL, DH, and JH segment is a corresponding signal sequence of a nonamer and a heptamer, again separated by an unconserved sequence (12 or 23 bases).

The heptameric and nonameric sequences following a VL, VH, or DH segment are complementary to those preceding the JL, DH, or JH segments (respectively) with which they recombine.

The 12 and 23 base spacers correspond to either one or two turns of the DNA helix (see Fig. 3.24).

Recombination sequences in immunoglobulin genes

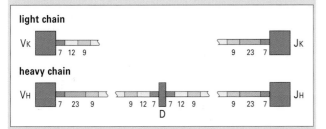

Fig. 3.24 The recombination sequences in the light chain genes (top) and heavy chain genes (bottom) consist of heptamers (7), 12 or 23 unconserved bases, and nonamers (9). The sequences of heptamers and nonamers are complementary and the nonamers act as signals for the recombination activating genes to form a synapsis between the adjoining exons. Similar recombination sequences are present in the T cell receptor V, D, and J segments (see Chapter 5).

The recombination process is mediated by the protein products of the two **recombination-activating genes (RAG-1 and RAG-2)**:

- a RAG-1–RAG-2 complex recognizes the RSS, bringing a 12-RSS and a 23-RSS together into a synaptic complex (Fig. 3.25);
- the RAG proteins initiate cleavage by introducing a nick in the area bordering the 5′ end of the signal heptamer and the coding region;
- the RAG proteins then convert this nick into a double-strand break, generating a hairpin at the coding end and a blunt cut at the signal sequence, resulting in a blunt signal end;
- the hairpinned coding end must be opened before the joining step, and usually undergoes further processing (the addition or deletion of nucleotides), resulting in an imprecise junction. The loss or addition of nucleotides during coding joint formation (termed '**junctional diversity**') creates additional diversity that is not encoded by the V, D, or J segments, and also contributes to the generation of nonproductive joints, since some of the modification create stop codons.

Signal ends, in contrast, are usually joined precisely to form circular signal joints that have no known immunological function and are lost from the cell (see Fig. 3.25).

Additional diversification is provided by the enzyme terminal deoxynucleotidyl transferase, which may add random nucleotides to the exposed cut ends of the DNA. Nucleotides may therefore be inserted between DH and JH, and between VH and DH, without need of a template (Figs 3.26 and 3.27).

Somatic hypermutation in antibody genes

The enormous size and sequence variability of the antigen-specific antibody repertoire could not be accommodated within the 'one gene, one polypeptide chain' dogma. Therefore, models of germline inheritance, 'genes in pieces' and somatic mutation were contemplated to account for the observed diversity.

It is now resolved that nature employs all three types of process to form the antibody repertoire. Libraries of germline gene segment sequences recombine, with a degree of junctional diversity, to generate the primary antibody repertoire, but this process does not account for the sequence diversity observed for antibodies that are generated during a secondary immune response.

The secondary response is characterized by the appearance of germinal centers, within the spleen, bone marrow and lymph glands, within which the recombined DNA encoding variable light and heavy chain sequences undergoes repeated rounds of random mutation (**somatic hypermutation**) to generate B cells expressing structurally distinct receptors (Fig. 3.28). Survival and expansion of these B cells requires that their receptors engage antigen presented to them by follicular dendritic cells in the lymphoid tissues:

- a majority will acquire a deleterious mutation and, in the absence of a survival signal, die;
- a minority bind antigen with increased affinity and compete with those of lower affinity (i.e. antibodies characteristic of the primary response).

Stages of V(D)J recombination

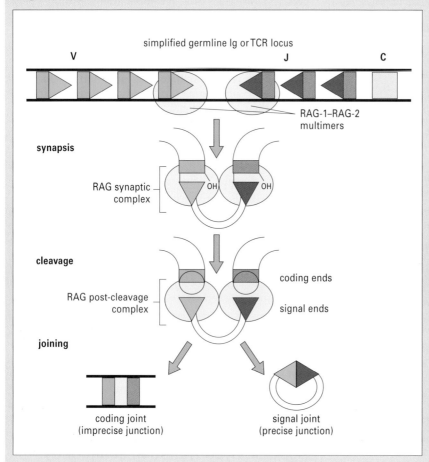

simplified germline Ig or TCR locus

Fig. 3.25 The recombination-activating genes (RAG-1–RAG-2) bind to two recombination signal sequences (RSS) – one 12-RSS and one 23-RSS – bringing them into a synaptic complex. Synapsis stimulates cleavage: first, one DNA strand is nicked, and the resulting 3′ OH group attacks the opposite strand, leaving two hairpinned coding ends and two blunt signal ends. After cleavage, these ends are held in the RAG post-cleavage complex and joined by the non-homologous end-joining (NHEJ) factors. The coding joint forms the new variable region exon; the signal ends are joined together to form a signal joint, often (but not always) as an excised circular product that is lost from the cell. The signal joint has no known immunological function.

Light chain diversity created by variable recombination

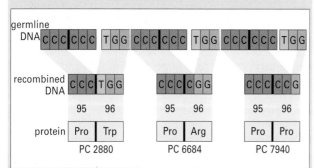

Fig. 3.26 The same Vκ21 and J1 sequences of the germline create three different amino acid sequences in the proteins PC2880, PC6684, and PC7940 by variable recombination. PC2880 has proline and tryptophan at positions 95 and 96, caused by recombination at the end of the CCC codon. Recombination one base down produces proline and arginine in PC6684. Recombination two bases down from the end of Vκ21 produces proline and proline in PC7940.

This process, called **affinity maturation**, is dependent on both T cells and germinal centers.

Athymic mice lacking T cells do not form germinal centers and show no affinity maturation.

Diversity is generated at several different levels

Antibody diversity therefore arises at several levels:

- there are multiple V genes recombining with D and J segments;
- VJ and VDJ recombination;
- recombinational inaccuracies and N-nucleotide addition;
- gene conversion (in some species – see Fig. 3.w6);
- the combination of different heavy and light chains; and
- somatic point mutation.

The structures of the first and second hypervariable regions (CDR-1 and CDR-2) of the primary antibody repertoire are encoded entirely by germline gene segments whereas CDR-3 diversity is generated by recombination events.

Heavy chain diversity created by variable recombination and N region diversity

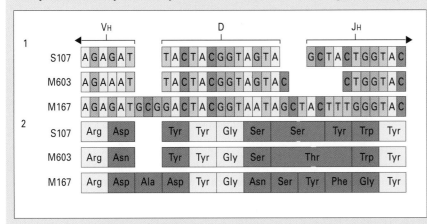

Fig. 3.27 The DNA sequence (**1**) and amino acid sequence (**2**) of three heavy chains of anti-phosphorylcholine are shown. Variable recombination between the germline, V, D, and J regions, and N region insertion causes variation (orange) in amino acid sequences. In some cases (e.g. M167) there appear to be additional inserted codons. However, these are in multiples of three, and do not alter the overall reading frame.

Mutations in the DNA of two heavy chain genes

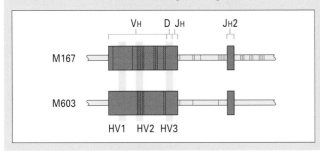

Fig. 3.28 DNA of two IgG antibodies to phosphorylcholine are illustrated. Both antibodies share the T15 idiotype. Black lines indicate positions where the sequence has mutated from the germline sequence. There are large numbers of mutations in both the introns and exons of both genes, but particularly in the second hypervariable region (HV2). By comparison, there are no mutations in the regions encoding the constant genes, implying that the mutational mechanism is highly localized.

CRITICAL THINKING: THE SPECIFICITY OF ANTIBODIES (SEE P. 433 FOR EXPLANATIONS)

The human rhinovirus HRV14 is formed from four different polypeptides: one of them (VP4) is associated with viral RNA in the core of the virus, while the other three polypeptides (VP1–VP3) make up the shell of the virus – the capsid.

1 When virus is propagated in the presence of neutralizing antiviral antiserum it is found that mutated forms of the virus develop. Mutations are detected in VP1, VP2, or VP3, but never in VP4. Why should this be so? The most effective neutralizing antibodies are directed against the protein VP1 – this is termed an immunodominant antigen. Two different monoclonal antibodies against VP1 were developed and used to

induce mutated forms of the virus. When the sequences of the mutated variants were compared with the original virus, it was found that only certain amino acid residues became mutated (see table below).

2 What can you tell about the epitopes that are recognized by the two different monoclonal antibodies?

3 When the binding of the antibody VP1-a is measured against the different mutant viruses, it is found that it binds with high affinity to the variant with glycine (Gly) at position 138, with low affinity to the variant with Gly at position 95, and does not bind to the variant with lysine (Lys) at position 95. How can you explain these observations?

Antibody	Amino acid number	Residue in wild type	Observed mutations
VP1-a	91	Glu	Ala, Asp, Gly, His, Asn, Val, Tyr
VP1-a	95	Asp	Gly, Lys
VP1-b	83	Gln	His
VP1-b	85	Lys	Asn
VP1-b	138	Glu	Asp, Gly
VP1-b	139	Ser	Pro

Further reading

Arnold JN, Wormald MR, Sim RB, et al. The Impact of Glycosylation on the Biological Function and Structure of Human Immunoglobulins. Annu Rev Immunol 2007;25:21–50.

Gould HJ, Sutton BJ. IgE in allergy and asthma today. Nat Rev Immunol 2008;8:205–217.

Jefferis R. Glycosylation as a strategy to improve antibody-based therapeutics. Nat Rev Drug Discov 2009;8:226–234.

Jefferis R, Lefranc M-P. Human immunoglobulin allotypes: possible implications for immunogenicity. MAbs 2009;1:332–338.

Litman GW, Rast JP, Fugmann SD. The origins of vertebrate adaptive immunity. Nat Rev Immunol 2010;10:543–553.

Monteiro RC. Role of IgA and IgA Fc receptors in inflammation. J Clin Immunol 2010;30:1–9.

Neuberger MS. Antibody diversification by somatic mutation: from Burnet onwards. Immunol Cell Biol 2008;86:124–132.

Reichert JM. Antibody-based therapeutics to watch in 2011. MAbs 2011;11:3.

Schroeder HW Jr., Cavacini L. Structure and function of immunoglobulins. J Allergy Clin Immunol 2010;125:S41–S52.

Shukla AA, Thömmes J. Recent advances in large-scale production of monoclonal antibodies and related proteins. Trends Biotechnol 2010;28:253–261.

Woof JM, Burton D. Human antibody-Fc receptor interactions illuminated by crystal structures. Nat Rev Immunol 2004;4:89–99.

Woof JM, Kerr MA. The function of immunoglobulin A in immunity. J Pathol 208:270–282.

Internet references

IMGT, the International ImMunoGeneTics Information System®. http://www.imgt.org/. An integrated knowledge resource for the immunoglobulins (IG), T cell receptors (TR), major histocompatibility complex (MHC), immunoglobulin superfamily and related proteins of the immune system of human and other vertebrate species.

Mike Clark's Immunoglobulin Structure/Function Home Page. http://www.path.cam.ac.uk/~mrc7/mikeimages.html. Provides a wealth of information, of his own generation and through access to many other related sites.

National Center for Biotechnology Information (NCBI). http://www.ncbi.nlm.nih.gov/. Established in 1988 as a national resource for molecular biology information, NCBI creates public databases, conducts research in computational biology, develops software tools for analyzing genome data, and disseminates biomedical information – all for the better understanding of molecular processes affecting human health and disease.

CD antigens. http://www.uniprot.org/docs/cdist.txt. Human cell differentiation molecules: CD nomenclature and list of entries.

Summary of Antibody Structures in the Protein Databank. http://acrmwww.biochem.ucl.ac.uk/abs/sacs/index.html.

CHAPTER 4

Complement

SUMMARY

- **Complement is central to the development of inflammatory reactions** and forms one of the major immune defense systems of the body. The complement system serves as one of the links between the innate and adaptive arms of the immune system.

- **Complement activation pathways have evolved to label pathogens for elimination.** The classical pathway links to the adaptive immune system through antibody. The alternative and lectin pathways provide antibody-independent 'innate' immunity, and the alternative pathway is linked to and amplifies the classical pathway.

- **The complement system is carefully controlled to protect the body from excessive or inappropriate inflammatory responses**. C1 inhibitor controls the classical and lectin pathways. C3 and C5 convertase activity are controlled by decay and enzymatic degradation. Membrane attack is inhibited on host cells by CD59.

- **The membrane attack pathway results in the formation of a lytic transmembrane pore.** Regulation of the membrane attack pathway by CD59 reduces the risk of 'bystander' damage to adjacent host cells.

- **Many cells express one or more membrane receptors for complement products.** Receptors for fragments of C3 are widely distributed on different leukocyte populations. Receptors for C1q are present on phagocytes, mast cells, and platelets. C5 fragment receptors are present on many cell types. The plasma complement regulator fH binds leukocyte surfaces.

- **Complement has a variety of functions.** Its principal functions include opsonization, chemotaxis and cell activation, lysis of target cells, and priming of the adaptive immune response.

- **Complement deficiencies illustrate the homeostatic roles of complement.** Classical pathway deficiencies result in tissue inflammation. Deficiencies of mannan-binding lectin (MBL) are associated with infections in infants and the immunosuppressed. Alternative pathway and C3 deficiencies are associated with bacterial infections. Terminal pathway deficiencies predispose to Gram-negative bacterial infections. C1 inhibitor deficiency leads to hereditary angioedema. Deficiencies in alternative pathway regulators produce a secondary loss of C3.

Complement and inflammation

The complement system was discovered at the end of the 19th century as a heat-labile component of serum that augmented (or 'complemented') its bactericidal properties.

Complement is now known to comprise some 16 plasma proteins, together constituting nearly 10% of the total serum proteins, and forming one of the major immune defense systems of the body (Fig. 4.1). In addition to serving as a key component of the innate immune system, complement also interfaces with and enhances adaptive immune responses. More than a dozen regulatory proteins are present in plasma and on cells to control complement. The functions of the complement system include:

- triggering and amplification of inflammatory reactions;
- attraction of phagocytes by chemotaxis;
- clearance of immune complexes and apoptotic cells;
- cellular activation for microbial killing;
- direct microbial killing; and
- an important role in the efficient development of antibody responses.

In evolutionary terms the complement system is very ancient and antedates the development of the adaptive immune system: even starfish and worms have a functional complement system.

The importance of complement in immune defense is readily apparent in individuals who lack particular components – for example, children who lack the central component **C3** are subject to overwhelming bacterial infections.

Like most elements of the immune system, when overactivated or activated in the wrong place, the complement system can cause harm.

Role of complement in inflammation

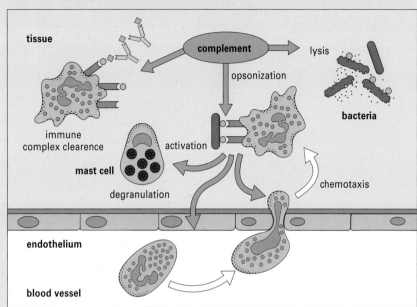

Fig. 4.1 Complement has a central role in inflammation causing chemotaxis of phagocytes, activation of mast cells and phagocytes, opsonization and lysis of pathogens, and clearance of immune complexes.

Complement is involved in the pathology of many diseases, provoking a search for therapies that control complement activation.

Complement activation pathways

One major function of complement is to label pathogens and other foreign or toxic bodies for elimination from the host. The complement activation pathways have evolved to serve this purpose, and the multiple ways in which activation can be triggered, together with intrinsic amplification mechanisms, ensure efficient recognition and clearance.

Moreover, there are several different ways to activate the complement system, so providing a large degree of flexibility in response (Fig. 4.2).

The first activation pathway to be discovered, now termed the **classical pathway**, is initiated by antibodies bound to the surface of the target. Although an efficient means of activation, it requires an adaptive immune response: that is, the host must have previously encountered the target microorganism in order for an antibody response to be generated.

The **alternative pathway**, described in the 1950s, provides an antibody-independent mechanism for complement activation on pathogen surfaces.

The **lectin pathway**, the most recently described activation pathway, also bypasses antibody to enable efficient activation on pathogens.

All three pathways – classical, alternative, and lectin pathways:

- involve the activation of C3, which is the most abundant and most important of the complement proteins;
- comprise a proteolytic cascade in which complexes of complement proteins create enzymes that cleave other complement proteins in an ordered manner to create new enzymes, thereby amplifying and perpetuating the activation cascade.

Complement activation pathways

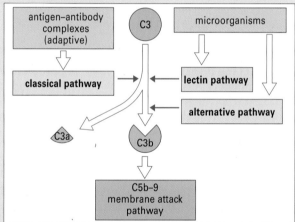

Fig. 4.2 Each of the activation pathways generates a C3 convertase, which converts C3 to C3b, the central event of the complement pathway. C3b in turn activates the terminal lytic membrane attack pathway. The first stage in the classical pathway is the binding of antigen to antibody. The alternative pathway does not require antibody and is initiated by the covalent binding of C3b to hydroxyl and amine groups on the surface of various microorganisms. The lectin pathway is also triggered by microorganisms in the absence of antibody, with sugar residues on the pathogen surface providing the binding sites. The alternative and lectin pathways provide antibody-independent 'innate' immunity, whereas the classical pathway represents a more recently evolved link to the adaptive immune system.

Thus a small initial stimulus can rapidly generate a large effect. Figure 4.3 summarizes how each of the pathways is activated.

All activation pathways converge on a common **terminal pathway** – a non-enzymatic system for causing membrane disruption and lytic killing of pathogens.

Summary of the activators of the classical, lectin, and alternative pathways

	immunoglobulins	microorganisms			other
		viruses	bacteria	other	
classical pathway	immune complexes containing IgM, IgG1, IgG2, or IgG3	HIV and other retroviruses, vesicular stomatitis virus		*Mycoplasma* spp.	polyanions, especially when bound to cations PO_4^{3-} (DNA, lipid A, cardiolipin) SO_4^{2-} (dextran sulfate, heparin, chondroitin sulfate)
lectin pathway		HIV and other retroviruses	many Gram-positive and Gram-negative organisms		arrays of terminal mannose groups acetylated sugars
alternative pathway	immune complexes containing IgG, IgA, or IgE (less efficient than the classical pathway)	some virus-infected cells (e.g. by Epstein–Barr virus)	many Gram-positive and Gram-negative organisms	trypanosomes, *Leishmania* spp., many fungi	dextran sulfate, heterologous erythrocytes, complex carbohydrates (e.g. zymosan)

Fig. 4.3 Summary of the activators of the classical, lectin, and alternative complement activation pathways.

The immune defense and pathological effects of complement activation are mediated by the fragments and complexes generated during activation:

- the small chemotactic and proinflammatory fragments **C3a** and **C5a**;
- the large opsonic fragments **C3b** and **C4b**; and
- the lytic **membrane attack complex (MAC)**.

The details of complement activation, the nomenclature, and the ways in which the pathways are controlled are shown in Figure 4.4.

The classical pathway links to the adaptive immune system

The classical pathway is activated by antibody bound to antigen and requires Ca^{2+}

Only surface-bound IgG and IgM antibodies can activate complement, and they do so via the classical pathway. Surface binding is the key:

- IgM is the most efficient activator, but unbound IgM in plasma does not activate complement;
- among IgG subclasses, IgG1 and IgG3 are strong complement activators, whereas IgG4 does not activate because it is unable to bind the first component of the classical pathway.

Q. What occurs when IgM binds to the surface of a bacterium that allows it to activate complement?
A. A transition occurs from a flat planar molecule to a staple form, which exposes binding sites for the first component of the complement system, C1 (see Fig. 3.6).

The first component of the pathway, **C1**, is a complex molecule comprising a large, 6-headed recognition unit termed **C1q** and two molecules each of **C1r** and **C1s**, the enzymatic units of the complex (Fig. 4.5). Assembly of the C1 complex is Ca^{2+}-dependent, and the classical pathway is therefore inactive if Ca^{2+} ions are absent.

C1 activation occurs only when several of the head groups of C1q are bound to antibody

C1q in the C1 complex binds through its globular head groups to the Fc regions of the immobilized antibody and undergoes changes in shape that trigger autocatalytic activation of the enzymatic unit C1r. Activated C1r then cleaves C1s at a single site in the protein to activate it.

Since C1 activation occurs only when several of the six head groups of C1q are bound to antibody, only surfaces that are densely coated with antibody will trigger the process. This limitation reduces the risk of inappropriate activation on host tissues.

C1s enzyme cleaves C4 and C2

The C1s enzyme has two substrates – C4 and C2 – which are the next two proteins in the classical pathway sequence. (Note that the complement components were named chronologically, according to the order of their discovery, rather than according to their position in the reaction.) C1s cleaves the abundant plasma protein **C4** at a single site in the molecule:

- releasing a small fragment, **C4a**; and
- exposing a labile thioester group in the large fragment **C4b**.

Through the highly reactive thioester, C4b becomes covalently linked to the activating surface (Fig. 4.6).

C4b binds the next component, **C2**, in a Mg^{2+}-dependent complex and presents it for cleavage by C1s in an adjacent C1 complex:

- the fragment **C2b** is released; and
- **C2a** remains associated with C4b on the surface.

$\overline{C4b2a}$ is the classical pathway C3 convertase

The complex of C4b and C2a (termed **$\overline{C4b2a}$** – the classical pathway C3 convertase) is the next activation enzyme. C2a in the $\overline{C4b2a}$ complex cleaves C3, the most abundant of the complement proteins:

Overview of the complement activation pathways

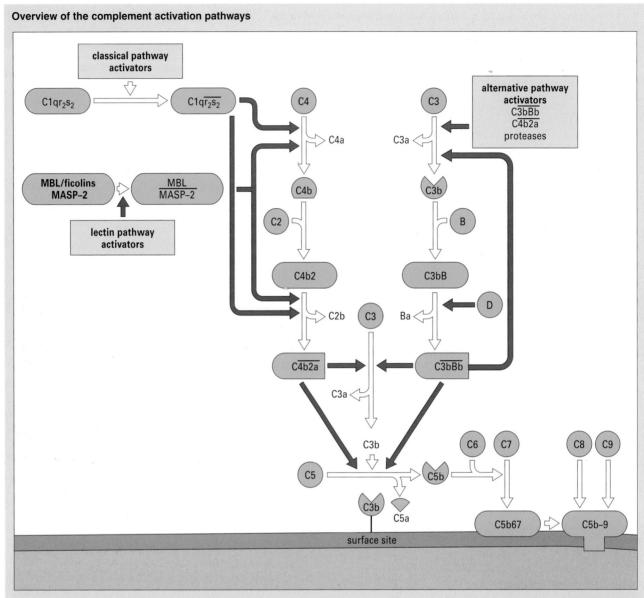

Fig. 4.4 The proteins of the classical and alternative pathways are assigned numbers (e.g. C1, C2). Many of these are zymogens (i.e. pro-enzymes that require proteolytic cleavage to become active). The cleavage products of complement proteins are distinguished from parent molecules by suffix letters (e.g. C3a, C3b). The proteins of the alternative pathway are called 'factors' and are identified by single letters (e.g. factor B, which may be abbreviated to fB or just 'B'). Components are shown in green, conversion steps as white arrows, and activation/cleavage steps as red arrows. The classical pathway is activated by the cleavage of C1r and C1s following association of C1qr₂s₂ with classical pathway activators (see Fig. 4.3), including immune complexes. Activated C1s cleaves C4 and C2 to form the classical pathway C3 convertase $\overline{C4b2a}$. Cleavage of C4 and C2 can also be effected via MASP-2 of the lectin pathway, which is associated with mannan-binding lectin (MBL) or ficolin. The alternative pathway is activated by the cleavage of C3 to C3b, which associates with factor B and is cleaved by factor D to generate the alternative pathway C3 convertase $\overline{C3bBb}$. The initial activation of C3 happens to some extent spontaneously, but this step can also be affected by classical or alternative pathway C3 convertases or a number of other serum or microbial proteases. Note that C3b generated in the alternative pathway can bind more factor B and generate a positive feedback loop to amplify activation on the surface. Note also that the activation pathways are functionally analogous, and the diagram emphasizes these similarities. For example, C3 and C4 are homologous, as are C2 and factor B. MASP-2 is homologous to C1r and C1s. Either the classical or alternative pathway C3 convertases may associate with C3b bound on a cell surface to form C5 convertases, $\overline{C4b2a3b}$, or $\overline{C3bBbC3b}$, which split C5. The larger fragment C5b associates with C6 and C7, which can then bind to plasma membranes. The complex of C5b67 assembles C8 and a number of molecules of C9 to form a membrane attack complex (MAC), C5b-9.

- releasing a small fragment, **C3a**; and
- exposing a labile thioester group in the large fragment **C3b**.

As described above for C4b, C3b covalently binds the activating surface.

$\overline{C4b2a3b}$ is the classical pathway C5 convertase

Some of the C3b formed will bind directly to $\overline{C4b2a}$, and the trimolecular complex formed, **$\overline{C4b2a3b}$** (the classical pathway C5 convertase), can bind **C5** and present it for cleavage by C2a:

Structure of C1

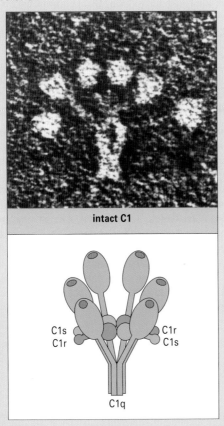

intact C1

C1s
C1r

C1r
C1s

C1q

Fig. 4.5 Electron micrograph of a human C1q molecule demonstrates six subunits. Each subunit contains three polypeptide chains, giving 18 in the whole molecule. The receptors for the Fc regions of IgG and IgM are in the globular heads. The connecting stalks contain regions of triple helix and the central core region contains collagen-like triple helix. The lower panel shows a model of intact C1 with two C1r and two C1s pro-enzymes positioned within the ring. The catalytic heads of C1r and C1s are closely apposed and conformational change induced in C1q following binding to complexed immunoglobulin causes mutual activation/cleavage of each C1r unit followed by cleavage of the two C1s units. The cohesion of the entire complex is dependent on Ca^{2+}. *(Electron micrograph, reproduced by courtesy of Dr N Hughes-Jones.)*

- a small fragment, **C5a**, is released; and
- the large fragment, **C5b**, remains associated with the $\overline{C4b2a3b}$ complex.

Cleavage of C5 is the final enzymatic step in the classical pathway.

The ability of C4b and C3b to bind surfaces is fundamental to complement function

C3 and C4 are homologous molecules that contain an unusual structural feature – an internal thioester bond between a glutamine and a cysteine residue that, in the intact molecule, is buried within the protein.

When either C3 or C4 is cleaved by the convertase enzyme, a conformational change takes place that exposes the internal thioester bond in C3b and C4b, making it very unstable and highly susceptible to attack by nucleophiles such as hydroxyl groups (-OH) and amine groups (-NH₂) in membrane proteins and carbohydrates. This reaction

Activation of the C3 thioester bond

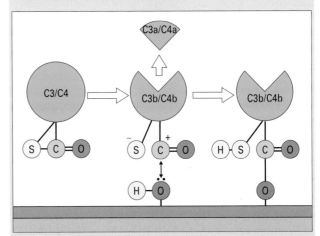

Fig. 4.6 The α chain of C3 contains a thioester bond formed between a cysteine and a glutamine residue, with the elimination of ammonia. Following cleavage of C3 into C3a and C3b, the bond becomes unstable and susceptible to nucleophilic attack by electrons on -OH and -NH₂ groups, allowing the C3b to form covalent bonds with proteins and carbohydrates – the active group decays rapidly by hydrolysis if such a bond does not form. C4 also contains an identical thioester bond, which becomes activated similarly when C4 is split into C4a and C4b.

creates a covalent bond between the complement fragment and the membrane ligand, locking C3b and C4b onto the surface (see Fig. 4.6).

The exposed thioester remains reactive for only a few milliseconds because it is susceptible to hydrolysis by water. This lability restricts the binding of C3b and C4b to the immediate vicinity of the activating enzyme and prevents damage to surrounding structures.

The alternative and lectin pathways provide antibody-independent 'innate' immunity

The lectin pathway is activated by microbial carbohydrates

The lectin pathway differs from the classical pathway only in the initial recognition and activation steps. Indeed, it can be argued that the lectin pathway should not be considered a separate pathway, but rather a route for classical pathway activation that bypasses the need for antibody.

The C1 complex is replaced by a structurally similar multimolecular complex, comprising a C1q-like recognition unit, either **mannan-binding lectin (MBL)** or **ficolin** (actually a family of three proteins in man), and several **MBL-associated serine proteases (MASPs)**. MASP-2 provides enzymatic activity. As in the classical pathway, assembly of this initiating complex is Ca^{2+}-dependent.

C1q and MBL are members of the collectin family of proteins characterized by globular head regions with binding activities and long collagenous tail regions with diverse roles (see Fig. 6.w3). Ficolins are structurally similar but the head regions comprise fibrinogen-like domains.

MBL binds the simple carbohydrates mannose and *N*-acetyl glucosamine, while ficolins bind acetylated sugars and other molecules; these ligands are abundant in the cell walls of diverse pathogens, including bacteria, yeast, fungi, and viruses, making them targets for lectin pathway activation. Binding induces shape changes in MBL and ficolins that in turn induce autocatalytic activation of MASP-2. This enzyme can then cleave C4 and C2 to continue activation exactly as in the classical pathway.

The lectin pathway is not the only means of activating the classical pathway in the absence of antibody. Apoptotic cells, released DNA, mitochondria and other products of cell damage can directly bind C1q, triggering complement activation and aiding the clearance of the dead and dying tissue.

Alternative pathway activation is accelerated by microbial surfaces and requires Mg^{2+}

The alternative pathway of complement activation also provides antibody-independent activation of complement on pathogen surfaces. This pathway is in a constant state of low-level activation (termed 'tickover').

C3 is hydrolyzed at a slow rate in plasma and the product, $C3(H_2O)$, has many of the properties of C3b, including the capacity to bind a **plasma protein factor B (fB)**, which is a close relative of the classical pathway protein C2. Formation of the complex between C3b (or $C3(H_2O)$) and fB is Mg^{2+}-dependent, so the alternative pathway is inactive in the absence of Mg^{2+} ions. (The differences in the ion requirements of the classical and alternative pathway are exploited in laboratory tests for complement activity.)

The C3bBb complex is the C3 convertase of the alternative pathway

Once bound to $C3(H_2O)$ or C3b, fB becomes a substrate for an intrinsically active plasma enzyme termed **factor D (fD)**. fD cuts fB in the C3bB complex:

- releasing a fragment, **Ba**;
- while the residual portion, **Bb**, becomes an active protease.

The **C3bBb** complex is the C3 cleaving enzyme (C3 convertase) of the alternative pathway. C3b generated by this convertase can be fed back into the pathway to create more C3 convertases, thus forming a positive feedback amplification loop (Fig. 4.7). Activation may occur in plasma or, more efficiently, on surfaces.

Q. What physiological advantages and problems can you see in a system with a positive feedback loop (i.e. where the presence of C3b leads to the production of an enzyme C3bBb that generates more C3b)?

A. The positive feedback amplification and 'always on' features of the alternative pathway are well suited to pathogen surveillance. For example, a small initial stimulus could produce the deposition of large amounts of C3b on a pathogen surface, thereby facilitating its phagocytosis. If unregulated, however, the system will continue to activate until all available C3 has been consumed. Self cells would also be subjected to complement activation and could be damaged or destroyed.

Specific features of host cell surfaces, including their surface carbohydrates and the presence of complement regulators (see below), act to protect the host cell from alternative pathway activation and risk of being destroyed, and such surfaces are termed non-activating.

On an activating surface such as a bacterial membrane, amplification will occur unimpeded and the surface will rapidly become coated with C3b (see Fig. 4.7). In a manner analogous to that seen in the classical pathway, C3b molecules binding to the C3 convertase will change the substrate specificity of the complex, creating a C5 cleaving enzyme, C3bBbC3b.

Regulation of the amplification loop

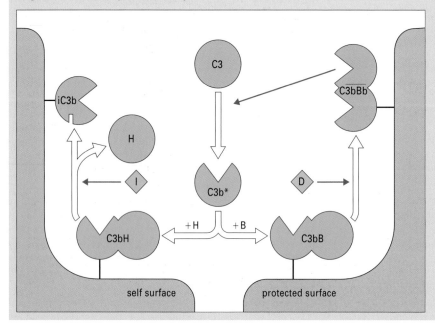

Fig. 4.7 Alternative pathway activation depends on the presence of activator surfaces. C3b bound to an activator surface recruits factor B, which is cleaved by factor D to produce the alternative pathway C3 convertase C3bBb, which drives the amplification loop, by cleaving more C3. However, on self surfaces the binding of factor H is favored and C3b is inactivated by factor I. Thus the binding of factor B or factor H controls the development of the alternative pathway reactions. In addition, proteins such as membrane cofactor protein (MCP) and decay accelerating factor (DAF) also limit complement activation on self cell membranes (see Fig. 4.9).

Cleavage of C5 is the last proteolytic step in the alternative pathway and the C5b fragment remains associated with the convertase.

The alternative pathway is linked to the classical pathway

The alternative pathway is inexorably linked to the classical pathway in that C3b generated through the classical pathway will feed into the alternative pathway to amplify activation. It therefore does not matter whether the initial C3b is generated by the classical, lectin, or alternative pathway – the amplification loop can ratchet up the reactions if they take place near an activator surface.

Complement protection systems

Control of the complement system is required to prevent the consumption of components through unregulated amplification and to protect the host. Complement activation poses a potential threat to host cells, because it could lead to cell opsonization or even lysis. To defend against this threat a family of regulators has evolved alongside the complement system to prevent uncontrolled activation and protect cells from attack.

C1 inhibitor controls the classical and lectin pathways

In the activation pathways, the regulators target the enzymes that drive amplification:

* activated C1 is controlled by a plasma serine protease inhibitor (serpin) termed C1 inhibitor (C1inh), which removes C1r and C1s from the complex, switching off classical pathway activation;
* C1inh also regulates the lectin pathway in a similar manner, removing the MASP-2 enzyme from the MBL or ficolin complex to switch off activation.

C3 and C5 convertase activity are controlled by decay and enzymatic degradation

The C3 and C5 convertase enzymes are heavily policed with plasma and cell membrane inhibitors to control activation. In the plasma:

* factor H (fH) and a related protein factor H-like 1 (fHL-1) destroy the convertase enzymes of the alternative pathway;
* C4 binding protein (C4bp) performs the same task in the classical pathway.

On membranes, two proteins, membrane cofactor protein (MCP) and decay accelerating factor (DAF), collaborate to destroy the convertases of both pathways (Fig. 4.8).

The regulators of the C3 and C5 convertases are structurally related molecules that have arisen by gene duplication in evolution. These duplicated genes are tightly linked in a cluster on chromosome 1, termed the regulators of complement activation (RCA) locus. This locus also encodes several of the complement receptors (see below).

Control of the convertases is mediated in two complementary ways

Decay acceleration –

The convertase complexes are labile, with a propensity to dissociate within a few minutes of creation. The regulators fH, fHL-1, and C4bp from the fluid phase and DAF on cell

C3 and C5 convertase regulators

	number of SCR domains*	dissociation of C3 and C5 convertases		cofactor for factor I on		localization
		classical pathway	alternative pathway	C4b	C3b	
C4b binding protein (C4bp)	52 or 56 in 7or 8 chains	+	–	+	–	plasma
factor H (fH)	20	–	+	–	+	plasma
decay accelerating factor (DAF) (CD55)	4	+	+	–	–	on most cells including blood cells, endothelia, and epithelia
membrane cofactor protein (MCP) (CD46)	4	–	–	+	+	on most cells including blood cells (but not erythrocytes), endothelia, and epithelia
complement receptor 1 (CR1) (CD35)	30	+	+	+	+	erythrocytes, B cells, follicular dendritic cells, macrophages

*SCR, short consensus repeat

Fig. 4.8 The five proteins listed are widely distributed and control aspects of C3b and C4b dissociation or breakdown. Each of these proteins contains a number of short consensus repeat (SCR) domains. They act either by enhancing the dissociation of C3 and C5 convertases or by acting as cofactors for the action of factor I on C3b or C4b.

membranes bind the convertase complex and markedly accelerate decay, displacing:

- C2a from the classical pathway convertase; and
- Bb from the alternative pathway enzyme (Fig. 4.9).

Cofactor activity –

Factor I (fI) is a fluid-phase enzyme that, in the presence of an appropriate cofactor, can cleave and irreversibly inactivate C4b and C3b (see Fig. 4.9). MCP is a cofactor for fI cleavage of both C4b and C3b, whereas:

- C4bp specifically catalyzes cleavage of C4b;
- fH/fHL-1 catalyzes cleavage of C3b.

It is interesting to note that, whereas the plasma regulators contain both activities in a single molecule, the two membrane regulators each contain only one activity.

Efficient regulation of the convertases on membranes therefore requires the concerted action of:

- DAF to dissociate the complex; and
- MCP to irreversibly inactivate it by catalyzing cleavage of the central component.

The alternative pathway also has a unique positive regulator, **properdin**, which stabilizes the C3 convertase and markedly increases its life span. Recent evidence has suggested an additional role of properdin as a catalyst for alternative pathway activation.

.Complement receptor 1 (CR1) is often included in the list of membrane regulators of C3 convertase activity, and, indeed, CR1 is a powerful regulator with both decay accelerating and cofactor activities in both pathways. Nevertheless, it is excluded from the above discussion because CR1 is primarily a receptor for complement-coated particles and does not have a role in protecting the host cell.

The two processes by which C3 convertase regulators inactivate the enzymes

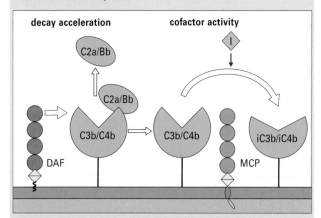

Fig. 4.9 DAF binds the enzyme complex, displacing the enzymatically active component (C2a or Bb). Membrane cofactor protein (MCP) binds the C3b/C4b unit released after decay and acts as a cofactor for factor I (fI) cleavage of C3b or C4b, resulting in the irreversible inactivation of the convertase.

The membrane attack pathway

Activation of the pathway results in the formation of a transmembrane pore

The **terminal or membrane attack pathway** involves a distinctive set of events whereby a group of five globular plasma proteins associate with one another and, in the process, acquire membrane-binding and pore-forming capacity to form the membrane attack complex (MAC).

The MAC is a transmembrane pore (Fig. 4.10). Cleavage of C5 creates the nidus for MAC assembly to begin. While still attached to the convertase enzyme, C5b binds first **C6** then **C7** from the plasma. Conformational changes occurring during assembly of this trimolecular **C5b67** complex:

- cause release from the convertase; and
- expose a labile hydrophobic site.

The complex can stably associate with a membrane through the labile hydrophobic site, though the process is inefficient and most of the C5b67 formed is inactivated in the fluid phase.

Membrane-bound C5b67 recruits **C8** from the plasma, and, finally, multiple copies of **C9** are incorporated in the complex to form the MAC.

The latter stages of assembly are accompanied by major conformational changes in the components with globular hydrophilic plasma proteins unfolding to reveal amphipathic regions that penetrate into and through the lipid bilayer.

The fully formed MAC creates a rigid pore in the membrane, the walls of which are formed from multiple copies of C9 (up to 12), arranged like barrel staves around a central cavity.

The MAC is clearly visible in electron microscopic images of complement lysed cells as doughnut-shaped protein-lined pores, first observed by Humphrey and Dourmashkin 40 years ago (see Fig. 4.10). The pore has an inner diameter approaching 10 nm:

- allowing the free flow of solutes and electrolytes across the cell membrane; and
- because of the high internal osmotic pressure, causing the cell to swell and sometimes burst.

Metabolically inert targets such as aged erythrocytes are readily lysed by even a small number of MAC lesions, whereas viable nucleated cells resist killing through a combination of ion pump activities and recovery processes that remove MAC lesions and plug membrane leaks.

Even in the absence of cell killing, MAC lesions may severely compromise cell function or cause cell activation.

Regulation of the membrane attack pathway reduces the risk of 'bystander' damage to adjacent cells

Although regulation in the activation pathways is the major way in which complement is controlled, there are further failsafe mechanisms to protect self cells from MAC damage and lysis.

The membrane attack pathway

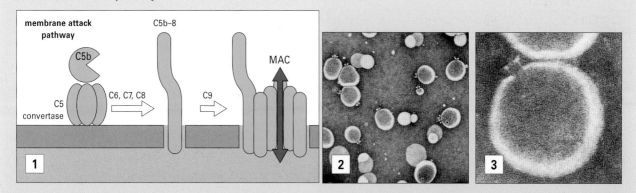

Fig. 4.10 (**1**) C5b, while still attached to the C5 convertase, binds C6 and C7 from the fluid phase. The trimolecular C5b–7 complex dissociates from the convertase and binds the target cell membrane. Binding of C8 and multiple copies of C9 generates a rigid protein-lined transmembrane channel, the membrane attack complex (MAC). (**2** and **3**) Electron micrographs of the MAC. The complex consists of a cylindrical pore in which the walls of the cylinder, formed by C9, traverse the cell membrane. In these micrographs the human C5b–9 complex has been incorporated into a lecithin liposomal membrane. × 234 000. *(Courtesy of Professor J Tranum-Jensen and Dr S Bhakdi.)*

First, the membrane binding site in C5b67 is labile. If the complex does not encounter a membrane within a fraction of a second after release from the convertase, the site is lost through:

- hydrolysis; or
- binding of one of the fluid-phase regulators of the terminal pathway – **S protein** (also termed **vitronectin**) or **clusterin** – both of which are multifunctional plasma proteins with diverse roles in homeostasis.

C8, an essential component of the MAC, also behaves as a regulator in that binding of C8 to C5b–7 in the fluid phase blocks the membrane binding site and prevents MAC formation.

The net effect of all these plasma controls is to limit MAC deposition to membranes in the immediate vicinity of the site of complement activation, so reducing risk of 'bystander' damage to adjacent cells.

CD59 protects host cells from complement-mediated damage

Complexes that do bind are further regulated on host cells by **CD59**, a membrane protein that locks into the MAC as it assembles and inhibits binding of C9, thereby preventing pore formation (Fig. 4.11). CD59 is a broadly expressed, glycolipid-anchored protein that is structurally unrelated to the complement regulators described above.

The importance of CD59 in protecting host cells from complement damage is well illustrated in the hemolytic disorder paroxysmal nocturnal hemoglobinuria (PNH), in which erythrocytes and other circulating cells are unable to make glycolipid anchors and as a consequence lack CD59 (and also DAF). The 'tickover' complement activation that occurs on all cells without much consequence is then sufficient in the absence of CD59 to cause low-grade hemolysis and hemolytic crises.

Role of CD59 in protecting host cells from complement damage

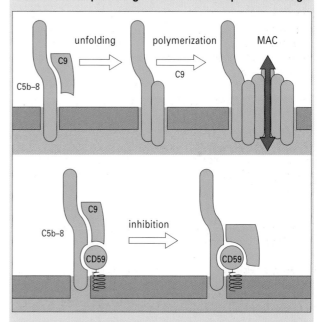

Fig. 4.11 The upper diagram models assembly of the MAC in the absence of the regulator CD59 – C9 binds C5b–8, unwinds, and traverses the membrane and recruits further C9 molecules, which in turn unfold and insert to form the MAC. In the lower diagram, CD59 binds the C5b–8 complex and prevents the unfolding and insertion of C9, which is essential for the initiation of MAC pore formation.

Membrane receptors for complement products

Receptors for fragments of C3 are widely distributed on different leukocyte populations

Many cells express one or more membrane receptors for complement products (Fig. 4.12). An understanding of the receptors is essential because the majority of the effects

Cell receptors for complement components and fragments

ligand	receptor	structure	function	location
C1q	cC1qR (C1q receptor enhancing phagocytosis)	acidic 100-kDa transmembrane glycoprotein	binds collagenous tail of C1q, enhances phagocytosis	myeloid cells, endothelia, platelets
	C1qRp (receptor for C1q globular heads)	acidic 33-kDa glycoprotein	binds globular heads of C1q, possible role in phagocytosis	all blood cells
C3, C4, and C5 fragments	CR1 (complement receptor 1 – CD35)	SCR-containing transmembrane glycoprotein, 30 SCRs	binds C3b and C4b, cofactor and decay accelerating activities, roles in immune complex handling	erythrocytes, B cells, FDCs, macrophages
	CR2 (complement receptor 2 – CD21)	SCR-containing transmembrane glycoprotein, 15 or 16 SCRs	binds C3d and iC3b, role in regulating B cell response to antigen	B cells, FDCs, some T cells, basophils, epithelia
	CR3 (complement receptor 3 – CD11b/CD18)	integrin family member, heterodimer	binds iC3b, roles in cell adhesion	myeloid cells, some B cells and NK cells
	CR4 (complement receptor 4 – CD11c/CD18)	integrin family member, heterodimer	binds iC3b, roles in cell adhesion	myeloid cells, FDCs, activated B cells
	C3aR (receptor for the C3a anaphylatoxin)	G protein-coupled 7-transmembrane spanning receptor	binds C3a, mediates cell activation	widely distributed on blood and tissue cells
	C5aR (receptor for the C5a anaphylatoxin – CD88).	G protein-coupled 7-transmembrane spanning receptor	binds C5a, mediates cell activation and chemotaxis	myeloid cells, smooth muscle, endothelia, epithelia
	C5L2	G-protein uncoupled 7-transmembrane	binds C3a, C3a-desArg, C5a, roles uncertain	leukocytes, adipose tissue

Fig. 4.12 Summary of information on the cell surface receptors for complement components and fragments and their biological roles. (FDC, follicular dendritic cell.)

of complement are mediated through these molecules. The best characterized of the complement receptors are those binding fragments of C3.

CR1, CR2, CR3, and CR4 bind fragments of C3 attached to activating surfaces

Four different receptors, termed complement receptors 1, 2, 3, and 4 (CR1, CR2, CR3, and CR4), bind fragments of C3 attached to activating surfaces:

- **CR1**, expressed on erythrocytes and leukocytes, binds the largest fragment C3b (and also C4b), an interaction that is crucial to the processing of immune complexes (see below);
- **CR2**, expressed mainly on B cells and follicular dendritic cells (FDCs), binds fragments derived from fI-mediated proteolysis of C3b – iC3b and C3d.

These interactions aid the B cell response to complement-coated particles.

Both CR1 and CR2 are structurally related to the C3 convertase regulators fH, C4bp, MCP, and DAF, and are encoded in the RCA (Regulators of Complement Activation) cluster on chromosome 1.

CR3 and **CR4**:

- belong to the integrin family of cell adhesion molecules;
- are expressed on the majority of leukocytes;
- bind the iC3b fragment, aiding adhesion of leukocytes to complement-coated particles and facilitating phagocytic ingestion of these particles.

Receptors for C3a and C5a mediate inflammation

C3a, the small fragment released during activation of C3, binds to a receptor (**C3aR**) expressed abundantly on eosinophils and basophils, and at much lower levels on neutrophils and many other cell types.

The C5a fragment released from C5 during activation is closely related to C3a and binds a distinct, but structurally related, receptor, the C5a receptor (**C5aR**), which is present on a wide variety of cell types, including all leukocytes.

The receptors for C3a and C5a are members of the large receptor family of seven-transmembrane segment receptors that associate with heterotrimeric G proteins. Receptors for chemokines belong to this same family and in many ways C3a and C5a behave like chemokines.

Together, C3aR and C5aR are important in orchestrating inflammatory responses and modulating antigen presentation and T cell activation (see below).

A third receptor, termed C5L2, expressed by leukocytes and in adipose tissue, has binding activity for C3a, its inactivation product C3a-desArg (see below) and C5a; however, this receptor is uncoupled from G proteins and its functional roles are currently the subject of active debate.

Receptors for C1q are present on phagocytes, mast cells, and platelets

Receptors for C1q are less well characterized than C3 receptors, but are increasingly recognized as important in homeostasis.

Receptors for the collagen tails (**cC1qR**):

- can recognize C1q attached through its globular head regions to complement-coated particles;
- are present on leukocytes, platelets, and some other cell types; and
- likely play roles in enhancing phagocytosis of C1q-labeled particles.

Receptors for the globular heads (**C1qRp**):

- bind C1q in an orientation that mimics antibody binding;
- are expressed principally on phagocytic cells, mast cells, and platelets; and
- may collaborate with cC1qR to mediate cell activation events.

The bulk of C1q in the circulation is, however, already complexed with C1r and C1s to form intact C1, and in this complex C1q does not interact with its receptors. This ensures that C1q receptors are activated only in specific circumstances, such as during complement activation when free C1q is available.

The plasma complement regulator fH binds cell surfaces

The plasma complement regulator fH binds host cell membranes via several heparin (or sugar) binding sites in the molecule. Surface-bound fH plays important roles in protecting self cells from complement attack. Indeed, a rare but fascinating disease, atypical hemolytic uremic syndrome (aHUS), which is typified by hemolysis, platelet destruction, and renal damage that may progress to renal failure, is caused in many cases by mutations in the C-terminus of fH that ablate a key heparin binding site causing loss of the surface binding capacity of fH. Uncontrolled complement activation due to the inability of the mutant fH lacking the membrane binding site to bind cells has been demonstrated in patients. Other patients with aHUS have mutations in complement components C3 or fB, or the membrane regulator MCP, demonstrating that this is a disease of alternative pathway dysregulation.

Some cells also bind fH through cell surface receptors – for example, CR3 on polymorphs binds fH and may contribute to polymorph pathogen recognition.

Many bacteria and other pathogens express specific receptors for fH, enabling them to hijack fH to protect themselves from complement attack in the plasma.

Complement functions

The principal functions of complement are:

- chemotaxis;
- opsonization and cell activation;
- lysis of target cells; and
- priming of the adaptive immune response.

C5a is chemotactic for macrophages and polymorphs

Polymorphs and macrophages express receptors for C3a and C5a. These small (~10 kDa) fragments (i.e. C3a and C5a) diffuse away from the site of activation, creating a chemical gradient along which the motile cells migrate to congregate at the site of activation (Fig. 4.13).

Binding of C3a and C5a to their receptors also causes cell activation:

- increasing adhesive properties;
- triggering extravasation; and
- priming phagocytes to release proinflammatory molecules including enzymes, vasoactive amines, reactive oxygen intermediates, and inflammatory cytokines.

C3a and C5a also enhance adhesion molecule expression on phagocytes, increasing cell stickiness, and may cause increased expression of the C3 fragment receptors CR1 and CR3.

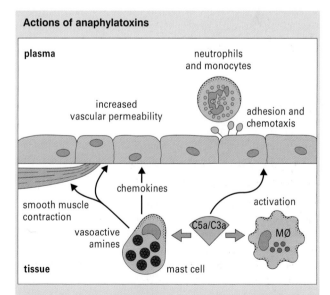

Actions of anaphylatoxins

Fig. 4.13 C5a and C3a both act on mast cells to cause degranulation and release of vasoactive amines, including histamine and 5-hydroxytryptamine, which enhance vascular permeability and local blood flow. The secondary release of chemokines from mast cells causes cellular accumulation, and C5a itself acts directly on receptors on monocytes and neutrophils to induce their migration to sites of acute inflammation and subsequent activation.

C3a and C5a activate mast cells and basophils

Tissue mast cells and basophils also express C3aR and C5aR, and binding of ligand triggers massive release of:

- histamine; and
- cytokines (see Fig. 4.13).

Together, these products cause local smooth muscle contraction and increased vascular permeability to generate the swelling, heat, and pain that typify the inflammatory response. These effects mirror on a local scale the more generalized and severe reactions that can occur in severe allergic or anaphylactic reactions, and for this reason C3a and C5a are sometimes referred to as **anaphylatoxins**.

The actions of C3a and C5a are limited temporally and spatially by the activity of a plasma enzyme, carboxypeptidase-N, which cleaves the carboxy terminal amino acid, arginine, from both of these fragments. The products, termed C3a-desArg and C5a-desArg (-desArg = without arginine), respectively, have either much reduced (C5a-desArg) or absent (C3a-desArg) anaphylatoxin activities.

The retention in C5a-desArg of some chemotactic activity enables the recruitment of phagocytes even from distant sites, making C5a and its metabolite the most important complement-derived chemotactic factor.

An important role for C3a-desArg in lipid handling has emerged. A mediator of increased lipid uptake and fat synthesis in adipose tissue, acylation stimulating protein (ASP), was shown to be identical to C3a-desArg, linking complement activation to lipid turnover. Of note, adipose tissue is the primary site for fD synthesis and also produces C3; a complete alternative pathway can thus be assembled locally to generate C3a-desArg/ASP.

C3b and iC3b are important opsonins

Complement activation and amplification cause complement fragments to efficiently coat activator surfaces of targets such as bacteria or immune complexes, enhancing their recognition by phagocytes (Fig. 4.14). Phagocytes and other cells carrying receptors for these complement fragments are then able to bind the target, triggering ingestion and cell activation. The key players here are the surface-bound fragments of C3 and the family of C3 fragment receptors described above.

The amplification inherent in the system ensures that bacteria and other activating surfaces rapidly become coated with C3b and its breakdown product **iC3b**, which enhances phagocytosis.

Phagocytes lured by the complement-derived chemotactic factors described above and activated to increase expression of CR1 and CR3 (receptors for C3b and iC3b, respectively) will bind the activating particle and engulf it for destruction in the phagosome system.

Opsonization, binding, and phagocytosis

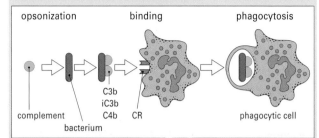

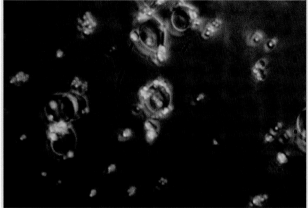

Fig. 4.14 A bacterium is sensitized by the covalent binding of C3b, iC3b, and C4b, which allow it to be recognized by complement receptors (CR) on neutrophils and mononuclear phagocytes. This promotes phagocytosis and activation of the phagocyte. In primates, erythrocytes also express CR1, which allows them to bind opsonized bacteria and immune complexes. In the lower panel fluoresceinated bacteria that have been opsonized with antibody and complement are seen adhering to human erythrocytes. *(Courtesy of Professor GD Ross.)*

The importance of complement opsonization for defense against pathogens is illustrated in individuals deficient in complement components. C3 deficiency in particular is always associated with repeated severe bacterial infections that without adequate prophylaxis inevitably lead to early death.

C3b disaggregates immune complexes and promotes their clearance

Immune complexes containing antigens derived either from pathogens or from the death of host cells form continuously in health and disease. Because they tend to grow by aggregation and acquisition of more components, they can cause disease by precipitating in capillary beds in the skin, kidney, and other organs, where they drive inflammation.

Complement activation on the immune complex via the classical pathway efficiently opsonizes the immune complex and helps prevent precipitation in tissues:

- first, coating with C3b masks the foreign antigens in the core of the immune complex, blocking further growth;

- second, coating with C3b disaggregates large immune complexes by disrupting interactions between antigen and antibody;
- third, C3b (and C4b) on immune complexes interacts with CR1 on erythrocytes, taking the immune complex out of the plasma – the **immune adherence phenomenon**.

Immune complex adherence to erythrocytes provides an efficient means of handling and transporting the hazardous cargo to sites of disposal (i.e. the resident macrophages in spleen and liver). Here the immune complex is:

- released from the erythrocyte; and
- captured by complement and immunoglobulin receptors on the macrophage, internalized, and destroyed.

The MAC damages some bacteria and enveloped viruses

Assembly of the MAC creates a pore that inserts into and through the lipid bilayer, breaching the membrane barrier (see Fig. 4.10). The consequences of MAC attack vary from target to target:

- for most pathogens, opsonization is the most important antibacterial action of complement;
- for Gram-negative bacteria, particularly organisms of the genus *Neisseria*, MAC attack is a major component of host defense, and individuals deficient in components of the MAC (e.g. patients with C6 deficiency, which is the second most common deficiency of complement) are susceptible to neisserial infection.

Gram-negative bacteria are protected by a double cell membrane separated by a peptidoglycan wall. Precisely how MAC traverses these protective structures to damage the inner bacterial membrane and causes osmotic lysis of these organisms remains unclear. The MAC:

- may also play roles in the efficient dispatching of other pathogens, including some viruses;
- can also damage or destroy host cells – in some instances, such as autoimmunity, the host cell is itself the target and complement is directly activated on the cell, leading to MAC attack.

> **Q. What term is applied to the deposition of MACs on cells near to but not directly the cause of complement activation, and what mechanism normally limits this process?**
>
> A. This event is called bystander lysis and is normally limited by the presence of CD59 and fluid phase regulators, and the inefficiency of C5b6 deposition.

Erythrocytes have only a limited capacity to resist and repair damage and can be lysed, as is seen in autoimmune hemolytic anemias and some other hemolytic disorders. Although nucleated host cells may escape lysis by MAC, the insertion of pores in the membrane is not without consequence. Ions, particularly Ca^{2+}, flow into the cell and cause activation events with diverse outcomes that may contribute to disease.

Immune complexes with bound C3b are very efficient in priming B cells

Complement is a key component of the innate immune response. However, it has recently become apparent that complement also plays important roles in adaptive immunity. This realization arose from studies in complement-depleted and complement-deficient mice in which antibody responses to foreign particles were markedly reduced. At least three linked mechanisms contribute to this effect (Fig. 4.15):

- first, immature B cells directly bind foreign particles through the B cell receptor (BCR) recognizing specific

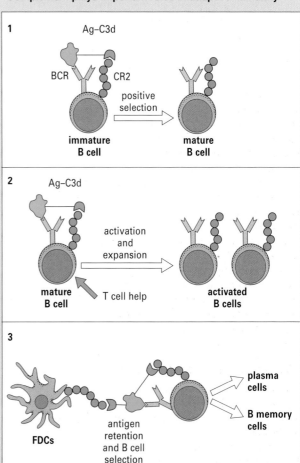

Complement plays important roles in adaptive immunity

Fig. 4.15 C3 fragments bound to antigen (Ag) bind complement receptors on B cells and follicular dendritic cells (FDCs), enhancing B cell development at multiple stages in the process. (**1**) B cells bind Ag through the B cell receptor (BCR) and bind Ag-attached C3d through CR2. The combined signals, delivered through these receptors and their co-receptors, markedly enhance positive selection of Ag-reactive B cells and subsequent maturation. (**2**) Binding of C3d-opsonized Ag to mature B cells in the lymphoid follicles (with appropriate T cell help) triggers B cell activation and proliferation. (**3**) In the spleen and bone marrow, C3d-opsonized Ag binds complement receptors on FDCs to retain Ag on the FDC, where it is efficiently presented to activated B cells. Ligation of BCR and C3d on the activated B cell triggers differentiation to plasma cells and B memory cells.

antigen in the particle, and through CR2 recognizing attached C3d – this co-ligation triggers B cell maturation, with the mature cells migrating to the lymphoid organs;

- second, while in the lymph nodes, mature B cells encounter opsonized antigen and, in the presence of B cell help, are induced to become activated and to proliferate;
- finally, in the lymphoid organs FDCs capture antigen through attached C3 fragments and use this bait to select the correct activated B cells and switch them on to further maturation and proliferation to form plasma cells and B memory cells (see Chapters 9 and 11).

The overriding principle of this 'adjuvant' effect of C3 opsonization is that simultaneous engagement of CR2 and BCR on the B cell, by recruiting signaling molecules to form an activation complex on the B cell surface, efficiently triggers the B cell response. As a consequence, complement-opsonized particles may be 1000-fold as active as the unopsonized particle in triggering antibody production.

More recently, roles for both C3a and C5a as modifiers of antigen presentation by FDC and other DCs have emerged; the physiological relevance of these interactions is not yet clear.

Complement deficiencies

Genetic deficiencies of each of the complement components and many of the regulators have been described and provide valuable 'experiments of nature' illustrating the homeostatic roles of complement. In general, complement deficiencies are rare, though some deficiencies are much more common in some racial groups.

A variety of assays (Method box 4.1) are available for detecting:

- the activity of different complement pathways;
- the functional activity of individual components;
- the total amount of individual components (functional or non-functional).

The consequences of a deficiency in part of the complement system depend upon the pathway(s) affected (Fig. 4.16).

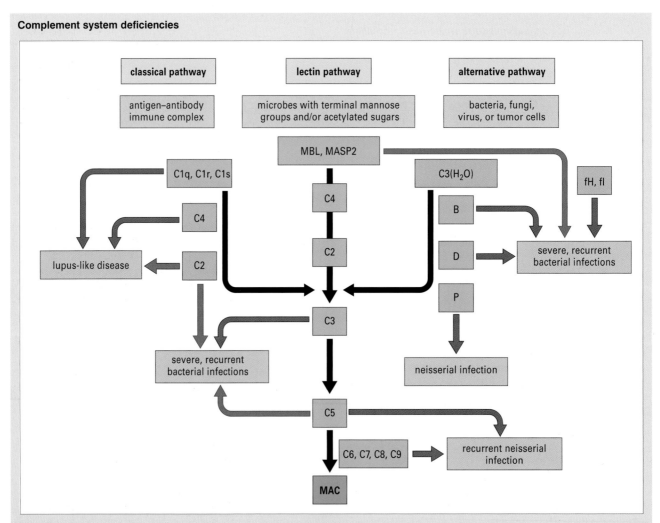

Fig. 4.16 A summary of the clinical consequences of the various complement deficiencies. Black arrows denote pathway, red arrows show strong effects, and blue arrows indicate weak effects.

Classical pathway deficiencies result in tissue inflammation

Deficiency of any of the components of the classical pathway (C1, C4, and C2) predisposes to a condition that closely resembles the autoimmune disease systemic lupus erythematosus (SLE), in which immune complexes become deposited in capillary networks, particularly in kidney, skin, and brain.

Deficiency of any of the C1 subunits (C1q, C1r, or C1s) invariably causes severe disease with typical SLE features including skin lesions and kidney damage. The disease usually manifests early in childhood and few patients reach adulthood.

C4 deficiency also causes severe SLE. Total deficiency of C4 is extremely rare because C4 is encoded by two separate genes (*C4A* and *C4B*), but partial deficiencies of C4 are relatively common and are associated with an increased incidence of SLE.

C2 deficiency is the commonest complement deficiency in Caucasians. Although it predisposes to SLE, the majority of C2-deficient individuals are healthy.

The large majority of cases of SLE are, however, not associated with complement deficiencies, and autoimmune SLE is discussed in Chapter 20. The historical view of immune complex disease in classical pathway deficiency was based upon defective immune complex handling.

Q. Why would a deficiency in the classical pathway lead to impaired handling of immune complexes?
A. Classical pathway activation and opsonization of immune complexes helps prevent precipitation in tissues and aids the carriage of immune complexes on erythrocytes. Classical pathway deficiencies would therefore result in a failure to maintain solubilization and permit the resultant precipitation of immune complexes in the tissues where they drive inflammation.

Although these mechanisms of immune complex handling undoubtedly contribute, a new perspective has recently developed that takes a different view of the role of complement in waste management.

Cells continually die by apoptosis in tissues and are removed silently by tissue macrophages. Complement contributes to this essential process because the apoptotic cell binds C1q and activates the classical pathway. In C1 deficiencies, apoptotic cells accumulate in the tissues and eventually undergo necrosis, which releases toxic cell contents and causes inflammation.

This recent observation, emerging from studies in complement deficiencies, has altered the way we think of the handling of waste in the body and moved complement to center-stage in this vital housekeeping role.

Deficiencies of MBL are associated with infection in infants

MBL is a complex multi-chain **collectin**. Each chain comprises a collagenous stalk linked to a globular carbohydrate recognition domain.

The plasma level of MBL is extremely variable in the population, and governed by a series of single nucleotide polymorphisms in the *MBL* gene, either in the promoter region or in the first exon, encoding part of the collagenous stalk:

- mutations in the promoter region alter the efficiency of gene transcription;
- mutations in the first exon disrupt the regular structure of the collagenous stalk, destabilizing complexes containing mutated chains, perhaps disrupting association with the MASP enzymes.

At least seven distinct haplotypes arise from mixing of these mutations, four of which yield very low plasma MBL levels. As a consequence, at least 10% of the population have MBL levels below 0.1 μg/mL and are considered to be MBL deficient.

MBL deficiency is associated in infants with increased susceptibility to bacterial infections. This tendency disappears as the individual ages and the other arms of immunity mature.

In adults, MBL deficiency is of little consequence unless there is an accompanying immunosuppression – for example, people with HIV infection who are MBL deficient appear to have more infections than those who have high levels of MBL.

Alternative pathway and C3 deficiencies are associated with bacterial infections

Deficiencies of either fB or fD prevent complement amplification through the alternative pathway amplification loop, markedly reducing the efficiency of opsonization of pathogens. As a consequence, deficient individuals are susceptible to bacterial infections and present with a history of severe recurrent infections with a variety of pyogenic (pus-forming) bacteria. Only a few families with each of these deficiencies have been identified, but the severity of the condition makes it imperative to identify affected families so that prophylactic antibiotic therapy can be initiated.

C3 is the cornerstone of complement, essential for all activation pathways and for MAC assembly, and is also the source of the major opsonic fragments C3b and iC3b. Individuals with **C3 deficiency** present early in childhood with a history of severe, recurrent bacterial infections affecting the respiratory system, gut, skin, and other organs. Untreated, all die before adulthood. When given broad-spectrum antibiotic prophylaxis, patients do reasonably well and survival into adulthood becomes the norm.

Total deficiency of the alternative pathway regulator, fH, results in dysregulation of the alternative pathway in the kidney and causes dense deposit disease (DDD), leading to renal failure.

Terminal pathway deficiencies predispose to Gram-negative bacterial infections

Deficiencies of any of the terminal complement components (C5, C6, C7, C8, or C9) predisposes to infections with Gram-negative bacteria, particularly those of the genus Neisseria. This genus includes the meningococci responsible for meningococcal meningitis and the gonococci responsible for gonorrhea.

Q. Why should these deficiencies be specifically associated with infection by Gram-negative bacteria and not with all bacterial infections?

A. Gram-negative bacteria have an outer phospholipid membrane, which may be targeted by the lytic pathway. Gram-positive bacteria have a thick bacterial cell wall on the outside.

Individuals with terminal pathway deficiencies usually present with meningitis, which is often recurrent and often accompanied by septicemia. Any patients with second or third episodes of meningococcal infection without obvious physical cause should be screened for complement deficiencies because prophylactic antibiotic therapy can be life-saving. Terminal pathway-deficient patients should also be intensively immunized with the best available meningococcal vaccines.

It is likely that terminal pathway deficiencies are relatively common and underascertained in most countries:

- in Caucasians and most other groups investigated, C6 deficiency is the most common;
- in the Japanese population, C9 deficiency is very common, with an incidence of more than 1 in 500 of the population.

C1 inhibitor deficiency causes hereditary angioedema

Deficiency of the classical pathway regulator C1inh is responsible for the syndrome **hereditary angioedema (HAE)**. C1inh regulates C1 in the classical pathway and MBL/MASP-2 (or ficolin-MASP-2) in the lectin pathway and also controls activation in the kinin pathway that leads to the generation of bradykinin and other active kinins. The condition and the underlying pathways are outlined in Chapter 16 (see Figs 16.14 & 16.15) and additional detail is given below.

Deficiencies in alternative pathway regulators cause a secondary loss of C3

fH or fI deficiency predisposes to bacterial infections

fH and fI collaborate to control activation of the alternative pathway amplification loop. Deficiency of either leads to uncontrolled activation of the loop and complete consumption of C3, which is the substrate of the loop. The resultant **acquired C3 deficiency** predisposes to bacterial infections and yields a clinical picture identical to that seen in primary C3 deficiency.

Properdin deficiency causes severe meningococcal meningitis

Properdin is a stabilizer of the alternative pathway C3 convertase that increases efficiency of the amplification loop. **Properdin deficiency** is inherited in an X-linked manner and is therefore seen exclusively in males. Boys deficient in properdin present with severe meningococcal meningitis, often with septicemia. The first attack is often fatal and survivors do not usually have recurrent infections because the acquisition of anti-meningococcal antibody enables a response via the classical pathway in the next encounter. Diagnosis is nevertheless important to identify affected relatives before they get disease – administration of meningococcal vaccine and antibiotic prophylaxis will prevent infection.

Autoantibodies against complement components, regulators and complexes also cause disease

The association of anti-C1inh autoantibodies with some cases of HAE was mentioned above. Autoantibodies against fH are frequently found in children (and less commonly in adults) with glomerulonephritis, likely causing disease by blocking fH activity. Autoantibodies against the C3 convertase enzyme, termed nephritic factors, are also found in rare patients with renal disease (a condition termed 'dense deposit disease' or DDD); these antibodies stabilize the convertase, increasing its lifetime and thereby causing complement dysregulation and disease.

Complement polymorphisms and disease

Common polymorphisms are found in almost all complement proteins and regulators; associations with inflammatory and infectious diseases have been reported, particularly with respect to alternative pathway proteins and regulators. Most strikingly, a common polymorphism in fH (fH_{Y402H}) is strongly associated with the common, blinding eye disease, age-related macular degeneration (AMD), homozygosity for the H allele increasing risk of disease up to 7-fold. Polymorphisms in C3 and fB are also linked to AMD, suggesting that dysregulation of the alternative pathway underlies the pathology in this disease.

CRITICAL THINKING: COMPLEMENT DEFICIENCY (SEE P. 434 FOR EXPLANATIONS)

A family has been identified in which three of the seven children have had repeated upper respiratory tract infections since early childhood. Of these, one has developed bacterial meningitis, and another a fatal septicemia. In all of the children the levels of antibodies in the serum are within the normal range. When an assay for hemolytic complement (CH50) is carried out, however, the three affected children are all found to be deficient in this functional assay.

1 Why would a deficiency in complement cause the children to be particularly susceptible to bacterial infections? Measurements are made of individual complement components of the classical and alternative pathways to determine which of the components is defective. The results are shown in the table.

Complement component	Normal concentration (μg/mL)	Levels in affected children (μg/mL)
C4	600	480–520
C2	20	15–22
C3	1300	10–80
factor B (fB)	210	not detectable
factor H (fH)	480	200–350
factor I (fI)	35	not detectable

2 Using knowledge of the complement reaction pathways, how can you explain the apparent combined deficiencies in C3, fB, and fI?

3 What is the fundamental deficiency in this family and how would you treat the affected children?

Further reading

Barrington R, Zhang M, Fischer M, Carroll MC. The role of complement in inflammation and adaptive immunity. Immunol Rev 2001;180:5–15.

Botto M, Kirschfink M, Macor P, et al. Complement in human diseases: lessons from complement deficiencies. Mol Immunol 2009;46:2774–2783.

Cole DS, Morgan BP. Beyond lysis: how complement influences cell fate. Clin Sci 2003;104:455–466.

Colten HR, Rosen FS. Complement deficiencies. Annu Rev Immunol 1992;10:809–834.

Davis AE 3rd. The pathogenesis of hereditary angioedema. Transfus Apher Sci 2003;39:195–203.

De Cordoba SR, de Jorge EJ. Genetics and disease associations of complement factor H. Clin Exp Immunol 2008;151:1–13.

Dodds AW, Ren XD, Willis AC, et al. The reaction mechanism of the internal thioester in the human complement component C4. Nature 1996;379:177–179.

Frank MM, Fries LF. The role of complement in inflammation and phagocytosis. Immunol Today 1991;12:322–326.

Gerard C, Gerard NP. C5a anaphylatoxin and its seven transmembrane-segment receptor. Annu Rev Immunol 1994;12:775–808.

Holmskov U, Malhotra R, Sim RB, et al. Collectins: collagenous C-type lectins of the innate immune defense system. Immunol Today 1994;14:67–74.

Hourcade D, Holers VM, Atkinson JP. The regulators of complement activation (RCA) gene cluster. Adv Immunol 1989;45:381–416.

Jack DL, Klein NJ, Turner MW. Mannose-binding lectin: targeting the microbial world for complement attack and opsonophagocytosis. Immunol Rev 2001;180:86–99.

Kavanagh D, Richards J, Atkinson J. Complement regulatory genes and hemolytic uremic syndromes. Annu Rev Med 2008;59:293–309.

Kemper C, Atkinson JP. T cell regulation: with complements from innate immunity. Nat Rev Immunol 2007;7:9–18.

Lambris JD, Reid KBM, Volanakis JE. The evolution, structure, biology and pathophysiology of complement. Immunol Today 1999;20:207–211.

Lambris JD, Ricklin D, Geisbrecht BV. Complement evasion by human pathogens. Nat Rev Microbiol 2008;6:132–142.

Liszewski MK, Farries TC, Lublin DM, et al. Control of the complement system. Adv Immunol 1996;61:201–283.

Manderson AP, Botto M, Walport MJ. The role of complement in the development of systemic lupus erythematosus. Annu Rev Immunol 2004;22:432–456.

Moffitt MC, Frank MM. Complement resistance in microbes. Springer Semin Immunopathol 1994;15:327–344.

Morgan BP. Complement regulatory molecules: application to therapy and transplantation. Immunol Today 1995;16:257–259.

Morgan BP. Complement in inflammation. In Rey K, ed. Physiology of inflammation, Oxford: Oxford University Press; 2001: 131–145.

Morgan BP. Hereditary angioedema: therapies old and new. N Engl J Med 2010;363:581–583.

Morgan BP, Harris CL. Complement therapeutics; history and current progress. Mol Immunol 2003;40:159–170.

Morgan BP, Meri S. Membrane proteins that protect against complement lysis. Springer Semin Immunopathol 1994;15:369–396.

Morgan BP, Walport MJ. Complement deficiency and disease. Immunol Today 1991;12:301–306.

Muller-Eberhard HJ. The membrane attack complex of complement. Annu Rev Immunol 1986;4:503–528.

Nonaka M, Yoshizaki F. Evolution of the complement system. Mol Immunol 2004;40:879–902.

Norris M, Remuzzi G. Atypical hemolytic-uremic syndrome. N Engl J Med 2009;361:1676–1687.

Ricklin D, Hajishengallis G, Yang J, Lambris JD. Complement: a key system for immunosurveillance and homeostasis. Nat Immunol 2010;11:785–797.

Walport MJ. Complement: first of two parts. N Engl J Med 2001;344:1058–1066.

Walport MJ. Complement: second of two parts. N Engl J Med 2001;344:1140–1144.

Zipfel PF, Skerka C. Complement regulators and inhibitory proteins. Nat Rev Immunol 2009;9:729–740.

CHAPTER 5

T Cell Receptors and MHC Molecules

SUMMARY

- **The T cell antigen receptor (TCR) is located on the surface of T cells and plays a critical role in the adaptive immune system.** Its major function is to recognize antigen and transmit a signal to the interior of the T cell, which generally results in activation of T cell responses.

- **TCRs are similar in many ways to immunoglobulin molecules.** Both are made up of pairs of subunits (α and β or γ and δ), which are themselves members of the immunoglobulin superfamily, and both recognize a wide variety of antigens via N terminal variable regions. These antigen recognition subunits are associated with the invariant chains of the T cell receptor, the CD3 complex, which perform critical signaling functions.

- **The two types of TCR may have distinct functions.** In humans and mice, the $\alpha\beta$ TCR predominates in most peripheral lymphoid tissues, whereas cells bearing the $\gamma\delta$ TCR are enriched at mucosal surfaces.

- **Like immunoglobulins, TCRs are encoded by several sets of genes,** and a large repertoire of TCR antigen-binding sites is generated by V(D)J recombination during T cell differentiation. Unlike immunoglobulins, TCRs are never secreted and do not undergo class switching or somatic hypermutation.

- **Antigen recognition by the $\alpha\beta$ TCR requires the antigen to be bound to a specialized antigen-presenting structure known as a major histocompatibility complex (MHC) molecule.** Unlike immunoglobulins, TCRs recognize antigen only in the context of a cell–cell interaction.

- **Class I and class II MHC molecules bind to peptides derived from different sources.** Class I MHC molecules bind to peptides derived from cytosolic (intracellular) proteins, known as **endogenous antigens.** Class II MHC molecules bind to peptides derived from extracellular proteins that have been brought into the cell by phagocytosis or endocytosis **(exogenous antigens).**

- **Class I and class II MHC present peptide antigens to the TCR in a cell–cell interaction** between an antigen-presenting cell (APC) and a T cell.

- **In humans the gene loci HLA-A, HLA-B, and HLA-C gene loci encode class I MHC molecules.**

- **HLA-DP, HLA-DQ, and HLA-DR gene loci encode class II MHC molecules.**

- **An individual's MHC haplotype affects susceptibility to disease.**

- **CD1 is an MHC class I-like molecule that presents lipid antigens.**

T cell receptors

As discussed in Chapter 1, the immune system of higher vertebrates can be divided into two components – humoral immunity and cell-mediated immunity.

Humoral immunity, of which antibodies are a key component, provides protection via the extracellular fluids. Antibodies deal quite effectively with extracellular pathogens:

- targeting them for phagocytosis or complement-mediated lysis;
- neutralizing receptors on the surface of bacteria and viruses; and
- inactivating circulating toxins.

If antibodies were our only defense, however, pathogens could escape immune surveillance simply by hiding within cells. In fact, many pathogens – all viruses, some bacteria, and certain parasites – do just that, carrying out substantial portions of their life cycles within host cells. Remarkably, some bacteria even thrive within macrophages after being phagocytosed. These considerations highlight the need for a second arm of the immune response – **cell-mediated immunity** – of which T cells are critical operatives.

T cells recognize antigen via specialized cell surface antigen receptors – T cell receptors (TCRs) – which are structurally and evolutionarily related to antibodies.

TCRs recognize antigen via variable regions generated through **V(D)J recombination** (see Chapter 3), much like immunoglobulins, but are much more restricted in their antigen recognition capabilities.

TCRs recognize peptides displayed by MHC molecules

T cells generally recognize fragments of degraded proteins (peptides), which must be bound to ('presented by') specialized antigen-presenting molecules encoded by the **major histocompatibility complex (MHC)**. In humans the MHC was first identified as the **human leukocyte antigen (HLA)** locus so the molecules may also be called HLA molecules.

MHC molecules can display a wide range of peptides, which have been derived from intracellular proteins, on the cell surface thereby alerting the immune system to the presence of intracellular invaders.

Because MHC molecules are expressed only on the cell surface, engagement of the TCR occurs only in the context of intimate cell–cell interactions.

When a primed T cell bearing an appropriate TCR (capable of recognizing, for example, a particular viral peptide) comes into contact with an infected cell, it can rapidly kill that cell and thereby limit the spread of the viral infection.

The requirement for cell–cell interaction also allows T cells to provide critical regulatory functions. T cells, for example, can couple signals from the innate immune system, such as those arising from 'professional' APCs (e.g. dendritic cells) with adaptive (T and B cell) responses, providing a critical layer of integration, coordination, and regulation.

TCRs are similar to immunoglobulin molecules

The TCR was identified much later than immunoglobulin, even though early theoretical considerations strongly suggested that T cells must bear cell surface antigen receptors. It is now clear that there are two varieties of TCR, termed αβ and γδ, and that both molecules:

- resemble immunoglobulins in several significant ways (Fig. 5.1);
- are made up of heterodimers (either α and β or γ and δ subunits), which are disulfide-linked;
- are integral membrane proteins with large extracellular domains and short cytoplasmic tails. The extracellular

portions are responsible for antigen recognition and contain variable N terminal regions, like antibodies. Both α and β (or γ and δ) subunits contribute to the antigen-binding sites.

The two types of TCR tend to populate different tissue sites and are thought to perform distinct functions.

The αβ heterodimer is the antigen recognition unit of the αβ TCR

The αβ TCR is the predominant receptor found in the thymus and peripheral lymphoid organs of mice and humans. It is a disulfide-linked heterodimer of α (40–50 kDa) and β (35–47 kDa) subunits and its structural features have been determined by X-ray crystallography (Fig. 5.2).

Each polypeptide chain of the αβ TCR contains two extracellular immunoglobulin-like domains of approximately 110 amino acids, anchored into the plasma membrane by a transmembrane domain that has a very short cytoplasmic tail.

Q. How can receptors that lack intracytoplasmic domains signal to the cell? Give some examples.
A. They signal by associating with other membrane molecules that do have intracytoplasmic domains. For example, immunoglobulin associates with Igα and Igβ (see Fig. 3.1), and FcγRI associates with its γ chain dimer (see Fig. 3.17).

The extracellular portions of the α and β chains fold into a structure that resembles the antigen-binding portion (Fab) of an antibody (see Fig. 3.9). Indeed, as in antibodies, the amino acid sequence variability of the TCR resides in the N terminal domains of the α and β (and also the γ and δ) chains.

The regions of greatest variability correspond to immunoglobulin hypervariable regions and are also known as **complementarity determining regions (CDRs)**. They are clustered together to form an antigen-binding site analogous to the corresponding site on antibodies (see Fig. 5.2). Note, however, that:

- the CDR3 loops (which are the most highly variable regions of the TCR, as they are generated by V(D)J recombination) from both the α and β chains lie at the center of the antigen-binding site, and make extensive contacts with antigen.

Similarities and differences between T cell receptors and immunoglobulins

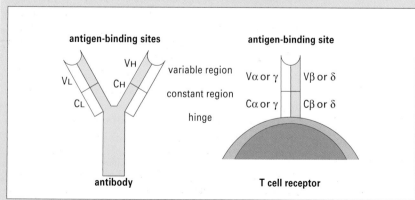

Fig. 5.1 TCRs are very similar to Fab fragments of B cell receptors. Both receptor types are composed of two different peptide chains and have variable regions for binding antigen, constant regions, and hinge regions. The principal differences are that TCRs remain membrane-bound and contain only a single antigen-binding site.

The T cell antigen receptor

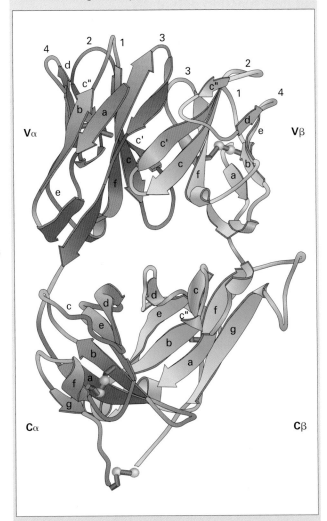

Fig. 5.2 Three-dimensional structure of an αβ TCR – only extracellular domains are shown. The α chain is colored blue (residues 1–213), and the β chain is colored green (residues 3–247). The β strands are represented as arrows and labeled according to the standard convention used for the immunoglobulin fold. The disulfide bonds (yellow balls for sulfur atoms) are shown within each domain and for the C terminal interchain disulfide. The complementarity determining regions (CDRs) lying at the top of the diagram are numerically labeled (1–4) for each chain. These form the binding site for antigen/MHC molecule.
(Adapted from Garcia KC, Degano M, Stanfield RL, et al. Science 1996;274:209–219. Copyright AAAS.)

The disulfide bond that links the α and β chains is in a peptide sequence located between the constant domain of the extracellular portion of the receptor and the transmembrane domain (shown as the C terminal residue in the α and β chain in Fig. 5.2).

One remarkable feature of the transmembrane portion of the receptor is the presence of positively charged residues in both the α and β chains. Unpaired charges would be unfavorable in a transmembrane segment. Indeed, these positive charges are neutralized by assembly of the complete TCR complex, which contains additional polypeptides bearing complementary negative charges (see below).

The CD3 complex associates with the antigen-binding αβ or γδ heterodimers to form the complete TCR

The αβ or γδ heterodimers must associate with a series of polypeptide chains collectively termed the **CD3 complex** for the antigen-binding domains of the TCR to form a complete, functional receptor that is stably expressed at the cell surface and is capable of transmitting a signal upon binding to antigen.

The four members of the CD3 complex (γ, δ, ε, and ζ) are sometimes termed the **invariant chains** of the TCR because they do not show variability in their amino acid sequences. (The γ and δ chains of the CD3 complex should not be confused with the quite distinct antigen-binding variable chains of the TCR that bear the same names.)

The CD3 chains are assembled as heterodimers of γε and δε subunits with a homodimer of ζ chains, giving an overall TCR stoichiometry of $(\alpha\beta)_2$, γ, δ, ε_2, ζ_2. Current data suggest that the TCR complex exists as a dimer (Fig. 5.3).

The CD3 γ, δ, and ε chains are the products of three closely linked genes, and similarities in their amino acid sequences suggest that they are evolutionarily related.

Indeed, all three are members of the immunoglobulin superfamily, each containing an external domain followed by a transmembrane region and a substantial, highly conserved, cytopasmic tail of 40 or more amino acids.

As with the transmembrane domains of the variable chains of the TCR, the membrane-spanning regions of these CD3 chains contain charged amino acids.

The negatively charged residues in the transmembrane region of the CD3 chains interact with (and neutralize) the positively charged amino acids in the αβ polypeptides, leading to the formation of a stable TCR complex (see Fig. 5.3).

The CD3ζ gene is on a different chromosome from the CD3γδε gene complex, and the ζ protein is structurally unrelated to the other CD3 components. The ζ chains possess:

- a small extracellular domain (nine amino acids);
- a transmembrane domain carrying a negative charge; and
- a large cytoplasmic tail.

An alternatively spliced form of CD3ζ, called CD3η, possesses an even larger cytoplasmic tail (42 amino acids longer at the C terminus).

The cytoplasmic portions of ζ and η chains contain ITAMs

The ζ and η chains may associate in all three possible combinations (ζζ, ζη, or ηη) and play a critical role in signal transduction through the TCR. The cytoplasmic portions of these subunits contain particular amino acid sequences called **immunoreceptor tyrosine-based activation motifs (ITAMs),** and each chain contains three of these motifs.

Q. Which other group of cell surface molecules contains ITAMs?
A. The Fcγ receptors, either as an intrinsic intracellular domain of the receptor, or because they associate with signaling molecules that have ITAMs (see Fig 3.17).

The conserved tyrosine residues in the ITAM motifs are targets for phosphorylation by specific protein kinases. When the TCR is bound to its cognate antigen–MHC complex, the

The T cell receptor complex

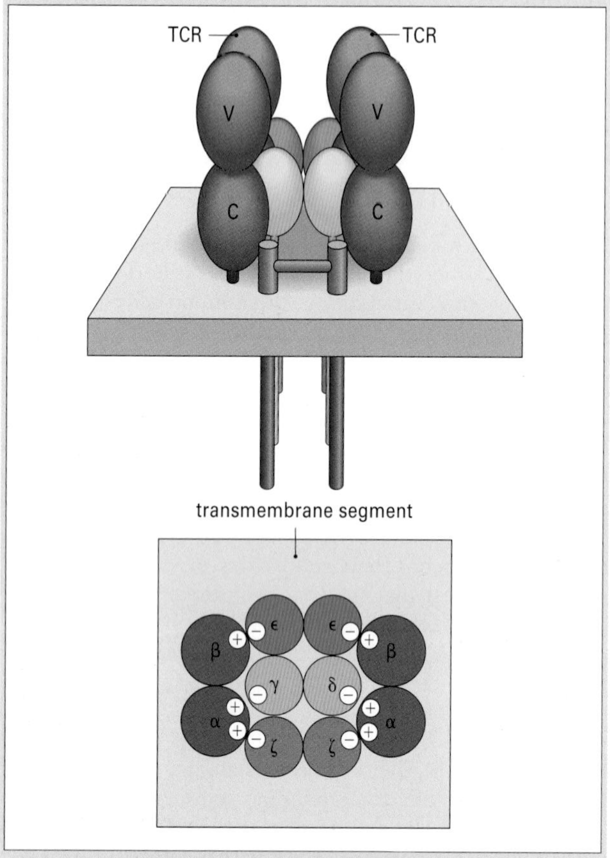

transmembrane segment

Fig. 5.3 The TCR α and β (or γ and δ) chains each comprise an external V and C domain, a transmembrane segment containing positively charged amino acids, and a short cytoplasmic tail. The two chains are disulfide linked on the membrane side of their C domains. The CD3 γ, δ, and ε chains comprise an external immunoglobulin-like C domain, a transmembrane segment containing a negatively charged amino acid, and a longer cytoplasmic tail. A dimer of ζζ, ηη, or ζη is also associated with the complex. Several lines of evidence support the notion that the TCR–CD3 complex exists at the cell surface as a dimer. The transmembrane charges are important for the assembly of the complex. A plausible arrangement that neutralizes opposite charges is shown.

ITAM motifs become phosphorylated within minutes in one of the first steps in T cell activation (see Fig. 8.w1). ITAMs:

- are essential for T cell activation, and mutational substitution of the tyrosines in the motif prevents activation;
- play critical roles in B cell activation, and are present in the B cell receptor chains, Igα and Igβ (see Fig. 3.1).

CD3ζ also functions in another signaling pathway, associating with the low-affinity FcγRIIIa receptor (CD16), which is involved in the activation of macrophages and natural killer (NK) cells (see Fig. 3.17).

Other subunits of the CD3 complex (γ, δ, ε), though lacking in ITAMs, may also become phosphorylated following TCR engagement. Phosphorylation of the CD3γ chain downregulates TCR expression on the cell surface via a mechanism involving increased receptor internalization.

The γδ TCR structurally resembles the αβ TCR but may function differently

The overall structure of the γδ TCR is similar to that of its αβ counterpart. Each chain is organized into:

- extracellular V and C domains;
- a transmembrane segment containing positively charged amino acids; and
- a short cytoplasmic tail.

One indication that the two types of T cell (i.e. T cells with αβ TCRs and T cells with γδ TCRs) might perform different functions comes from their anatomic distribution:

- in humans and mice, αβ TCRs are present on more than 95% of peripheral blood T cells and on the majority of thymocytes;
- T cells bearing γδ TCRs are relatively rare in spleen, lymph nodes, and peripheral blood but predominate at epithelial surfaces – they are common in skin and in the epithelial linings of the reproductive tract and are especially numerous in the intestine, where they are found as **intraepithelial lymphocytes.**

It is further believed that there are distinct subsets of γδ T cells that can perform different functions.

Antigen recognition by γδ T cells is unlike that of their αβ counterparts

The fact that γδ T cells are rare in anatomic locations known to support the classical mechanisms of antigen presentation and lymphocyte clonal expansion suggests the possibility that γδ cells might not need to rely upon normal antigen presentation mechanisms for their activation.

Several lines of evidence support the hypothesis that γδ T cells can recognize antigen in an MHC-independent fashion, for example:

- γδ T cells can be found in normal numbers in MHC class I and class II-deficient mice;
- their cognate antigens are not necessarily peptides, and do not require classical processing – indeed, some murine γδ T cells have been found to recognize proteins directly, including MHC molecules and viral proteins, in a manner that requires neither antigen processing nor presentation by MHC.

γδ T cells therefore appear to be able to follow a different paradigm for T cell recognition of antigen than that employed by αβ T cells.

γδ T cells recognize at least two classes of ligand:

- molecules that signal the presence of cellular stress; and
- small organic molecules that serve as signifiers of infection.

For example, human intraepithelial γδ T cells have been found to respond to MHC class I-related antigens (MICA and MICB) expressed on the surface of stressed cells.

In addition, some human γδ T cells recognize small organic compounds secreted by mycobacteria, such as monoethylphosphate and isopentenyl pyrophosphate. These ligands are secreted by a number of bacteria and may also be produced by some eukaryotic pathogens.

The γδ T cell arm of the adaptive immune system therefore appears to share some key characteristics of innate immune responses.

γδ T cells have a variety of biological roles

γδ T cells:

- are essential for primary immune responses to certain viral and bacterial pathogens in mouse models, but in many cases their contribution to the primary response can be substituted by αβ T cells, and they rarely contribute to memory responses;
- interact with a variety of lymphocytes, and have been implicated in stimulating immunoglobulin class switch recombination by B cells in response to T-dependent antigens;
- provide regulatory signals to αβ T cells and have been implicated in shaping immune responses (e.g. γδ cells appear to be involved in downregulating inflammation and in this role may be responding to epithelial cells stressed by inflammatory processes rather than to specific antigens borne by pathogens).

The unique ability of γδ T cells to sense tissue damage and to recognize antigens without the normal constraints of antigen processing/MHC restriction (see below), may allow them to fill several key biological roles such as immunoregulation. In particular, γδ T cells may downregulate potentially damaging inflammatory responses, providing immune protection:

- when MHC function is compromised by, for example, viral infections that downregulate MHC;
- in early life when αβ T cell function is immature and when the antigen processing and antigen sampling systems have not yet matured.

TCR variable region gene diversity is generated by V(D)J recombination

As with antibody genes, a highly diverse repertoire of TCR variable region genes is generated during T cell differentiation by a process of somatic gene rearrangement termed V(D)J recombination (see Chapter 3). Variable (V), joining (J), and sometimes diversity (D) gene segments are joined together to form a completed variable region gene.

Junctional diversity (imprecise joining of V, D, and J with loss and/or addition of nucleotides) contributes an enormous amount of variability to the TCR repertoire in addition to the variation that results from combinatorial assortment of the various gene segments.

The mechanism of V(D)J recombination is the same in both T cells and B cells

The TCR genes are flanked by recombination signal sequences, just like their immunoglobulin cousins (see Fig. 3.24), and the same recombination machinery (the RAG proteins) operates in both B and T cells. Indeed, experiments have shown that TCR Dβ and Jγ genes can rearrange appropriately even if transfected into B cells.

Analysis of the amino acid sequences of many different TCRs shows that the greatest diversity lies within the third CDR (CDR3), which is also the case for B cell receptors. Addition of N regions (non-templated nucleotides added to the junctions by terminal deoxynucleotidyl transferase, TdT) is much more pronounced in TCRs, however. It is important to note, too, that neither somatic hypermutation nor class switching occur in T cells.

Q. Why is it that, unlike B cells, T cells have not evolved a class switching mechanism?
A. Class switching is irrelevant because there is no secreted form of the TCR and hence no interaction analogous to that of immunoglobulin and FcR.

Recombination yields great diversity

Hunkapiller and Hood have calculated that it is possible to construct about:

- 4.4×10^{13} different forms of TCR Vβ; and
- 8.5×10^{12} forms of TCR Vα.

They estimate that if only 1% of the sequences coded for viable proteins this would still give 2.9×10^{22} receptors. Even if 99% of these viable receptors were rejected due to autoreactivity or other defects, recombination would still yield 2.9×10^{20} possible murine TCRs. This would seem to be more than enough potential diversity, given that the thymus produces fewer than 10^9 thymocytes over the lifetime of a mouse.

TCR V genes used in the responses against different antigens

A major area of research in recent years has been to determine which sets of TCR V genes are used in the responses against different antigens. Because T cells recognize antigenic peptides bound to a particular MHC molecule this depends on:

- the antigen; and
- the MHC molecules expressed by an individual.

Once the TCRs have been generated, T cells are subjected to thymic selection and may be further selected by interactions with APCs in the periphery. For these reasons, even if TCRs are generated by random recombination of gene segments, the expressed repertoire will be skewed toward the use of particular gene segments. Furthermore, the preference for different V gene segments by distinct T cell subsets may reflect their ontogeny. For example:

- γδ T cells residing in mouse skin (dendritic epidermal cells or DECs) express only the Vγ3 and Vδ1 segments;
- intraepithelial lymphocytes from the gut express Vγ5 almost exclusively (in combination with Vδ4–7).

It is thought that these populations arise at distinct stages of intrathymic T cell development, and they appear to have distinct functions.

MHC molecules

Recognition by the αβ TCR requires antigen to be bound to an MHC molecule

As discussed in Chapter 3, antibodies recognize intact proteins, binding either to linear epitopes derived from contiguous amino acids or discontinuous epitopes produced by amino acids that are not near one another in the primary structure but are brought together in the three dimensional structure of the protein. In contrast, T cell receptors only recognize linear epitopes present in the form of short peptides which are generated by degradation of intact proteins within the cell (a process termed **antigen processing**). This property of T cell receptors is critical to the way the immune system recognizes intracellular pathogens and tumor antigens. Such antigens present a special challenge to the immune system: intracellular antigens are hidden within the cell, and are not available for recognition by antibodies. How can intracellular antigens be recognized by extracellular receptors? The immune system has solved this problem by evolving an elegant means of displaying internal antigens (including those of intracellular pathogens) on the cell surface, allowing their recognition by T cells:

- proteins from within the cell (either produced by the cell or taken into the cell) are digested into short peptide fragments;
- peptides derived from proteins produced within the cell are displayed on the cell surface through binding to specialized antigen-presenting molecules termed **MHC class I** molecules, which are present on all nucleated cells of the body;
- in a similar fashion, peptides derived from proteins ingested from the extracellular environment by phagocytosis are presented by **MHC class II** molecules, which are present only on professional antigen presenting cells;
- the peptide–MHC complexes serve as ligands for TCRs.

This antigen processing and presentation pathway, upon which both activation and regulation of the immune response rests, is a complex and fascinating subject (see Chapter 8).

In humans the MHC is known as the HLA

The proteins responsible for presenting antigens to T cells, MHC class I and class II proteins, were originally discovered as histocompatibility (transplantation) antigens. Histocompatibility refers to the ability to accept tissue grafts from an unrelated donor.

The major histocompatibility complex locus (MHC) comprises over 100 separate genes and was discovered when it was recognized that both donor and recipient had to possess the same MHC haplotype to avoid graft rejection.

The principal moieties that determine rejection were identified as MHC class I and class II molecules (see below), but we know now that the main purpose of the MHC is not

to prevent graft rejection. The remaining genes in the MHC (sometimes called class III) are very diverse. Some encode:

- complement system molecules (C4, C2, factor B);
- cytokines (e.g. tumor necrosis factor);
- enzymes;
- heat-shock proteins; and
- other molecules involved in antigen processing.

There are no functional or structural similarities between these other gene products.

All mammalian species possess the MHC, though details of the complex vary from one species to the next. In humans the locus is known as the **HLA** (an abbreviation for **human leukocyte antigen**); in mice it is known as the **H-2 locus** (Fig. 5.4).

MHC molecules provide a sophisticated surveillance system for intracellular antigens

From a cell's perspective, there are two types of antigen that must be dealt with:

- **endogenous** antigens (antigenic peptides from viruses or other pathogens that inhabit the cell);
- **exogenous** antigens (antigenic peptides from extracellular pathogens that have been taken up by a professional APC).

Q. How are antigens taken up by APCs?
A. They are internalized by phagocytosis or pinocytosis, either by directly binding to receptors on the surface of the APC (see Fig. 1.11) or following opsonization by antibody and/or complement (see Fig. 4.14).

MHC class I molecules handle endogenous (or **intrinsic**) antigens, while MHC class II molecules handle exogenous (**extrinsic**) antigens. In both cases, the antigenic peptides are produced by proteolytic processing of proteins.

In general:

- MHC class I molecules present antigen to cytotoxic T cells, which are important in controlling viral infections by lysing infected cells;

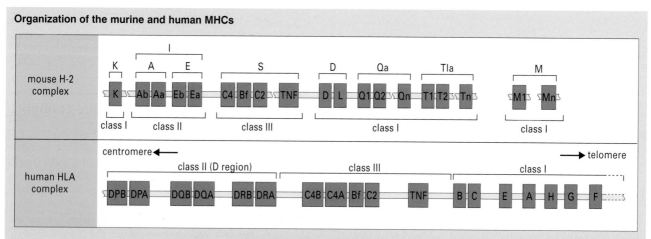

Organization of the murine and human MHCs

Fig. 5.4 Diagram showing the locations of subregions of the murine and human MHCs and the positions of the major genes within these subregions. The human organization pattern, in which the class II loci are positioned between the centromere and the class I loci, occurs in every other mammalian species so far examined. The regions span 3–4 Mbp of DNA.

• MHC class II molecules present antigen to helper T cells, which aid B cells in generating antibody responses to extracellular protein antigens.

MHC class I molecules consist of an MHC-encoded heavy chain bound to β₂-microglobulin

The overall structure of the extracellular portion of an MHC class I molecule is depicted in Figure 5.5. It comprises a glycosylated heavy chain (45 kDa) non-covalently associated with β₂-microglobulin (12 kDa), which is a polypeptide that is also found free in serum.

The class I heavy chain consists of:

• three extracellular domains, designated α_1 (N terminal), α_2, and α_3;
• a transmembrane region; and
• a cytoplasmic tail.

The three extracellular domains each comprise about 90 amino acids:

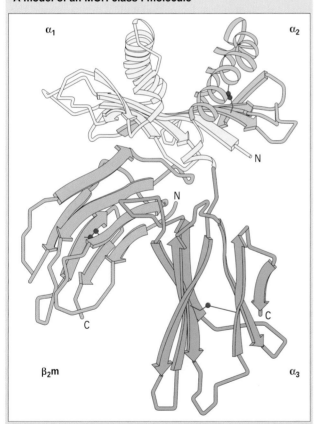

A model of an MCH class I molecule

Fig. 5.5 The peptide backbone of the extracellular portion of HLA-A2 is shown. The three globular domains (α_1, α_2, and α_3) of the heavy chain are shown in green or turquoise and are closely associated with the non-MHC-encoded peptide, β₂-microglobulin (β₂m, gray). β₂-Microglobulin is stabilized by an intrachain disulfide bond (red) and has a similar tertiary structure to an immunoglobulin domain. The groove formed by the α_1 and α_2 domains is clearly visible.

• the α_2 and α_3 domains both have intrachain disulfide bonds enclosing loops of 63 and 86 amino acids, respectively;
• the α_3 domain is structurally homologous to the immunoglobulin constant region domain (C) and contains a site that interacts with CD8 on cytotoxic T cells.

The extracellular portion of the class I heavy chain is glycosylated, the degree of glycosylation depending on the species and haplotype.

The predominantly hydrophobic transmembrane region comprises 25 amino acid residues and traverses the lipid bilayer, most probably in an α-helical conformation.

The hydrophilic cytoplasmic domain, 30–40 residues long, may be phosphorylated in vivo.

β2-Microglobulin is essential for expression of MHC class I molecules

β₂-Microglobulin:

• is non-polymorphic in humans, but dimorphic in mice (because of a single amino acid change);
• like the α_3 domain, has the structure of an immunoglobulin constant region domain;
• associates with a number of other class I-like molecules, such as the products of the *CD1* genes on chromosome 1 in humans (see below) and the Fc receptor, which mediates the uptake of IgG from milk in neonatal rat intestinal cells (see Fig. 3.18). These class I-like molecules, which have a structural similarity to the products of the MHC class I genes, are encoded by genes located in the class I loci and are referred to as **class Ib molecules;**
• is essential for the expression of all class I molecules at the cell surface – mutant mice lacking β₂-microglobulin do not express MHC class I molecules and are severely defective in presenting intrinsic antigens to T cells.

Heavy chain α1, and α2 domains form the antigen-binding groove

X-ray crystallography has shown that the α_1 and α_2 domains constitute a platform of eight antiparallel β strands supporting two α helices (Fig. 5.6). The disulfide bond in the α_2 domain connects the N terminal β strand to the α helix of the α_2 domain. A long groove separates the a helices of the α_1 and α_2 domains.

The original crystal structure of the HLA-A2 molecule revealed diffuse extra electron density in the groove, suggesting the presence of bound peptide antigen. This interpretation was supported by the observation that the majority of polymorphic residues and T cell epitopes on class I molecules are located in or near the groove.

Variations in amino acid sequence change the shape of the binding groove

Comparison of the structures of HLA-A2 and HLA-Aw68 have further refined our understanding of the structural basis for the binding of peptide to class I antigens.

The antigen-binding site of the MHC class I molecule HLA-A2

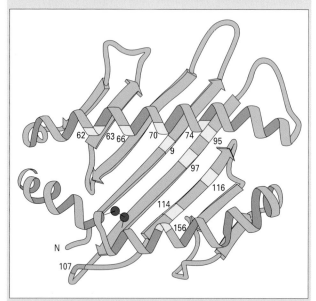

Fig. 5.6 The view of the peptide antigen-binding groove in HLA-A2 as 'seen' by the TCR. The α_1 and α_2 domains each consist of four antiparallel β strands followed by a long helical region. The domains pair to form a single eight-stranded β sheet topped by α helices. The locations of the most polymorphic residues are highlighted. Residues around the binding site are highly polymorphic. For example, HLA-2 and HLA-Aw68 differ from each other by 13 amino acid residues. Ten of these differences occur around the antigen-binding site (yellow). *(Modified from Bjorkman et al. Nature 1987;329:512–516, with additional data from Parham P. Nature 1989;342:617–618.)*

Peptide-binding grooves of HLA-Aw68 and HLA-A2

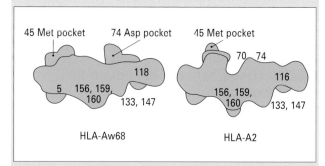

Fig. 5.7 The shapes of the antigen-binding groove on each molecule are illustrated. Differences in amino acids around the groove create different antigen-binding sites. For example, residues around position 45 produce a methionine-binding pocket in both molecules, but the aspartate-binding pocket around residue 74 is present only in HLA-Aw68.

These products are heterodimers of heavy (α) and light (β) glycoprotein chains, and both chains are encoded in the MHC:

- the α chains have molecular weights of 30–34 kDa;
- the β chains range from 26–29 kDa, depending on the locus involved.

A number of lines of evidence indicate that the α and β chains have the same overall structures. An extracellular portion comprising two domains (α_1 and α_2 or β_1 and β_2) is connected by a short sequence to a transmembrane region of about 30 residues and a cytoplasmic domain of about 10 to 15 residues.

The α_2 and β_2 domains are similar to the class I α_3 domain and β_2-microglobulin, possessing the structural characteristics of immunoglobulin constant domains.

The β_1 domain contains a disulfide bond, which generates a 64 amino acid loop.

The difference in molecular weights of the class II α and β chains is due primarily to differential glycosylation:

- the α_1, α_2, and β_1 domains are N-glycosylated;
- the β_2 domain is not N-glycosylated.

The β_2 domain does, however, contain a binding site for CD4, and MHC class II molecules on APCs interact with CD4 on T cells in a manner analogous to the interaction of MHC class I molecules with CD8. CD4 and CD8 are important elements in the recruitment of kinases that signal T cell activation.

Despite the differences in length and organization of the polypeptide chains, the overall three-dimensional structure of MHC class II molecules is very similar to that of MHC class I molecules (Fig. 5.8).

The differences between HLA-A2 and HLA-Aw68 result from amino acid side-chain differences at 13 positions:

- six in α_1;
- six in α_2; and
- one (residue 245, which contributes to interactions with CD8) in α_3.

Ten of the twelve differences between HLA-A2 and HLA-Aw68 are at positions lining the floor and side of the peptide-binding groove (see Fig. 5.6). These differences give rise to dramatic differences in the shape of the groove and on the antigen peptides that it will bind.

Seen in detail, the peptide-binding groove forms a number of ridges and pockets with which amino acid side chains can interact. Typically the groove of an MHC class I molecule will accommodate peptides of eight or nine residues.

Amino acid variations within the peptide-binding groove can vary the positions of the pockets, providing the structural basis for differences in peptide-binding affinity that in turn govern exactly what is presented to a T cell (Fig. 5.7).

MHC class II molecules resemble MHC class I molecules in their overall structure

The products of the MHC class II genes are:

- HLA-DP, -DQ, and -DR in humans;
- H-2A and E in the mouse.

Peptide binding properties of MHC molecules

The MHC class II binding groove accommodates longer peptides than MHC class I

The structures of MHC class I and class II molecules reflect their functional differences.

Comparison of the extracellular domains of class I and class II molecules

HLA-Aw68 (class I)

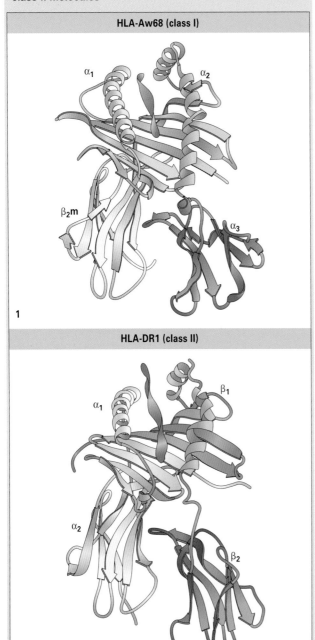

HLA-DR1 (class II)

Fig. 5.8 Ribbon diagrams of the extracellular domains of class I HLA-Aw68 (**1**) and class II HLA-DR1 (**2**) MHC molecules. The binding cleft is shown with a resident peptide. These diagrams emphasize the similarity in the three-dimensional structures of class I and class II molecules. *(Redrawn from Stern LJ. Structure 1994;2:245–251. Copyright 1994 with permission from Elsevier.)*

Peptide-binding sites of class I (H-2K^b) and class I (HLA-DR1) MHC molecules

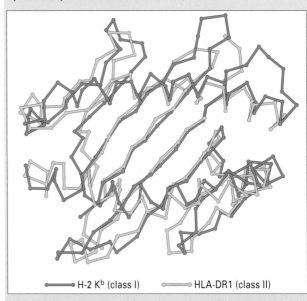

H-2 K^b (class I)   HLA-DR1 (class II)

Fig. 5.9 The peptide binding sites of class I (H-2K^b) and class II (HLA-DR1) MHC molecules are shown as α carbon atom traces in a top view of the peptide-binding clefts. The similarities between the two sites can clearly be seen, but there are also some differences, some of which account for the difference in peptide length preference between class I (8–10 amino acid residues) and class II (>12 amino acid residues). *(Redrawn from Stern LJ. Structure 1994;2:245–251. Copyright 1994 with permission from Elsevier.)*

- MHC class II molecules bind peptides of 13 to 24 amino acids.

The structural features of the class II antigen-binding site have been illuminated by determination of the crystal structure of HLA-DR1 complexed with an influenza virus peptide. Pockets clearly visible within the peptide-binding site accommodate five side chains of the bound peptide and explain the peptide specificity of HLA-DR1.

The precise topology of the MHC peptide-binding groove depends partly on the nature of the amino acids within the groove, and thus varies from one haplotype to the next.

Which peptide can bind to a particular MHC molecule depends on the nature of the side chains of the peptide and their complementarity with the MHC molecule's binding groove. Some amino acid side chains of the peptide stick out of the groove and are available to contact the TCR.

Peptides are held in MHC molecule binding grooves by characteristic anchor residues

It is possible to purify and sequence peptides that have been generated by a cell and then bound by MHC molecules at the cell surface. These peptides include:

- foreign peptides from internalized antigens or viral particles; and
- self molecules produced within the cell or endocytosed from extracellular fluids.

The binding groove of MHC class II molecules is more open than that of MHC class I molecules, to accommodate longer peptides (Figs 5.9 and 5.10):

- MHC class I molecules bind short fragments of eight to ten amino acids; whereas

Peptides bind non-covalently within the antigen-binding groove

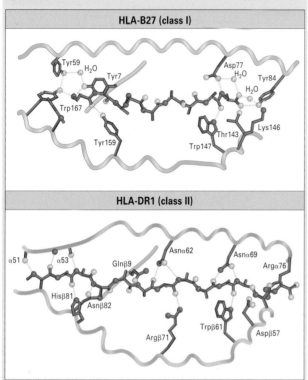

Fig. 5.10 The hydrogen bonds made by the main chain of a bound peptide with class I (HLA-B27) or class II MHC molecules (HLA-DR1) are shown. The major difference between the two hydrogen-bonding patterns is the clustering of conserved class I hydrogen bonds at the ends of the peptide. By contrast, conserved class II hydrogen bonds are distributed throughout the length of the peptide. *(Redrawn from Stern LJ. Structure 1994;2:245–251. Copyright 1994 with permission from Elsevier.)*

Interactions at the N and C termini confine peptides to the binding groove of MHC class I molecules

A number of peptides bound by particular MHC molecules have been sequenced, and characteristic residues identified – one at the C terminus and another close to the N terminus of the peptide. These characteristic motifs distinguish sets of binding peptides for different MHC class I molecules (Fig. 5.11).

The significance of the conserved residues has become clear by analysis of the three-dimensional structures of several MHC class I molecules, which have generated a clear picture of the peptide residing in the binding groove:

- the ends of the peptide-binding groove are closed;
- the peptide is an extended (not α-helical) chain of nine amino acids and the N and C terminals are buried at the ends of the groove;
- some of the side chains extend into the pockets formed within the variable region of the class I heavy chain;
- numerous hydrogen bonds are formed between residues in the class I molecule and those of the peptide along its length;
- in particular, tyrosine residues commonly found at the N terminus of the peptide and a conserved lysine in the MHC class I molecule binding groove stabilize peptide binding (see Fig. 5.10);

Allele-specific motifs in peptides eluted from MHC class I molecules

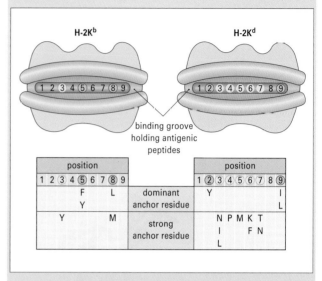

Fig. 5.11 Class I MHC molecules from either H-2K[b] or H-2K[d] haplotypes were immunoprecipitated. Peptides bound to these molecules were purified and sequenced. Amino acid residues commonly found at a particular position are classified as 'dominant' anchor residues. Residues that are fairly common at a site are shown as 'strong'. Positions for which no amino acid is shown could be occupied by several different amino acids with equal frequency. The one-letter amino acid code is used. The diagram represents the class I MHC molecule binding groove, viewed from above with anchor positions of each haplotype highlighted.

- the centers of the peptides bulge out of the groove, so presenting different structures to TCRs.

This picture is consistent with the characteristic motifs found at the ends of peptides eluted from class I molecules.

Peptides may extend beyond the ends of the binding groove of MHC class II molecules

The binding groove of the MHC class II molecule:

- also incorporates a number of binding pockets, though the locations are somewhat different from that on class I molecules;
- is not closed at the ends, so bound peptides extend out of the ends of the groove.

Consistent with this observation, peptides eluted from MHC class II molecules tend to be longer (over 15 residues).

Conserved anchor residues in peptides eluted from MHC class II molecules have been identified (Fig. 5.12).

Peptides binding MHC class II are less uniform in size than those binding MHC class I molecules

A major difference between MHC class I and class II molecules occurs at the ends of the peptide-binding groove:

- for MHC class I molecules, interactions at the N and C terminals confine the peptide to the cleft;
- for MHC class II molecules, peptides may extend beyond the ends of the cleft.

Allele-specific motifs in peptides eluted from MHC class II molecules

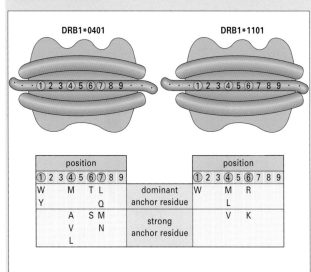

position						position			
①2 3 ④5 ⑥⑦8 9					①2 3 ④5 ⑥7 8 9				
W	M	T L	dominant anchor residue		W	M	R		
Y		Q					L		
	A	S M	strong anchor residue				V K		
	V	N							
	L								

Columns labelled DRB1*0401 (left) and DRB1*1101 (right).

Fig. 5.12 HLA-DR molecules of two haplotypes (DRB1*0401 and DRB1*1101) were purified and incubated with a library of peptides (generated in phage M13). After multiple rounds of selection, peptides that bound effectively to the MHC class II molecules were identified and sequenced. Residues having a frequency greater than 20% are shown as 'dominant' anchor residues. Other fairly common residues are shown as 'strong'. Note that the binding site on MHC class II molecules accommodates longer peptides than that on MHC class I molecules. *(Data abstracted from Hammer J, Valsasnini P, Tolba K, et al. Cell 1993;74:197–203.)*

The peptides that bind to MHC class I molecules come from endogenous proteins synthesized within the cell, which are broken down and transported to the endoplasmic reticulum. The mechanism of antigen processing is explained fully in Chapter 8, but it should be noted here that the internal antigen processing pathways generally produce peptides of an appropriate size to occupy the MHC class I molecule antigen-binding groove.

Peptides that bind to MHC class II molecules come from exogenous antigens – proteins that have been internalized by the cell and then degraded. These peptides are less uniform in size than those that bind to MHC class I molecules and may be trimmed once they have found their way to the MHC class II molecule.

The MHC class II molecule antigen processing pathway is quite distinct from the MHC class I molecule pathway (see Chapter 7).

Antigen presentation by MHC molecules

Once the structures of the TCR and the MHC–peptide complex had been established, the next question was to determine how they interacted.

The first crystallographic data were derived using a co-crystal of a mouse MHC class I molecule bound to an endogenous cellular peptide and αβ TCR (Fig. 5.13). This structure showed that the axis of the TCR was roughly

Interaction of a T cell receptor and MHC-peptide complex

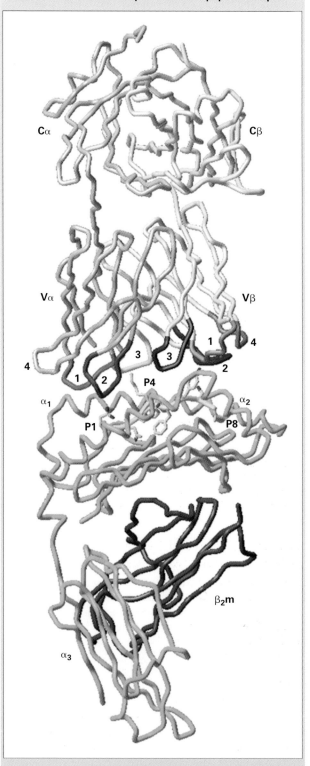

Fig. 5.13 The structure of an MHC class I molecule (H-2K^b) complexed to an octapeptide (yellow tube) is shown bound to an αβ TCR. The six CDRs that contact the peptide (1, 2, 3, 3, 1, 2) are highlighted in deeper colors. Residues from αHV4 (pink) and βHV4 (orange) are not positioned to take part in the intermolecular interactions. *(Illustration kindly provided by Dr Christopher Garcia, from Science 1996;274:209–219. Copyright 1996 AAAS.)*

aligned with the peptide-binding groove on the MHC molecule, but set at 20–30° askew. This means that:

- the first and second CDRs of the TCR α and β chains (see Fig. 5.2) are positioned over residues near the N and C terminals of the presented polypeptide; and
- the most variable CDRs of each chain (CDR3), lying at the center of the TCR binding site, are positioned over the central residues of the peptide that protrude from the groove. Residues from each of the CDRs are positioned to interact with residues from the MHC molecule.

Q. What advantage is there in having CDR3 segments at the center of the TCR binding site?

A. CDR3 demonstrates the greatest diversity of the TCR CDRs (because it is generated by gene recombination). It is therefore better suited than CDR1 and CDR2 for interactions with diverse antigenic peptides.

The molecular structure therefore underpins the experimental findings that T cells recognize antigenic peptides bound to particular MHC molecules.

This arrangement of TCR and MHC–antigen is broadly comparable to those found with the small number of receptors so far analyzed by X-ray crystallography.

Aggregation of TCRs initiates T cell activation

Although basic models of T cell activation by antigen–MHC show one receptor being triggered by one complex (e.g. Fig. 1.12), this is simplistic.

Each T cell may express 10^5 receptors and each APC has a similar number of MHC molecules. If a T cell engages an APC, only a tiny proportion of the MHC–antigen complexes on its surface will be of the correct type to be recognized by the T cell.

What, then, is the minimum signal for T cell activation? In practice:

- only a few peptide–MHC–TCR interactions are needed – perhaps 100 specific interactions, involving about 0.1% of the MHC molecules on the APC;
- moreover, the interactions can take place over a period of time – it is not necessary for all 100 TCRs to be engaged simultaneously.

The model of the TCR shown in Figure 5.3 suggests that it can form a dimeric structure clustered around the signaling molecules of the CD3 complex.

Interestingly, there is some evidence that MHC molecules can also dimerize, and that TCRs bound to MHC–peptide complexes tend to form dimers or aggregates. These observations have led to the view that T cell activation requires the cooperative aggregation of specific TCRs with MHC–peptide complexes.

The auxiliary molecules CD4 and CD8 are also important in T cell activation, and the presence of CD4 or CD8 can help stabilize the interaction of the TCR and MHC–peptide. In addition, kinases associated with these molecules are brought into proximity with CD3 so they can phosphorylate the ζζ dimer that initiates activation (Fig. 5.14). The ensuing steps are described in Chapter 8.

The role of CD4 and CD8 in T cell activation

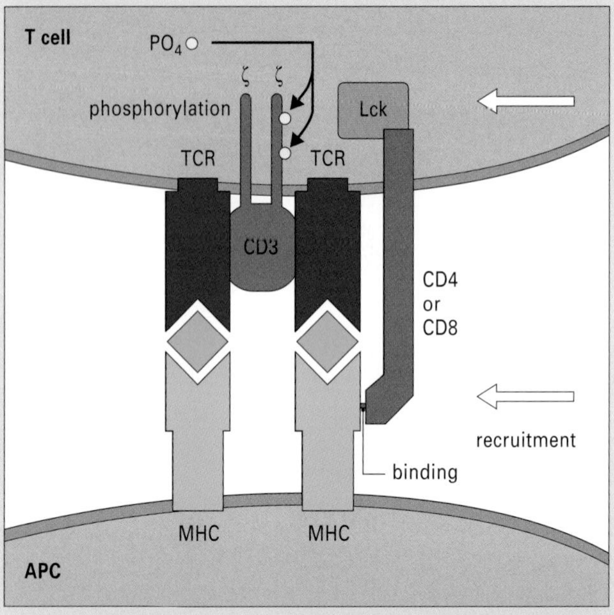

Fig. 5.14 After aggregation of MHC–peptide on the APC with the TCR, either CD4 or CD8 can join the complex. CD4 binds to MHC class II molecules and CD8 to MHC class I molecules. The kinase Lck is attached to the intracytoplasmic portion of CD4 or CD8. Binding of the CD4 or CD8 molecules to specific sites of the MHC molecules brings the kinase into proximity with the ITAMs on the CD3 ζζ dimer (see Fig. 5.3). The kinase phosphorylates the motifs, as the first step in T cell activation.

Antigenic peptides can induce or antagonize T cell activation

The affinity of TCRs for antigen peptide–MHC, expressed as an association constant, is typically of the order of 10^{-5} to 10^{-6} M, which is much lower than the typical affinity of an antibody for its epitope.

The affinity of antigen–MHC for the TCR is especially important because it determines the degree to which the T cell becomes activated. Peptides that activate a T cell are called **agonist peptides.** By changing one or two amino acids in an agonist peptide, it is possible to generate peptides that antagonize the normal activation by the original peptide. The **antagonist peptides** typically have a lower affinity for the TCR than the original agonist peptide and are thought to act by either:

- interfering with the binding of the agonist peptide to the MHC molecule; or
- binding less effectively to the TCR.

Occasionally, a modified peptide will be more effective than the agonist in activating the T cell. These **strong agonist (or superagonist) peptides** produce higher affinity binding in the TCR–MHC–peptide complex.

The distinctions between these three different types of peptide (agonist, antagonist, and strong agonist) have biological ramifications. Researchers are attempting, for example, to use antagonist peptides to block adverse immune responses.

Understanding TCR affinity could provide insight into how T cells become tolerant to self antigens during development (see Chapter 19).

What constitutes T cell specificity?

Finally we should consider the question of what constitutes T cell specificity. When the specificity of lymphocytes was first explained in Chapter 1, it was stated that each lymphocyte binds to just one antigen using its receptor. Although this is a useful starting point for understanding immune responses, it is not strictly true.

In Chapter 3 it was seen that immunoglobulins could bind to different antigens if they had epitopes that were sufficiently similar. This chapter has shown that antigenic peptides can be mutated and still bind and trigger T cell activation.

One question, then, is how far a peptide can be mutated and still bind to its own TCR. In some cases it has been possible to individually change each amino acid in a peptide without destroying its ability to bind to the MHC molecule or the TCR.

Provided the peptide can form part of the TCR–MHC–peptide complex and provide sufficient binding energy, its precise amino acid sequence does not matter. This is a very important observation.

Later, when we consider how antigenic peptides from microorganisms can trigger autoimmune diseases (see Chapter 20), we learn that one possible mechanism is that a self peptide and a foreign peptide are sufficiently similar to bind to the same T cell, so causing a breakdown in self tolerance. One conclusion from the work cited above is that such peptides do not have to be identical to be cross-reactive.

Genetic organization of the MHC

The number of gene loci for MHC class I and class II molecules varies between species and between different haplotypes within each species, and many polymorphic variants have been described at each of the loci.

Much of the original work on the MHC was done using mice and what has been learned from these studies has been broadly applicable to humans.

The three principal human MHC class I loci are HLA-A, HLA-B, and HLA-C

The human MHC class I region contains three principal class I loci – called HLA-A, HLA-B, and HLA-C. Each locus encodes the heavy chain of a classical MHC class I molecule and the whole region:

- extends over 1.8 million bases of DNA; and
- includes 118 genes (Fig. 5.15).

Closer analysis of this region has revealed multiple additional MHC class I genes.

HLA-E, HLA-F, HLA-G, and HLA-H are class Ib genes

The *HLA-E*, *HLA-F*, *HLA-G*, and *HLA-H* genes also encode MHC class I proteins, and are called class Ib genes. They are much less polymorphic than the A, B, and C locus gene products, and recent work has ascribed various functions to them. For example, *HLA-E and HLA-G* gene products can bind to antigenic peptides, but are involved in recognition by NK cells.

Human MHC class II genes are located in the HLA-D region

The human MHC class II region spans about 1000 kb of DNA, and the order and orientation of the various loci are similar to that of the homologous loci in the mouse MHC class II region.

The HLA-D region encodes at least six α and ten β chain genes for MHC class II molecules (Fig. 5.16). Three loci (DR, DQ, and DP) encode the major expressed products of the human MHC class II region, but additional genes have also been identified:

- the DR family comprises a single α gene (DRA) and up to nine β genes (DRB1–9), including pseudogenes and several different gene arrangements occur within the locus;
- the DQ and DP families each have one expressed gene for α and β chains and an additional pair of pseudogenes.

DR, DQ, and DP α chains associate in the cell primarily with β chains of their own loci. For example:

- the *DPA1* and *DPB1* gene products associate to generate the HLA-DP class II molecules detected using specific antibodies;
- similarly, *DQA1* and *DQB1* encode the HLA-DQ antigens.

The organization and length of the DRB region varies in different haplotypes (Fig. 5.17), with different numbers of β chains expressed.

The MHC class II region also contains genes that encode proteins involved in antigen presentation that are not expressed at the cell surface (see Chapter 8).

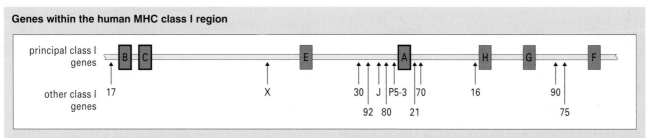

Genes within the human MHC class I region

Fig. 5.15   The human MHC class I region lies telomeric to the MHC class II region (see Fig. 5.5). In addition to the genes encoding the classic transplantation antigens (*HLA-A*, *HLA-B*, and *HLA-C*), several other principal class I-like genes have been identified (*HLA-E*, *HLA-F*, and *HLA-G*). Mutations in the *HLA-H* gene are associated with hemochromatosis, a disorder that causes the body to absorb excessive amounts of iron from the diet. A number of other non-classical class I genes and pseudogenes are present, mostly with unknown functions.

Genes within the human and mouse class II regions

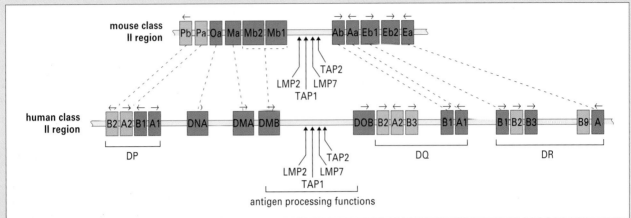

Fig. 5.16 The arrangement of the genes within the human and murine MHCs is shown. Homologous genes between the two species are indicated. Expressed genes are colored orange and pseudogenes are shown yellow. Mice of the b, s, f, and q haplotypes fail to express class II-E molecules. The b and s haplotypes fail to transcribe the Ea gene, but make normal cytoplasmic levels of Eb chain. Mice of f and q haplotypes fail to make both Ea and Eb chains.

The number of DRB loci varies with different haplotypes

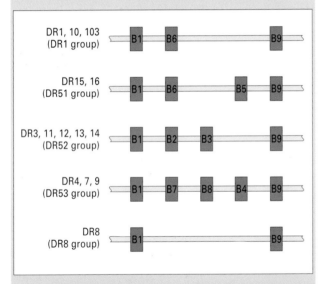

Fig. 5.17 The numbers of DRB loci varies between individuals. For example, a person who has a haplotype producing molecules of the type DR1 (see Appendix 1) has three loci for DRB (top line). Not all of these loci produce mRNA for DR β chains.

MHC polymorphism is concentrated in and around the peptide-binding cleft

A hallmark of the MHC is the extreme degree of polymorphism (structural variability) of the molecules encoded within it. The class Ib molecules are much less polymorphic than the classical class I and II molecules. New allelic variants are identified frequently and logged on dedicated databases (see Internet references).

Within a particular MHC class I or class II molecule, the structural polymorphisms are clustered in particular regions. The amino acid sequence variability in class I molecules is clustered in three main regions of the α_1 and α_2 domains. The α_3 domain appears to be much more conserved.

> **Q. Correlate the domains that show structural variability and structural conservation with the molecules that they interact with.**
>
> A. The α_1 and α_2 domains interact with the variable antigen peptides and the TCR (see Fig. 5.13), while the α_3 domain interacts with the monomorphic CD8 molecule (see Fig. 5.14).

In MHC class II molecules, the extent of variability depends on the subregion and on the polypeptide chain. For example:

- most polymorphism occurs in DRβ and DQβ chains, whereas DPβ chains are slightly less polymorphic;
- DQα is polymorphic whereas DRα chains are virtually invariant, being represented by just two alleles.

In outbred populations in which individuals have two MHC haplotypes, hybrid class II molecules with one chain from each haplotype can be produced. This generates additional structural diversity in the expressed molecules.

Most of the polymorphic amino acids in MHC class I and class II molecules are clustered on top of the molecule around the peptide-binding site (see Fig. 5.6). Variation is therefore centered in the base of the antigen-binding groove or pointing in from the sides of the α helices. This polymorphism affects the ability of the different MHC molecules to bind antigenic peptides.

MHC haplotype and disease susceptibility

Genetic variations in MHC molecules affect:

- the ability to make immune responses, including the level of antibody production;
- resistance or susceptibility to infectious diseases;
- resistance or susceptibility to autoimmune diseases and allergies.

Knowing this, we can start to answer the question of why the MHC is so polymorphic. The immune system must handle many different pathogens. By having several different MHC molecules, an individual can present a diverse range of antigens and is therefore likely to be able to mount an effective immune response. There is therefore a selective advantage in having different MHC molecules.

Going beyond this, we know that different pathogens are prevalent in different areas of the world, so evolutionary pressures from pathogens will tend to select for different MHC molecules in different regions.

Q. The haplotype HLA-B53 is associated with protection against childhood malaria, a disease that is prevalent in equatorial regions. In which country would you expect to find the highest frequency of the HLA-B53 allele – China, Ghana, or South Africa?
A. The gene frequency is around 40% in Ghana and 1–2% in China and South Africa, which are outside the equatorial regions affected by malaria.

All nucleated cells of the body express MHC class I molecules

The function of MHC class I molecules is to present antigens that have entered the cell, such as viral peptides. Because any cell of the body may become infected with a virus or intracellular pathogen, all cells need to sample their internal molecules and present them at the cell surface to cytotoxic T cells.

By contrast, MHC class II molecules are used by APCs to present antigens to helper T cells. Consequently the distribution of class II molecules is much more limited (see Fig. 8.4).

MHC molecules are co-dominantly expressed

This means that, in one individual, all of the principal MHC gene loci are expressed from both the maternal and paternal chromosomes. As there are three MHC class I loci in humans (HLA-A, HLA-B, and HLA-C), each of which is highly polymorphic, most individuals will have genes for six different class I molecules, all of which will be present at the cell surface. Each MHC molecule will have:

- a slightly different shape; and
- present a different set of antigenic peptides.

A similar logic applies to MHC class II molecules. There are three principal class II loci in humans (HLA-DP, HLA-DQ, and HLA-DR), all of which are polymorphic. At first sight, it would appear that an APC could express six different class II molecules as well as its class I molecules. However, this is probably an underestimate. As noted above, hybrid class II molecules (using one polypeptide encoded by the maternal chromosome and one by the paternal chromosome) also occur.

The specificity of the TCR and MHC explains genetic restrictions in antigen presentation

Much of the original work on antigen presentation was carried out using strains of mice that had been inbred to the point where both maternal and paternal chromosomes were

identical. Any offspring therefore inherited the same set of autosomes from each parent, and the offspring were genetically identical to their parents. Clearly the level of diversity in the MHC molecules was much less than in an outbred human population.

The artificial simplicity of the inbred mouse system, however, allowed immunologists to dissect how antigens were presented to T cells in a whole animal, when the molecular structures of the MHC molecules and the TCR were completely unknown.

The key experiment that demonstrated the importance of the MHC in antigen presentation revealed a phenomenon called **genetic restriction** (also known as **MHC restriction**). In essence, it was noted that cytotoxic T cells from a mouse infected with a virus are primed to kill cells of the same H-2 haplotype infected with that virus; they do not kill cells of a different haplotype infected with the same virus (Fig. 5.18).

These data, and similar experiments using APCs and helper T cells, showed that T cells that have been primed to recognize antigen presented on MHC molecules of one haplotype will normally respond again only when they see the same antigen on the same MHC molecule.

Q. Interpret these findings in relation to the way in which T cells recognize antigen.
A. The TCR interacts with residues from both the antigenic peptide and the associated MHC molecule. In other words, the T cell recognizes the specific combination of MHC molecule plus peptide.

MHC restriction of cytotoxic T cells

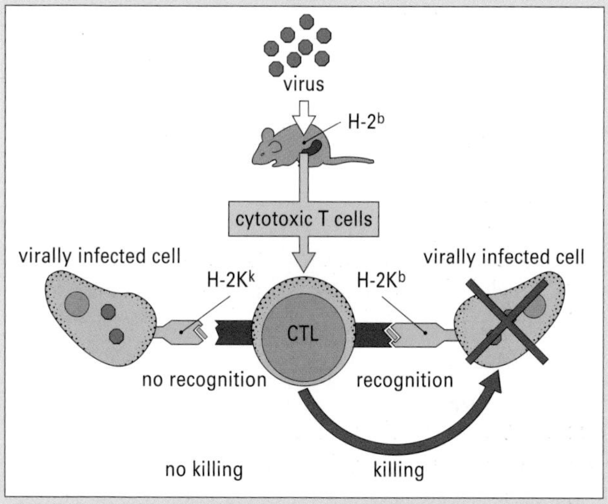

Fig. 5.18 A mouse of the H-2^b haplotype is primed with virus and the cytotoxic T cells thus generated are isolated and tested for their ability to kill H-2^b and H-2^k cells infected with the same virus. The cytotoxic T cells kill H-2^b, but not H-2^k cells. In this instance, it is the H-2K class I gene product presenting the antigen to the T cells. The T cell is recognizing a specific structure produced by the association of a specific MHC molecule with a specific viral antigen.

Peter Doherty and Rolf Zinkernagel performed the key experiments delineating the phenomenon of MHC restriction of T cell responses in the mid 1970s and were awarded the Nobel Prize in Physiology or Medicine in 1996 for this work.

Presentation of lipid antigens by CD1

CD1 molecules are structurally related to MHC class I molecules and are non-covalently bound to β_2-microglobulin.

The genes encoding CD1 molecules are located outside the MHC and are not polymorphic. In humans, they consist of five closely linked genes, of which four are expressed (Fig. 5.19), encoding proteins that fall into two separate groups:

- group 1 molecules in humans include CD1a, CD1b, and CD1c;
- CD1d proteins form the second group.

Murine CD1b has been crystallized and analyzed by X-ray crystallography. This shows that the molecule has a deep electrostatically neutral antigen-binding groove, which is highly hydrophobic and can accommodate lipid or glycolipid

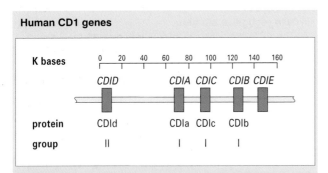

Human CD1 genes

Fig. 5.19 The genes of the human CD1 cluster extend over 160 kilobases on chromosome 1. A gene product for *CD1E* has not yet been identified.

antigens (see Fig. 5.w3). One model for the binding places hydrophobic acyl groups of the lipids into the large hydrophobic pockets, leaving the more polar groups of the antigens such as phosphate and carbohydrate on the top, where they can interact with the TCR.

The binding requirements of the hydrophobic pockets on CD1 are fairly tolerant because they will accommodate acyl groups of different lengths, but the interactions with the TCR are much more specific – small changes in the structure of the carbohydrate moiety will destroy the ability to stimulate a T cell.

The antigens presented by the group I CD1 molecules and CD1d are different. For example, group I molecules present lipoarabinomannan, a component of the cell wall of mycobacteria (see Fig. 14.1), whereas CD1d cannot do this.

Another difference between CD1 and conventional MHC molecules is the way in which antigen is loaded into the antigen-binding groove:

- MHC class I molecules are loaded with antigenic peptides in the endoplasmic reticulum, and this requires transport of the peptides from the cytoplasm (see Chapter 8).
- group I CD1 molecules appear to be loaded in an acidic endosomal compartment because they do not bind to lipid antigens unless they are partially unfolded at low pH.

There is some debate about the physiological functions of the CD1 molecules in host defense:

- group I CD1 molecules present lipids from mycobacteria and *Haemophilus influenzae* and can stimulate both $CD4^+$ and $CD8^+$ cytotoxic T cells, and therefore appear to have a role in antimicrobial defense.
- most CD1d molecules appear to bind self antigens, though they also present lipids from parasites such as *Plasmodium falciparum* and *Trypanosoma brucei* (see Chapter 15) to T cells that use a restricted group of TCRs, indicating a role in defense against single-celled protozoal parasites.

CRITICAL THINKING: SOMATIC HYPERMUTATION (SEE P. 434 FOR EXPLANATION)

1 Can you think of reasons why TCRs do not undergo somatic hypermutation?

The specificity of T cells (see p. 434 for explanation)

SM/J mice of the haplotype H-2^v were immunized with the λ repressor protein, a molecule with 102 amino acid residues. After 1 week, T cells were isolated from the animals and set up in culture with APCs and antigen. The ability of APCs to activate the T cells was determined in a lymphocyte proliferation assay.

It was found that when APCs from SM/J mice were used in the culture the T cells were activated, but that when APCs from Balb/c mice were used (H-2^d) they were not activated. APCs from F1 (SM/J•Balb/c) mice were able to activate the T cells just as well as the APCs from the parental SM/J strain.

2 Explain why the SM/J cells and the F1 cells can present antigen to the T cells, but the Balb/c cells cannot.

Using the primed T cells from the SM/J mouse and APCs from the same strain, the investigation continues, but peptides of the λ repressor protein are used instead of intact antigen. It is found that a peptide corresponding to residues 80–94 of the intact protein is able to stimulate the T cells, but that other peptides are much less effective or ineffective. The table below shows the sequences of some of these peptides and their ability to activate the T cells when included in the culture at a concentration of 10 μM.

Continued

CRITICAL THINKING: SOMATIC HYPERMUTATION (SEE P. 434 FOR EXPLANATION) CONT.

Peptide	Amino acid sequence	T cell activation
12–36	QLEDARRLKAIYEKKKNELGLSQESV	–
80–102	SPSIAREIYEMYEAVSMQPSLRS	+++
73–88	ILKVSVEEFSPSIAREIY	–
80–94	SPSIAREIYEMYEAVS	++
84–98	AREIYEMYEAVSMQP	–

3 Explain why peptides 80–102 and 80–94 activate the T cells while the others do not.

In a final experiment the T cells are stimulated with a mutated variant of peptide 80–94 with aspartate (D) substituted for isoleucine (I) at position 87 (bold type). It is found that the mutated peptide is able to stimulate the T cells as well as the original peptide, even when present at lower concentrations (1 μM).

4 What term is used to describe this kind of mutated peptide? What would you predict about the binding affinity of this peptide within the TCR–MHC–peptide complex?

Further reading

Bentley GA, Mariuzza RA. The structure of the T cell antigen receptor. Annu Rev Immunol 1996;14:563–590.

Bjorkman PJ, Parham P. Structure, function and diversity of class I major histocompatibility complex molecules. Annu Rev Biochem 1990;59:253–288.

Bjorkman PJ, Saper MA, Samraoui B, et al. The structure of the human class I histocompatibility antigen HLA-A2. Nature 1987;329:506–512.

Bjorkman PJ, Samraoui B, Bennett WS, et al. The foreign antigen binding site and T-cell recognition regions of class I histocompatibility antigens. Nature 1987;329:512–516.

Bodmer JG, Marsh SE, Albert ED, et al. Nomenclature for factors of the HLA system, 1994. Tissue Antigens 1994;44:1–18.

Brenner MB, MacLean J, Dialynas DP, et al. Identification of a putative second T-cell receptor. Nature 1986;322:145–149.

Brown JH, Jardetzky TS, Gorga JC, et al. Three-dimensional structure of the human class II histocompatibility antigen HLA-DR1. Nature 1993;364:33–39.

Burdin N, Kronenberg M. CD1-mediated immune responses to glycolipids. Curr Opin Immunol 1999;111:326–331.

Carosella ED, Dausett J, Kirzenbaum H. HLA-G revisited. Immunol Today 1996;17:407–409.

Chien Y-H, Jores R, Crowley MP. Recognition by γδ T cells. Annu Rev Immunol 1996;14:511–532.

Davis MM, Bjorkman PJ. T-cell antigen receptor genes and T-cell recognition. Nature 1988;334:395–402.

Davis MM, Boniface JJ, Reich Z, et al. Ligand recognition by αβ T cells. Annu Rev Immunol 1998;16:523–544.

Garcia KC, Degano M, Stanfield RL, et al. An αβ T cell receptor structure at 2.5Å and its orientation in the TCR–MHC. Complex Sci 1996;274:209–219.

Garcia KC, Teyton GL, Wilson IA. Structural basis of T cell recognition. Annu Rev Immunol 1999;17:369–398.

Garratt TPJ, Saper MA, Bjorkman PJ, et al. Specificity pockets for the side chains of peptide antigens in HLA-w68. Nature 1989;342:692–696.

Hass W, Pereira P, Tonegawa S. Gamma/delta cells. Annu Rev Immunol 1993;11:637–685.

Hayday AC. γδ cells: a right time and a right place for a conserved third way of protection. Annu Rev Immunol 2000;18:975–1026.

Hunkapiller T, Hood L. Diversity of the immunoglobulin gene superfamily. Adv Immunol 1989;44:1–63.

Lefranc M-P, Rabbitts TH. The human T-cell receptor γ (TRG) genes. Trends Biochem Sci 1989;14:214–218.

Leiden JM. Transcriptional regulation of T cell receptor genes. Annu Rev Immunol 1993;11:539–570.

Madden DR, Gorga JC, Strominger L, et al. The structure of HLA-B27 reveals nonamer self-peptides bound in an extended conformation. Nature 1991;353:321–325.

Manning TC, Kranz DM. Binding energetics of T-cell receptors: correlation with immunological consequences. Immunol Today 1999;20:417–422.

Porcelli SA, Segelke BW, Sugita M, et al. The CD1 family of lipid antigen-presenting molecules. Immunol Today 1998;19:362–368.

Powis SH, Trowsdale J. Human major histocompatibility complex genes. Behring Inst Mitt 1994;94:17–25.

Raulet DH. How γδ T cells make a living. Curr Biol 1994;4:246–251.

Roth DB. Generating antigen receptor diversity, 2005: In Lewin B, ed. Immunology module of Virtual Text, www.ergito.com Chapter 5.

Salter RD, Benjamin RJ, Wesley PK, et al. A binding site for the T-cell co-receptor CD8 on the α_3 domain of HLA-A2. Nature 1990;345:41–46.

San José E, Sahuquillo AG, Bragado R, Alarcón B. Assembly of the TCR/CD3 complex: CD3 epsilon/delta and CD3 epsilon/gamma dimers associate indistinctly with both TCR alpha and TCR beta chains. Evidence for a double TCR heterodimer model. Eur J Immunol 1998;28:12–21.

Sloan-Lancaster J, Allen PM. Altered peptide–ligand induced partial T cell activation: molecular mechanisms and role in T cell biology. Annu Rev Immunol 1996;14:1–27.

Stern LJ, Wiley DC. Antigenic peptide binding by class I and class II histocompatibility proteins. Structure 1994;2:245–251.

Stern LJ, Brown JH, Jardetzky TS, et al. Crystal structure of the human class II MHC protein HLA-DR1 complexed with an influenza virus peptide. Nature 1994;368:215–221.

Weiss A, Littman DR. Signal transduction by lymphocyte antigen receptor. Cell 1994;76:263–274.

Zeng ZH, Castaño LH, Segelke B, et al. The crystal structure of mouse CD1: an MHC-like fold with a large hydrophobic binding groove. Science 1997;277:339–345.

Internet references

HLA Nomenclature. Nomenclature for Factors of the HLA System. http://hla.alleles.org/nomenclature/updates/200911.html.

Modes of Immune Response

CHAPTER 6

Mechanisms of Innate Immunity

SUMMARY

- **Innate immune responses do not depend on immune recognition by lymphocytes, but have co-evolved with and are functionally integrated with the adaptive elements of the immune system.**

- **The body's responses to damage include inflammation, phagocytosis, and clearance of debris and pathogens, and remodeling and regeneration of tissues.** Inflammation is a response that brings leukocytes and plasma molecules to sites of infection or tissue damage.

- **The phased arrival of leukocytes in inflammation depends on chemokines and adhesion molecules expressed on the endothelium.** Adhesion molecules fall into families that are structurally related. They include the cell adhesion molecules (CAMs) of the immunoglobulin supergene family (which interact with leukocyte integrins), and the selectins (which interact with carbohydrate ligands).

- **Leukocyte migration to lymphoid tissues is also controlled by chemokines.** Chemokines are a large group of signaling molecules that initiate chemotaxis and/or cellular activation. Most chemokines act on more than one receptor, and most receptors respond to more than one chemokine.

- **Plasma enzyme systems modulate inflammation and tissue remodeling.** The kinin system and mediators from mast cells including histamine contribute to the enhanced blood supply and increased vascular permeability at sites of inflammation.

- **Pathogen-associated molecular patterns (PAMPs) or microbial-associated molecular patterns (MAMPs) are distinctive biological macromolecules that can be recognized by the innate immune system.** Innate antimicrobial defenses include molecules of the collectin, ficolin, and pentraxin families, which can act as opsonins, either directly or by activating the complement system. Macrophages have cell-surface scavenger-receptors and lectin-like receptors, which allow them to directly bind to pathogens and cell debris.

- **Toll like receptors (TLRs) are a family of receptors that recognize PAMPs from bacteria, viruses and fungi.** They are present on many cell types, and can activate macrophages, using signaling systems that are closely related to those used by inflammatory cytokines TNFα and IL-1.

- **Intracytoplasmic pattern recognition receptors (PRRS) recognize products of intracellular pathogens.** Receptors of the Nod family recognize bacterial products, while the RLH receptors can recognize products of viral replication.

Innate immune responses

The immune system deals with pathogens by means of a great variety of different types of immune response, but these can be broadly divided into:

- adaptive responses; and
- innate immunity.

The adaptive immune responses depend on the recognition of antigen by lymphocytes, a cell type that has evolved relatively recently – lymphocytes are present in all vertebrates, but not invertebrates, although lymphocyte-like cells are present in closely related phyla, including the tunicates and echinoderms (Fig. 6.1).

Q. What are the two key characteristics of adaptive immune responses?
A. They display a high level of specificity for the particular pathogen, and the responses show long-lasting memory.

Before the evolution of lymphocytes, and the emergence of specific antigen receptors (antibodies and the TCR), different types of immune defense were already present in precursor organisms. Many of these systems have been retained in vertebrates and have continued to evolve alongside the adaptive immune system. Hence, in present-day mammals we see an integrated immune system in which different types of defense work in concert.

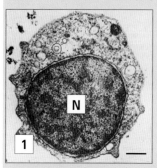
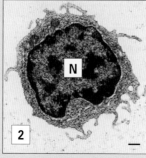

Electron micrographs of lymphocyte-like cells

Fig. 6.1 Electron micrographs of lymphocyte-like cells from the tunicate *Ciona intestinalis* (**1**), and from a fish, the blenny, *Blennius pholis* (**2**). Note the similar morphology – both cells have a large nucleus and a thin rim of undifferentiated cytoplasm. Scale bar 0.5 μm. (*Courtesy of Dr AF Rowley from Endeavour 1989;13;72–77. Copyright 1989 with permission from Elsevier.*)

In reality it is quite artificial to try to segregate adaptive and innate immune responses. For example a macrophage:

- displays the very primitive immune defense of phagocytosis; but also
- expresses MHC molecules and acts as an antigen-presenting cell, a function that makes sense only in relation to the evolution of T cells.

We can identify some of the ancient innate immune defense systems because related systems are seen in distant phyla. For example, the family of **Toll-like receptors (TLRs,** see Fig. 6.21) were first identified in insects. We can therefore infer that the distant ancestor of mammals and insects had a receptor molecule of this type that probably recognized microbial components.

Q. Why would it be a mistake to think that the immune system seen in insects or worms was the precursor of the immune system seen in present-day vertebrates
A. Both have evolved separately for millions of years. The immune systems of worms and insects have developed to cope with the pathogens that they encounter in the context of their life cycles.

Having stated how the functional distinction between adaptive and immune systems is essentially artificial, this chapter outlines some of the immune defenses that do not depend on immune recognition by lymphocytes.

Inflammation – a response to tissue damage

The body's response to tissue damage depends on:

- what has caused the damage;
- its location; and
- its severity.

In many cases damage can be caused by physical means, and does not involve infection or an adaptive immune response.

However, if an infection is present, the body's innate systems for limiting damage and repairing tissues work in concert with the adaptive immune responses. The overall process involves a number of overlapping stages, which typically take place over a number of days or weeks. These may include some or all of the following:

- stopping bleeding;
- acute inflammation;
- killing of pathogens, neutralizing toxins, limiting pathogen spread;
- phagocytosis of debris, pathogens, and dead cells;
- proliferation and mobilization of fibroblasts or other tissue cells to contain an infection and/or repair damage;
- removal or dissolution of blood clots and remodeling of the components of the extracellular matrix;
- regeneration of cells of the tissue and re-establishing normal structure and function.

Inflammation brings leukocytes to sites of infection or tissue damage

Many immune responses lead to the complete elimination of a pathogen (sterile immunity), followed by resolution of the damage, disappearance of leukocytes from the tissue and full regeneration of tissue function – the response in such cases is referred to as **acute inflammation**.

Q. What three principal changes occur in the tissue during an acute inflammatory response?
A. An increased blood supply to the affected area, an increase in capillary permeability allowing larger serum molecules to enter the tissue and an increase in leukocyte migration into the tissue (see Chapter 1).

In some cases an infection is not cleared completely. Most pathogenic organisms have developed systems to deflect the immune responses that would eliminate them. In this case the body often tries to contain the infection or minimize the damage it causes; nevertheless, the persistent antigenic stimulus and the cytotoxic effects of the pathogen itself lead to ongoing **chronic inflammation**.

The cells seen in acute and chronic inflammation are quite different, and reflect the phased arrival of different populations of leukocytes into a site of infection (Fig. 6.2). Consequently:

- sites of acute inflammation tend to have higher numbers of neutrophils and activated helper T cells; whereas
- sites of chronic inflammation have a higher proportion of macrophages, cytotoxic T cells, and even B cells.

The phased arrival of different populations of leukocytes at a site of inflammation is dependent on **chemokines** expressed on the endothelium (see below). These chemokines activate distinct leukocyte populations causing them to migrate into the tissue.

The cell types seen in sites of damage and the capacity of the tissue for repair and regeneration also depend greatly on the tissue involved. For example, in the brain the capacity for cell regeneration is very limited, so in chronic inflammatory diseases, such as multiple sclerosis, the area of damage often becomes occupied by scar tissue formed primarily by a specialized CNS cell type, the astrocyte.

The following sections explain the general principles of how inflammation develops, though the specific details depend on:

- the type of infection;
- the tissue; and
- the immune status of the individual.

The phased arrival of different populations of leukocytes into a site of infection

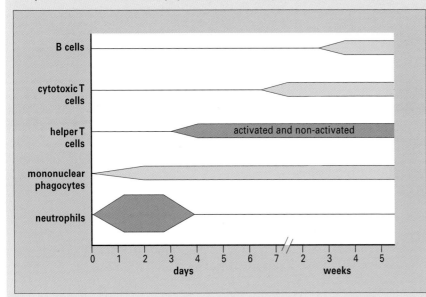

Fig. 6.2 Leukocytes enter sites of infection in phases. Sites of chronic inflammation have more macrophages and T cells.

Cytokines control the movement of leukocytes into tissues

Tissue damage leads to the release of a number of inflammatory cytokines, either from:

- patrolling leukocytes; or
- cells within the tissue, including resident mononuclear phagocytes.

The cytokines **tumor necrosis factor-α (TNFα)**, IL-1 and **interferon-γ (IFNγ)** are particularly important in this respect. TNFα is produced primarily by macrophages and other mononuclear phagocytes and has many functions in the development of inflammation and the activation of other leukocytes (Fig. 6.3). Notably, TNFα induces the adhesion molecules and chemokines on the endothelium, which are required for the accumulation of leukocytes. TNFα and the related cytokines, the **lymphotoxins**, act on a family of receptors causing the activation of the transcription factor **NF-κB** (Fig. 6.4), which has been described as a master-switch of the immune system. NF-κB is, in fact, a group of related transcription factors, which can also be activated by Toll-like receptors and IL-1. The activation of vascular endothelium by TNFα or IL-1 causes chemokine production and adhesion molecules to be expressed on the endothelial surface.

Once an immune reaction has developed in tissue, leukocytes generate their own cytokines (e.g. IFNγ, is produced by active Th1 cells), which also activate the endothelium and promote further leukocyte migration. The chemokines that are produced at the site depends on the type of immune response that is occurring within the tissue, and this in turn affects which leukocytes migrate into the tissue. This partly explains why different patterns of leukocyte migration and inflammation are seen in different diseases.

Leukocytes migrate across the endothelium of microvessels

The mechanisms that control leukocyte migration into inflamed tissues have been carefully studied because of their biological and medical importance. These mechanisms are also applicable in principle to the cell movement that occurs between lymphoid tissues during development and normal life.

The routes that leukocytes take as they move around the body are determined by interactions between:

- circulating cells; and
- the endothelium of blood vessels.

Leukocyte migration is controlled by signaling molecules, which are expressed on the surface of the endothelium, and occurs principally in venules (Fig. 6.5). There are three reasons for this:

- the signaling molecules and adhesion molecules that control migration are selectively expressed in venules;
- the hemodynamic shear force in the venules is relatively low, and this allows time for leukocytes to receive signals from the endothelium and allows adhesion molecules on the two cell types to interact effectively;
- the endothelial surface charge is lower in venules (Fig. 6.6).

Although the patterns of leukocyte migration are complex, the basic mechanism appears to be universal. The initial interactions are set out in a three-step model (Fig. 6.7):

- Step-1 leukocytes are slowed as they pass through a venule and roll on the surface of the endothelium before being halted – this is mediated primarily by adhesion molecules called **selectins** interacting with carbohydrates on glycoproteins;
- Step-2 the slowed leukocytes now have the opportunity to respond to signaling molecules held at the endothelial surface – particularly important is the large group of cytokines called **chemokines**, which activate particular populations of leukocytes expressing the appropriate chemokine receptors;
- Step-3 activation upregulates the affinity of the leukocytes' **integrins**, which now engage the cellular adhesion molecules on the endothelium to cause firm adhesion and initiate a program of migration.

TNFα is a cytokine with many functions

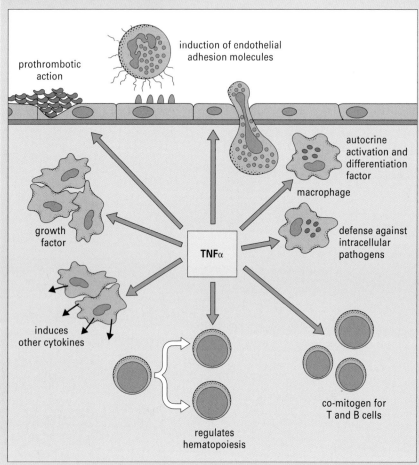

Fig. 6.3 TNFα has several functions in inflammation. It is prothrombotic and promotes leukocyte adhesion and migration (top). It has an important role in the regulation of macrophage activation and immune responses in tissues (center), and it also modulates hematopoiesis and lymphocyte development (bottom).

Transendothelial migration is an active process involving both leukocytes and endothelial cells (Fig. 6.8). Generally leukocytes migrate through the junctions between cells, but in specialized tissues such as the brain and thymus, where the endothelium is connected by continuous tight junctions, lymphocytes migrate across the endothelium in vacuoles, near the intercellular junctions, which do not break apart.

Migrating cells extend pseudopods down to the basement membrane and move beneath the endothelium using new sets of adhesion molecules. Enzymes are now released that digest the collagen and other components of the basement membrane, allowing cells to migrate into the tissue. Once there, the cells can respond to new sets of chemotactic stimuli, which allow them to position themselves appropriately in the tissue.

Leukocyte traffic into tissues is determined by adhesion molecules and signaling molecules

Intercellular adhesion molecules are membrane-bound proteins that allow one cell to interact with another. Often these molecules traverse the membrane and are linked to the cytoskeleton.

Q. Why is it important that cell adhesion molecules (CAMs) interact with the cytoskeleton?
A. By binding to the cytoskeleton the adhesion molecules allow a cell to gain traction on another cell or on the extracellular matrix, which allows the cell to move through tissues.

In many cases, a particular adhesion molecule can bind to more than one ligand, using different binding sites. Although the binding affinity of individual adhesion molecules to their ligands is usually low, clustering of the molecules in patches on the cell surface means that the avidity of the interaction can be high.

Cells can modulate their interactions with other cell types by increasing the numbers of adhesion molecules on the surface or altering their affinity and avidity. They can alter the level of expression of adhesion molecules in two ways:

- many cells retain large intracellular stores of these molecules in vesicles, which can be directed to the cell surface within minutes following cellular activation;
- alternatively, new molecules can be synthesized and transported to the cell surface, a process that usually takes several hours.

Intracellular signaling pathways induced by TNFα

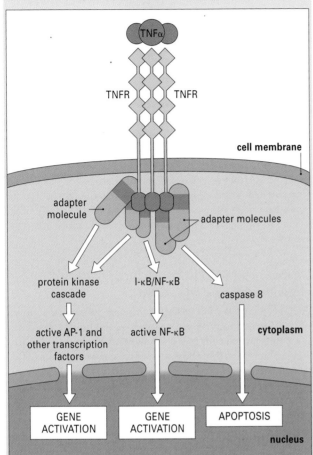

Fig. 6.4 TNFα induces the trimerization of the TNF receptor (TNFR), which causes adapter molecules to be recruited to the receptor complex. One pathway leads to the activation of caspase 8 and apoptosis. Other pathways lead to the activation of transcription factors AP1 and NF-κB, which activate many genes involved in adaptive and innate immune responses.

Leukocytes adhering to the wall of a venule

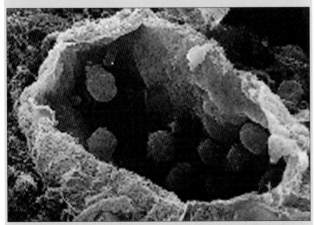

Fig. 6.5 Scanning electron micrograph showing leukocytes adhering to the wall of a venule in inflamed tissue. × 16 000. *(Courtesy of Professor MJ Karnovsky.)*

Leukocyte migration across endothelium

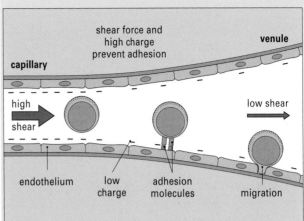

Fig. 6.6 Leukocytes circulating through a vascular bed may interact with venular endothelium via sets of surface adhesion molecules. In the venules, hemodynamic shear is low, surface charge on the endothelium is lower, and adhesion molecules are selectively expressed.

Three-step model of leukocyte adhesion

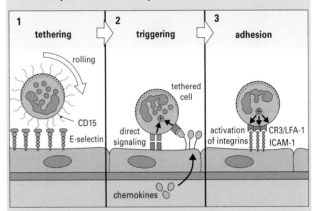

Fig. 6.7 The three-step model of leukocyte adhesion and activation is illustrated by a neutrophil, though different sets of adhesion molecules would be used by other leukocytes in different situations. (**1**) Tethering – the neutrophil is slowed in the circulation by interactions between E-selectin and carbohydrate groups on CD15, causing it to roll along the endothelial surface. (**2**) Triggering – the neutrophil can now receive signals from chemokines bound to the endothelial surface or by direct signaling from endothelial surface molecules. The longer a cell rolls along the endothelium, the longer it has to receive sufficient signal to trigger migration. (**3**) Adhesion – the triggering upregulates integrins (CR3 and LFA-1) so that they bind to ICAM-1 induced on the endothelium by inflammatory cytokines.

Selectins bind to carbohydrates to slow the circulating leukocytes

Selectins are involved in the first-step of transendothelial migration. The selectins include the molecules:

- E-selectin and P-selectin, which are expressed predominantly on endothelium and platelets; and
- L-selectin, which is expressed on some leukocytes (Fig. 6.9).

Lymphocyte migration

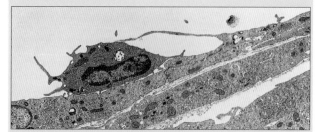

Fig. 6.8 Electron micrograph showing a lymphocyte adhering to brain endothelium close to the interendothelial cell junction in an animal with experimental allergic encephalomyelitis. Adhesion precedes transendothelial migration into inflammatory sites. *(Courtesy of Dr C Hawkins.)*

Selectins

carbohydrate ligands expressed on:		
platelets, endothelium, neutrophils	leukocytes	HEV, endothelium
EGF-R domain / CCP domain	lectin domain	
P-selectin platelet, endothelium	**E-selectin** endothelium	**L-selectin** leukocytes

Fig. 6.9 The structures of three selectins are shown. They have terminal lectin domains, which bind to carbohydrates on the cells listed. The EGF-R domain is homologous to a segment in the epidermal growth factor receptor. The CCP domains are homologous to domains found in complement control proteins, such as factor H, decay accelerating factor, and membrane cofactor protein.

Selectins are transmembrane molecules; their N terminal domain has lectin-like properties (i.e. it binds to carbohydrate residues), hence the name selectins. When tissue is damaged, TNFα or IL-1, induce synthesis and expression of E-selectin on endothelium. P-selectin acts similarly to E-selectin, but is held ready-made in the Weibel–Palade bodies of endothelium and released to the cell surface if the endothelium becomes activated or damaged. Both E-selectin and P-selectin can slow circulating platelets or leukocytes.

The carbohydrate ligands for the selectins may be associated with several different proteins:

- at sites of inflammation, E-selectin and P-selectin, which are induced on activated endothelium, bind to the sialyl Lewis-X carbohydrate associated with CD15, present on many leukocytes;

- some of the selectin ligands are selectively expressed on particular populations of leukocytes, for example the molecule PSGL-1 (P-selectin glycoprotein ligand) present on TH1 cells binds to E- and P-selectin, but a variant found on TH2 cells does not.

When selectins bind to their ligands the circulating cells are slowed within the venules. Video pictures of cell migration show that the cells stagger along the endothelium. During this time the leukocytes have the opportunity of receiving migration signals from the endothelium. This is a process of signal integration – the more time the cell spends in the venule, the longer it has to receive sufficient signals to activate migration. If a leukocyte is not activated it detaches from the endothelium and returns to the venous circulation. A leukocyte may therefore circulate many times before it finds an appropriate place to migrate into the tissues.

Chemokines and other chemotactic molecules trigger the tethered leukocytes

The chemokines are a group of at least 50 small cytokines involved in cell migration, activation, and chemotaxis. They determine which cells will cross the endothelium and where they will move within the tissue. Most chemokines have two binding sites:

- one for their specific receptors; and
- a second for carbohydrate groups on proteoglycans (such as heparan sulfate), which allows them to attach to the luminal surface of endothelium (blood side), ready to trigger any tethered leukocytes (Fig. 6.10).

The chemokines may be produced by the endothelium itself. This depends on several factors including:

- the tissue;
- the presence of inflammatory cytokines; and
- hemodynamic forces.

In addition chemokines produced by cells in the tissues can be transported to the luminal side of the endothelium, by the process of transcytosis. Immune reactions or events occurring within the tissue can therefore induce the release of chemokines, which signal the inward migration of populations of leukocytes.

Q. What advantage is there in having different types of inflammation occurring in different tissues?
A. What constitutes an appropriate immune response depends on the pathogen, the amount of damage it is causing in a particular tissue, and the capacity of that tissue to repair and regenerate.

Chemokines fall into four different families, based on the spacing of two conserved cysteine (C) residues. For example:

- α-chemokines have a CXC structure, where 'X' is any amino acid residue; and
- β-chemokines a CC structure, where the cysteines are directly linked.

A single chemokine CX3CL1 is produced as a cell surface molecule, and it doubles-up as an adhesion molecule.

Chemokines

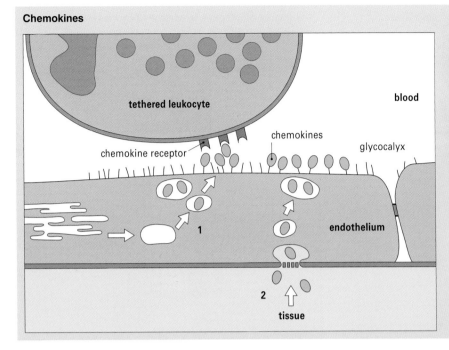

tethered leukocyte

blood

chemokine receptor

chemokines

glycocalyx

endothelium

1

2

tissue

Fig. 6.10 Chemokines bind to glycosaminoglycans on endothelium via one binding site while a second site interacts with chemokine receptors expressed on the surface of the leukocyte. Chemokines may be synthesized by the endothelial cell and stored in vesicles (Weibel–Palade bodies) to be released to the luminal surface (blood side) following activation (**1**). Alternatively chemokines may be produced by cells in the tissues and transported across the endothelium (**2**). Cells in the tissue can therefore signal either directly or indirectly to circulating leukocytes.

Chemokines receptors have promiscuous binding properties

All chemokines act via receptors that have seven transmembrane segments (**7tm receptors**) linked to GTP-binding proteins (**G-proteins**), which cause cell activation. There are also three non-signalling, scavenger receptors, which bind and clear chemokines, thereby helping to maintain chemotactic gradients.

Most chemokines act on more than one receptor, and most receptors will respond to several chemokines. Because of this complexity, it is easiest to understand what chemokines do by considering their receptors:

- the receptors for the CXC chemokines are called CXCR1, CXCR2, and so on; while
- the receptors for the CC chemokines are called CCR1, CCR2, etc.

Originally most chemokines had a descriptive name and acronym such as macrophage chemotactic protein-1 (MCP-1). The current nomenclature describes them according to their type, hence MCP-1 is CCL2, meaning that it is a **ligand** for the CC family of chemokine receptors (Fig. 6.11).

The chemokine receptors are selectively expressed on particular populations of leukocytes (see Fig. 6.11) and this determines which cells can respond to signals coming from the tissues. The profile of chemokine receptors on a cell depends on its type and state of differentiation. For example:

- all T cells express CCR1;
- TH2 cells preferentially express CCR3; and
- TH1 cells preferentially express CCR5 and CXCR3. After activation in lymph nodes, the levels of CXCR3 on a T cell increase, so that it becomes more responsive for the IFNγ-inducible chemokines CXCL9, CXCL10, and CXCL11, which activate CXCR3. As a consequence, antigen-activated lymphocytes are more readily triggered to enter sites of inflammation where these chemokines are expressed.

Other molecules are also chemotactic for neutrophils and macrophages

Several other molecules are chemotactic for neutrophils and macrophages, both of which have an f.Met-Leu-Phe (f.MLP) receptor. This receptor binds to peptides blocked at the N terminus by formylated methionine – prokaryotes (i.e. bacteria) initiate all protein translation with this amino acid, whereas eukaryotes do not.

Neutrophils and macrophages also have receptors for:

- C5a, which is a fragment of a complement component generated at sites of inflammation following complement activation; and
- LTB4 (leukotriene-B4), a product of arachidonic acid, which is generated at sites of inflammation, particularly by macrophages and mast cells.

In addition, molecules generated by the blood clotting system, notably fibrin peptide B and thrombin, attract phagocytes, though many molecules such as these only act indirectly by inducing chemokines.

The first leukocytes to arrive at a site of inflammation, if activated, are able to release chemokines that attract others. For example:

- CXCL8 released by activated monocytes can induce neutrophil and basophil chemotaxis;
- similarly, macrophage activation leads to release of LTB4.

All of these chemotactic molecules act via 7tm receptors which activate trimeric G-proteins.

Q. Which of the chemotactic molecules described above has a microbial-associated molecular pattern (MAMP)?
A. fMLP. It is the only molecule that comes from bacteria; all other chemotactic molecules are produced by cells of the body.

Some chemokine receptors and their principal ligands

	T H1	MØ	T H2	eosinophil	basophil	neutrophil
	(CCR1)	CCR1		(CCR1)	CCR1	(CCR1)
	CCR2	CCR2	CCR2	CCR2	CCR2	
	CCR5↔CCR5		CCR3↔CCR3↔CCR3			CXCR1
	CXCR3					CXCR2
CCL3	+	+		+	+	+
CCL4	+	+				
CCL5	+	+	+	+	+	+
CCL2	+	+	+	+	+	
CCL7,8	+	+	+	+	+	+
CCL13	+	+	+	+	+	
CCL11			+	+	+	
CXCL8						+
CXCL1,2,3						+
CXCL9,10,11	+					

Fig. 6.11 Some of the chemokine receptors found on particular leukocytes and the chemokines they respond to are listed. The cells are grouped according the principal types of effector response. Note that T H1 cells and mononuclear phagocytes both express chemokine receptor CCR5, which allows them to respond to chemokine CCL3, while T H2 cells, eosinophils, and basophils express CCR3, which allows them to respond to CCL11. This allows selective recruitment of sets of leukocytes into areas with particular types of immune/inflammatory response. Both groups of cells express chemokine receptors CCR1 and CCR2, which allow responses to macrophage chemotactic proteins (CCL2, CCL7, CCL8, and CCL13). Neutrophils express chemokine receptors CXCR1 and CXCR2, which allow them to respond to CXCL8 (IL-8) and CXCL1 and CXCL2. Bracketed entries indicate that only a subset of cells express that receptor.

The affinity of integrins is controlled by inside-out signaling

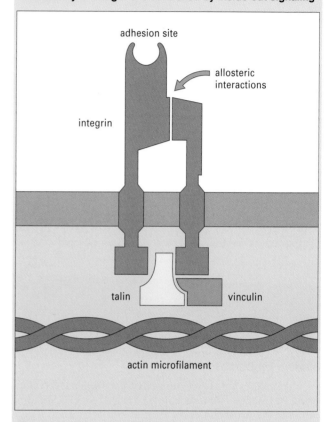

Fig. 6.12 Activation of the cell causes a change in the position of the two chains of the integrin, which become linked to the cytoskeleton via the adapter molecules vinculin and talin. The association produces an allosteric change in the extracellular portion of the molecule, causing the binding site to open and allowing the integrin to attach to its ligand.

Integrins on the leukocytes bind to CAMs on the endothelium

Activation of leukocytes via their chemokine receptors initiates the next stage of migration.

Leukocytes and many other cells in the body interact with other cells and components of the extracellular matrix using a group of adhesion molecules called integrins.

In the third step of leukocyte migration (see Fig. 6.7), the leukocytes use their integrins to bind firmly to cell-adhesion molecules (CAMs) on the endothelium. Leukocyte activation promotes this step in three ways:

- it can cause integrins to be released from intracellular stores;
- it can cause clustering of integrins on the cell surface into high-avidity patches;
- most importantly, the cell activation induced by the chemokines causes the integrins to become associated with the cytoskeleton and can switch them into a high-affinity form (Fig. 6.12) – this is referred to as 'inside-out signaling' because activation inside the cell causes a change in the position and affinity of the extracellular portion of the integrin.

Normally the binding affinity of integrins for the CAMs on the endothelium is relatively weak, but when sufficient interactions take place, the cells adhere firmly.

Many of the CAMs on the endothelium belong to the immunoglobulin superfamily. Some of them (e.g. ICAM-1 – intercellular adhesion molecule-1 and VCAM-1 – vascular cell adhesion molecule-1) are induced on endothelium at sites of inflammation, by inflammatory cytokines while others (e.g. ICAM-2) are constitutively expressed and not inducible (Fig. 6.13). Specific integrins bind to particular CAMs (Fig. 6.14), and since integrins vary between leukocytes and CAMs vary between endothelium in different tissues, the adhesion-step also affects which leukocytes will enter the tissue.

Expression and induction of endothelial adhesion molecules

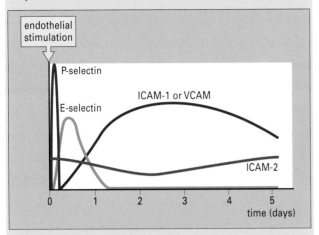

Fig. 6.13 The graph shows the time course of induction of different endothelial molecules on human umbilical vein endothelium in vitro following stimulation by TNFα.

Endothelial cell adhesion molecules

integrin ligands			
LFA-1 and CR3	LFA-1	VLA-4, LPAM-1	LPAM-1 = $\alpha_4\beta_7$
ICAM-1	ICAM-2	VCAM-1	MAdCAM-1
			endothelial cell

Fig. 6.14 The molecules ICAM-1, ICAM-2, VCAM-1, and MAdCAM-1 are illustrated diagrammatically with their immunoglobulin-like domains. Their integrin ligands (see Fig. 6.w1) are listed above. MAdCAM-1 also has a heavily glycosylated segment, which binds L-selectin.

Leukocyte migration varies with the tissue and the inflammatory stimulus

Although the 3-stage mechanism described above applies to all leukocyte migration, distinct patterns of leukocyte accumulation are seen in different sites of inflammation, depending on:

- the state of activation of the lymphocytes or phagocytes – the expression of adhesion molecules and their functional affinity vary depending on the type of cell and whether

it has been activated by antigen, cytokines, or cellular interactions. For example, activation of T cells induces both the chemokine receptor CXCR3, and the adhesion molecule LFA-1, which therefore promotes migration of activated cells into inflamed tissues.
- the types of adhesion molecule expressed by the vascular endothelium, which is related to its anatomical site and whether it has been activated by cytokines. For example: ICAM-1 is expressed at higher levels on brain endothelium than VCAM-1, whereas they are equally expressed on skin endothelium.
- the particular chemotactic molecules and cytokines present; receptors vary between leukocyte populations so that particular chemotactic agents act selectively.

Different chemokines cause different types of leukocyte to accumulate

In the second step of migration, neutrophils are triggered by chemokines such as CXCL8 synthesized by cells in the tissue, or by the endothelium itself. CXCL8 acts on two different chemokine receptors – CXCR1 and CXCR2 (see Fig. 6.11) – to initiate neutrophil migration.

In some tissues different sets of chemokines cause the local accumulation of other groups of leukocytes. For example:

- in the bronchi of individuals with asthma, CCL11 (eotaxin) is released, which causes the accumulation of eosinophils – CCL11 acts on CCR3, which is also present on TH2 cells and basophils, so by releasing one chemokine, the tissue can signal to three different kinds of cell to migrate into the tissue and this particular set of cells is characteristic of the cellular infiltrates in asthma;
- in sites of chronic inflammation, the chemokines CXCL10 and CCL2 are released by endothelium in response to IFNγ and TNFα – CXCL10 acts on activated TH1 cells (via CXCR3), while CCL2 acts on macrophages (via CCR5); consequently macrophages and TH1 cells tend to accumulate at sites of chronic inflammation.

> **Q. In what type of inflammatory reaction would you expect to see the production of CXCL10 and the accumulation of activated macrophages?**
> A. In chronic inflammatory reactions.

Preventing leukocyte adhesion can be used therapeutically

The importance of leukocyte adhesion has been pinpointed in a group of patients who have leukocyte adhesion deficiency (LAD) syndrome due to the absence of all β_2-integrins; they suffer from severe infections. The mechanism was confirmed by studies using antibodies to CR3 in experimental animals, which inhibit phagocyte migration into tissues.

A number of antibodies against adhesion molecules are now used therapeutically to treat inflammatory diseases. For example, antibodies against VLA-4 (the ligand for VCAM-1) are used to treat patients with multiple sclerosis, where the aim is to limit the migration of active T cells into the CNS.

Leukocyte migration to lymphoid tissues

Migration of leukocytes into lymphoid tissues is also controlled by chemokines and adhesion molecules on the endothelium.

Q. What is distinctive about the endothelium in secondary lymphoid tissues?

A. These tissues have high endothelial venules (HEVs) with columnar endothelial cells (see Figs. 2.53 & 2.54) that express high levels of sulfated glycoproteins and distinctive sets of adhesion molecules.

Up to 25% of lymphocytes that enter a lymph node via the blood may be diverted across the HEV. In contrast, only a tiny proportion of those circulating through other tissues will cross the regular venular endothelium at each transit. HEVs are therefore particularly important in controlling lymphocyte recirculation. Normally they are only present in the secondary lymphoid tissues, but they may be induced at sites of chronic inflammation.

In addition to their peculiar shape, HEV cells express distinct sets of heavily glycosylated sulfated adhesion molecules, which bind to circulating T cells and direct them to the lymphoid tissue.

The HEVs in different lymphoid tissues have different sets of adhesion molecules. In particular, there are separate molecules controlling migration to:

- Peyer's patches;
- mucosal lymph nodes; and
- other lymph nodes.

These molecules were previously called vascular addressins, and their expression on different HEVs partly explains how lymphocytes relocalize to their own lymphoid tissue.

Naive lymphocytes express L-selectin, which contributes to their attachment to carbohydrate ligands on HEVs in mucosal and peripheral lymph nodes. Once they have stopped on the HEV, migrating lymphocytes may use the integrin $\alpha_4\beta_7$ (LPAM-1, see Fig. 6.14) to bind to MAdCAM on the HEV of mucosal lymph nodes or Peyer's patches.

Because the expression of $\alpha_4\beta_7$ allows migration to mucosal lymphoid tissue, whereas $\alpha_4\beta_1$ allows attachment to VCAM-1 on activated endothelium or fibronectin in tissues, expression of one or other of these molecules can alternately be used by naive lymphocytes migrating to lymphoid tissue or by activated T cells migrating to inflammatory sites.

Chemokines are important in controlling cell traffic to lymphoid tissues

Chemokines are also important in controlling cell traffic to lymphoid tissues. Naive T cells express CXCR4 and CCR7, which allows them to respond to chemokines expressed in lymphoid tissues. Initially, they recognize CCL21 on the endothelium and subsequently CCL19 produced by dendritic cells, which is thought to direct them to the appropriate T cell areas of the lymph node where dendritic cells can present antigen to them.

Once T cells have been activated they lose CXCR4 and CCR7, but gain new chemokine receptors (see Fig. 6.11), which allow them to respond to chemokines produced at sites of inflammation.

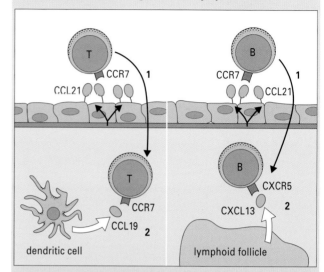

Chemokines and cell migration into lymphoid tissue

Fig. 6.15 Cell migration occurs in stages. Naive T cells express CCR7, which allows them to respond to CCL21 expressed by secondary lymphoid tissues (**1**). Once the cells have migrated across the endothelium, the same receptor can respond to signals from CCL19 produced by dendritic cells (**2**), which promotes interactions with the T cells in the paracortex (T cell area) of the lymph node. B cells also express CCR7 and use similar mechanisms to migrate into the lymphoid tissues (**1**). However, they also express CXCR5, which allows them to respond to CXCL13, a chemokine produced in lymphoid follicles (**2**) – B cells are therefore directed to the B cell areas of the node. Mice lacking CXCR5 do not develop normal lymphoid follicles.

Naive B cells express CCR7 and CXCR5, a receptor for CXCL13, which is required for localization to lymphoid follicles within the lymph nodes. A subset of T cells, which are required to help B cell differentiation, also express CXCR5 causing them to colocalize with B cells in lymphoid follicles. Cells moving into lymphoid tissue therefore respond sequentially to signals on the endothelium and signals from the different areas within the tissue (Fig. 6.15).

Mediators of inflammation

Increased vascular permeability is another important component of inflammation. However, whereas cell migration occurs across venules, serum exudation occurs primarily across capillaries where blood pressure is higher and the vessel wall is thinnest. This event is controlled in two ways:

- blood supply to the area increases;
- there is an increase in capillary permeability caused by retraction of the endothelial cells and increased vesicular transport across the endothelium – this permits larger molecules to traverse the endothelium than would ordinarily be capable of doing so, and so allows antibody and molecules of the plasma enzyme systems to reach the inflammatory site.

The four major plasma enzyme systems that have an important role in hemostasis and control of inflammation are the:

- clotting system;
- fibrinolytic (plasmin) system;
- kinin system; and
- complement system (see Chapter 4).

Activation of the kinin system

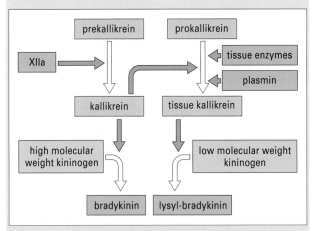

Fig. 6.16 Activated Hageman factor (XIIa) acts on prekallikrein to generate kallikrein, which in turn releases bradykinin from high molecular weight kininogen (HMWK). Prekallikrein and HMWK circulate together in a complex. Various enzymes activate prokallikrein to tissue kallikrein, which releases lysyl-bradykinin from low molecular weight kininogen. Bradykinin and lysyl-bradykinin are both extremely powerful vasodilators.

The plasmin system

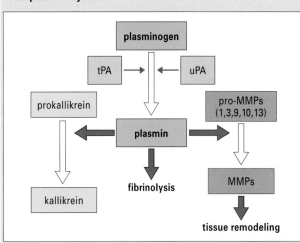

Fig. 6.17 Plasmin is generated by the enzymatic activity of plasminogen activators. (MMP, matrix metalloproteinase; tPA, tissue plasminogen activator; uPA, urokinase plasminogen activator.)

The kinin system generates powerful vasoactive mediators

The kinin system generates the mediators bradykinin and lysyl-bradykinin (kallidin). Bradykinin is a very powerful vasoactive nonapeptide that causes:

- venular dilation due to release of nitric oxide (NO);
- increased vascular permeability; and
- smooth muscle contraction.

Bradykinin is generated following the activation of Hageman factor (XII) of the blood clotting system, whereas tissue kallikrein is generated following activation of the plasmin system or by enzymes released from damaged tissues (Fig. 6.16).

The plasmin system is important in tissue remodeling and regeneration

The plasmin system can be activated by a soluble or a tissue-derived plasminogen activator, which leads to the enzymatic conversion of plasminogen into plasmin. Plasmin itself was originally identified by its ability to dissolve fibrin but it has several other activities, in particular it activates some matrix metalloproteases (MMPs), enzymes that are required for the breakdown and remodeling of collagen (Fig. 6.17). Additionally, it can promote angiogenesis (the formation of new blood vessels) by causing the release of cytokines that induce proliferation and migration of endothelial cells.

Mast cells, basophils and platelets release a variety of inflammatory mediators

Auxiliary cells, including mast cells, basophils, and platelets, are also very important in the initiation and development of acute inflammation. They act as sources of the vasoactive mediators

histamine and 5-hydroxytryptamine (serotonin), which produce vasodilation and increased vascular permeability.

Many of the proinflammatory effects of C3a and C5a result from their ability to trigger mast cell granule release, because they can be blocked by antihistamines. Mast cells and basophils are also a route by which the adaptive immune system can trigger inflammation – IgE sensitizes these cells by binding to their IgE receptors and the cells can then be activated by antigen. They are an important source of slow-reacting inflammatory mediators, including the leukotrienes and prostaglandins, which contribute to a delayed component of acute inflammation and are synthesized and act some hours after mediators like histamine, which are pre-formed and released immediately following mast cell activation.

Figure 6.18 lists the principal mediators of acute inflammation. The interaction of the immune system with complement and other inflammatory systems is shown in Figure 6.19.

Platelets may be activated by:

- immune complexes; or
- platelet activating factor (PAF) from neutrophils, basophils, and macrophages.

Activated platelets release mediators which are important in type II and type III hypersensitivity reactions (see Chapters 24 and 25).

Pain is associated with mediators released from damaged or activated cells

The substances released from damaged cells, mast cells and basophils are also important in producing the sensation of pain. Platelet activating factor (PAF), histamine, serotonin, prostaglandins and leukotrienes act on C-fibers which are responsible for the poorly localized, dull-aching pain associated with inflammation. Substance-P released from activated nerve fibers further contributes to the feeling of

Inflammatory mediators

mediator	main source	actions
histamine	mast cells, basophils	increased vascular permeability, smooth muscle contraction, chemokinesis
5-hydroxytryptamine (5HT – serotonin)	platelets, mast cells (rodent)	increased vascular permeability, smooth muscle contraction
platelet activating factor (PAF)	basophils, neutrophils, macrophages	mediator release from platelets, increased vascular permeability, smooth muscle contraction, neutrophil activation
IL-8 (CXCL8)	mast cells, endothelium, monocytes and lymphocytes	polymorph and monocyte localization
C3a	complement C3	mast cell degranulation, smooth muscle contraction
C5a	complement C5	mast cell degranulation, neutrophil and macrophage chemotaxis, neutrophil activation, smooth muscle contraction, increased capillary permeability
bradykinin	kinin system (kininogen)	vasodilation, smooth muscle contraction, increased capillary permeability, pain
fibrinopeptides and fibrin breakdown products	clotting system	increased vascular permeability, neutrophil and macrophage chemotaxis
prostaglandin E_2 (PGE$_2$)	cyclo-oxygenase pathway, mast cells	vasodilation, potentiates increased vascular permeability produced by histamine and bradykinin
leukotriene B_4 (LTB$_4$)	lipoxygenase pathway, mast cells	neutrophil chemotaxis, synergizes with PGE$_2$ in increasing vascular permeability
leukotriene D_4 (LTD$_4$)	lipoxygenase pathway	smooth muscle contraction, increasing vascular permeability

Fig. 6.18 The major inflammatory mediators that control blood supply and vascular permeability or modulate cell movement.

pain. Various types of mechanical and physical damage can all also lead to the release of these mediators from the tissue cells, resulting in pain.

Lymphocytes and monocytes release mediators that control the accumulation and activation of other cells

Once lymphocytes and monocytes have arrived at a site of infection or inflammation, they can also release mediators, which control the later accumulation and activation of other cells. For example:

- activated macrophages release the chemokine CCL3 and leukotriene-B$_4$, both of which are chemotactic and encourage further monocyte migration;
- lymphocytes can modulate later lymphocyte traffic by the release of chemokines and inflammatory cytokines, particularly IFNγ.

Q. What determines whether an immune response is acute or chronic?

A. Ultimately the outcome of an acute inflammatory response is related to the fate of the antigen. If the initiating antigen or pathogen persists, then leukocyte accumulation continues and a chronic inflammatory reaction develops. If the antigen is cleared then no further leukocyte activation occurs and the inflammation resolves.

In recurrent inflammatory reactions and in chronic inflammation the patterns of cell migration are different from those seen in an acute response. We now know that the patterns of inflammatory cytokines and chemokines vary over the course of an inflammatory reaction and this can be related to the successive waves of migration of different types of leukocyte into the inflamed tissue.

Chronic inflammation is characteristic of sites of persistent infection and occurs in autoimmune reactions where the antigen cannot ultimately be eradicated (see Chapter 20).

Pathogen-associated molecular patterns

Before the evolutionary development of B cells and T cells, organisms still needed to recognize and react against microbial pathogens. Hence, a variety of soluble molecules and cell surface receptors developed which were capable of recognizing distinctive molecular structures on pathogens. Such structures are called **pathogen-associated molecular patterns (PAMPs)** and the proteins which recognize them are **pattern recognition receptors (PRRs)**. Typical examples of PAMPs are carbohydrates, lipoproteins and lipopolysaccharide components of bacterial and fungal cell walls while some of the PRRs recognize the distinctive nucleic acids (e.g. dsRNA) formed during viral replication.

The immune system in acute inflammation

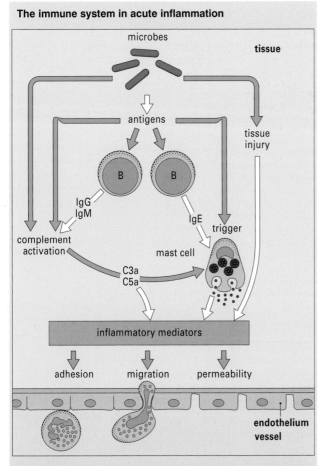

Fig. 6.19 The adaptive immune system modulates inflammatory processes via the complement system. Antigens (e.g. from microorganisms) stimulate B cells to produce antibodies including IgE, which binds to mast cells, while IgG and IgM activate complement. Complement can also be activated directly via the alternative pathway (see Fig. 4.4). When triggered by antigen, sensitized mast cells release their granule-associated mediators and eicosanoids (products of arachidonic acid metabolism, including prostaglandins and leukotrienes). In association with complement (which can also trigger mast cells via C3a and C5a), the mediators induce local inflammation, facilitating the arrival of leukocytes and more plasma enzyme system molecules.

Strictly speaking, many of these molecules are found on non-pathogenic organisms, so some authors prefer to call them **microbe-associated molecules patterns (MAMPs)**, and distinguish them from products of damaged cells, **damage-associated molecular patterns (DAMPs)**.

Many of the PRRs that evolved in invertebrates have been retained in vertebrates and work alongside the adaptive immune system to recognize pathogens. However, the importance of different PRRs often differs between different species of mammals.

There are three main types of PRR:

- secreted molecules, present in serum and body fluids;
- receptors, present on the cell surface and on endocytic vesicles; and
- intra-cytoplasmic recognition molecules.

The intra-cytoplasmic recognition molecules are particularly important for macrophage-mediated recognition of internalized pathogens. The functions of the secreted molecules and the cell surface receptors are explained below. They are divided into families according to structure.

Some of the secreted molecules are **acute phase proteins** (i.e. they are present in the blood and their levels increase during infection). Indeed the first of these molecules to be recognized was C-reactive protein, which can increase by more than 1000-fold in serum, during infection or inflammation. This protein has been used as a clinical marker of inflammation for more than 70 years.

PRRs allow phagocytes to recognize pathogens

In many cases, the innate recognition mechanisms allow phagocytes to bind and internalize the pathogens and this is often associated with activation of the phagocytes, which enhances their microbicidal activity.

The binding of the pathogen to the phagocyte can be direct or indirect:

- direct recognition involves the surface receptors on the phagocyte directly recognizing surface molecules on the pathogen;
- indirect recognition involves the deposition of serum-derived molecules onto the pathogen surface and their subsequent binding to receptors on the phagocyte (i.e. the process of opsonization) (Fig. 6.20).

Q. Give an example of an innate immune recognition system that allows macrophages to recognize and phagocytose bacteria

A. Complement C3b can become deposited on bacteria following activation of either the lectin pathway or the alternative pathway (see Fig. 4.4). The deposited C3b acts as an opsonin and is recognized by the receptors CR1, CR3, and CR4 on macrophages (see Fig. 4.12).

Opsonins come from a number of different families of proteins and include pentraxins, collectins and ficolins.

Phagocytes have receptors that recognize pathogens directly

Even in the absence of opsonins, phagocytes have a number of receptors that allow them to recognize PAMPs. These include:

- scavenger receptors;
- carbohydrate receptors;
- Toll-like receptors (TLRs).

The scavenger receptors and carbohydrate receptors are primarily expressed on mononuclear phagocytes, and will be described more fully in Chapter 7.

Q. Why do bacteria not just mutate their MAMPs so that they cannot be recognized by the innate immune system – after all, protein antigens of pathogens often mutate?

A. This is a difficult question because it requires deep insight into the evolutionary history of microbes, but many of the MAMPs are so fundamental to the structure of the bacterial or fungal cell walls that it is difficult to see how they could be altered without destroying the integrity of the microbe.

The binding of pathogen to the macrophage can be direct or indirect

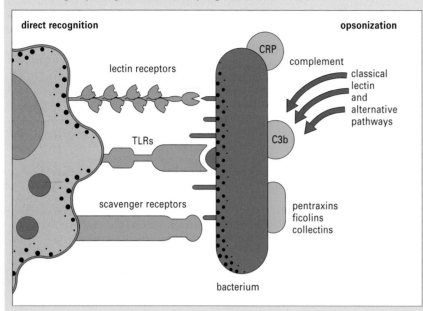

direct recognition

opsonization

CRP

complement

lectin receptors

classical
lectin
and
alternative
pathways

C3b

TLRs

scavenger receptors

pentraxins
ficolins
collectins

bacterium

Fig. 6.20 Macrophages can recognize PAMPs either directly or following opsonization with serum molecules.

Toll-like receptors

Receptor	Location	Ligand	Pathogen
TLR1	Cell surface	Lipopeptides	Gram-negative bacteria mycobacteria
TLR1/TLR2	Cell surface	Tri-acyl lipoprotein	Bacteria
TLR2	Cell surface	Lipoteichoic acid Lipoarabinomannan Zymosan Glycoinositol-phospholipids	Gram-positive bacteria Mycobacteria Fungi *T. cruzi*
TLR2/TLR6	Cell surface	Di-acyl lipoprotein	Bacteria
TLR3	Endosome or Cell surface	dsRNA	Viruses
TLR4	Cell surface	LPS	Gram-negative bacteria
TLR5	Cell surface	flagellin	Bacteria
TLR6	Cell surface	Di-acyl lipopeptides	Mycobacteria
TLR7	Endosome	ssRNA	Viruses
TLR8	Endosome	ssRNA	Viruses
TLR9	Endosome	Unmethylated CpG DNA	Bacteria

Fig. 6.21 Toll-like receptors recognize a variety of PAMPs. Gene duplication of the TLR precursor and divergence of function has led to a family of molecules capable of recognizing different types of pathogen.

Toll-like receptors activate phagocytes and inflammatory reactions

The transmembrane protein Toll was first identified in the fruit fly *Drosophila* as a molecule required during embryogenesis. It was also noted that mutants lacking Toll were highly susceptible to infections with fungi and Gram-positive bacteria, suggesting that the molecule might be involved in immune defence. Subsequently a series of Toll-like receptors (TLRs) was identified in mammals that had very similar intracellular portions to the receptor in the flies.

The intracellular signaling pathways activated by the TLRs and the receptor for IL-1 are very similar and lead to activation of the transcription factor NK-κB.

The family of TLRs include ten different receptors, in humans, many of which are capable of recognizing different microbial components (Fig. 6.21). All of the TLRs are present on phagocytic cells, and some are also expressed on dendritic cells, mast cells, and B cells. Indeed, most tissues of the body express at least one TLR.

Q. TLR5 is present on the basal surface of epithelia in the gut, but not on the apical surface. What consequence might this have for immune reactions in the gut?
A. Bacteria within the gut would not stimulate the cell, whereas any microbes that have invaded the epithelial layer may do so. This may explain why non-pathogenic commensal bacteria in the gut do not elicit an inflammatory reaction, whereas pathogenic bacteria that have invaded the tissue do.

Expression of many of the TLRs is increased by inflammatory cytokines (e.g. TNFα, IFNγ) and elevated expression is seen in conditions such as inflammatory bowel disease. The functional importance of the TLRs has been demonstrated in mouse strains lacking individual receptors. Depending on the TLR involved, such animals fail to secrete inflammatory cytokines in response to pathogens and the microbicidal activity of phagocytes is not stimulated. These results show that the TLRs are primarily important in activating phagocytes in addition to any role they may have in endocytosis. Occasionally humans are deficient in individual TLRs.

For example, TLR3 deficiency is associated with susceptibility to *Herpes simplex*, and a variant of TLR7 is associated with higher viral load and disease progression in HIV infection.

The TLRs make an important link between the innate and adaptive immune systems because their activation leads to the expression of co-stimulatory molecules on the phagocytes, which convert them into effective antigen-presenting cells. The binding of microbial components to the TLRs effectively acts as a danger signal to increase the microbicidal activity of the phagocytes and allows them to activate T cells.

CRITICAL THINKING: THE ROLE OF ADHESION MOLECULES IN T CELL MIGRATION (SEE P. 434 FOR EXPLANATIONS)

An experiment has been carried out to determine which CAMs mediate the migration of antigen-activated T cells across brain endothelium using a monolayer of endothelium overlaid with lymphocytes in vitro. The endothelium is either unstimulated or has been stimulated for 24 hours before the experiment with IL-1. In some cases the co-cultures were treated with blocking antibodies to different adhesion molecules. The results shown in the table below indicate the percentage of T cells that migrate across the endothelium in a 2-hour period.

Blocking antibody	Percentage of T cells migrating in 2 hours	
	Unstimulated endothelium	IL-1-stimulated endothelium
none	18	48
anti-ICAM-1	3	16
anti-VCAM-1	19	28
anti-$\alpha_L\beta_2$-integrin (LFA-1)	2	14
anti-$\alpha_4\beta_1$-integrin (VLA-4)	17	32

1 Why does treatment of the endothelium with IL-1 cause an increase in the percentage of migrating cells in the absence of any blocking antibody?

2 Why does it require 24 hours of treatment with IL-1 to enhance the migration (1 hour of treatment does not produce this effect)?

3 Which adhesion molecules are important in mediating T cell migration across unstimulated endothelium?

4 Which adhesion molecules are important in mediating T cell migration across IL-1-activated endothelium?

CHAPTER 7

Mononuclear Phagocytes in Immune Defense

SUMMARY

- **Macrophages: The 'big eaters'.** Macrophages are endowed with a remarkable capacity to internalize material through phagocytosis.

- **Macrophages differentiate from circulating blood monocytes and are widely distributed throughout the body.** Macrophages belong to the family of mononuclear phagocytes, which also comprise monocytes, osteoclasts, and dendritic cells. These cells share a common hematopoietic precursor that cannot differentiate into neutrophils. Phenotypically distinct populations of macrophages are present in each organ.

- **Macrophages are highly effective endocytic and phagocytic cells.** Macrophages have a highly developed endocytic compartment that mediates the uptake of a wide range of stimuli and targets them for degradation in lysosomes.

- **Macrophages sample their environment through opsonic and non-opsonic receptors.** Macrophages express a wide range of receptors that act as sensors of the physiological status of organs, including the presence of infection.

- **Clearance of apoptotic cells by macrophages produces anti-inflammatory signals.** Macrophages produce IL-10 and TGF-β upon internalization of apoptotic cells.

- **Macrophages coordinate the inflammatory response.** Recognition of necrotic cells and microbial compounds by macrophages initiates inflammation leading to the recruitment of neutrophils. Monocyte recruitment to sites of inflammation is promoted by activated neutrophils and there is a collaborative effort between macrophages and neutrophils to eliminate the triggering insult. Macrophages are actively involved in the resolution of the inflammatory reaction.

- **There are different pathways of macrophage activation.** TH1 cytokines such as IFNγ enhance inflammation and anti-microbial activity. TH2 cytokines induce an alternate activation that promotes tissue repair. TGFβ, corticosteroids and IL-10 can induce an anti-inflammatory phenotype.

Macrophages: the 'big eaters'

Macrophages are cells of hematopoietic origin widely distributed throughout lymphoid and non-lymphoid tissues. They are endowed with a remarkable capacity to internalize material through phagocytosis, which makes them key players in both homeostasis and immune defense. Macrophages clear approximately 2×10^{11} erythrocytes a day and are also implicated in the removal of cell debris and apoptotic cells, processes critical for normal development and physiology. The machinery mediating this homeostatic uptake also enables macrophages to recognize and internalize invading microorganisms, a process that facilitates clearance of infectious agents and elicits inflammation. Macrophages are highly heterogeneous and differentiate according to the environmental cues and physiological conditions present in tissues including the presence of microbes or cellular damage.

Macrophages differentiate from blood monocytes

Macrophages belong to the family of mononuclear phagocytes, which also comprise monocytes, osteoclasts, and dendritic cells. These cells share a common hematopoietic precursor that cannot differentiate into neutrophils or other cells of myeloid lineage. Monocytes circulate through the blood stream and are the precursors of macrophages in all tissues of the body, including secondary lymphoid organs even in the absence of an overt inflammatory stimulus. Monocytes may also develop into dendritic cells at sites of inflammation.

Monocytes are immune effector cells in their own right capable of detecting and internalizing pathogens and triggering inflammation. Recently, subpopulations of monocytes have been described in human and mouse blood. These subpopulations display differential expression of chemokine

Differentiation of mononuclear phagocytes

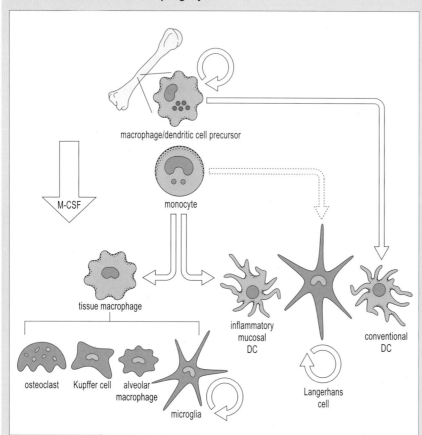

osteoclast   Kupffer cell   alveolar macrophage

microglia

tissue macrophage

M-CSF

monocyte

macrophage/dendritic cell precursor

inflammatory mucosal DC

Langerhans cell

conventional DC

Fig. 7.1 Mononuclear phagocytes and some dendritic cells differentiate from a precursor in the bone marrow. Differentiation into monocytes and tissue macrophages is driven by M-CSF. Inflammatory dendritic cells and Langerhans' cells also appear to belong to this lineage although Langerhans' cells may be directly bone-marrow derived. They are effective in presenting antigen to naive T cells. Some of the populations, indicated by a circular arrow, have some capacity for self renewal.

receptors and respond differently to stimulation indicating that they play distinct roles during inflammation with each subset implicated in either promotion or resolution of inflammation.

Within tissues the mononuclear phagocytes undergo maturation, adapt to their local microenvironment, and differentiate into various cell types (Fig. 7.1). Distinctive populations of resident macrophages are found in most tissues of the body; they differ in their life span, morphology, and phenotype, for example the microglial cells in the brain appear quite unlike mononuclear phagocytes in other tissues (Fig. 7.2). Resident cells have usually ceased to proliferate, but may remain as relatively long-lived cells, with low turnover, unlike neutrophils.

M-CSF is required for macrophage differentiation

Macrophage colony stimulating factor (M-CSF) is a major growth, differentiation, and survival factor, selective for monocytes and macrophages. It is produced constitutively by fibroblasts, stromal cells, endothelial cells, macrophages and smooth muscle. Most members of the mononuclear phagocyte family express the receptor for M-CSF, CD115 and mice deficient in M-CSF have major defects in different macrophage populations, including osteoclasts.

In contrast, granulocyte-macrophage colony stimulating factor (GM-CSF) primarily regulates myeloid cell production.

Microglia in mouse brain stained for F4/80

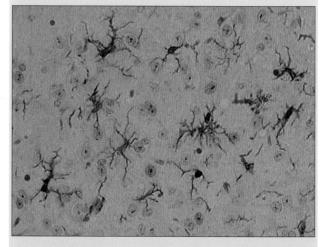

Fig. 7.2 Microglia are widely distributed in non-overlapping fields and show a dendritic morphology – mouse brain stained with antibody to F4/80. *(Courtesy of Dr Payam Rezaie.)*

It is only produced after cell activation and mice deficient in GM-CSF have no major defects in macrophage populations, with only the maturation of alveolar macrophage being altered leading to pulmonary alveolar proteinosis.

Differentiation and distribution of macrophages

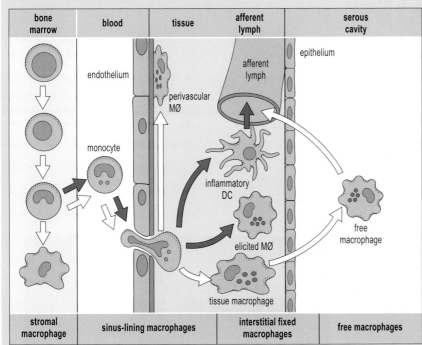

Fig. 7.3 Blood monocytes are derived from bone marrow and enter tissues initially as extravascular macrophages or tissue macrophages which may subsequently migrate into the serous cavities. At sites of inflammation monocytes may develop into elicited inflammatory macrophages or dendritic cells which can migrate through afferent lymph to the local lymph nodes. White arrows indicate recruitment during steady state conditions. Red arrows denote recruitment during inflammation.

The tissue environment controls differentiation of resident macrophages

It is possible to reconstruct a constitutive migration pathway in which monocytes become endothelial-like and line vascular sinusoids, as in the liver (Kupffer cells, see Fig. 2.3), or penetrate between endothelial cells. They underlie endothelia or epithelia or enter the interstitial space or serosal cavities (Fig. 7.3). The molecular mechanisms of constitutive macrophage distribution and induced migration are beginning to be defined, and involve cellular adhesion molecules, cytokines, and growth factors, as well as chemokines and chemokine receptors.

Mature macrophages are themselves part of the stromal microenvironment in bone marrow. They associate with developing hematopoietic cells to perform poorly defined non-phagocytic trophic functions, as well as removing effete cells and erythroid nuclei. In bone, osteoclasts, highly specialized multinucleated cells of monocytic origin, mediate bone resorption and their deficency leads to osteopetrosis.

Secondary lymphoid organs contain several distinct types of macrophages. These macrophages have been better characterized in the mouse (Fig. 7.4) and subsets involved in the clearance of apoptotic lymphocytes (tingible body macrophages) or presentation of naive antigens to B cells (subcapsular sinus macrophages) have been identified. Anatomical differences between human and mouse spleen, such as the absence of a well defined marginal sinus, correlates with phenotypical differences in splenic macrophages (see Fig. 7.4)

Macrophages can act as antigen-presenting cells

Although macrophages are often regarded as sessile cells, they readily migrate to draining lymph nodes after an inflammatory stimulus and become arrested there. They are therefore absent from efferent lymph and do not, as a rule, re-enter the circulation.

Q. Why is there no advantage for the immune system in the recirculation of macrophages, whereas recirculation of lymphocytes is a central element in immune defense?

A. Macrophages do not develop an immunological memory, and do not undergo the selective clonal expansion of antigen-stimulated lymphocytes that occurs in lymphoid tissues. Therefore there is no advantage in having macrophages return to the circulation from lymphoid tissues.

Macrophages, like dendritic cells, have all the machinery required for antigen processing and presentation of exogenous peptides and endogenous peptides on MHC class II and class I, respectively. Cross-presentation, a process by which peptides of exogenous origin are presented on MHC class I, also takes place in macrophages. While dendritic cells are uniquely suited for stimulating naive T cells in secondary lymphoid organs, macrophages present antigen in the periphery to activated (already primed) T cells. This interaction makes macrophages important effector cells during adaptive immunity (Fig. 7.5). The specialization of dendritic cells for antigen presentation correlates with a reduced degradative capacity that facilitates the generation of MHC-peptide complexes.

Macrophages act as sentinels within the tissues

Macrophages react to a wide range of environmental influences that help to fulfill their role as sentinels of the innate immune system (Fig. 7.6). The presence of cells within tissues with the potential to initiate inflammation through the release of cytokines and chemokines and to cause tissue damage through the production of reactive oxygen species

Macrophages in secondary lymphoid tissues

Fig. 7.4 Heterogeneity of macrophages in secondary lymphoid organs of mouse and human. (**1**) Red pulp of spleen stained for F4/80. Macrophages stain strongly positive. (**2**) Mouse spleen stained with antibody to sialoadhesin. The marginal metallophils of spleen are strongly sialoadhesin (CD169) positive. (**3**) Human spleen stained for CD68 and (**4**) immunofluorescence staining with anti-CD68 (green), and for the mannose receptor (red) indicates staining along sinusoids but most CD68+ macrophages lack the mannose receptor. Nuclei are stained blue. (*(1) Courtesy of Dr DA Hume. (2) Courtesy of Dr PR Crocker.*)

requires control systems capable of downmodulating macrophage activation. One of these systems involves the molecule CD200L, which is an inhibitory receptor expressed by myeloid cells. CD200L inhibitory signaling is triggered through interaction with CD200 expressed by non-hematopoietic cells as well as macrophages. The CD200–CD200L interaction is important for the control of macrophage activation by other cells present in tissues.

Phagocytosis and endocytosis

Soluble compounds are internalized by endocytosis

Macrophages play a key role in the clearance of altered forms of lipoproteins (e.g. acetylated lipoproteins) or glycoproteins (e.g. asialylated mannosylated proteins or proteins bearing advanced glycan products), damaged or apoptotic cells, pollutant particles and microbes. For this purpose, macrophages have a highly developed endocytic compartment that mediates the uptake of a wide range of stimuli and targets them for degradation in lysosomes. Soluble

Comparison of the functions of macrophages and dendritic cells

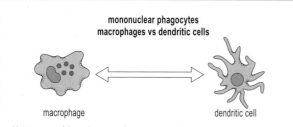

mononuclear phagocytes
macrophages vs dendritic cells

macrophage   dendritic cell

- Maintenance of tissue homeostasis
- Antigen presentation to activated T cells
- Effector cells during cell mediated immunity with enhanced microbicidal properties in the presence of IFNγ
- Key role in restoring tissue homeostasis after inflammation by clearing apoptotic neutrophils and promoting wound repair

- Antigen presentation to naïve T cells
- Modulation of T cell differentiation
- Poor lysosomal degradative capacity

Fig. 7.5 Comparison of the functions of macrophages and dendritic cells.

Macrophage phenotype and function

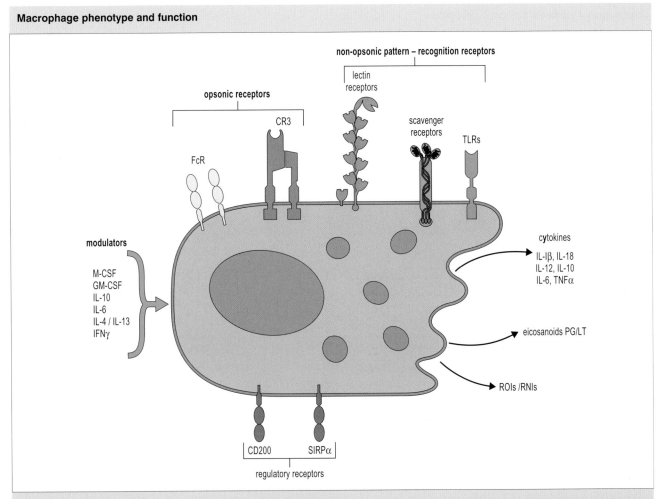

Fig. 7.6 Macrophage phenotype and function are modulated by the cytokines shown left. And they can sense their environment via opsonic receptors for antibody (FcR) and complement C3b (CR3) and via pattern-recognition receptors. They are also negatively regulated via CD200 and SIRPα (signal regulatory protein-alpha). Macrophages secrete cytokines and eicosanoids (prostaglandins and leukotrienes) and may release reactive oxygen and nitrogen intermediates (ROIs, RNIs) at sites of inflammation.

compounds are internalized through fluid phase or receptor-mediated endocytosis (see below) leading to the generation of vesicles called endosomes. Endosomes mature by fusing with different endocytic vesicles from the early and late endocytic compartments and finally the endocytosed material is targeted to lysosomes. This endosomal trafficking is also characterized by a reduction in the luminal pH which facilitates the action of acid hydrolases and degradation of the endosomal content.

Large particles are internalized by phagocytosis

Phagocytosis involves the uptake of particulate material (>0.5 µm) after recognition by opsonic or non-opsonic receptors (see Fig 7.6), its engulfment through the generation of pseudopodia and the formation of phagosomes. Phagosomes follow a similar maturation process to endosomes through the fusion with components of the early and late endocytic compartments so that maturing phagosomes sequentially adopt characteristics of early and late endosomes; this process culminates in the fusion of phagosomes to

lysosomes to form phagolysosomes (Fig. 7.7). Phagosomal maturation is accompanied by acidification of the lumen (from 6.1–6.5 in early phagosomes to 4.5 in phagolysosomes), which controls membrane traffic and has a direct effect on microbial growth. Other microbicidal mechanisms associated with phagosome maturation are the generation of reactive oxygen and nitrogen species and the presence of antimicrobial proteins and peptides.

Host cells control the phagocytic activity of macrophages by displaying the 'don't eat me' signal CD47. CD47 engages a receptor in macrophages called SIRPα that through its immunoreceptor tyrosine-based inhibitory motif (ITIM) motif inhibits the uptake process. CD47 expression by tumor cells has been proposed as an immunosurveillance escape mechanism.

Macrophages sample their environment through opsonic and non-opsonic receptors

Macrophages are endowed with a wide range of receptors that act as sensors of the physiological status of organs, including the presence of infection. These receptors can be

Phagocytosis mediated by opsonic receptors

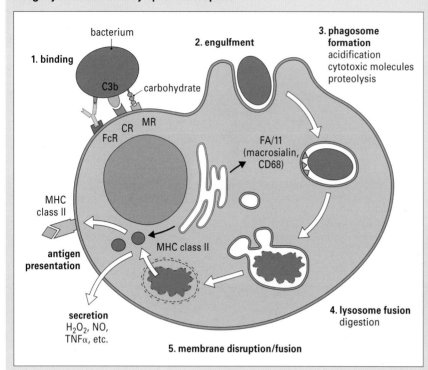

Fig. 7.7 (**1**) Pathogens, such as bacteria or fungi, are taken up by binding to opsonic receptors including the Fc receptor, complement receptors, and receptors for carbohydrate e.g. mannose receptor (MR) or dectin-1. (**2**) The particle is engulfed and the phagosome forms (**3**). Acidification of the phagosome follows as toxic molecules (reactive oxygen and nitrogen intermediates) are pumped into the phagosome. The marker CD68 is located in the phagosome membrane. (**4**) Lysosomes fuse with the phagosome, releasing proteolytic enzymes into the phagolysosome, which digest the pathogen. (**5**) On completion the membrane of the phagolysosome is disrupted. Antigenic fragments may become diverted to the acidic endosome compartment for interaction with MHC class II molecules and antigen presentation. The process induces secretion of toxic molecules and cytokines.

categorized as opsonic or non-opsonic depending on their capacity to interact directly with the stimuli or their need for a bridging molecule such as antibody or fragments of the complement component C3, which act as opsonins.

Opsonic receptors require antibody or complement to recognize the target

Bacteria opsonized by C3 fragments or antibody engage complement receptors (CR) or Fc receptors (FcR). CR-dependent phagocytosis is not an automatic process but requires additional stimulation such as inflammation. Monocytes and macrophages express a range of receptors (CR1, CR3, CR4) for C3 cleavage products that may become bound to pathogens, immune complexes or other complement activators. The role of CR3 role in regulated phagocytosis has been well studied, and the mechanism of CR3-mediated ingestion differs strikingly from that mediated by Fc receptors.

Q. What other function does CR3 have, unrelated to its role as an opsonic receptor?
A. CR3 is an adhesion molecule, which also has a role in cell migration by binding to ICAM-1 on endothelium or fibrinogen in the extracellular matrix (see Fig. 6.13).

FcRs belong to the immunoglobulin superfamily (see Fig. 3.17). The best characterized FcR is CD64 (FcγRI), the high affinity receptor for IgG which signals through the common γ chain that contains an immunoreceptor tyrosine based activation motif (ITAM). The common γ chain is also used by some non-opsonic receptors that bind carbohydrates (see below) and it signals through the key kinase

Syk. In humans other activating receptors for IgG are low affinity FcγRIIa (CD32) and FcγRIII (CD16), which require the recognition of immune complexes for inducing internalisation. IgG-opsonized material is readily internalized by macrophages and leads to the production of reactive oxygen species and cellular activation. The activating effect of ITAM-associated FcγRs is regulated by the presence of the inhibitory form of CD32 (FcγRIIb), which bears an ITIM.

The mechanism for ingestion of antibody-coated particles is distinct from that mediated by CR3 (Fig. 7.8). FcR-mediated uptake proceeds by a zipper-like process where sequential attachment between receptors and ligands guides pseudopod flow around the circumference of the particle. In contrast, CR3 contact sites are discontinuous for complement-coated particles which 'sink' into the macrophage cytoplasm. Small GTPases play distinct roles in actin cytoskeleton engagement by each receptor-mediated process.

The best characterized non-opsonic receptors are the Toll-like receptors (TLRs)

Non-opsonic receptors or pattern recognition receptors (PRRs) recognize unusual features characteristic of damaged, malfunctioning or infected tissues and their general characteristics are described in Chapter 6.

TLRs are membrane glycoproteins with an extracellular region responsible for ligand binding and a cytoplasmic domain responsible for triggering an intracellular signaling cascade. They can form hetero- or homo-dimers with each other or complex with other receptors in order to detect a wide range of microbial components. They are located at the cell surface or within endosomes. In humans there are 10 of

Zipper model of phagocytosis

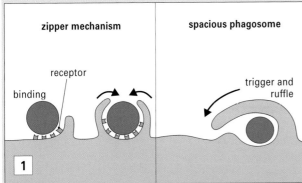

| zipper mechanism | spacious phagosome |

receptor

binding

trigger and ruffle

1

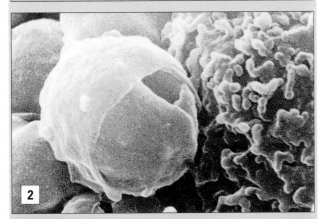

2

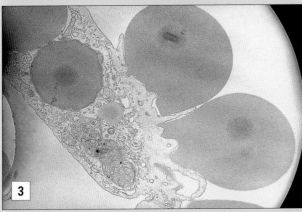

3

Fig. 7.8 (**1**) During phagocytosis, receptor–ligand interactions guide the extension of tightly apposed pseudopods around the particle's total circumference until a fusion of the plasma membrane occurs at the tip. This is known as the zipper mechanism. Alternative 'trigger' mechanisms, in which spacious phagosomes result from flipping over of ruffles back onto the plasma membrane, have also been described. The cytoskeleton of phagocytes plays a key role in engulfment, during which there is extensive remodeling of actin filaments. Some microorganisms and intracellular parasites induce novel mechanisms to recruit cell membranes during entry into phagocytes. (**2** and **3**) Electron micrographs of ingestion of antibody (IgG)-coated sheep erythrocytes by peritoneal macrophage by the zipper mechanism. (Scanning electron micrograph (**2**), courtesy of Dr GG MacPherson. Transmission electron micrograph (**3**), courtesy of Dr SC Silverstein.)

Activation of macrophages by lipopolysaccharide and IL-1

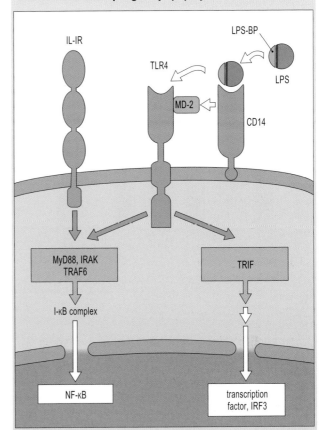

Fig. 7.9 LPS binds leukocyte CD14 (which is GPI-anchored to the membrane) through LPS binding protein (LPS-BP) and interacts with transmembrane TLRs, by transferring LPS to MD-2 to initiate signal transduction. Signaling pathways of the receptor share elements with the IL-1R pathway (e.g. IRAK – IL-1R-associated kinase). Cell activation proceeds via both the mitogen-activated protein (MAP) kinase pathways and the induction of NF-κB. (IL-1R, IL-1 receptor.)

these receptors and together they are able to recognize a wide range of microbes including Gram-positive bacteria and mycobacteria (see Fig. 6.20). For example, TLR4 detects Gram-negative bacteria because of its ability to recognize endotoxin. It then signals to the cell using similar systems to those mediated by IL-1 (Fig. 7.9). It can also activate the macrophage by a second pathway that is initiated by Trif, which leads to a secondary production of IFNβ and autocrine activation of additional macrophage genes.

CD14 is a GPI-linked membrane protein that facilitates the recognition of LPS by TLR4 so that it increases LPS sensitivity (see Fig. 7.9). Recently CD14 has also been shown to facilitate recognition of ligands by TLR2 and TLR3, which opens the possibility of CD14 acting as a multifunctional adaptor protein.

TLR4 also recognizes degraded extracellular matrix and the nuclear protein high mobility group 1 protein (HMGB1) which can be released by necrotic cells, an example of damage-associated molecules.

Class A and related scavenger receptors

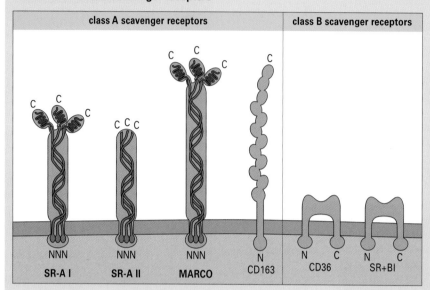

Fig. 7.10 Selected scavenger receptors are shown. Scavenger receptors of macrophages are responsible for the uptake of apoptotic cells, modified lipoproteins, and other polyanionic ligands (e.g. LPS and lipoteichoic acids [LTA]), as well as selected bacteria such as *Neisseria* spp. CD163 is involved in endocytosis of hemoglobin–haptoglobin complexes.

Lectin and scavenger receptors are non-opsonic receptors that recognize carbohydrates and modified proteins directly

In the plasma membrane, members of the scavenger receptor and lectin families mediate the recognition of modified lipoproteins and carbohydrates. Most of these receptors have signaling and internalisation motifs in their cytoplasmic region and are capable of mediating endocytosis and phagocytosis in isolation but their role is largely confined to the fine-tuning of TLR signaling.

Scavenger receptors (SR) (Fig. 7.10) such as **SR-A** are involved in LPS clearance, and may serve to downregulate responses induced via the TLR4-CD14 pathway (see Fig. 7.9) and therefore limit the systemic release of TNFα and resultant septic shock. SR-A has also been involved in bacterial uptake. Another member of this family, CD36, collaborates with TLR2 in the recognition of *S. aureus* and *M. tuberculosis*.

Dectin-1 (Fig. 7.11), a lectin with a single lectin-like domain and an intracellular ITAM-like motif, is highly specific for the fungi-derived compound β-glucan (Fig. 7.12). Dectin-1-mediated effects are largely mediated by the kinase, Syk and Card 9 Dectin-1 mediates phagocytosis of β-glucan particles and synergizes with TLRs to boost immune responses. It also has a role in Th cell differentiation and β-glucan treated dendritic cells promote the development of TH17 cells. Humans deficient in dectin-1 are more susceptible to mucosal candidiasis.

The mannose receptor (MR) may play a unique role in tissue homeostasis as well as host defense (see Fig. 7.11). Endogenous ligands include lysosomal hydrolases and myeloperoxidase. The N terminal cysteine-rich domain of the MR is a distinct lectin for sulfated glycoconjugates highly expressed in secondary lymphoid organs. The cysteine-rich domain also contributes to the clearance of hormones such as lutropin. MR can internalize collagen, which is recognized through the fibronectin type II domain and recent evidence suggests that MR promotes TH2 responses, which correlates

with its capacity to interact with multiple glycosylated allergens and secreted helminth products.

DC-SIGN, another mannose-binding C-type lectin (see Fig. 7.11), is expressed on some macrophages. It forms tetramers and lacks obvious signaling motifs at its cytoplasmic region. It has been implicated in interactions between APCs and T cells and in microbial recognition. DC-SIGN has been shown to modulate TLR signaling to promote transcription of various cytokine genes, particularly *IL-10* and *IL-8*.

Other lectin receptors are langerin and dectin-2, which have mannose specificity, and Mincle, which recognizes ligands expressed by necrotic cells in addition to fungal pathogens. Dectin-2 and Mincle (see Fig. 7.11) signal through the common γ-chain that also mediates signaling by the FcR CD64.

DCIR is the only single lectin receptor bearing an ITIM. Animals deficient in DCIR have altered DC numbers and increased susceptibility to autoimmune diseases.

Cytosolic receptors recognize intracellular pathogens

Cytosolic receptors include two families of molecules that recognize intracellular bacteria and viruses:

- the nucleotide binding and oligomerization domain (NOD)-like receptors (NLR) recognize, among others, bacterial compounds such as peptidoglycan; and
- the retinoic acid-inducible gene I (RIG-I)-like helicases (RLHs) recognize nucleic acids such as dsRNA which are produced during viral replication (Fig. 7.13).

Some of the NLRs form part of a multi-protein complex, the **inflammasome**, which is assembled in the cytoplasm and triggers inflammatory cell death (pyroptosis) of the infected cell. Pyroptosis causes release of cell contents and induces inflammation. Caspase I also processes the precursors of IL-1 and IL-18 to produce the active inflammatory cytokines. The composition of the inflammasome varies depending on the initiating stimulus as the NLRs responsible for the formation of the inflammasome complex are activated by different agents.

Lectin receptors

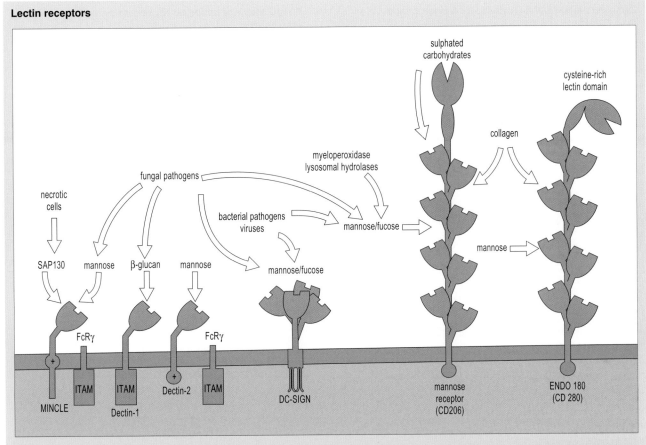

Fig. 7.11 The mannose receptor contains eight C-type lectin domains involved in binding to mannosylated carbohydrates and related glycoconjugates. It is related to a more broadly expressed endocytic receptor, ENDO 180. A distinct lectin domain located in the distal (C terminal) segment binds sulfated glycoconjugates. The β-glucan receptor (dectin-1) contains a single lectin domain and an intracellular immunoreceptor tyrosine-based activation motif (ITAM). Both dectin-2 and MINCLE recognize mannose and are associated with the common γ-chain that is associated with Fc receptors. DC-SIGN recognizes mannose and fucose through four associated lectin domains. '+' indicates charged amino acid residues.

The two RLH proteins RIG-1 and MDA5 both recognize RNA viruses, but they have different specificity. For example RIG-1 is important in recognition of influenza virus, whereas MDA5 recognizes polio virus. Both, RIG-1 and MDA-5 are involved in the recognition of Dengue virus. There are also cytosolic receptors able to recognize DNA.

Q. What other non-opsonic receptors can recognize products of viral replication?
A. The Toll-like receptors TLR3, TLR7 and TLR8 also recognize RNA molecules (see Fig. 6.20).

Functions of phagocytic cells

Clearance of apoptotic cells by macrophages produces anti-inflammatory signals

To maintain appropriate cell numbers during development, normal tissue homeostasis and pathological responses, cells die naturally by apoptosis, which involves activation of non-inflammatory caspases.

Q. Give an example in the immune system where macrophages phagocytose apoptotic cells.
A. Thymocytes that fail the processes of positive and negative selection die by apoptosis and are phagocytosed

by thymic macrophages (Chapter 2). Also B cells that die within lymphoid follicles are taken up by tingible body macrophages as described in Chapter 9.

Cellular and biochemical pathways resulting in apoptosis are conserved in evolution and apoptotic cells are rapidly and efficiently cleared by macrophages (Fig. 7.14), although they can also be engulfed by non-professional phagocytes. The appearance of phosphatidylserine (PS) in the outer leaflet of the plasma membrane is characteristic of apoptotic cells. PS recognition by PS-binding proteins stimulates the uptake of apoptotic cells and the production of anti-inflammatory mediators, especially TGFβ, which inhibit production of proinflammatory chemokines and cytokines.

There is redundancy in the receptors involved in apoptotic cell recognition. These include a range of scavenger receptors (SR-AI, CD36), T-cell immunoglobulin receptors (Tim) 3 and 4 and stabilin-2, and the complement component C1q which directly recognize the 'eat-me' signals displayed by the apoptotic cells.

Inefficient clearance of apoptotic cells may also contribute to autoimmune disorders such as systemic lupus erythematosus, and may explain their association with genetic deficiencies of complement components.

Zymosan particles phagocytosed by a macrophage

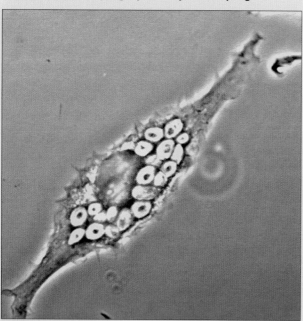

Fig. 7.12 The micrograph shows zymosan (yeast) particles phagocytosed by a macrophage, a process dependent on dectin-1. Truncation of the cytoplasmic tail prevents phagocytosis.

Phagocytosis of apoptotic thymocyte by thymic macrophage

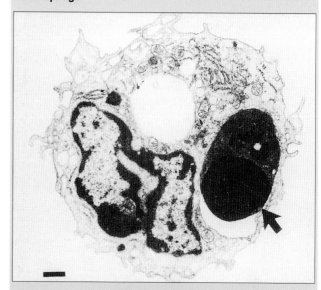

Fig. 7.14 Thymic macrophages phagocytose the large numbers of thymocytes that die by apoptosis during T cell development. The arrow indicates the nucleus of a phagocytosed thymocyte.

Intracellular PRRs

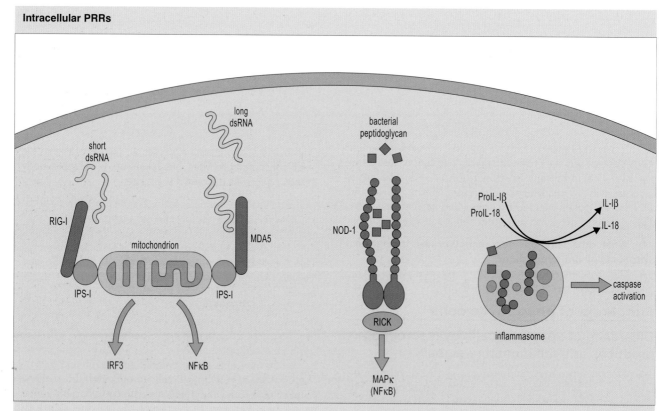

Fig. 7.13 Viral nucleic acids are recognized by RIG-1 and MDA-5, which assemble with the adapter protein IPS-1 onto the mitochondrial outer membrane and activate the transcription factors IRF3 and NFκB, which induce genes involved in inflammation. Bacterial peptidoglycans are detected by NOD-1 and NOD-2, which signal through RICK to activate NFκB and the MAP-kinase pathway. Molecules of this type form inflammasomes that can lead to the induction of caspases and production of IL-1β and, IL-18.

Secretory products of macrophages

category	example	function
low molec-ular weight metabolites	reactive oxygen intermediates reactive nitrogen intermediates eicosanoids – prostaglandins, leukotrienes platelet-activating factor (PAF)	killing, inflammation killing, inflammation regulation of inflammation clotting
cytokines	IL-1β, TNFα, IL-6 IFNα/IFNβ IL-10 IL-12, IL-18 TGFβ CCL2, CCL3, CCL4, CCL5, CXCL8	local and systemic inflammation antiviral, innate immunity, immunomodulation deactivation of MØ, B cell activation IFNγ production by NK and T cells repair, modulation, inflammation chemokines
adhesion molecules	fibronectin thrombospondin	opsonization, matrix adhesion, phagocytosis of apoptotic cells
complement	C3, all others	local opsonization
procoagulant	tissue factor	clotting cascade
enzymes	lysozyme urokinase (plasminogen activator) collagenase elastase	Gram-positive bacterial lysis fibrinolysis matrix catabolism matrix catabolism

Fig. 7.15 Macrophages produce a wide range of secreted molecules.

Macrophages coordinate the inflammatory response

Recognition of necrotic cells and microbial compounds by macrophages initiates inflammation

In contrast to the recognition of apoptotic cells, uptake of microbial products and necrotic cells by resident macrophages promotes cellular activation leading to the production of secreted molecules (Fig. 7.15). Recognition of PAMPS and molecules from damaged cells through PRRs leads to the activation of the NFκB pathway (see Fig. 7.w4) and the production of cytokines and chemokines. The activation of cytosolic phospholipase A2 causes the release of arachidonic acid, the precursor of prostaglandins and leukotrienes, through the actions of the cyclooxygenase and lipoxygenase pathways, respectively. Proinflammatory prostaglandins control blood flow and vascular dilation and permeability at sites of inflammation. Trafficking of lymphocytes and neutrophils into tissues is induced by leukotriene-B4 (see Figs. 6.17 & 6.18).

Resident macrophages recruit neutrophils to inflammatory sites

Neutrophils are the first cells recruited to the site of inflammation and play a key role in elimination of the inflammatory insult (Fig. 7.16). Appropriate neutrophil recruitment is essential for successful resolution of the inflammatory response as deficiencies in the clearance of the triggering stimuli will result in chronic inflammation and tissue dysfunction (Fig. 7.17). Although macrophages and neutrophils share the capacity to mediate phagocytosis and intracellular killing, there are key differences between them:

- neutrophils are short lived, store a wide range of antimicrobial polypeptides in intracellular granules and readily produce oxygen radicals;
- resident macrophages are long lived, less microbicidal and cytotoxic, and display a higher degree of specificity which makes them better suited as sentinels of the immune system.

Activated tissue macrophages produce chemokines CXCL5 and CXCL8 that promote neutrophil recruitment (see Fig. 7.16) and neutrophil extravasation is also promoted through proteolytic cleavage of chemokines by metalloproteases (MMP8 and MMP9), which enhance their chemotactic activity. The primary role of neutrophils in a wound is to eliminate invading pathogens. To aid this goal recruited neutrophils that fail to encounter bacteria in a short period of time will soon release their microbicidal compounds leading to the liquefaction of tissue and the formation of pus. Tissue destruction facilitates bacterial clearance by eliminating collagen fibrils that limit cellular movement.

Monocyte recruitment to sites of inflammation is promoted by activated neutrophils

There is a transition from neutrophil recruitment to monocyte influx that is prompted by the shedding of IL6Rα from the surface of neutrophils after activation. sIL6Rα complexed with IL6, produced by macrophages and endothelial cells, is recognized by gp130 on endothelial cells leading to the expression of VCAM-1 (a ligand for the integrin VLA-4 expressed by monocytes) and CCL2.

The role of mononuclear phagocytes in inflammation

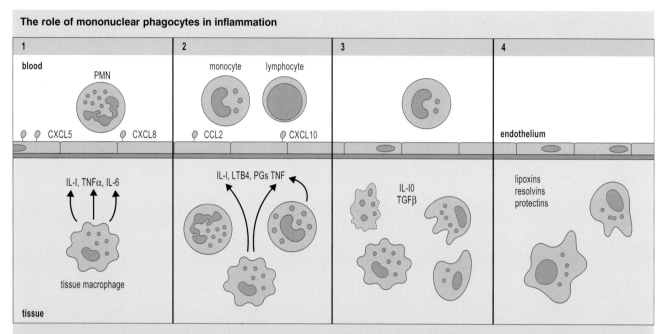

Fig. 7.16 (1) Tissue-resident macrophages respond to injury by the release of IL-1, TNFα and IL-6, which attract neutrophils from the blood. (2) As the inflammatory reaction develops the release of leukotrienes, prostaglandins and chemokines attracts monocytes and lymphocytes. (3) As the inflammation resolves dead neutrophils are phagocytosed by mononuclear phagocytes and the profile of cytokines switches towards production of IL-10 and TGFβ. (4) The production of lipoxins, protectins and resolvins is associated with restoration of normal function, and termination of the inflammatory response.

Crohn's disease

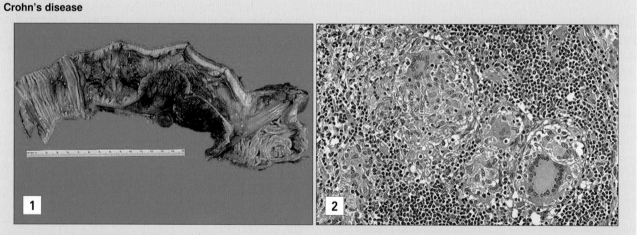

Fig. 7.17 A section of the gut wall from a patient with Crohn's disease, showing the intense inflammation of the tissue (1). The histological section shows a granulomatous reaction with lymphocyte and macrophage infiltration and the formation of giant cells (2).

Q. What effect will the expression of VCAM-1 and CCL2 have at a site of inflammation?

A. VCAM-1 is an adhesion molecule that binds to the integrin VLA-4 expressed on some monocytes and lymphocytes. CCL2 is a chemokine that attracts monocytes by its interaction with CCR2. Their expression will therefore enhance monocyte and lymphocyte transendothelial migration.

Shedding of IL6Rα by neutrophils is also induced by apoptosis. Additionally, serine proteases released by neutrophils are capable of modifying chemokines to increase their affinity for CCR1 and promote the recruitment of inflammatory monocytes.

Macrophages and neutrophils have complementary microbicidal actions

Macrophages and neutrophils complement each other in the clearance of pathogens. Following extravasation neutrophils release preformed proteins stored in granules, in three phases:

- secretory vesicles loaded with membrane-bound receptors are mobilized to the plasma membrane;
- secondary and tertiary granules containing lactoferrin, lipocalin, lysozyme and LL37 are released. These granules also contain matrix metalloproteases MMP-8, -9 and -25, that digest extracellular matrix and facilitate tissue destruction;

Oxygen-dependent microbicidal activity

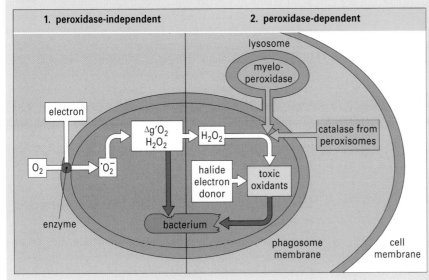

Fig. 7.18 **(1)** An enzyme (NADPH oxidase) in the phagosome membrane reduces oxygen to the superoxide anion ($^{\bullet}O_2^-$). This can give rise to hydroxyl radicals ($^{\bullet}OH$), singlet oxygen ($\Delta g'O_2$), and hydrogen peroxide (H_2O_2), all of which are potentially toxic. Lysosome fusion is not required for these parts of the pathway, and the reaction takes place spontaneously following formation of the phagosome. **(2)** If lysosome fusion occurs, myeloperoxidase (or, under some circumstances, catalase from peroxisomes) acts on peroxides in the presence of halides (preferably iodide). Then additional toxic oxidants, such as hypohalites (HIO, HClO), are generated.

- primary or azurophilic granules containing defensins (see below) and myeloperoxidase are released – myeloperoxidase converts H_2O_2 to hypochlorous acid which reacts with amines to produce anti-bacterial chloramines (Fig. 7.18).

The defensins are a group of highly cationic polypeptides which contribute to antibacterial activities. The defensins:

- are small peptides (30–33 amino acids) found in some macrophages of many species and specifically in human neutrophils, where they comprise up to 50% of the granule proteins;
- form ion-permeable channels in lipid bilayers and probably act before acidification of the phagolysosome;
- are able to kill a range of pathogens, including bacteria (*S. aureus, Pseudomonas aeruginosa, E. coli*), fungi (*Cryptococcus neoformans*), and enveloped viruses (*Herpes simplex*).

Q. What other molecule can generate ion-permeable channels in lipid bilayers?
A. The final component of the lytic complement pathway, C9 (see Chapter 4).

The primary granules also contain BPI (LPS-binding bactericidal permeability increasing protein) and serprocidins that include 3 serine proteases which in addition to their microbicidal activity, cause tissue destruction.

Cytosolic and nuclear components of neutrophils can also contribute to antimicrobial activity – chromatin from neutrophils forms extracellular nets that associate with proteases from the azurophil granules.

Phagocytes kill pathogens with reactive oxygen and nitrogen intermediates

Phagocytes mediate microbial killing through a wide range of mechanisms including acidification of the phagosome, through the formation of a H^+ ion gradient by V-ATPase. Acidification has direct microbicidal activity and facilitates the action of enzymes that have acidic pH optima.

Additionally the H^+ ion gradient facilitates the extrusion of nutrients needed by the microbes.

Macrophages and neutrophils can also kill pathogens by secreting highly toxic reactive oxygen intermediates (ROIs) and reactive nitrogen intermediates (RNIs) into the phagosome (see Fig. 7.18). The NOX2 NADPH oxidase located at the phagosomal membrane generates ROIs and this property is most prominent in neutrophils. This oxidase transfers electrons from cytosolic NADPH to molecular oxygen releasing O_2^- into the lumen. ROIs can interact with macromolecules (for instance through sulfur groups) rendering them inactive. Patients with chronic granulomatous disease lacking essential oxidase components suffer from repeated bacterial infections.

One major difference between resting and activated macrophages is the ability to generate hydrogen peroxide (H_2O_2), and other metabolites generated by the respiratory burst. Whereas neutrophils are readily endowed with microbicidal properties, macrophages require activation through the engagement of activating PRRs, reaching maximal microbicidal activity in the presence of IFNγ, which triggers classical activation (see below). Failure of macrophage activation in AIDS contributes to opportunistic pathogen infections and persistence of HIV, as well as reactivation of latent tuberculosis.

Q. Some people have a defect in the type-2 IFN receptor – the condition is very rare. What effect do you think it would have on their resistance to different types of pathogen?
A. It makes them very susceptible to infection by intracellular bacteria.

Macrophages can also be activated by IFNγ to express high levels of **inducible nitric oxide synthase (i-NOS, NOS2)**, which catalyzes the production of nitric oxide (NO) from arginine (Fig. 7.19). ROIs and RNIs can interact to produce peroxynitrites and these reactive species all act within the phagosome to cause toxic effects on intraphagosomal pathogens; they interact with thiols, metal centers and tyrosines,

The nitric oxide pathway

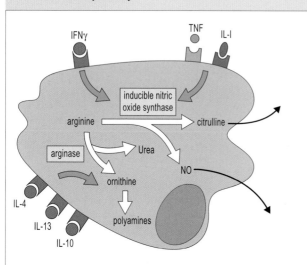

Fig. 7.19 IFNγ and other inflammatory cytokines cause production of inducible nitric oxide synthase (i-NOS, also known as NOS2) which combines oxygen with guanidino nitrogen of L-arginine to give nitric oxide (NO•), which is toxic for bacteria and tumor cells. Toxicity may be increased by interactions with products of the oxygen reduction pathway, leading to the formation of peroxynitrites. Cell activation by TH2-type cytokines promotes breakdown of arginine to ornithine and urea. Polyamines are products of ornithine which promote collagen synthesis and cell proliferation.

damaging nucleic acids and converting lipids through oxidative damage. In this way bacterial metabolism and replication are impaired.

Q. Describe four roles of IFNγ in the development of the immune response, each modulating a different group of cells.

A. IFNγ induces MHC molecules and co-stimulatory molecules on APCs, and induces adhesion molecules and chemokines on endothelium. It also activates macrophage microbicidal activity, modulates class switching by B cells (see Chapter 9), and regulates the balance between TH1 and TH2 populations of T cells. It has some capacity to induce production of anti-viral proteins.

Another mechanism that limits bacterial growth involves the sequestration of key nutrients by lactoferrin (Fe^{2+}) or NRAMP1, which extrudes Fe^{2+}, Zn^{2+} and Mn^{2+} from the lumen. Additionally, phagosomes contain endopeptidases, exopeptidases, and hydrolases, which break down the pathogens. The proteases are delivered by different granules at different stages during the maturation of the phagosome.

Some pathogens avoid phagocytosis or escape damage

Some pathogens have developed elaborate mechanisms to evade killing within phagosomes. These include the escape of the bacteria from the phagosome (*Listeria monocytogenes*), promotion of fusion to the endoplasmic reticulum

(*Legionella*) and inhibition (*M. tuberculosis*) or delay (*C. burnetii*) of phagosome maturation. This will depend on the mechanism used for internalization; while direct recognition of the pathogen through non-opsonic receptors has limited activating capacity and enables the pathogen to exploit particular escape mechanisms, internalization of antibody-coated pathogens leads to enhanced cellular activation and triggering of microbicidal mechanisms. Macrophages once activated through PRRs such as TLRs induce autophagy which mediates degradation of vacuolar *M. tuberculosis* and *Toxoplasma gondii*. Autophagy is also used by macrophages to sequester and degrade cytosolic pathogens such as *Francisella tularensis* and *Salmonella enterica*.

Resolution of inflammation by macrophages is an active process

Complete removal of the inflammatory trigger initiates the resolution of inflammation, in which neutrophil infiltration stops and apoptotic neutrophils are phagocytozed. A key event in this process is 'lipid mediator class-switch' in which prostaglandin and leukotriene synthesis is replaced by the synthesis of **lipoxins**, **resolvins** and **protectins** (see Fig. 7.16). Intriguingly, the signaling pathways leading to the proinflammatory prostaglandins E2 and D2, synthesized early during inflammation, also lead to the transcription of the enzyme responsible for lipoxin synthesis. Lipoxin synthesis by neutrophils occurs through their interaction with platelets and epithelial cells that provide metabolic precursors through a process called **transcellular biosynthesis**. In the case of macrophages, lipoxin synthesis is triggered by uptake of apoptotic cells. Lipoxin A4 reduces neutrophil activity, increases the migration of monocytes, favors uptake of apoptotic neutrophils and inhibits the synthesis of CXCL8. Resolvin E1 and protectin D1 increase the expression of CXCR5 on the surface of apoptotic neutrophils which facilitates clearance of CXCL3 and CXCL5 (neutrophil chemoattractants) from the inflammatory site. Apoptotic neutrophils produce 'find me' signals (e.g. lysophosphatidylcholine) that attract macrophages. Uptake of these neutrophils by macrophages inhibits production of IL-23, a cytokine involved in promoting granulopoiesis. As described above, recognition of apoptotic cells by macrophages also leads to the production of the anti-inflammatory cytokines IL-10 and TGFβ that together with factors such as vascular endothelial growth factor promote tissue repair.

Different pathways of macrophage activation

Previous sections have hinted at the capacity of macrophages to adapt to their surroundings (i.e. macrophages in different anatomical compartments display distinct phenotypes and resident macrophages have lower microbicidal activity compared to recruited macrophages, even after activation). Study of the phenotype of macrophages exposed in culture to different combinations of cytokines further illustrated the plasticity of these cells. Broadly, macrophages can follow classical (M1) or alternative (M2) activation profiles though it is possible to encounter intermediate phenotypes:

- M1 activation refers to macrophages with enhanced microbicidal activity that can be generated in culture by

Modulation of macrophage activation

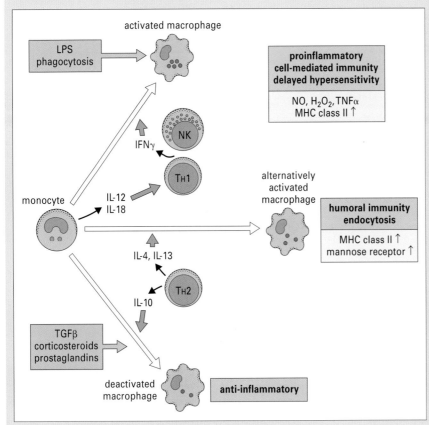

Fig. 7.20 Signals from microbial products, phagocytosis, and cytokines result in changes to the surface and secretory properties of macrophages, which can be classified as activated, deactivated, or alternatively activated. (NO, nitric oxide; TGFβ, transforming growth factor-β.)

treating with selected TLR ligands or pathogens in the presence (classical activation) or absence (innate activation) of IFNγ;

- M2 activation generally refers to macrophages exposed to IL-4 or IL-13 although within the spectrum of M2 activation, macrophages with a regulatory phenotype can also be obtained in response to immunocomplexes and TLR engagement (Fig. 7.20).

Major attempts are being made to correlate the phenotypes observed *in vitro* with patterns of differentiation *in vivo* through the analysis of signature markers, some of them having been identified during parasite infection in mice (Fig. 7.21). Classical activation appears to be consistent with the role of macrophages as effector cells during the course of cell-mediated immune responses where IFNγ produced by TH1 T cells will enable the elimination of intracellular pathogens by macrophages (see above). Additionally M1 macrophages promote TH1 responses by producing IL-12, and secreting CXCL9 and CXCL10 which selectively recruit TH1 T cells.

Macrophages treated with IL-4 and IL-13 have a more developed endocytic compartment, produce reduced levels of proinflammatory cytokines and IL-12, increased levels of IL-10 and the decoy receptor IL1RA and can recruit Tregs and TH2 cells, eosinophils and basophils through the production of CCL17, CCL22 and CCL24, thereby amplifying TH2-type responses. M2 macrophages are less efficient in producing ROIs and RNIs. In these cells arginine is processed into ornithine and polyamines through activation

of arginase. Arginase activity has been proposed as a way of controlling T cell activation (see Fig. 7.19).

In the absence of T cells, other cells at the site of injury collaborate to modulate the phenotype of macrophages. For example, natural killer cells activated by TNF-α and IL-12 produced by macrophages will synthesize IFNγ and under certain conditions, mast cells or early recruited eosinophils will produce IL-4 at sites of inflammation.

While the damaging effects of unregulated classical activation are widely illustrated and mediate the pathology of autoimmune diseases, examples of M2-like activation under selective pathological processes have also been described. For example, chronic exposure to LPS, leads to a state of tolerance that has been associated with immunosuppression during sepsis and is considered a state of M2 activation.

There are numerous reports of a role for M2 in parasitic disease models where they exert a regulatory, protective role probably due to their capacity to promote tissue repair. Interestingly, some microbes (e.g. *Francisella tularensis*) exploit the reduced microbicidal activity of M2 macrophages and alter the macrophage activation profile towards this path in order to minimize bacterial killing. Tumor-associated macrophages have also been shown to often display a M2-like phenotype, which promotes tumor survival through their capacity to produce IL-10 and angiogenic mediators.

The macrophage has so many functions in normal physiology and immune defense that it is not surprising that macrophage phenotypes vary both with location in the tissues and in response to cytokines produced in different types of inflammation.

Regulation of macrophage phenotype

	TH1 type	TH2 types		significance
	IFNγ	**IL-4/IL-13**	**IL-10**	
MHC class II molecule (Ia)	++	+	−	immune cell interactions
respiratory burst NO	++ ++	(−) (−)	− −	cell-mediated immunity tissue injury (e.g. tuberculosis)
TNFα IL-1 IL-6	++	(−)	−	proinflammatory
mannose receptor	−	++	+	phagocytosis/endocytosis (e.g. antigens)
growth	−	++	0	local growth of MØ in immune lesions
fusion	0	++	0	giant cell formation–granulomas
growth factor secretion	−	++	+	healing of lesions

Fig. 7.21 TH1 and TH2 cytokines act on macrophages to induce distinctive functions, which can be described classical 'activation' (TH1-type), 'alternative activation', or deactivation (TH2-type). (+, increase; −, decrease; 0, no effect.)

CRITICAL THINKING: THE ROLE OF MACROPHAGES IN TOXIC SHOCK SYNDROME (SEE P. 435 FOR EXPLANATIONS)

In an experimental model of septic shock, mice are infected systemically with bacille Calmette–Guérin (BCG), a non-lethal vaccine strain of mycobacteria. After 12 days, the mice are challenged intraperitoneally with graded doses of lipopolysaccharide (LPS). Blood samples are taken at 2 hours and the clinical condition of the mice is monitored for up to 24 hours. Experiments are terminated earlier if mice show severe signs of distress.

1 What cytokines would you measure in the 2-hour serum sample?

2 What clinical signs would be indicative of incipient septic shock?

3 What mechanisms contribute to septic shock?

4 What outcome would you expect if the following knockout mouse strains were used instead of wild-type controls: CD14, scavenger receptor class A (SR-A), IFNγ?

5 Interpret your results.

6 Suggest further experiments.

7 What is the clinical significance of this experiment?

The distinction between inflammatory responses and housekeeping of apoptotic cells

Mouse peritoneal macrophages are fed a meal of apoptotic cells in culture, and then challenged with an intracellular pathogen, *Trypanosoma cruzi*. Subsequent single cell analysis of parasite survival shows that *T. cruzi* growth is enhanced by prior uptake of apoptotic cells, but not of necrotic cells or control particles.

8 How would you investigate the macrophage surface receptors responsible for apoptotic cell uptake?

9 Suggest a possible mechanism by which apoptotic cell uptake promotes *T. cruzi* survival.

10 How would you investigate this experimental model?

11 What is the possible in vivo and clinical significance of this observation?

The role of macrophages in TH1 and TH2 responses

Isolated mouse peritoneal macrophages are treated for 2 days with selected cytokines (IFNγ, IL-4, IL-13, IL-10) in culture and a range of assays for cell activation is employed. It is found that IFNγ enhances the respiratory burst (after LPS challenge), MHC class II expression, and proinflammatory cytokine production, but downregulates mannose receptor (MR)-mediated endocytosis. IL-10 is an efficient antagonist of the above effects. IL-4 and IL-13 are weak antagonists of respiratory burst and proinflammatory cytokine production and markedly induce MHC class II molecules and MR activity.

12 Interpret the significance and possible functional relevance of these results in relation to concepts of TH1/TH2 differentiation.

13 What further work could be done to investigate the possibility that macrophage activation could by analogy be classified as M1/M2?

14 How would you investigate the role of macrophages and dendritic cells as possible inducers of CD4+ T cell subset differentiation?

Further reading - reviews

Allen J, Wynn T. Evolution of TH2 immunity: a rapid repair response to tissue destructive pathogens. PLOS Pathogens 2011;7:e1002003.

Auffray C, Sieweke MH, Geissmann F. Blood monocytes: development, heterogeneity, and relationship with dendritic cells. Annu Rev Immunol 2009;27:669–692.

Bergsbaken T, Fink SL, Cookson BT. Pyroptosis: host cell death and inflammation. Nat Rev Microbiol 2009;7:99–109.

Biswas SK, Lopez-Collazo E. Endotoxin tolerance: new mechanisms, molecules and clinical significance. Trends Immunol 2009;30:475–487.

Biswas SK, Mantovani A. Macrophage plasticity and interaction with lymphocyte subsets: cancer as a paradigm. Nat Immunol 2010;11:889–896.

Burdette DL, Monroe KM, Sotelo-Troha K, et al. STING is a direct innate immune sensor of cyclic di-GMP. Nature 2011;478: 515–518.

Elliott MR, Ravichandran KS. Clearance of apoptotic cells: implications in health and disease. J Cell Biol 2010;189:1059–1070.

Flannagan RS, Cosio G, Grinstein S. Antimicrobial mechanisms of phagocytes and bacterial evasion strategies. Nat Rev Microbiol 2009;7:355–366.

Geijtenbeek TB, Gringhuis SI. Signalling through C-type lectin receptors: shaping immune responses. Nat Rev Immunol 2009;9:465–479.

Geissmann F, Gordon S, Hume DA, et al. Unravelling mononuclear phagocyte heterogeneity. Nat Rev Immunol 2010;10:453–460.

Geissmann F, Manz MG, Jung S, et al. Development of monocytes, macrophages, and dendritic cells. Science 2010;327:656–661.

Gordon S, Martinez FO. Alternative activation of macrophages: mechanism and functions. Immunity 2010;32:593–604.

Hamilton JA. Colony-stimulating factors in inflammation and autoimmunity. Nat Rev Immunol 2008;8:533–544.

Hampton MB, Kettle AJ, Winterbourn CC. Inside the neutrophil phagosome: oxidants, myeloperoxidase, and bacterial killing. Blood 1998;92:3007–3017.

Hornung V, Latz E. Intracellular DNA recognition. Nat Rev Immunol 2010;10:123–130.

Kerrigan A, Brown GD. Syk-coupled C-type lectins in immunity. Trends Immunol 2011;32:151–156.

Lawrence T, Gilroy DW. Chronic inflammation: a failure of resolution? Int J Exp Pathol 2007;88:85–94.

Levine B, Mizushima N, Virgin HW. Autophagy in immunity and inflammation. Nature 2011;469:323–335.

Martinez FO, Helming L, Gordon S. Alternative activation of macrophages: an immunologic functional perspective. Annu Rev Immunol 2009;27:451–483.

Mosser DM, Edwards JP. Exploring the full spectrum of macrophage activation. Nat Rev Immunol 2008;8:958–969.

Nathan C. Neutrophils and immunity: challenges and opportunities. Nat Rev Immunol 2006;6:173–182.

Nathan C. Ding A. Nonresolving inflammation. Cell 2010;140:871–882.

Nguyen KD, Qiu Y, Cui X, et al. Alternatively activated macrophages produce catecholamines to sustain adaptive thermogenesis. Nature 2011;480:104–109.

Olefsky JM, Glass CK. Macrophages, inflammation, and insulin resistance. Annu Rev Physiol 2010;72:219–246.

O'Neill LA, Bowie AG. The family of five: TIR-domain-containing adaptors in Toll-like receptor signalling. Nat Rev Immunol 2007;7:353–364.

O'Neill LA, Bowie AG. Sensing and signaling in antiviral innate immunity. Curr Biol 2010;20:R328–R333.

Peiser L, Mukhopadhyay S, Gordon S. Scavenger receptors in innate immunity. Curr Opin Immunol 2002;14:123–128.

Ray K, Marteyn B, Sansonetti PJ, Tang CM. Life on the inside: the intracellular lifestyle of cytosolic bacteria. Nat Rev Microbiol 2009;7:333–340.

Robinson MJ, Sancho D, Slack EC, et al. Myeloid C-type lectins in innate immunity. Nat Immunol 2006;7:1258–1265.

Schroder K. Tschopp J. The inflammasomes. Cell 2010;140:821–832.

Serhan CN, Savill J. Resolution of inflammation: the beginning programs the end. Nat Immunol 2005;6:1191–1197.

Serhan CN, Yacoubian S, Yang R. Anti-inflammatory and proresolving lipid mediators. Annu Rev Pathol 2008;3:279–312.

Soehnlein O, Lindbom L. Phagocyte partnership during the onset and resolution of inflammation. Nat Rev Immunol 2010;10:427–439.

Soehnlein O, Lindbom L, Weber C. Mechanisms underlying neutrophil-mediated monocyte recruitment. Blood 2009;114:4613–4623.

Taylor PR, Gordon S, Martinez-Pomares L. The mannose receptor: linking homeostasis and immunity through sugar recognition. Trends Immunol 2005;26:104–110.

Taylor PR, Martinez-Pomares L, Stacey M, et al. Macrophage receptors and immune recognition. Annu Rev Immunol 2005;23:901–944.

Vieira OV, Botelho RJ, Grinstein S. Phagosome maturation: aging gracefully. Biochem J 2002;366:689–704.

Woodward JJ, Iavarone AT, Portnoy DA. c-di-AMP secreted by intracellular *Listeria monocytogenes* activates a host type I interferon response. Science 2010;328:1703–1705.

Selected references

Emara M, Royer PJ, Abbas Z, et al. Recognition of the major cat allergen Fel d 1 through the cysteine-rich domain of the mannose receptor determines its allergenicity. J Biol Chem 2011;286:13033–13040.

Ferwerda B, Ferwerda G, Plantinga TS, et al. Human dectin-1 deficiency and mucocutaneous fungal infections. N Engl J Med 2009;361:1760–1767.

Heinsbroek SE, Taylor PR, Martinez FO, et al. Stage-specific sampling by pattern recognition receptors during Candida albicans phagocytosis. PLoS Pathog 2008;4:e1000218.

Krausgruber T, Blazek K, Smallie T, et al. IRF5 promotes inflammatory macrophage polarization and TH1-TH17 responses. Nat Immunol 2011;12:231–238.

LeibundGut-Landmann S, Gross O, et al. Syk- and CARD9-dependent coupling of innate immunity to the induction of T helper cells that produce interleukin 17. Nat Immunol 2007;8:630–638.

Liu Y, Stewart KN, Bishop E, et al. Unique expression of suppressor of cytokine signaling 3 is essential for classical macrophage activation in rodents in vitro and in vivo. J Immunol 2008;180:6270–6278.

Pesce JT, Ramalingam TR, Mentink-Kane MM, et al. Arginase-1-expressing macrophages suppress Th2 cytokine-driven inflammation and fibrosis. PLoS Pathog 2009;5:e1000371.

Royer PJ, Emara M, Yang C, et al. The mannose receptor mediates the uptake of diverse native allergens by dendritic cells and determines allergen-induced T cell polarization through modulation of IDO activity. J Immunol 2010;185:1522–1531.

Satoh T, Takeuchi O, Vandenbon A, et al. The Jmjd3-Irf4 axis regulates M2 macrophage polarization and host responses against helminth infection. Nat Immunol 2010;11:936–944.

Smith AM, Rahman FZ, Hayee B, et al. Disordered macrophage cytokine secretion underlies impaired acute inflammation and bacterial clearance in Crohn's disease. J Exp Med 2009;206:1883–1897.

CHAPTER 8

Antigen Presentation

SUMMARY

- **T cells survey proteins derived from intracellular or extracellular pathogens by recognizing peptide fragments that have been processed and become bound to major histocompatibility complex (MHC) class I or II molecules, respectively.** These MHC–antigen complexes are presented at the cell surface.

- **MHC class I molecules associate with endogenously synthesized peptides, produced by degradation of the cells' internal molecules.** This type of antigen processing is carried out by proteasomes, which cleave the proteins and transporters, which take the fragments to the endoplasmic reticulum (ER).

- **MHC class II molecules bind to peptides produced following the breakdown of proteins that the cell has endocytosed.** The peptides produced by degradation of these external antigens are loaded onto MHC class II molecules in a specialized endosomal compartment called MIIC.

- **The highly ordered area of contact between the T cell and APC is an immunological synapse.** TCRs and costimulatory receptors occupy the center of the synapse. Adhesion molecules are found in the periphery.

- **Costimulatory molecules are essential for T cell activation.** Molecules such as B7 (CD80/86) on the APC bind to CD28 on the T cell to cause activation. Antigens presented without costimulation usually induce T cell anergy. Intercellular adhesion molecules also contribute to the interaction between a T cell and an antigen-presenting cell (APC). Interactions between intercellular cell adhesion molecule-1 (ICAM-1) and leukocyte functional antigen-1 (LFA-1) and between CD2 and its ligands extend the interaction between T cells and APCs.

- **CD4 binds to MHC class II and CD8 to MHC class I molecules.** These interactions increase the affinity of T cell binding to the appropriate MHC–antigen complex and bring kinases to the TCR complex.

- **Binding of CTLA-4 or PD-1 on the T cell limits activation.** Both of these ligands inhibit the costimulatory signal that the T cell receives from CD28.

- **T cell activation induces enzyme cascades, leading to the production of interleukin-2 (IL-2) and the high-affinity IL-2 receptor on the T cell.** IL-2 is required to drive T cell division.

- **Antigen presentation affects the subsequent course of an immune response.** The immune system responds to clues that an infection has taken place before responding strongly to antigens.

Antigen presenting cells

T cells only recognize antigen peptides bound to MHC-encoded molecules. Endogenous peptides, derived from intracellular sources such as replicating viruses, are presented on MHC class-I molecules to $CD8^+$ T cells, while exogenous peptides, derived from extracellular sources such as microbes, are presented on MHC class-II molecules to $CD4^+$ T cells. Before peptides can associate with the MHC molecules they are generated by partial proteolysis from the original protein antigen. Antigen processing refers to the degradation of antigen into peptide fragments, which may become bound to MHC class I or class II molecules (see Chapter 5). Whether a peptide binds to an MHC molecule depends on the amino-acid sequence of the peptide and on whether a suitable binding MHC molecule is available, which depends on the set of MHC molecules present in the individual. Broadly speaking, a single T cell recognizes a specific peptide(s) bound in the peptide-binding groove of a specific MHC molecule. However there are instances where T cells can respond to a different MHC/peptide combination, and this is equivalent to the cross-reactivity that may occur when antibodies bind to cross-reactive antigens.

Antigen presentation plays a central role in initiating and maintaining an appropriate immune response to antigen. The process is tightly controlled at several levels as follows:

- different types of antigen-presenting cell (APC) are brought into play depending on the situation. Dendritic cells (DCs) are particularly crucial for initiating responses;
- the interaction between the TCR, and the MHC/peptide complex is highly specific;
- another level of control is exerted by **costimulatory molecules** on APCs, resulting in T cell activation only when appropriate, such as in an infection;
- adhesion molecules on the interacting cells also contribute to the stable binding of the cells, which promotes effective antigen presentation;
- signals from the cell surface are then transmitted by a series of signal transduction pathways that regulate gene expression including cytokine production;
- in the final stages the actions of cytokines on the lymphocytes drive cell division.

The four stages of antigen presentation are outlined in Figure 8.1. In lymphoid organs, all four stages of the process can occur, resulting in T cell proliferation. However, antigen presentation can also occur to a more limited degree in tissues, resulting in cytokine production, but with little T cell division.

Interactions with antigen-presenting cells direct T cell activation

The way in which a T cell first encounters antigen largely dictates how it will react subsequently. A wide spectrum of cells can present antigen, depending on how and where the antigen is first encountered by cells of the immune system. In a lymphoid organ, the three main types of APC are:

- DCs which are most effective at presentation to naive T cells;
- macrophages; and
- B cells (Fig. 8.2).

Activation of naive T cells on first encounter with antigen on the surface of an APC is called **priming**, to distinguish it from the responses of effector T cells to antigen on the surface of their target cells and the responses of primed memory T cells.

Dendritic cells are crucial for priming T cells

Dendritic cells which are found in abundance in the T cell areas of lymph nodes and spleen, are the most effective cells for the initial activation of naive T cells. They pick up antigens in peripheral tissues, then migrate to lymph nodes, where they express high levels of adhesion and costimulatory molecules, as well as MHC class II molecules, which allow them to interact with CD4⁺ TH cells.

Once they have migrated, DCs stop synthesizing MHC class II molecules, but maintain high levels of MHC class II molecules containing peptides from antigens derived from the tissue where they originated. Interdigitating DCs are believed to be the major APCs involved in primary immune responses because they induce T cell proliferation more effectively than any other APC.

The majority of dendritic cells enter lymph nodes via afferent lymphatics. Originally it was thought that these cells were mostly derived from Langerhans' cells in the skin, but it now appears that a substantial proportion of the early migrating DCs in afferent lymph are dermal dendritic cells (they do not express langerin (CD207) a marker of Langerhans' cells). Moreover DCs derived from Langerhans' cells tend to localize in the paracortex of the lymph node, whereas dermal DCs remain near lymphoid follicles. Dendritic cells arriving from the periphery of the body transport antigen to the lymph node and process it for presentation to T cells. A minor proportion of the DCs in lymph nodes, arrive from the blood across the HEV, using the same route as T cells and B cells (see Fig. 6.15), however these cells have not acquired antigen in the periphery and they can only acquire it from lymph or transfer from other cells. As they mature, dendritic cells express CCR7 which allows them to localize to the lymphoid tissues. There is also some evidence that DCs from skin and the gut have distinctive chemokine receptors, which allow them to selectively recirculate to their own lymphoid organs. As they mature, DCs also increase expression of key costimulatory molecules, including CD40, CD80 and CD86 (B7-1 and B7-2).

Macrophages and B cells present antigen to primed T cells

Macrophages and B cells are less effective than DCs at antigen presentation to naive T cells, partly because they only express appropriate costimulatory molecules upon infection or contact with microbial products. Although they migrate to lymph nodes, the numbers of macrophages in afferent lymph is relatively few by comparison with DCs and this

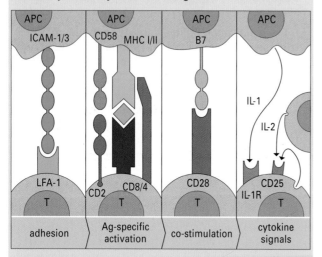

Summary of the key intercellular signals in T cell activation

APC	APC	APC	APC
ICAM-1/3	CD58 MHC I/II	B7	
			IL-1
			IL-2
LFA-1	CD2 CD8/4	CD28	CD25 IL-1R
T	T	T	T
adhesion	Ag-specific activation	co-stimulation	cytokine signals

Fig. 8.1 Association of APCs and T cells first involves non-specific, reversible binding through adhesion molecules, such as LFA-1 with ICAM-1 or ICAM-3. Antigen-specific recognition of the peptide antigen in the MHC molecule by the TCR, provides the specificity of the interaction, and results in prolonged cell–cell contact. A second signal (costimulation) is necessary for the T cell to respond efficiently, otherwise tolerance may result. Cytokine signals result in upregulation of cytokines and their receptors, including IL-2 and the IL-2 receptor (CD25) which drive T cell division. Expression of IL-2 receptor is enhanced by IL-1 from the APC.

Localization of antigen-presenting cells (APCs) in lymph nodes

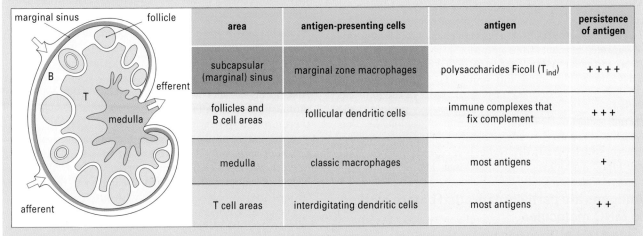

area	antigen-presenting cells	antigen	persistence of antigen
subcapsular (marginal) sinus	marginal zone macrophages	polysaccharides Ficoll (T_{ind})	+ + + +
follicles and B cell areas	follicular dendritic cells	immune complexes that fix complement	+ + +
medulla	classic macrophages	most antigens	+
T cell areas	interdigitating dendritic cells	most antigens	+ +

Fig. 8.2 A lymph node represented schematically showing afferent and efferent lymphatics, follicles, the outer cortical B cell area, and the paracortical T cell area. Different APCs predominate in these areas and selectively take up different types of antigen, which then persist on the surface of the cells for variable periods. Polysaccharides are preferentially taken up by marginal zone macrophages and may persist for months or years, whereas antigens on recirculating macrophages in the medulla may last for only a few days or weeks. The recirculating 'veiled' cells (Langerhans' cells and dermal dendritic cells), which originally come from the skin, change their morphology to become interdigitating dendritic cells within the lymph node. Both these cells and the follicular dendritic cells have long processes, which are in intimate contact with lymphocytes.

too limits their effectiveness in activating naive T cells. Macrophages:

- ingest microbes and particulate antigens;
- digest them in phagolysosomes; and
- present fragments at the cell surface on MHC molecules.

Q. A number of bacterial components enhance the expression of MHC molecules and costimulatory molecules on macrophages. What effect would you expect this to have on the immune response? Would it be advantageous for the individual?

A. In the presence of infection, the action of the microbial components would enhance the ability of macrophages to present antigen to T cells. This would generally be advantageous because it would allow the immune system to respond more effectively to the infection. However, in some circumstances it might be disadvantageous because microbial components would also enhance unwanted immune responses such as autoimmune reactions.

B cells can:

- bind to a specific antigen through surface IgM or IgD;
- internalize it; and
- then degrade it into peptides, which associate with MHC class II molecules.

If antigen concentrations are very low, B cells with high-affinity antigen receptors (IgM or IgD) are the most effective APC because other APCs simply cannot capture enough antigen. Therefore, for secondary responses, when the number of antigen-specific B cells is high, B cells may be a major APC.

The properties and functions of some APCs are summarized in Figures 8.3 and 8.4.

Antigen presentation

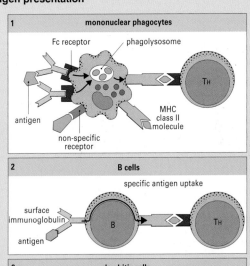
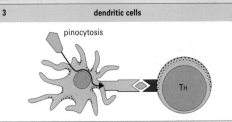

Fig. 8.3 Mononuclear phagocytes (**1**), B cells (**2**), and DCs (**3**) can all present antigen to MHC class II restricted T_H cells. Macrophages take up bacteria or particulate antigen via non-specific receptors or as immune complexes, process it, and return fragments to the cell surface in association with MHC class II molecules. Activated B cells can take up antigen via their surface immunoglobulin and present it to T cells associated with their MHC class II molecules. DCs constitutively express MHC class II molecules and take up antigen by pinocytosis.

Antigen processing

Antigen processing involves degrading the antigen into peptide fragments. The vast majority of epitopes recognized by T cells are fragments from a peptide chain. Only a minority of peptide fragments from a protein antigen are able to bind to a particular MHC molecule. Furthermore, different MHC molecules bind different sets of peptides (see Chapter 5). For example, the great majority of the immune response in humans against the HIV matrix protein is directed against a single **immunodominant region**, i.e. one which is recognized by a large number of T cells. However, exactly which part of this region is recognized, depends on the MHC haplotypes of the individual (Fig. 8.5).

Antigens are partially degraded before binding to MHC molecules

The processing of antigens to generate peptides that can bind to MHC class II molecules occurs in intracellular organelles. Phagosomes containing endocytosed proteins fuse with lysosomes where a number of proteases are involved in breaking down the proteins to smaller fragments. The proteases include:

- cathepsins B and D;
- an acidic thiol reductase, γ-interferon-inducible lysosomal thiol reductase (GILT), which acts on disulfide-bonded proteins.

Alkaline agents such as chloroquine or ammonium chloride diminish the activity of proteases in the phagolysosomes and therefore interfere with antigen processing.

In laboratory studies, the requirement for internal degradation of antigen by APCs can be circumvented by the use of synthetic peptides. This ability to use synthesized peptides of known sequences has enabled researchers to readily identify epitopes recognized by T cells with different specificities.

The relative importance of different amino acids within a defined epitope can also be investigated by amino acid replacements at different sites to identify residues that bind to the MHC molecule and those that bind to the TCR.

MHC class I pathway

MHC class I-restricted T cells (CTLs) recognize endogenous antigens synthesized within the target cell, whereas class II-restricted T cells (TH) recognize exogenous antigen.

Manipulation of the location of a protein can determine whether it elicits an MHC class I- or class II-restricted response. For example:

- influenza virus hemagglutinin (HA), a glycoprotein associated with the membrane of an infected host cell, normally elicits only a weak CTL response, but influenza virus HA can be generated in the cytoplasm by deleting that part of its sequence that encodes the N terminal signal peptide (required for translation across the membrane of the endoplasmic reticulum [ER]) and, when this is done, there is a strong CTL response to HA;

Antigen-presenting cells

	phago-cytosis	type	location	class II expression
phagocytes (monocyte/ macrophage lineage)	+	monocytes	blood	(+)→+++ inducible
		macrophages	tissue	
		marginal zone macrophages	spleen and lymph node	
		Kupffer cells	liver	
		microglia	brain	
non-phagocytic constitutive APCs	−	Langerhans' cells	skin	++ constitutive
		interdigitating DCs (IDCs)	lymphoid tissue	
		follicular dendritic cells	lymphoid tissue	−
lymphocytes	−	B cells and T cells	lymphoid tissues and at sites of immune reactions	−→++ inducible
facultative APCs	+	astrocytes	brain	inducible
		follicular cells	thyroid	inducible
	−	endothelium	vascular and lymphoid tissue	−→++ inducible
		fibroblasts	connective tissue	
		other types in appropriate tissue		

Fig. 8.4 Many APCs are unable to phagocytose antigen, but can take it up in other ways, such as by pinocytosis. Endothelial cells (not normally considered to be APCs) that have been induced to express MHC class II molecules by interferon-γ (IFNγ) are also capable of acting as APCs, as are some epithelial cells. Another example is the thyroid follicular cell, which acts as an APC in the pathogenesis of Graves' autoimmune thyroiditis.

Recognition of HIV protein gag

Recognition of HIV protein gag	HLA-restriction
LQTGSEELRSLYNTVATLYCVHQRI	A*29 B*44
LQTGSEELRSLYNTVATLYCVHQRI	A*02
LQTGSEELRSLYNTVATLYCVHQRI	A*01
LQTGSEELRSLYNTVATLYCVHQRI	A*11
LQTGSEELRSLYNTVATLYCVHQRI	B*08

Fig. 8.5 Overlapping polypeptide fragments from an immunodominant region of the matrix protein (p17) of the HIV protein Gag, are presented by different variant MHC molecules. The amino acid sequence is given in single letter code and the peptide presented by each MHC molecule is shaded in blue.

- the introduction of ovalbumin into the cytoplasm of a target cell (using an osmotic shock technique) generates CTLs recognizing ovalbumin, whereas the addition of exogenous ovalbumin generates an exclusively TH cell response.

Proteasomes are cytoplasmic organelles that degrade cytoplasmic proteins

Although the assembly of MHC class I molecules occurs in the ER of the cell, peptides destined to be presented by MHC class I molecules are generated from cytosolic proteins. The initial step in this process involves an organelle called the proteasome – a multi-protein complex which forms a barrel-like structure (Fig. 8.6).

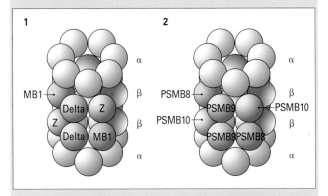

Generation of immunoproteasomes by replacement of active subunits

Fig. 8.6 The 20 S proteasome, shown in cartoon form, is composed of four stacked disks, two identical outer disks of α subunits, and two similar inner disks comprised of β subunits. Each disk has seven different subunits. Peptides enter into the body of the proteasome for cleavage into peptides. Only three of the β subunits are active. In normal proteasomes, these are called MB1, delta, and Z (**1**). Interferon-γ treatment of cells results in replacement of these three subunits by the two MHC-encoded proteins, PSMB8 and PSMB9, as well as a third inducible protein, PSMB10 (**2**). These subunits are shown adjacent to each other here, whereas they are actually in separate parts of the β ring and some would be hidden at the back of the structure shown.

Proteasomes provide the major proteolytic activity of the cytosol. They have a range of different endopeptidase activities and they degrade denatured or ubiquitinated proteins to peptides of about 5–15 amino acids (ubiquitin is a protein that tags other proteins for degradation).

Two genes, *PSMB8* and *PSMB9* located in the class II region of the MHC (Fig. 8.7), encode proteasome components that subtly modify the range of peptides produced by proteasomes. The expression of these genes is induced by interferon-γ (IFNγ). The proteins displace constitutive subunits of the proteasome and along with a third inducible proteasome component (*PSMB10* encoded on a different chromosome) influence processing of peptides by creating a wider range of peptide fragments suitable for binding MHC class I molecules. Additional subunits associate with the ends of core (20 S) proteasomes and may influence antigen processing. These include interferon-inducible PA28 (proteasome-activator-28) molecules as well as a complex of proteins that result in a larger 26 S particle.

Proteasomes may not be the only proteases involved in producing peptides for presentation by MHC class I molecules. There is evidence for the involvement of enzymes, such as the giant tripeptidyl aminopeptidase II (TPPII) complex.

Transporters move peptides to the ER

The products of two genes, *TAP1* and *TAP2*, that map in the MHC (see Fig. 8.7), function as a heterodimeric transporter that translocates peptides into the lumen of the ER. TAP is a member of the large ATP-binding cassette (ABC) family of transporters localized in the ER membrane. Microsomes from cells lacking TAP1 or TAP2 could not take up peptide in experiments in vitro. Using a similar system it was shown that the most efficient transport occurred with peptide substrates of 8–15 amino acids. Although this size is close to the length preference of MHC class I molecule binding sites, it suggests that some additional trimming may be required by enzymes in the lumen of the ER, particularly ERAAP (ER-associated aminopeptidase).

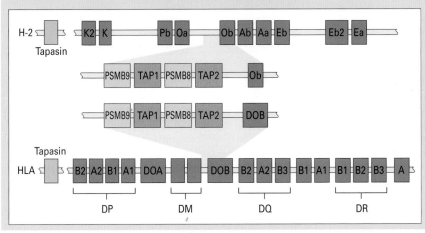

MHC genes involved in antigen processing and presentation

Fig. 8.7 Genes encoding the two subunits of the peptide transporter (TAP) and two components (PSMB8 and 9) of the multisubunit proteasome (see Fig. 8.6) are located in the murine and human class II regions. The Tapasin gene is located just centromeric of the MHC.

Peptide loading onto MHC class-I molecules

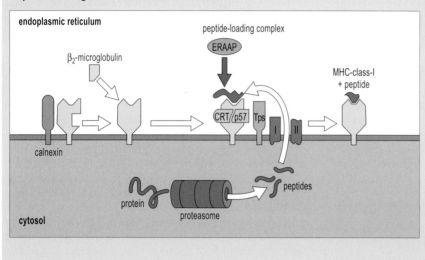

Fig. 8.8 MHC class-I alpha chains (α) are initially held in the endoplasmic reticulum associated with the chaperone protein calnexin. After combining with β2-microglobulin, to form a complete MHC class-I molecule, they are released from calnexin and join a peptide loading complex, consisting of tapasin (Tps), ER-protein-p57 and calreticulin (CRT). Tapasin also associates with the TAP transporters (I and II). Proteins are degraded in the cytosol by proteasomes to produce polypeptides which are transported into the ER and loaded onto the MHC class-I molecule. The peptides may be trimmed by ER-associated aminopeptidases (ERAAP). The MHC class-I molecule with a bound peptide is finally released from the peptide loading complex, to be transported to the plasma membrane.

A multi-component complex loads peptides onto MHC class-I molecules

MHC class-I α-chains are initially associated with the chaperone, calnexin. Once released from calnexin they bind to β2-microglobulin to form a complete MHC class-I molecule, which is incorporated into a peptide-loading complex associated with the TAP transporters (Fig. 8.8). MHC class I molecule complexes lacking peptide are unstable, ensuring that only functionally useful complexes are available for interaction with TCRs.

Antigen processing affects which peptides are presented

Originally it was thought that the MHC haplotype of an individual largely controlled which sets of antigenic peptides would be presented to T cells. We now know that antigen processing is at least as important: The availability of peptides to load onto MHC class-I molecules in the ER is dependent on:

- the efficiency of the proteasome in generating different peptides, which varies if the proteasome contains interferon-inducible components;
- the efficiency of the transporters in taking peptides from the cytosol to the ER;
- whether the peptides can be trimmed by ERAAP.

Each one of these factors also depend on the amino-acid sequence of the original protein (Fig. 8.9), and to some extent on genetic variations in molecules involved in antigen processing (Fig. 8.10). All of these considerations are important in developing vaccines, where the aim is to identify an immunodominant region of a pathogen to stimulate T cells; but it is not enough for a peptide to bind to MHC molecules, it must also be processed properly if it is to be immunogenic.

Cross-presentation can occur if exogenous antigen is presented on class-I molecules

Cross-presentation is a phenomenon which may occur when exogenous peptides are presented by MHC class I molecules. This is an exception to the principle that endogenously synthesized proteins are the source of peptides for MHC class I, and its mechanism and physiological importance is debated. However it could allow antigen-presenting cells to present viral antigens on their own MHC class-I molecules and activate Tc cells, even if they had not themselves been infected.

Some class I-like molecules can present limited sets of antigens

In addition to the standard MHC class I molecules (class Ia), a number of class I-like molecules (class Ib), encoded in the MHC or elsewhere on the genome, can present very limited sets of antigens.

HLA-E-signal peptide complex interacts with the NKG2A inhibitory receptor on NK cells

HLA-E molecules bind a restricted set of peptides consisting of hydrophobic leader sequence peptides from class Ia molecules. Intriguingly, though these leader sequences are generated by signal peptidase within the ER, HLA-E is dependent on TAP transporters. By binding and presenting sequences from class Ia molecules HLA-E signals the fact that MHC expression has not been downregulated (e.g. by a virus).

The HLA-E–signal peptide complex interacts with the NKG2A inhibitory receptor on NK cells (see Fig. 10.6). A cell that expresses HLA-E is therefore not killed by NK cells.

Production of antigenic peptides

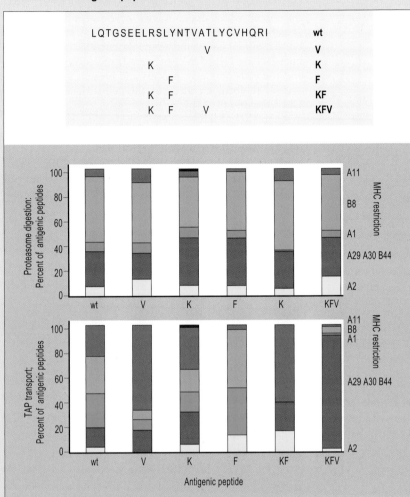

Fig 8.9 Production of antigenic peptides by the proteasome and their transport to the ER varies depending on the amino acid sequence of the epitope. The upper diagram shows the amino acid sequence of an immunodominant epitope of HIV matrix protein p17, and 5 mutants that often emerge during HIV infection. The sequence is shown in single amino acid code, and the variants indicate single, double or triple mutations in the wild-type sequence (wt). The lower diagram shows how efficiently these different mutants are digested by proteasomes and transported to the ER by binding to TAP transporters. The bars show the proportion of peptides generated which are presented by different MHC molecules (A11, B8, etc.). For example the KFV mutant produces peptides (red, recognized by HLA-A29, -A30 and -B44) that have a high affinity for the transporters and are transported well to the ER. Conversely the KFV mutant generates some HLA-11-binding peptides (dark blue) but they are not well transported, compared with peptides of the wild-type sequence. *(Based on data from Tenzer et al., 2009, Nature Immunology, 10, 636–646.)*

Linkage of *TAP* and class I alleles

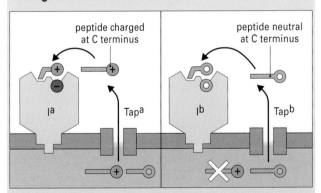

Fig. 8.10 Different MHC class I molecules in rats can accommodate peptides (blue bars) with either a positive charge at the C terminus (+) or a neutral amino acid (o). Similarly, TAP molecules (orange) come in two forms, which differ in the types of peptide they preferentially transport into the ER. Most rat strains have the appropriate *TAP* allele on the same haplotype as the class I gene that it serves best.

Q. Why would conventional HLA-A, HLA-B, or HLA-C molecules be less well suited to the presentation of signal peptide to receptors on NK cells than HLA-E?

A. The conventional MHC molecules have evolved as highly diverse molecules that present the great range of microbial polypeptides to the diverse repertoire of T cell receptors. In contrast HLA-E molecules have a single function – to present well-defined signal peptides to a monomorphic receptor.

CD1 molecules present lipids and glycolipids

CD1 molecules, encoded on chromosome 1, present lipids and glycolipids to T cells. Humans have five *CD1* genes and mice have two. CD1b presents the bacterial lipid mycolic acid to T cells with αβ TCRs. Other CD1 molecules are recognized by γδ T cells or NK cells.

The intracellular trafficking pathways of CD1 involve recycling between the plasma membrane and endosomes, which is similar to MHC class-II molecules (see below) however the pathways are distinct. Immature dendritic cells can present antigens on CD1, but unlike the class-II pathway, presentation does not improve as the cell matures.

Why are antigen-processing genes located in the MHC?

The finding of a cassette of antigen-processing genes such as PSMBs and TAPs in the class II region of the MHC is striking. There is some evidence, especially from studies in rats, that particular alleles of *TAP* are genetically linked with alleles of class I genes that are most suited to receive the kind of peptides preferentially transported by the products of that *TAP* allele (see Fig. 8.10). The clustering of antigen processing and presenting genes in the MHC of most vertebrate species may not be fortuitous. It may help to coordinate co-evolution of some molecules as well as facilitating exchange of sequences between loci.

MHC class II pathway

Class II molecules are loaded with exogenous peptides

MHC class II molecules are produced in the ER, complexed to a polypeptide called the invariant chain (Ii) (encoded outside the MHC), which stabilizes the complex and prevents the inappropriate binding of antigen. The αβ–Ii complex is transported from the Golgi to an antigen processing compartment which appears as a multivesicular body (also called the MIIC compartment), specialized for the transport and loading of MHC class II molecules. The compartment has characteristics of both endosomes and lysosomes with an onion-skin appearance under the electron microscope, comprising multiple membrane structures (Fig. 8.11). The αβ complex spends 1–3 hours in this compartment before reaching the cell surface (Fig. 8.12).

Exogenous antigens reach the MIIC compartment from acidic endosomes, where they have been partly degraded by the actions of proteases and chaperone proteins. The Ii chain is cleaved by cathepsins into small fragments, one of which, termed CLIP (class II-associated invariant peptide), is located in the groove of the class II molecule until replaced by peptides destined for presentation. The exchange of CLIP for other peptides is orchestrated by

HLA-DM, an MHC class-II-like chaperone protein, consisting of α and β chains both encoded within the MHC class II region, but which does not itself have a peptide binding site (Fig. 8.13). HLA-DM binds to the αβ-CLIP complex to stabilize it until it has bound a suitable antigenic peptide. In cell lines lacking HLA-DM, the class II molecules are unstable and the cells no longer process and present proteins. Their class II molecules end up at the cell surface occupied by CLIP fragments of the invariant chain.

A further MHC-encoded molecule, HLA-DO (see Fig. 8.7), which associates with DM, regulates peptide loading. Like conventional MHC class II molecules, HLA-DO is a heterodimer, consisting of the DOA and DOB chains.

Peptide loading is also affected by the amount of antigenic peptide supplied to the MIIC compartment which varies

MHC class II molecule processing compartment

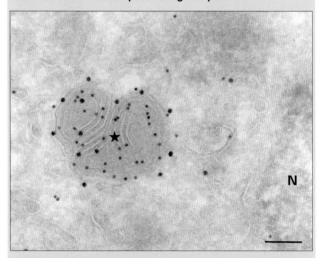

Fig. 8.11 Electron micrograph of ultrathin cryosections from B cells showing a multilaminar MIIC vesicle. The bar represents 100 nm. MHC class II molecules are revealed by antibodies coupled to 10 nm gold particles and HLA-DM by large gold particles (15 nm). *(Courtesy of Dr Monique Kleijmeer.)*

Pathways of MHC class-II protein traffic

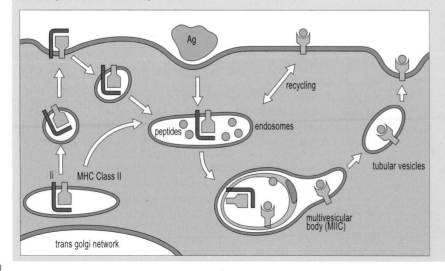

Fig. 8.12 Newly synthesized MHC class II molecules in the trans-Golgi network are associated with a protein Ii which prevents loading with peptide and contains sequences that enable the MHC class II molecule to exit the ER. Class II molecules move to an acidic endosome compartment, either via the cell surface or directly, where they encounter antigen that has been internalized and partly degraded into peptides. The endosomes form multivesicular bodies (MIIC) where the Ii protein is replaced by an antigenic peptide. Tubular vesicles bud from the multivesicular bodies carrying MHC class-II molecules loaded with peptide to the cell surface. These cell surface complexes may subsequently recycle through endosomes.

depending on the cell-type. Macrophages are more efficient at degrading antigen than dendritic cells, and are therefore less efficient at antigen presentation.

MHC-II peptide complexes recycle from the plasma membrane

Class-II/peptide complexes are released from the multivesicular bodies as tubular/vesicular structures that fuse with the plasma membrane. The complexes tend to cluster on the cell surface in lipid rafts, which probably favors formation of the immunological synapse (see below). There is a continuous recycling of complexes from the plasma membrane to endosomal compartments, and the proportion of complex that is present on the plasma membrane is regulated by ubiquitinylation, which varies between cells. For example, mature dendritic cells tend to maintain more of the class-II/peptide complexes on the cell surface than immature dendritic cells.

T cell interaction with APCS

The interactions between a T cell and an antigen presenting cell develops over time, in three phases.

The initial encounter of T cells with APCs is by non-specific binding through adhesion molecules, particularly ICAM-1 (CD54) on the APC and the integrin LFA-1 (CD11/18), present on all immune cells. Transient binding permits the T cell to interact with many APCs; T cells *in vivo* are highly active and a single T cell may contact up to 5000 dendritic cells in one hour. Adhesion between the cells is enhanced by the interaction of CD2 (LFA-2) on the T cell with CD58 (LFA-3) on the APC (in rodents, CD48 performs a similar function to CD58). CD2 contributes towards the initial activation signal for the T cell, but more importantly, it allows the TCR time to recognize specific MHC/peptide on the APC. The initial phase of antigen presentation may last for several hours, but in the absence of a specific interaction, the APC and T cell dissociate.

When the T cell encounters the appropriate MHC/peptide, a conformational change in LFA-1 on the T cell, signaled via the TCR, results in tighter binding to ICAM-1 and prolonged cell–cell contact. (Fig. 8.14) The joined cells can exist as a pair for up to 12 hours, and this marks the

second phase of interaction. At this stage an 'immunological synapse' forms and the T cell may be activated (Fig. 8.15).

In the third phase, the APC and T cell dissociate and the activated T cell undergoes several rounds of division and differentiation.

The immunological synapse is a highly ordered signaling structure

The interactions between APCs and T cells have been studied extensively in vitro, where the cells form a 'bulls-eye' structure at the point of contact (see Fig. 8.14). This 'immunological synapse' is thought to reflect, in idealized

Color-enhanced reconstruction of an immunological synapse

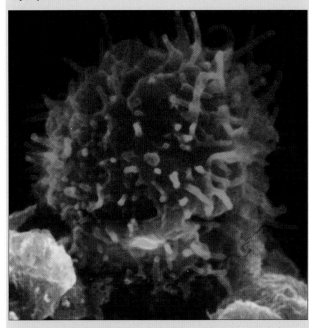

Fig. 8.14 A live-cell fluorescence image, showing the peripheral zone of adhesion molecules (red) surrounding the core containing TCRs (green), is superimposed on a scanning electron micrograph of a T cell (purple) interacting with a DC (dark green). *(Courtesy of Dr Mike Dustin and Science.)*

HLA-DM acts like a catalyst to influence binding of peptides in exchange for CLIP

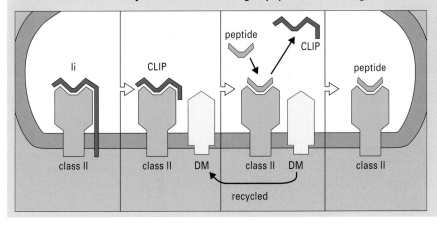

Fig. 8.13 An MHC class II molecule is shown loaded with the Ii chain. The Ii chain is cleaved to the CLIP fragment. Association of the complex with HLA-DM then allows CLIP to be exchanged for other peptides derived from endocytosed proteins present in MIIC vesicles.

conditions, the events that occur within a lymph node when T cells and dendritic cells interact; in vitro high doses of antigen may be used, and it is known that the size of the synapse relates to the amount of antigen present.

In the synapse, TCRs cluster in a patch on the cell surface and are surrounded by a ring of adhesion molecules. The movement of TCRs to the center of the synapse is a dynamic process and as few as 10 cognate interactions between a TCR and MHC/peptide can initiate synapse formation and T-cell activation. The final configuration of the synapse has TCRs at the hub of the synapse ringed by ICAM-1–LFA-1 interactions. Large CD45 molecules, a phosphatase which is 'leukocyte common antigen', are relegated to an outer ring.

The majority of work on immunological synapses has been done using CD4+ TH cells. TC cells form similar structures when they recognize their targets, but with a distinct secretory domain. Lytic granules from the cytotoxic cell are shifted towards the synapse along microtubules and accumulate just below the plasma membrane, before the granule contents are released into the inter-cellular space by exocytosis.

Costimulation by B7 binding to CD28 is essential for T cell activation

Productive T cell proliferation appears to depend on the formation of a stable central cluster of TCRs interacting with MHC molecules. The affinity of the binding of a single TCR molecule to its specific MHC/peptide is not high, and the formation of the immunological synapse requires the concerted interactions of a number of additional molecules, including CD4 which enhances binding of TH cells to MHC class-II molecules and CD8 to MHC class-I molecules. These molecules increase the sensitivity of a T cell for its target antigen by ~100fold. Although signaling efficiency for CD8+ T cells and thymocytes relates closely to the affinity of their TCR for the MHC/peptide, this is only partly true for the CD4+ T cells.

The specific MHC/peptide/TCR interaction, though necessary, is not sufficient to fully activate the T cell. A second signal, referred to as costimulation, is of crucial importance for T cell activation. The most potent costimulatory molecules are B7s, which are homodimeric members of the immunoglobulin superfamily molecules; they include B7–1 (CD80) and B7–2 (CD86). They are constitutively expressed on DCs, but can be upregulated on monocytes, B cells, and other APCs, particularly when stimulated by inflammatory cytokines and by interaction of microbial products with Toll-like receptors on the APC.

The B7 co-receptors bind to CD28 and its homolog CTLA-4 (CD152), which is expressed after T cell activation. CD28 is the main costimulatory ligand expressed on naive T cells. CD28 stimulation:

- prolongs and augments the production of IL-2 and other cytokines; and
- is probably important in preventing the induction of tolerance, a condition where the T cell is not activated and is put into a state of **anergy**, i.e. it is unable to respond subsequently.

Many cells in the tissues can be induced to express MHC class-II molecules and present antigenic peptides to CD4+ T cells, however, they are mostly ineffective in inducing T cell activation and proliferation, because they lack the necessary costimulatory molecules (Fig. 8.16).

Ligation of CTLA-4 inhibits T cell activation

CTLA-4 (CD152) is an alternative ligand for B7, with higher affinity than CD28. It is an inhibitory receptor limiting T cell activation, resulting in less IL-2 production. CTLA-4 appears to act by reducing the time for interaction between the APC and the T cell, so a stronger activation signal is needed otherwise incomplete signaling will occur. As a T cell matures, it expresses higher levels of CTLA-4 and hence requires stronger activation stimuli to continue division (Fig. 8.17).

> **Q. What effect would you expect to see in mice that have the CTLA-4 gene knocked out?**
> A. They suffer from an aggressive lymphoproliferative disorder, because their T cells are not inactivated.

CTLA-4 is a member of a family of molecules that control lymphocyte activation

Another inhibitory receptor on T cells is PD-1 (Programmed-Death-1, CD279), which belongs to the same family as CD28 and CTLA-4. It is associated with the 'exhausted' T-cell phenotype, i.e. cells that are incapable of producing cytokines and undergoing further division. PD-1 is ligated by PD-L1 and PD-L2 (CD273 and CD274) on antigen presenting cells,

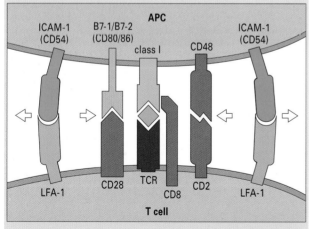

Diagram of an immunological synapse

Fig. 8.15 Molecular interactions in the immunological synapse. TCR–peptide–MHC, CD2–CD48 and CD28–CD80/86 all contribute to the formation of a synapse. The TCR assembles with MHC molecule–antigen peptide molecules and moves with the costimulatory molecules to the centre of the synapse, while the adhesion molecules LFA-1–ICAM-1 move to the periphery. The diagram shows presentation by an MHC class-I molecule, but similar structures occur in MHC class-II mediated antigen presentation.

which inhibits the costimulatory signal from CD28. There is therefore a balance in the costimulatory signals that a T cell receives, which determine whether it remains in an activated state.

Both PD-1 and another inhibitory receptor BTLA-4 (CD272) are also found on activated B cells, and their ligands are not confined to antigen presenting cells, hence the functions of this family probably extend to more general control of cell division within the body.

Intracellular signaling pathways activate transcription factors

An appropriate stimulatory signal initiates a cascade of intracellular signals, leading to the activation of transcription factors and expression of genes required for cell division. Two widely-used immunosuppressive drugs, cyclosporin and tacrolimus, interfere with the activation pathways.

Interleukin-2 drives T cell division

T cell activation leads to the production of IL-2 and IL-2 receptors, so a T cell can act on itself and surrounding cells. In most CD4$^+$ cells and some CD8$^+$ T cells, there is a transient production of IL-2 for 1–2 days. During this time the interaction of IL-2 with the high-affinity IL-2R results in T cell division.

On resting T cells, the IL-2R is predominantly present as a low-affinity form consisting of two polypeptide chains, a β chain (p75) that binds IL-2 and a common γc chain that signals to the cell. When the T cell is activated, it produces an α chain (CD25), which contributes to IL-2 binding and, together with the β and γc chains, forms the high-affinity receptor (Fig. 8.18). IL-2 is internalized within 10–20 minutes and the β and γc chains are degraded in

Dual signaling is necessary for full T cell activation

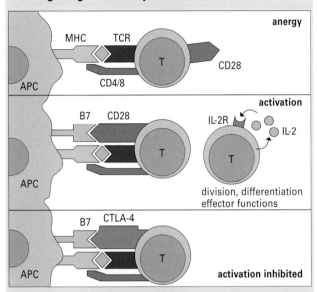

Fig. 8.16 A T cell requires signals from both the TCR and CD28 for activation. In the absence of costimulatory molecules inactivation or anergy results. If CD28 is bound by B7 on the surface of a professional APC, the T cell is activated and produces IL-2 and its receptor (IL-2R). The cell divides and differentiates into an effector T cell, which no longer requires signal 2 for its effector function. However, if CTLA-4 on the T cell binds to B7, activation is inhibited.

Role of CTLA-4 in controlling T cell activation

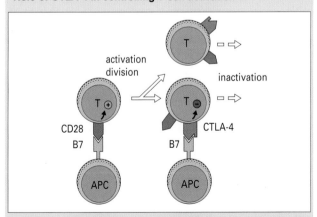

Fig. 8.17 Before activation, T cells express CD28, which ligates B7–1 and B7–2 on APCs (e.g. dendritic cells). After activation, CTLA-4 is expressed, which is an alternative high-affinity ligand for B7. CTLA-4 ligates B7, so the T cells no longer receive an activation signal.

Expression of the high-affinity IL-2 receptor on T cells

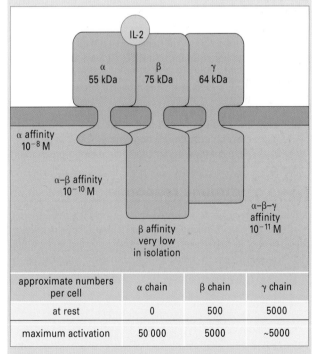

approximate numbers per cell	α chain	β chain	γ chain
at rest	0	500	5000
maximum activation	50 000	5000	~5000

Fig. 8.18 The high-affinity IL-2R consists of three polypeptide chains, shown schematically. Resting T cells do not express the α chain, but after activation they may express up to 50 000 α chains per cell. Some of these associate with the β chain to form the high-affinity IL-2R. (The γc chain is a common signaling chain of several cytokine receptors.)

lysosomes while the α chain is recycled to the cell surface. Sustained signaling by IL-2 over several hours is needed to drive T-cell division.

The transient expression of the high-affinity IL-2R for about 1 week after stimulation of the T cell, together with the induction of CTLA-4, helps limit T cell division. In the absence of positive signals, the T cells will start to die by apoptosis.

In view of the importance of IL-2 in T cell division, it was surprising that the rare patients who lack CD25 (and IL-2 receptor knockout mice) develop an immunoproliferative condition. These observations lead to an awareness that IL-2 also has a regulatory function in T cell development – regulatory T cells (Tregs) are characterized by high CD25 expression, and IL-2 is required for their generation in the thymus and maintenance in the periphery (see Chapter 11).

Other cytokines contribute to activation and division

As T cell division and immune responses are not ablated in mice lacking the IL-2 or IL-2R genes, it suggests that other cytokines may support T-cell division. The cytokine IL-15 is structurally similar to IL-2; it acts on a receptor which shares the β and γc chains of the IL-2 receptor and it causes expansion of T cells and some NK cell populations. IL-15 is made by APCs and may therefore be very important in initial T cell activation before IL-2 is produced.

Although it was originally identified as a B cell growth and differentiation factor IL-4 can also induce division of naive T cells. The relative importance of these other cytokines will vary depending on the state of T cell, and these cytokines may partly overlap the function of IL-2.

Other cytokines contribute indirectly to T cell proliferation. For example, IL-1 and IL-6 induce the expression of IL-2R on resting T cells and thus may enhance their responsiveness to IL-2.

Q. Which cells generate IL-1 and IL-6?
A. Mononuclear phagocytes among others. Thus the production of these cytokines enhances their antigen-presenting function.

Types of immune response

APCs may be activated rapidly in an immune response, for example by the immunogenic entity itself, in the case of bacteria and some viruses. Antigen presentation is not a unidirectional process. T cells, as they become activated:

- release cytokines such as IFNγ and granulocyte–macrophage colony stimulating factor (GM–CSF);

- express surface molecules such as CD154 which binds to the costimulatory molecule CD40 on antigen presenting cells.

When APCs are activated, they express more MHC class I and II molecules, Fc receptors, and costimulatory adhesion molecules, including B7–1 and B7–2, CD11a/b/c, ICAM-1, and ICAM-3. They also produce numerous cytokines (e.g. IL-1, IL-6, TNFα), enzymes, and other mediators.

Activation of lymphocytes leads to two partially competing processes:

- cell proliferation; and
- cell differentiation into effector cells.

The fate of lymphocytes responding to antigen is varied; some can persist for a long time as memory cells – the life span of memory cells can be more than 40 years in humans. Other lymphocytes have a short life span, which explains why moderate antigenic stimulation does not lead to lymphoid enlargement – this is nevertheless sufficient for generating effective cell-mediated and antibody responses. Apoptosis is critically important for disposing of unwanted cells after an immune response.

Danger signals enhance antigen presentation

For appropriate immune responses to be generated, APCs must respond to infection, but not to high levels of harmless substances that may fluctuate in the environment. Mucosal tissue in the gut are in contact with high concentrations of harmless food antigens, while respiratory mucosa contacts many airborne antigens such as pollen, but strong immune responses against these antigens are undesirable.

APC activation is generally a response to infection, or at least the presence of substances, such as constituents of bacterial cell walls, characteristic of infection. This requirement explains the action of **adjuvants** derived from bacterial components, which are used to enhance immune responses in vaccines.

The concept of immune activation only in response to infection (or adjuvant as a surrogate for infection), and not to other antigens, has been promoted as the 'danger' hypothesis. This idea proposes that the immune system does not merely distinguish self from non-self, but responds to clues that an infection has taken place before responding strongly to antigens.

In other words, foreign substances may be innocuous or invisible to the immune system unless accompanied by danger signals, such as infection. These danger signals are provided by receptors for microbial products on APCs, such as the Toll-like receptors (TLRs, see Fig. 6.21).

CRITICAL THINKING: ANTIGEN PROCESSING AND PRESENTATION (SEE P. 435 FOR EXPLANATIONS)

Two T cell clones have been produced from a mouse infected with influenza virus. One of the clones reacts to a virus peptide when it is presented on APCs that have the same MHC class I (H-2 K) locus as the original mouse (i.e. the clone is MHC class I restricted). The other clone is MHC class II restricted. The two clones are stimulated in tissue culture using syngeneic macrophages as APCs. The macrophages have been either infected with live influenza virus or treated with inactivated virus. The patterns of reactivity of the two clones are shown in the table below. In the last two lines of the table the macrophages are pretreated with either emetine or chloroquine before they are infected with virus. Emetine is a protein synthesis inhibitor. Chloroquine inhibits the fusion of lysosomes with phagosomes.

Antigen	APCs treated with	Reactivity of clone	
		Clone 1	Clone 2
none	–	–	–
live virus	–	+	+
inactivated virus	–	–	+
live virus	emetine	–	+
live virus	chloroquine	+	–

1 Why are macrophages used as APCs in this experiment? Would you get the same results if you used infected fibroblasts?

2 Why does the live influenza virus stimulate both clones whereas the inactivated virus stimulates only the MHC class II-restricted clone?

3 Why does emetine prevent the macrophages from presenting antigen to the MHC class I-restricted T cells whereas chloroquine prevents them from presenting to MHC class II-restricted cells?

4 One of these clones expresses CD4 and the other CD8. Which way round is it?

Further reading

Ackerman AL, Cresswell P. Cellular mechanisms governing cross-presentation of exogenous antigens. Nat Immunol 2004;5:678–684.

Bell D, Young JW, Banchereau J. Dendritic cells. Annu Rev Immunol 1999;17:255–305.

Berger AC, Roche PA. MHC class II transport at a glance. J Cell Sci 2009;122:1–4.

Boes M, Ploegh HL. Translating cell biology in vitro to immunity in vivo. Nature 2004;430:264–271.

Brocke P, Garbi N, Momburg F, Hammerling GJ. HLA-DM, HLA-DO and tapasin: functional similarities and differences. Curr Opin Immunol 2002;14:22–29.

Cresswell P, Ackerman AL, Giodin A, et al. Mechanisms of MHC class-I restricted antigen processing and cross presentation. Imm Revs 205;207:145–157.

Fooksman DR, Vardhana S, Vasiliver-Shamis G, et al. Functional anatomy of T cell activation and synapse formation. Ann Revs Immunol 2010;28:79–106.

Kloetzel PM. Generation of MHC class I antigens: functional interplay between proteasomes and TPPII. Nat Immunol 2004;5:661–669.

Okazaki T, Honjo T. PD-1 and PD-1 ligands: from discovery to clinical application. Int Immunol 2007;19:813–824.

Randolph G, Orchando J, Partida-Sanchez S. Migration of dendritic cell subsets and their precursors. Ann Revs Immunol 2008;26:293–316.

Tenzer S, Wee E, Burgevin A, et al. Antigen processing influences HIV-specific cytotoxic lymphocyte immunodominance. Nat Immunol 2009;10:636–646.

Watts C, Powis S. Pathways of antigen processing and presentation. Rev Immunogenet 1999;1:60–74.

CHAPTER 9

Cell Cooperation in the Antibody Response

SUMMARY

- **The primary development of B cells is antigen independent.** Pre-B cells recombine genes for immunoglobulin heavy and light chains to generate their surface receptor for antigen.

- **T-independent antigens activate B cells without requiring T-cell help.** They can be divided into two groups. TI-1 antigens can act as polyclonal stimulators, while TI-2 antigens are polymers which activate by cross-linking the B-cell receptor.

- **T-dependent antigens are taken up by B cells, processed and presented to TH cells.** T cells and B cells usually recognize different parts of an antigen.

- **B-cell activation requires signals from the B-cell receptor and costimulation.** CD40 is the most important costimulatory molecule on B cells. Ligation of the B-cell–coreceptor complex can lower the threshold of antigen needed to trigger the B cell.

- Intracellular signaling pathways are analogous in B cells and T cells.

- **Activated B cells proliferate and differentiate into antibody-forming cells.** Cytokines from TH cells control the process of division, differentiation and class switching.

- **Somatic hypermutation of immunoglobulin genes, followed by selection of high-affinity clones is the basis of affinity maturation.** These processes occur in germinal centers.

- **Class switching is effected by somatic recombination occurring within the heavy chain genes.** Somatic hypermutation and class-switching by recombination are linked processes, which require selective targeting of DNA-modification and DNA-repair enzymes to the heavy chain gene locus.

The antibody response is the culmination of a series of cellular and molecular interactions occurring in an orderly sequence between a B cell and a variety of other cells of the immune system. This chapter discusses the principles of B-cell development, activation, proliferation and differentiation leading to the generation of plasma cells and memory cells. In addition, the consequences of these interactions, including affinity maturation and class switching, are examined.

In adults, B cell development occurs in the bone marrow and does not require contact with antigen. During this time the B cells rearrange the genes for their heavy and light chains, and synthesize cell surface IgM which acts as their antigen receptor (BCR). The BCR complex includes:

- membrane-bound immunoglobulin (mIg);
- the signaling chains Igα and Igβ (CD79a and CD79b).

Immature transitional B-cells exit the bone marrow and enter the periphery where they further mature in secondary lymphoid organs. If these cells do not encounter antigen, they soon die within a few weeks by apoptosis. If, however, these mature B cells encounter specific antigen, they undergo activation, proliferation and differentiation leading to the generation of plasma cells and memory B cells.

B cell activation

T-independent antigens do not require T cell help to stimulate B cells

The immune response to most antigens depends on both T cells and B cells recognizing the antigen in a linked fashion. This type of antigen is called a **T-dependent (TD) antigen**.

A small number of antigens, however, can activate B cells without MHC class II-restricted T cell help and are referred to as **T-independent (TI) antigens** (Fig. 9.1).

Importantly, many TI antigens are particularly resistant to degradation. TI antigens can be divided into two groups (TI-1 and TI-2) based on the manner in which they activate B cells:

- TI-1 antigens are predominantly bacterial cell wall components – the prototypical TI-1 antigen is lipopolysaccharide (LPS), a component of the cell wall of Gram-negative bacteria;
- TI-2 antigens are predominantly large polysaccharide molecules with repeating antigenic determinants (e.g. Ficoll, dextran, polymeric bacterial flagellin, and poliomyelitis virus).

T-independent antigens

antigen	polymeric	polyclonal activation	resistance to degradation
lipopolysaccharide (LPS)	+	+ + +	+
Ficoll	+ + +	–	+ + +
dextran	+ +	+	+ +
levan	+ +	+	+ +
poly-D amino acids	+ + +	–	+ + +
polymeric bacterial flagellin	+ +	+ +	+

Fig. 9.1 The major common properties of some of the main T-independent antigens are listed. T-independent antigens induce the production of cytokines IL-1, TNFα and IL-6 by macrophages. (Note: both poly-L amino acids and monomeric bacterial flagellin are T-dependent antigens, demonstrating the role of antigen structure in determining T-independent properties.)

Q. What common characteristic can you see in many of the TI antigens, and how are such antigens recognized by the immune system?

A. Many TI antigens have pathogen-associated molecular patterns (PAMPs) recognized by Toll-like receptors. They therefore have an intrinsic ability to activate the immune system irrespective of their ability to bind to the specific antigen receptor on individual B cell clones.

Many TI-1 antigens possess the ability in high concentrations to activate B cell clones that are specific for other antigens – a phenomenon known as polyclonal B cell activation. However, in lower concentrations they only activate B cells specific for themselves. TI-1 antigens do not require a second signal.

TI-2 antigens, on the other hand, are thought to activate B cells by clustering and cross-linking immunoglobulin molecules on the B cell surface, leading to prolonged and persistent signaling. TI-2 antigens require residual non-cognate T cell help, such as cytokines.

Several signal transduction molecules are necessary for mediating TI antigen responses in B cells. These include CD19, HS1 protein and Lyn.

T-independent antigens induce poor memory

Primary antibody responses to TI antigens *in vitro* are generally slightly weaker than those to TD antigens. They peak fractionally earlier and both generate mainly IgM. However, the secondary responses to TD and TI antigens differ greatly. The secondary response to TI antigens resembles the primary response, whereas the secondary response to TD antigens is far stronger and has a large IgG component (Fig. 9.2). It seems, therefore, that TI antigens do not usually induce the maturation of a response leading to class switching or to an increase in antibody affinity, as seen with TD antigens. This is most likely due to the lack of CD40 activation (see below). Memory induction to TI antigens is also relatively poor.

Comparison of the secondary immune response to T-dependent and T-independent antigens in vitro

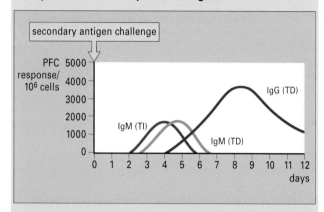

Fig. 9.2 The secondary response to T-dependent antigens is stronger and induces a greater number of IgG-producing cells, as measured by plaque-forming cells (see Method box 9.1).

There are potential survival advantages if the immune response to bacteria does not depend on complex cell interactions, as it could be more rapid. Many bacterial antigens bypass T-cell help because they are very effective inducers of cytokine production by macrophages – they induce IL-1, IL-6 and tumor necrosis factor-α (TNFα) from macrophages. The short-lived response and lack of IgG may also be due to lack of costimulation via CD40L and lack of IL-2, IL-4 and IL-5, which T cells produce in response to TD antigens.

It is possible to convert TI antigens into T-dependent antigens by altering their structure. For example, pneumococcal polysaccharides are TI antigens and do not induce immunological memory or antibodies in infants. However, conjugation of pneumococcal polysaccharides to a carrier protein induces polysaccharide-specific antibody in infants, and memory similar to T-dependent antigens (see Method boxes 9.1 and 2.1).

T-independent antigens tend to activate the CD5+ subset of B cells

TI antigens predominantly activate the B-1 subset of B cells found mainly in the peritoneum. These B-1 cells can be identified by their expression of CD5, which is induced upon binding of TI antigens. In contrast to conventional B cells, B-1 cells have the ability to replenish themselves.

Activation of B cells by T-dependent antigens

T cells and B cells recognize different parts of antigens

In the late 1960s and early 1970s, studies by Mitchison and others, using chemically modified proteins, led to significant advances in understanding of the different functions of T cells and B cells. To induce an optimal secondary antibody response to a small chemical group or hapten (which is immunogenic only if bound to a protein carrier), it was found that the experimental animal must be immunized and then challenged using the same hapten–carrier conjugate – not just the same hapten. This was referred to as the carrier effect.

Cell cooperation in the antibody response

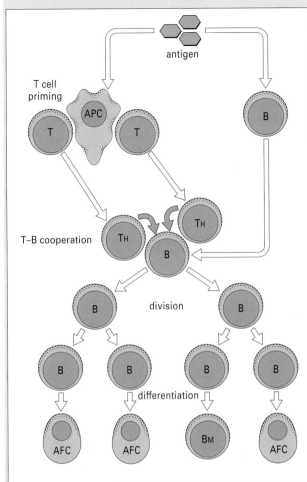

Fig. 9.3 Antigen is presented to virgin T cells by antigen-presenting cells (APCs) such as dendritic cells. B cells also take up antigen and present it to the T cells, receiving signals from the T cells to divide and differentiate into antibody-forming cells (AFCs) and memory B (Bm) cells.

Intracellular signaling in B cell activation

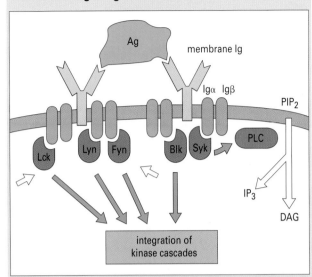

Fig. 9.4 B-cell activation is similar to T-cell activation. If membrane Ig becomes cross-linked (e.g. by a T-independent antigen), tyrosine kinases, including Lck, Lyn, Fyn and Blk, become activated. They phosphorylate the ITAM domains in the Igα and Igβ chains of the receptor complex. These can then bind another kinase, Syk, which activates phospholipase C. This acts on membrane PIP_2 to generate IP_3 and diacyl glycerol (DAG) which activates protein kinase C. Signals from the other kinases are transduced to activate nuclear transcription factors.

antigen entering the body is processed by cells that present the antigen in a highly immunogenic form to the TH and B cells. The T cells recognize determinants on the antigen that are distinct from those recognized by the B cells, which differentiate and divide into antibody-forming cells (AFCs). Therefore two processes are required to activate a B cell:

- antigen interacting with B cell immunoglobulin receptors – this involves 'native' antigen;
- stimulating signal(s) from TH cells that respond to processed antigen bound to MHC class II molecules.

B-cell activation and T-cell activation follow similar patterns

In B cells, the signaling function of CD3 is carried out by a heterodimer of Igα and Igβ. Two molecules of the Igα/Igβ heterodimer associate with surface Ig to form the B-cell receptor (BCR). The cytoplasmic tails of Igα and Igβ carry **immunoreceptor tyrosine activation motifs (ITAM)**.

Cross-linking of surface Ig leads to activation of the src family kinases, which in B cells are Fyn, Lyn, and Blk. Syk is analogous to ZAP-70 in T cells, and binds to the phosphorylated ITAMs of Igα and Igβ (Fig. 9.4). This leads to activation of a kinase cascade and translocation of nuclear transcription factors analogous to the process that occurs in T cells.

B-cell activation is also markedly augmented by the 'co-receptor complex' comprising three proteins:

- CD21 (complement receptor-2, CR2);
- CD19; and
- CD81 (target of anti-proliferative antibody, TAPA-1) (Fig. 9.5).

By manipulating the cell populations in these experiments, it was shown that:

- TH cells are responsible for recognizing the carrier; whereas
- the B cells recognize hapten.

These experiments were later reinforced by details of how:

- B cells use antibody to recognize epitopes; while
- T cells recognize processed antigen fragments.

One consequence of this system is that an individual B cell can receive help from T cells specific for different antigenic peptides provided that the B cell can present those determinants to each T cell.

In an immune response in vivo, it is believed that the interactions between T and B cells that drive B cell division and differentiation involve T cells that have already been stimulated by contact with the antigen on other antigen-presenting cells (APCs), for example dendritic cells.

This has led to the basic scheme for cell interactions in the antibody response set out in Figure 9.3. It is proposed that

B cell–co-receptor complex

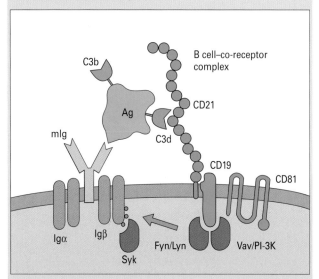

Fig. 9.5 The B cell–co-receptor complex consists of CD21 (the complement receptor type-2), CD19 and CD81 (a molecule with four transmembrane segments). Antigen with covalently bound C3b or C3d can cross-link the membrane Ig to CD21 of the co-receptor complex. This greatly reduces the cell's requirement for antigen to activate it. CD19 can associate with tyrosine kinases including Lyn, Fyn, Vav and PI-3 kinase (PI-3 K). Compare this with CD28 on the T cell. Receptor cross-linking causes phosphorylation of the Igα and Igβ chains of the antigen–receptor complex and recruitment and activation of Syk.

Follicular dendritic cells are known to retain antigen on their surface for prolonged periods of time as immune complexes (**iccosomes**). The antigen in such complexes can bind to:

- CD21 (via the complement molecule C3d); and
- surface Ig on the B cells.

Phosphorylation of the cytoplasmic tail of CD19 can then occur, leading to binding and activation of Lyn. It is likely that these kinases enhance the activation signal through the phospholipase C and phosphatidylinositol 3-kinase pathways, particularly when antigen concentration is low.

Q. If an animal was depleted of complement C3 during the primary immune response, what effect do you think this would have on the development of the secondary antibody response?

A. Lack of C3 means that immune complexes containing C3b and C3d do not form. Therefore they cannot bind to follicular dendritic cells (FDCs) via CR2 or engage with B cells via the B cell co-receptor complex (see Fig. 9.5); consequently B cell activation and the development of the secondary immune response is greatly impaired. (These experiments have been done by depleting mice of C3 using cobra venom factor.)

Direct interaction of B cells and T cells involves costimulatory molecules

Antigen-specific T-cell populations can be obtained by growing and cloning T cells with antigens, APCs and IL-2. It is thus possible to visualize directly B-cell and T-cell clusters interacting *in vitro*:

Cell surface molecules involved in the interaction between B and TH cells

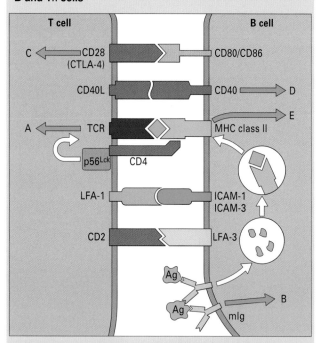

Fig. 9.6 Membrane immunoglobulin (mIg) takes up antigen (Ag) into an intracellular compartment where it is degraded and peptides can combine with MHC class II molecules. Other arrows show the discrete signal transduction events that have been established. A and B are the antigen–receptor signal transduction events involving tyrosine phosphorylation and phosphoinositide breakdown. The antigen receptors also regulate LFA-1 affinity for ICAM-1 and ICAM-3, possibly through the signal transduction events. In the T cell, CD28 also sends a unique signal to the T cell (C). In the later phases of the response CTLA-4 can supplant CD28 to cause downregulation. In the B cell, stimulation via CD40 is the most potent activating signal (D). In addition, class II MHC molecules appear to induce distinct signaling events (E). Not shown is the exchange of soluble interleukins and binding to the corresponding receptors on the other cell. (*Adapted with permission from DeFranco A, Nature 1991; 351: 603–5.*)

- the T cells become polarized, with the T-cell receptors concentrated on the B-cell side;
- the B cells also become polarized and express most of their MHC class II molecules and ICAM-1 in proximity to the T cells.

The interactions in these clusters strongly suggest an intense exchange of information, which leads to two important events in the B-cell life cycle:

- induction of proliferation; and
- differentiation into APCS.

The initial interaction between a naive B cell and a cognate antigen via the BCR in the presence of cytokines or other growth stimuli induces activation and proliferation of the B cell. This then leads to processing of the T-dependent antigen and presentation to T cells. The interaction between B cells and T cells is a two-way process in which B cells present antigen to T cells and receive signals from the T cells for division and differentiation (Fig. 9.6).

Cytokines and B cell development

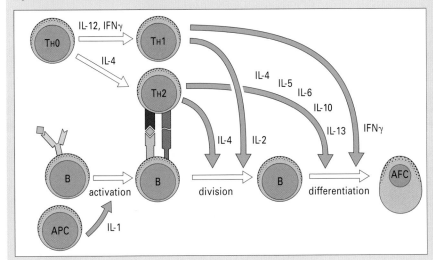

Fig. 9.7 B cell development is influenced by cytokines from T cells and APCs, and by direct interactions with TH2 cells. IL-4 is most important in promoting cell division, and a variety of other cytokines including IL-4, IL-5, IL-6, IL-10 and IFNγ, influence development into antibody-forming cells (AFCs) and affect the isotype of antibody that will be produced.

The central, antigen-specific interaction is that between the MHC class II–antigen complex and the TCR. This interaction is augmented by interactions between LFA-3 and CD2 and between ICAM-1 or ICAM-3 and LFA-1.

Q. Which costimulatory molecules, present on B cells and other APCs, promote T cell proliferation? What mechanisms are involved?
A. B7–1 (CD80) and B7–2 (CD86) act on antigen-activated T cells by ligating CD28, leading to expression of the high-affinity IL-2 receptor (see Fig. 8.1).

The interaction between B and T cells is a two-way event as follows:

- CD40, a member of the TNF receptor family, delivers a strong activating signal to B cells, more potent even than signals transmitted via surface immunoglobulin;
- upon activation, T cells transiently express a ligand, termed CD40L (a member of the TNF family), which interacts with CD40;
- CD40–CD40L interaction helps to drive B cells into cell cycle;
- transduction of signals through CD40 induces upregulation of CD80/CD86 and therefore helps to provide further costimulatory signals to the responding T cells.

Signaling through CD40 is also essential for germinal center development and antibody responses to TD antigens.

Q. Some individuals have a mutation that produces a non-functional variant of CD40L. In its homozygous form, what effect would you expect this mutation to have on serum antibody levels?
A. The mutation produces hyper-IgM syndrome, with high serum IgM and low IgG, IgA, and IgE levels, due to lack of germinal centers and failure of the B cells to switch isotype.

Cytokine secretion is important in B-cell proliferation and differentiation

Recent work has shown that CD4+ T cells in both mouse and man can be divided into different subsets, depending on their cytokine profile (see Fig. 11.4). During B-cell–T-cell interaction, T cells can secrete a number of cytokines that have a powerful effect on B cells (Fig. 9.7). IL-2, for example, is an inducer of proliferation for B cells as well as T cells.

In particular, cytokines produced by TH2 cells strongly promote B cell activation and the production of IgG1 and IgE. These cytokines include IL-4, IL-5, IL-6, IL-10 and IL-13:

- IL-4 acts on B cells to induce activation and differentiation. It also acts on T cells as a growth factor and promotes differentiation of TH2 cells, thus reinforcing the antibody response; excess IL-4 plays a part in allergic disease, causing production of IgE;
- IL-5 in humans is chiefly a growth and activation factor for eosinophils and is responsible for the eosinophilia of parasitic disease. In the mouse it also acts on B cells to induce growth and differentiation;
- IL-6 is produced by many cells including T cells, macrophages, B cells, fibroblasts and endothelial cells and acts on many cell types, but is particularly important in inducing B cells to differentiate into AFCs. IL-6 is considered to be an important growth factor for multiple myeloma, a malignancy of plasma cells;
- IL-10 acts as a growth and differentiation factor for B cells in addition to modulating cytokine production by TH1 cells;
- IL-13, which shares a receptor component and signaling pathways with IL-4, acts on B cells to produce IgE.

Additional TH subsets have been identified having distinct developmental programs and cytokine profiles. TH17 cells secrete IL-17 and are associated with immunity against extracellular bacteria and fungi, chronic inflammatory disease, and autoimmunity. Another T cell subset that helps B cells is the T follicular helper (TFH) cell, characterized by the expression of the chemokine receptor CXCR5 and localized to developing germinal centers. TFH cells help provide instructive signals that lead to Ig class switching and somatic mutation. TFH cells also produce high levels of IL-21, a cytokine that is critical for germinal center formation.

Q. Give three different ways in which IL-4 can reinforce the TH2-type response

A. It promotes differentiation of TH2 cells. It acts on B cells to promote their division and differentiation. It acts on endothelium and tissue cells to promote the synthesis of chemokines that selectively attract TH2 cells.

Cytokines can also influence antibody affinity. Antibody affinity to most TD antigens increases during an immune response, and a similar effect can be produced by certain immunization protocols. For example, high-affinity antibody subpopulations are potentiated after immunization with antigen and IFNγ (Fig. 9.8). A number of adjuvants are capable of enhancing levels of antibody, but few also potentiate affinity. As affinity markedly influences the biological effectiveness of antibodies, IFNγ may be an important adjuvant for use in vaccines.

In addition to the effects of cytokines on B-cell proliferation and differentiation, cytokines are capable of influencing the class switch from IgM to other immunoglobulin classes.

Cytokine receptors guide B-cell growth and differentiation

Receptors for the many growth and differentiation factors required to drive the B cells through early stages of development are expressed at various stages of B-cell differentiation. Receptors for IL-7, IL-3 and low-molecular-weight B-cell growth factor are important in the initial stages of B-cell differentiation, whereas other receptors are more important in the later stages (Fig. 9.9).

A recently identified cytokine, B-lymphocyte stimulator (BlyS), secreted by a variety of cells including monocytes and dendritic cells, is important in both the early development of B cells and their subsequent development and survival in germinal centers. BlyS acts through the receptor BR3 which appears to be important in T-dependent responses, whereas an alternative receptor TAC1 is more important in T-independent responses. BlyS is one of a pair of related cytokines belonging to the TNF family, which signal through these receptors to promote B cell differentiation.

B-cell–T-cell interaction may either activate or inactivate (anergize)

The description of B-cell–T-cell interaction suggests that the only possible outcome is activation of the B cell. However, this is not the case. It has already been seen that APC–T-cell interaction may yield two diametrically opposing results, namely activation or inactivation (clonal anergy). In the same way, B cells frequently become anergic. This is an important

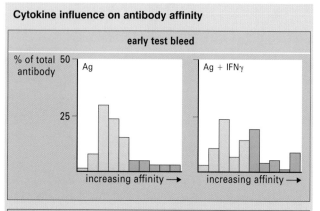

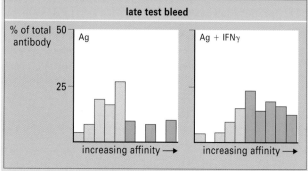

Fig. 9.8 Mice were immunized either with antigen alone (Ag) or with antigen plus 30 000 units of IFNγ (Ag + IFNγ). The affinity of the antibodies was measured either early or late after immunization. Mice receiving IFNγ show more high-affinity antibody (darker bars) in both the early and late bleeds than those mice that received antigen alone. *(Adapted from Holland, Holland & Steward. Clin Exp Immunol 1990;82:221–226.)*

Cytokine receptor expression during B cell development

markers	lymphoid stem cell	pro-B cell (progenitor)	pre-B cell	immature B cell	mature B cell	activated/blast B cell	memory B cell	plasma cell
IL-1R						◁▷		
IL-2R						◁▷		
IL-3R	◁━━━━━━━▷							
IL-4R				◁━━━━━━━━━━━▷				
IL-5R						◁▷		
IL-6R						◁▷		◁▷
IL-7R	◁━━━━━━▷							

Fig. 9.9 The whole life history of B cells from stem cell to mature plasma cell is regulated by cytokines present in their environment. Receptors for these cytokines are selectively expressed by B cells at different stages of development. Some of these receptors now have CD designation.

process because affinity maturation of B cells during the immune response, as a result of rapid mutation in the genes encoding the antibody variable regions, could easily result in high-affinity autoantibodies.

Clonal anergy and other forms of tolerance in the periphery are important for silencing these potentially damaging clones. However, the molecular details of this process are still unclear. Moreover, the respective roles of IgM and IgD, the two cell-surface receptors for antigen on B cells, are also not understood in terms of activation or inactivation.

B cell differentiation and the antibody response

Following activation, antigen-specific B cells can follow either of two separate developmental pathways:

- the first pathway involves proliferation and differentiation into antibody forming cells (AFCs) in the lymph nodes or in the periarteriolar lymphoid sheath of the spleen. These AFCs function to rapidly clear antigen. However, the great majority of these cells die via apoptosis within 2 weeks. Therefore, it is unlikely that these AFCs are responsible for long-term antibody production;
- in the second pathway some members of the expanded B-cell population migrate into adjacent follicles to form germinal centers before differentiating into memory B cells.

The mechanism that determines which path a B cell takes is unknown. However, it is likely that the decision can be influenced by the nature of the naive B cells initially recruited, the affinity and specificity of the BCR, the type of antigen driving the response, and the levels of T-cell help.

Q. Which type of APC is specifically located in the germinal center?
A. Follicular dendritic cells, which are very important in driving B cell development.

B cell affinity maturation occurs in germinal centers

The germinal center is important in that it provides a microenvironment where B cells can undergo developmental events that ultimately result in an affinity-matured, long-lived memory B-cell compartment (Fig. 9.10). These developmental events come about due to complex interactions between B cells, CD4$^+$ TH cells, and follicular dendritic cells. These events include:

- clonal proliferation;
- antibody variable region somatic hypermutation;
- receptor editing;
- isotype switch recombination;
- affinity maturation;
- positive selection.

The germinal center initially contains only dividing centroblasts. Shortly thereafter, it polarizes into a dark zone containing centroblasts and a light zone containing nondividing (resting) centrocytes (Figs 9.11 & 9.12). Centroblasts proliferate rapidly in the dark zone and downregulate the expression of their surface immunoglobulin. **Somatic hypermutation** then occurs to diversify the rearranged variable region genes (see Chapter 3, Fig. 3.28). Somatic hypermutation allows a single B cell to give rise to variants with different affinities for the antigen.

Isotype switch recombination occurs following somatic hypermutation and requires cell cycling. Receptor editing of immunoglobulin light chain genes also occurs in centroblasts.

B cell development in germinal centers

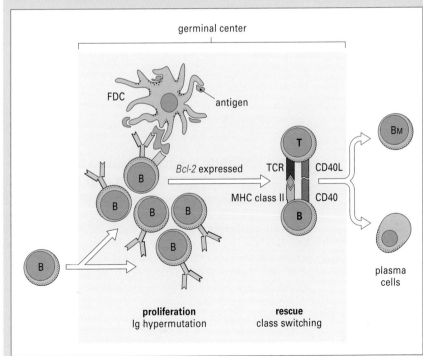

germinal center

FDC
antigen

Bcl-2 expressed
T
TCR   CD40L
MHC class II   CD40
B

B
B
B   B
B
B

BM

plasma cells

proliferation
Ig hypermutation

rescue
class switching

Fig. 9.10 A B cell enters a germinal center and undergoes rapid proliferation and hypermutation of its immunoglobulin genes. Antigen is presented by the follicular dendritic cell (FDC), but only B cells with high-affinity receptors will compete effectively for this antigen. B cells, which do have a higher-affinity immunoglobulin, express Bcl-2 and are rescued from apoptosis by interaction with T cells (i.e. the B-cell-presenting antigen to the T cell). Interaction with T cells promotes class switching. The class switch that takes place depends on the T cells present, which partly relates to the particular secondary lymphoid tissue and the type of immune response current (TH1 versus TH2). B cells leave the germinal center to become either plasma cells or B memory cells (Bm).

Schematic organization of the germinal center

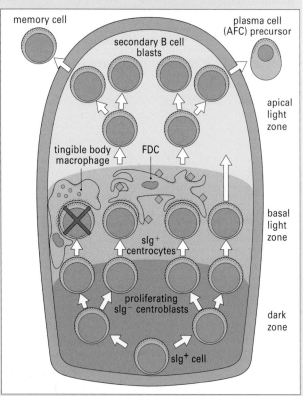

Fig. 9.11 The functions of the germinal center are clonal proliferation, somatic hypermutation of Ig receptors, receptor editing, isotype class switching, affinity maturation and selection by antigen. In this model, the germinal center is composed of three major zones: a dark zone, a basal light zone and an apical light zone. These zones are predominantly occupied by centroblasts, centrocytes, and secondary blasts, respectively. Primary B-cell blasts carrying surface immunoglobulin receptors (sIg⁺) enter the follicle and leave as memory B cells or AFCs. Antigen-presenting follicular dendritic cells (FDCs) are mainly found in the two deeper zones, and cell death by apoptosis occurs primarily in the basal light zone where tingible body macrophages are also located. Blue squares are iccosomes on FDC. *(Adapted from Roitt IM. Essential Immunology, 7th edn. Oxford: Blackwell Scientific Press, 1991.)*

Zoning of the germinal center of a lymph node

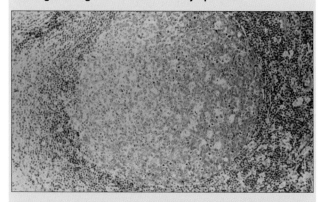

Fig. 9.12 The Giemsa-stained section (×40) shows the light zone (left) and the more actively proliferating dark zone (right). There is a well-developed mantle of small resting lymphocytes which have less cytoplasm and therefore appear more densely packed. *(Courtesy of Dr K McLennan.)*

Self-reactive B cells generated by somatic mutation are deleted

Centrocytes that respond to soluble antigen or do not receive T-cell help are negatively selected and undergo Fas-independent apoptosis. In this way, selection provides a mechanism for elimination of self-reactive antibodies that may be generated during somatic hypermutation.

Positively selected centrocytes can re-enter the dark zone for successive rounds of expansion, diversification and selection. Somatic hypermutation and selection improve the average affinity of the germinal center B-cell population for presented antigen.

Following these B-cell developmental stages, the centrocytes exit the germinal center and lose their susceptibility to apoptosis by downregulating Fas and increasing the expression of Bcl-2. Three possible outcomes are associated with exit from the germinal center:

- antibody-secreting bone marrow homing effector B cells;
- marginal zone memory B cells;
- recirculating memory B cells.

The factors that regulate the decision to exit the germinal center are poorly understood.

In-vivo antibody responses show isotype switching, affinity maturation and memory

The earliest studies on antibody responses *in vivo* identified different phases in the response. Following primary antigenic challenge, there is an initial lag phase when no antibody can be detected. This is followed by phases in which the antibody titer increases logarithmically to a plateau and then declines. The decline occurs because the antibodies are either naturally catabolized or bind to the antigen and are cleared from the circulation (Fig. 9.13).

It is now possible to understand the features of the antibody response *in vivo* in terms of the underlying cellular events, although the events can best be understood by viewing the B-cell population as a whole, rather than as a

Following these developmental changes, the centroblasts migrate to the follicular dendritic cell- (FDC-) light zone of the germinal center and give rise to centrocytes which then re-express surface immunoglobulin BCR. In the light zone, centrocytes encounter antigen bound to the FDCs and antigen-specific TH2 cells. FDCs and T cells interact with centrocytes through:

- surface molecules such as the BCR, CD40, CD80 (B7-1), CD86 (B7-2), LFA-1, VLA-4, CD54 (ICAM-1); and
- cytokines such as IL-2, IL-4, IL-5, IL-6, IL-10, IL-13 and lymphotoxin-α.

After the centrocytes have stopped dividing, they are selected according to their ability to bind antigen. Those with high-affinity receptors for foreign antigen are positively selected, while those without adequate affinity are induced to undergo apoptosis by ligation of the surface molecule Fas.

The four phases of a primary antibody response

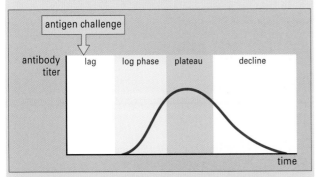

Fig. 9.13 After antigen challenge, the antibody response proceeds in four phases: a lag phase when no antibody is detected; a log phase when the antibody titre increases logarithmically; a plateau phase during which the antibody titre stabilizes and a decline phase during which the antibody is cleared or catabolized.

Primary and secondary antibody responses

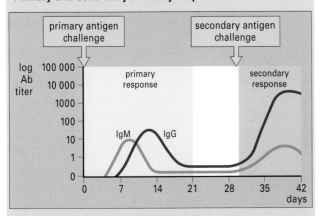

Fig. 9.14 In comparison with the antibody response after primary antigenic challenge, the antibody level after secondary antigenic challenge in a typical immune response appears more quickly, persists for a longer period of time, attains a higher titre and consists predominantly of IgG.

Affinity maturation

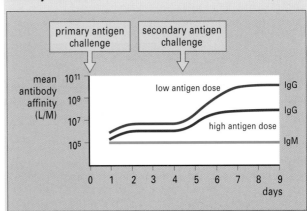

Fig. 9.15 The average affinity of the IgM and IgG antibody responses after primary and secondary challenge with a T-dependent antigen is shown. The affinity of the IgM response is constant throughout. The affinity maturation of the IgG response depends on the dose of the secondary antigen. Low antigen doses produce higher-affinity immunoglobulin than do high antigen doses, because the high-affinity clones compete effectively for the limiting amount of antigen.

Antibody class –
IgM antibodies form a major proportion of the primary response, whereas the secondary response consists almost entirely of IgG, with very little IgM.

Antibody affinity –
The affinity of the antibodies in the secondary response is usually much higher. This is referred to as 'affinity maturation'.

Affinity maturation depends on cell selection

The antibodies produced in a primary response to a TD antigen generally have a low average affinity. However, during the course of the response, the average affinity of the antibodies increases or 'matures.' As antigen becomes limiting, the clones with the higher affinity will have a selective advantage. This process is called **affinity maturation**.

The degree of affinity maturation is inversely related to the dose of antigen administered. High antigen doses produce poor maturation compared with low antigen doses (Fig. 9.15). It is thought that:

- in the presence of low antigen concentrations, only B cells with high-affinity receptors bind sufficient antigen and are triggered to divide and differentiate;
- in the presence of high antigen concentrations, there is sufficient antigen to bind and trigger both high- and low-affinity B cells.

Although individual B cells do not usually change their overall specificity, the affinity of the antibody produced by a clone may be altered. Affinity maturation is achieved through two processes:

- somatic hypermutation of the region including the recombined VDJ gene segment which encodes the variable domain of the heavy chain;
- antigen-driven selection and expansion of mutant clones expressing higher affinity antibodies.

collection of individual cells. Features of the antibody response *in vivo* include:

- the enhanced secondary response;
- isotype switching;
- affinity maturation;
- the development of memory.

The responses following primary and secondary antigenic challenge are shown in Figure 9.14 and they differ in four major respects.

Time course –
The secondary response has a shorter lag phase and an extended plateau and decline.

Antibody titre –
The plateau levels of antibody are much greater in the secondary response, typically 10-fold or more than plateau levels in the primary response.

Constant-region genes of mouse

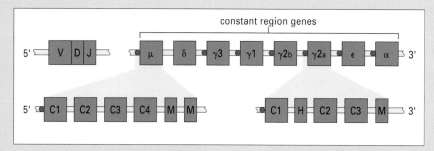

Fig. 9.16 The constant-region genes of the mouse are arranged 8.5 kb downstream from the recombined VDJ segment. Each C gene (except Cδ) has one or more switching sequences at its start (red circles), which correspond to a sequence at the 5′ end of the μ gene. This allows any of the C genes to be expressed together with the VDJ segment. δ genes appear to use the same switching sequences as μ, but the μ gene transcript is lost in RNA processing to produce IgD (see Fig. 9.19). The C genes (expanded below for μ and γ2a) contain introns separating the exons for each domain (C1, C2, etc.). The γ genes also have a separate exon coding for the hinge (H), and all the genes have one or more exons coding for membrane-bound immunoglobulin (M).

The mechanism by which affinity maturation occurs is thought to involve B-cell progeny binding to antigen on follicular dendritic cells (FDCs) in order to proliferate and differentiate further. Unprocessed antigen in immune complexes is captured by the FDCs via their Fc and complement receptors and held there. As B cells encounter the antigen, there is competition for space on the surface of the FDC, leading to selection. When a cell with higher affinity arises, it will stay there longer and be given a stronger signal. B cells with higher affinity will thus have a selective advantage.

An alternative theory is that B cells with higher affinity receptors will compete more effectively to bind and internalize antigen and therefore they have a greater potential of presenting antigen to T cells, and receiving T-cell help.

B cell isotype switching and somatic hypermutation

Somatic hypermutation is a common event in antibody-forming cells during T-dependent responses and is important in the generation of high-affinity antibodies. Somatic hypermutation introduces point mutations at a very high rate into the variable regions of the rearranged heavy and light chain genes (see Fig. 3.28). This results in mutated immunoglobulin molecules on the surface of the B cell. Mutants that bind antigen with higher affinity than the original surface immunoglobulin provide the raw material for the selection processes mentioned above.

Receptor editing is another mechanism by which diversity can be introduced into B cells during affinity maturation. Secondary V(D)J recombination can occur in immature B cells whose antigen receptors bind self antigen. The resulting immunoglobulin rearrangement converts these cells into non-self-reactive cells. In this way, specificity for foreign antigens can be improved and self-reactivity avoided.

Somatic hypermutation occurs at the same time as isotype switching and both processes involve an enzyme, **activation-induced cytidine deaminase (AID)**, which is highly expressed in germinal centers and is induced by

IL-4 and ligation of CD40. Animals lacking this enzyme have deficient somatic hypermutation and class switch recombination. The mechanisms involved in isotype switching and somatic hypermutation are described below.

B cells recombine their heavy chain genes to switch immunoglobulin isotype

B cells produce antibodies of five major classes – IgM, IgD, IgG, IgA, and IgE. In humans, there are also four subclasses of IgG and two of IgA (see Chapter 3). Each terminally differentiated plasma cell is derived from a specific B cell and produces antibodies of just one class or subclass (isotype).

The first B cells to appear during development carry surface IgM as their antigen receptor. Upon activation, other classes of immunoglobulin are seen, each associated with different effector functions. When a mature AFC switches antibody class, all that changes is the constant region of the heavy chain. The expressed V(D)J region and light chain do not change. Antigen specificity is therefore retained.

The arrangement of the constant genes in mouse and humans is shown in Figures 9.16 and 9.17. Upstream of the μ genes is a switch sequence (S), which is repeated upstream to each of the other constant region genes except δ. These sequences are important in the recombination events that occur during class switching, as explained below.

Class switching occurs during maturation and proliferation

Most class switching occurs during proliferation. However, it can also take place before encounter with exogenous antigen during early clonal expansion and maturation of the B cells (Fig. 9.18). This is known because some of the progeny of immature B cells synthesize antibodies of other immunoglobulin classes, including IgG and IgA.

Further evidence that some class switching occurs independently of antigen comes from experiments with vertebrates raised in gnotobiotic (virtually sterile) environments where exposure to exogenous antigens is severely restricted.

Constant-region genes and class switching in humans

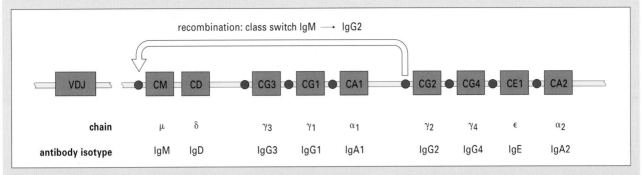

Fig. 9.17 The human immunoglobulin heavy chain gene locus (IGH) is shown. Initially, B cells transcribe a VDJ gene and a μ heavy chain that is spliced to produce mRNA for IgM. Under the influence of T cells and cytokines, class switching may occur, illustrated here as a switch from IgM to IgG2. Each heavy chain gene except CD (which encodes IgD) is preceded by a switch region. When class switching occurs, recombination between these regions takes place, with the loss of the intervening C genes – in this case CM, CD, CG3, CG1 and CA1. (Note that pseudogenes have been omitted from this diagram.)

B cell differentiation – class diversity

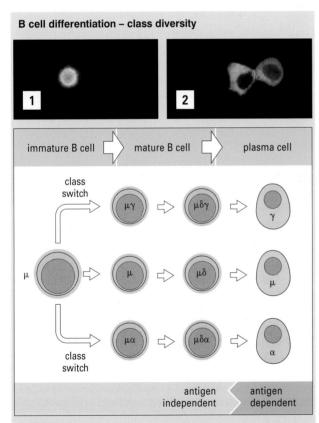

Fig. 9.18 Immature B cells produce IgM only, but mature B cells can express more than one cell surface antibody, because mRNA and cell surface immunoglobulin remain after a class switch. IgD is also expressed during clonal maturation. Maturation can occur in the absence of antigen, but the development into plasma cells (which have little surface immunoglobulin but much cytoplasmic immunoglobulin) requires antigen and (usually) T-cell help. The photographs show B cells stained for surface IgM (green, 1) and plasma cells stained for cytoplasmic IgM and IgG (green and red, 2). IgM is stained with fluorescent anti-μ chain and IgG with rhodaminated anti-γ chain.

Isotype switching by differential RNA splicing

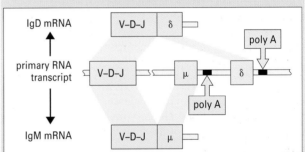

Fig. 9.19 Single B cells produce more than one antibody isotype from a single long primary RNA transcript. A transcript containing μ and δ is shown here. Polyadenylation can occur at different sites, leading to different forms of splicing, producing mRNA for IgD (top) or IgM (bottom). Even within this region, there are additional polyadenylation sites that determine whether the translated immunoglobulin is the secreted or membrane-bound form.

Class switching may be achieved by differential splicing of mRNA

Initially, a complete section of DNA that includes the recombined VDJ region and the δ and μ constant regions is transcribed. Two mRNA molecules may then be produced by differential splicing, each with the same VDJ segment, but having either μ or δ constant regions.

It is suggested that much larger stretches of DNA are sometimes also transcribed together, with differential splicing giving other immunoglobulin classes sharing Vh regions (Fig. 9.19). This has been observed in cells simultaneously producing IgM and IgE.

Class switching is mostly achieved by gene recombination

The principal mechanism of class switching is by recombination. B cells switch from IgM to the other immunoglobulin classes or subclasses by an intrachromosomal deletion

Class switching by gene recombination

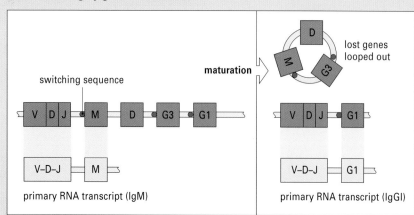

switching sequence

primary RNA transcript (IgM)

maturation

lost genes looped out

primary RNA transcript (IgGl)

Fig. 9.20 Initially the VDJ region is transcribed together with the M gene for the IgM heavy chain (left). After removal of introns during processing, mRNA for secreted IgM is produced. During B-cell maturation, class-switch recombination occurs between the Sµ recombination region and a downstream switch region (G1 in this example). The intervening region (containing genes for IgM, IgD and IgG3 in this instance) is looped out and then cut, with deletion of the intervening regions and joining of the two switch regions.

process which involves the excision of intervening genetic material between highly repetitive switch regions 5′ to each chain (Fig. 9.20).

Switching involves cytokine-dependent transcription of DNA in the region of the new constant region, reflecting changes in the chromatin in that region. This occurs before recombination of the 5′ switch regions that precede the genes for each of the heavy chain isotype constant region domains.

The mechanism of recombination involves the deamination of cytosine residues in the switch sequences by the enzyme AID, to leave uracil residues which are excised to leave abasic DNA strands. These regions are now targeted by an endonuclease to cause double-stranded breaks in the DNA, which are then rejoined (with the loss of the intervening loop) by DNA repair enzymes.

AID is also involved in the process of hypermutation. Uracil residues and abasic sites introduced into the variable region exon are scanned by enzymes that mediate mismatch repair and base-excision repair. These enzymes are normally involved in correcting DNA-replication errors preceding cell division, but in the germinal center they are diverted to the process of variable region hypermutation. The DNA polymerases that correct the mismatches and abasic sites introduced by AID are error-prone. Hence the high level of mutation that occurs.

Both recombination and hypermutation require that the enzyme AID is selectively targeted to the actively-transcribing immunoglobulin heavy chain genes. How this occurs is uncertain, however it may involve secondary structure in the DNA of the heavy chain genes, or additional DNA-binding proteins, that recognize sequences in the switch regions and variable region exons.

Immunoglobulin class expression is influenced by cytokines and type of antigenic stimulus

During a TD immune response, there is a progressive change in the predominant immunoglobulin class of the specific antibody produced, usually to IgG. This class switch is not seen in TI responses, in which the predominant immunoglobulin usually remains IgM.

Isotype regulation by mouse T cell cytokines

TH	cytokines	immunoglobulin isotypes					
		IgG1	IgE	IgA	IgG3	IgG2b	IgG2a
TH2	IL-4	↑	↑	↓	↓	↓	↓
	IL-5	=	=	↑	=	=	=
TH1	IFNγ	↓	↓	↓	↓	↓	↑

Fig. 9.21 The effects of IFNγ (product of TH1 cells) and IL-4 and IL-5 (products of TH2 cells) which result in an increase (↑), a decrease (↓) or no change (=) in the frequency of isotype-specific B cells after stimulation with the polyclonal activator LPS, *in vitro*.

There is now considerable evidence for the involvement of T cells and their cytokines in the de-novo isotype switching:

- in mice, T cells in mucosal sites have been shown to stimulate IgA production;
- IL-4 preferentially switches B cells that have been either polyclonally activated (by lipopolysaccharide) or specifically activated by antigen to the IgG1 or IgE isotype, with concomitant suppression of other isotypes, and in a similar system IL-5 induces a 5–10-fold increase in IgA production with no change in other isotypes;
- IFNγ enhances IgG2a responses in mice, but suppresses all other isotypes (Fig. 9.21).

It is interesting that IL-4 and IFNγ, which act as reciprocal regulatory cytokines for the expression of antibody isotypes, are derived from different TH subsets. In addition, IL-12 and IL-18 stimulation of mouse T cells can induce the production of IFNγ. These cells can therefore act as immunoregulatory cells by differentially inducing IgG2a expression, while inhibiting IgG1, IgE, and IgG2b expression. Transforming growth factor-β (TGFβ) induces the switch to IgA or IgG2b. In humans, the situation is somewhat different:

- IL-4 induces the expression of IgG4 and IgE; and
- TGFβ induces the expression of IgA alone.

Isotype switching is greatly affected by the tissue environment; cells in the tissue can affect isotype switching directly by release of cytokines, but more importantly they selectively attract particular lymphocyte subsets into the tissue, by release of appropriate chemokines.

CRITICAL THINKING: DEVELOPMENT OF THE ANTIBODY RESPONSE (SEE P. 436 FOR EXPLANATIONS)

A project is underway to develop a vaccine against mouse hepatitis virus, a pathogen of mice, which may become a serious problem in colonies of mice. The vaccine consists of capsid protein of the virus, which is injected subcutaneously as a depot in alum on day 0. At days 5 and 14, the group of six mice is bled and the serum is tested for the presence of antibodies against the viral capsid protein. Separate assays are done for each of the immunoglobulin classes, IgM, IgG and IgA. The amounts, expressed in μg/mL of antibody, are shown in Figure 9.22.

When the data is analyzed it appears that two of the animals (green spots) have high titres of antibody particularly of IgG and IgA, at both days 5 and 14.

1 Why do the titres of IgG antibodies increase more rapidly between days 5 and 14 than do IgM antibodies, in all animals?

2 Propose an explanation for the high titres of IgG antibodies in the two animals indicated at day 5. Can this explanation also account for the relatively high levels of IgA antibodies also seen in these mice?

    The spleens from mice taken at day 14 are used to produce B cells making monoclonal antibodies against the viral protein. Of the clones produced, 15 produce IgG, three produce IgM and none produce IgA.

3 Why do you suppose there are no IgA-producing clones, despite the good IgA response?

4 You want a high-affinity antibody for use in an assay. Which of the clones you have produced are likely to be of higher affinity?

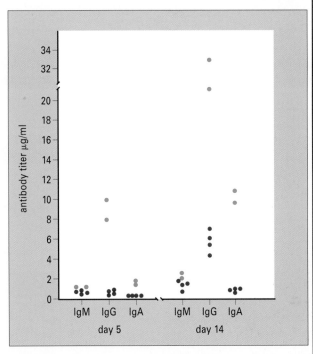

Fig. 9.22 Antibody titres in immunized mice.

Further reading

Hardy RR, Hayakawa K. B cell development pathways. Annu Rev Immunol 2001;19:595–621.

Peled JU, Kuang FL, Iglesias-Ussel MD, et al. The biochemistry of somatic hypermutation. Ann Rev Immunol 2008;26:481–511.

Smith KG, Fearon DT. Receptor modulators of B cell receptor signaling – CD19/CD22. Curr Top Microbiol Immunol 2000;245:195–212.

Stavenezer J, Guikema JEJ, Schrader CE. Mechanisms and regulation of class switch recombination. Ann Rev Immunol 2008;26:261–292.

CHAPTER 10

Cell-mediated Cytotoxicity

SUMMARY

- **Cell-mediated cytoxicity is an essential defence against intracellular pathogens, including viruses, some bacteria and some parasites.**

- **CTLs and NK cells are the lymphoid effectors of cytotoxicity.** Most CTLs are CD8$^+$ and respond to non-self antigens presented on MHC class I molecules. Some virally infected and cancerous cells try to evade the CTL response by downregulating MHC class I. NK cells recognize these MHC class I negative targets.

- **NK cells recognize cells that fail to express MHC class I.** NK cells express a variety of inhibitory receptors that recognize MHC class I molecules. When these receptors are not engaged, the NK cell is activated. Killer Immunoglobulin-like Receptors (KIRs) recognize classical MHC class I molecules. CD94 interacts with HLA-E. LILRB1 recognizes a wide range of class I molecules.

- **Cancerous and virally infected cells express ligands for the activating receptor NKG2D.** Stressed cells, including cancerous and virally infected cells, upregulate ULBP1–3, MICA and MICB, which are ligands for NKG2D. This results in NK cell activation.

- **NK cells can also mediate ADCC.**

- **The balance of inhibitory and activating signals determines NK cell activation.**

- **Cytotoxicity is effected by direct cellular interactions, granule exocytosis and cytokine production.** Fas ligand and TNF can induce apoptosis in the target cell. Granules containing perforin and granzymes are also released. Perforin forms a pore in the cell membrane, allowing granzymes access to the cytosol. Granzymes trigger the cell's intrinsic apoptosis pathways.

- **Macrophages, neutrophils and eosinophils are non-lymphoid cytotoxic effectors.** Macrophages and neutrophils usually destroy pathogens by phagocytosis, but can also sometimes release the contents of their granules into the extracellular environment. Eosinophils release cytotoxic granules in response to antibody-coated cells.

Cytotoxic lymphocytes

Cytotoxicity describes the ways in which leukocytes can recognize and destroy other cells. It is an essential defense against intracellular pathogens, including:

- viruses;
- some bacteria; and
- some parasites.

Tumor cells and even normal host cells may also become the targets of cytotoxic cells. Cytotoxicity is important in the destruction of allogeneic tissue grafts.

Several types of cells have cytotoxic potential, including:

- cytotoxic T lymphocytes (CTLs);
- natural killer (NK) cells; and
- some myeloid cells.

The two cytotoxic lymphoid effector cells recognize their targets in different ways, but use similar mechanisms to kill them. The myeloid cells use different recognition and killing mechanisms from the lymphoid cells, and indeed these also differ between different types of myeloid cell.

CTLs and NK cells mediate cytotoxicity

T cells and NK cells belong to the lymphoid lineage, and are more closely related to each other than they are to B cells. CTLs and NK cells both induce apoptosis in their targets by production of TNF family molecules, cytokines and cytotoxic granules, but they recognize their targets in different ways. CTLs recognize foreign antigens being presented on MHC class I, whereas NK cells respond to cells that fail to express class I. NK cells are also able to recognize stressed or antibody-coated targets directly (Fig. 10.1).

CTLs and NK cells mediate cytotoxicity

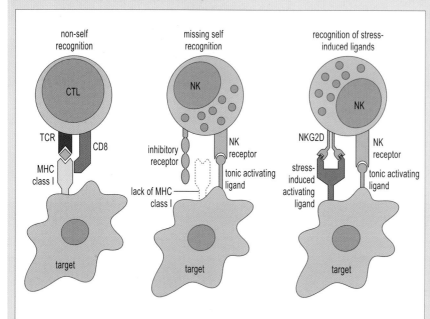

Fig. 10.1 CTLs recognize processed antigen presented on the target cell by MHC molecules, using their T cell receptor (TCR). Most CTLs are CD8+ and recognize antigen presented by MHC class I molecules, but a minority are CD4+ and recognize antigen presented on MHC class II molecules. In contrast, NK cells have receptors that recognize MHC class I on the target and inhibit cytotoxicity. NK cells also express a number of activating receptors to identify their targets positively, including NKG2D and their Fc receptor (CD16).

Effector CTLs home to peripheral organs and sites of inflammation

Naive CTLs circulate in the blood and lymphatic system, but in order to kill specific target cells, they must be activated and become effector cells. This process is mediated by APCs in the lymph nodes. Naive T cells in the lymph nodes use their T cell receptor (TCR) to recognize specific antigens being presented by MHC molecules on APCs. Most CTLs are CD8+ and therefore recognize antigen presented on MHC class I molecules, although some CD4+ cells are cytotoxic and so recognize antigen presented on MHC class II molecules.

If, in addition to signaling through the TCR, the APC also delivers a costimulatory signal through CD28, the CTL becomes activated and proliferates. Activated CTLs downregulate sphingosine phosphate receptor, allowing them to exit the lymph node. They also downregulate molecules associated with homing to the lymph node, such as L-selectin and CCR7, and upregulate molecules that allow them to home to sites of inflammation, such as CD44 and LFA-1. Effector T cells may also express adhesion molecules that allow them to home to specific tissues. CD8+ memory T cells appear to preferentially migrate to the tissue in which they first encountered their antigen.

CTLs recognize antigen presented on MHC class I molecules

The most important role of CTLs is the elimination of virally infected cells. CTLs recognize specific antigens (e.g. viral peptides on infected cells) presented by MHC class I molecules, which are expressed by nearly all nucleated cells. Cellular molecules that have been partly degraded by the proteasome are transported to the endoplasmic reticulum, where they become associated with MHC class I molecules and are transported to the cell surface. Normal cells

therefore present a sample of all the antigens they produce to CD8+ T cells.

Q. How does a virus-infected cell know which molecules are viral antigens and should therefore be presented to CTLs?

A. It does not. Each cell samples its own molecules and presents them for review by CD8+ T cells. Both the cell's own molecules and those of intracellular pathogens will be presented in this way. It is the T cells that distinguish self from non-self antigens, not the infected cell.

Additional interactions may be required to stabilize the bond between a CTL and its target. Like CD4+ T cells, CD8+ CTLs form an immunological synapse with their target. Signaling molecules including the TCR and CD3 are found in the central zone of the supra-molecular activation cluster (cSMAC), while adhesion molecules segregate in the peripheral zone (pSMAC). In contrast to CD4+ T cells, the cSMAC of CTLs and NK cells is divided into signaling and secretory domains (Fig. 10.2). After signaling has occurred, the microtubule organizing center polarizes towards the synapse, directing cytotoxic granules to the secretory domain of the cSMAC. Early CTL signaling occurs within ten seconds of cell–cell contact and granule release follows some two minutes later.

CTLs and NK cells are complementary in the defense against virally infected and cancerous cells

Natural killer (NK) cells were first identified as a subset of immune cells that were able to kill tumor cells *in vitro* without prior immunization of the host, even in T cell deficient mice. In 1981 Klas Kärre made the seminal observation that targets killed by NK cells tend to be spared by T cells and *vice versa*. From this, he reasoned that NK cells must recognize targets that are not expressing a full complement

Some interactions involved in the CTL synapse

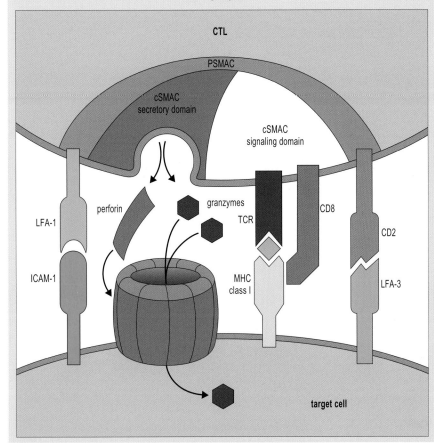

Fig. 10.2 The TCR and CD8 localize to the signaling domain in the center of the synapse (cSMAC); degranulation occurs in the secretory domain. Adhesion molecules that stabilize the cell–cell interactions are located at the periphery of the supramolecular activation complex (pSMAC).

of 'self' molecules. Kärre's 'missing self' hypothesis postulates that unlike T cells, which recognize 'non-self' (foreign peptide or foreign MHC), NK cells respond to the absence of MHC class I.

Several viruses (particularly herpes viruses) have evolved mechanisms to avoid recognition by CTLs. They reduce the expression of MHC class I molecules on the cell surface to reduce the likelihood that processed viral peptides can be presented to CTLs. Cancerous cells may evade the CTL response in a similar way. NK cells specifically recognize cells that have lost their MHC class I molecules. Therefore, NK cells and CTLs act in a complementary way. In effect:

- NK cells check that cells of the body are carrying their identity card (MHC class I);
- CTLs check the specific identity (antigen specificity) on the card.

Not all NK cells mediate cytotoxicity

In humans, most NK cells are CD56⁺CD3⁻ cells. However, not all cells with this phenotype are effective killers:

- 90% of blood NK cells are CD56^{low} (i.e. they have low expression of CD56). These cells contain cytotoxic granules and are effective killers;
- 10% of blood NK cells are CD56^{hi} (i.e. they express high levels of CD56). These cells do not contain cytotoxic

granules, but can respond to target cells by producing the TH1 cytokine IFNγ;
- NK cells present in the lymph nodes, liver, and lungs are also less cytotoxic than CD56^{low} blood NK cells;
- NK cells found in the uterus do contain cytotoxic granules, but do not degranulate in response to target cells. Their function is likely to be the production of angiogenic factors and mediation of placental implantation;
- a recently described subset of NK-like cells found in MALT are not cytotoxic but do produce IL-22, which is important for mucosal integrity.

NK cell receptors

NK cells recognize cells that fail to express MHC class I

NK cells express inhibitory receptors that bind to MHC class I molecules. When they encounter a target cell that is not expressing MHC class I, this inhibitory signal is lost and tonic activating signals cause the NK cell to degranulate or produce cytokines in response to the target cell. Interestingly, many of the inhibitory receptors expressed by NK cells also have activating counterparts, many of which recognize the same ligands but with lower affinity. The function of these activating receptors is not known (Fig. 10.3).

NK cell receptors with well-defined ligands

family	receptor	ligand	
KIR	KIR2DL1	HLA-C2	inhibitory
	KIR2DS1	HLA-C2	activating
	KIR3DL1	HLA-Bw4	inhibitory
	KIR3DL2	HLA-A3 and A11	inhibitory
	KIR2DL2/3	HLA-C1	inhibitory
c-type lectin-like	CD94-NKG2A	HLA-E	inhibitory
	CD94-NKG2C	HLA-E	activating
	CD94-NKG2E	HLA-E	activating
	NKG2D	ULBPs, MICA/B	activating
LILR	LILRB1	broad MHC-I	inhibitory
NCRs	NKp44	viral hemagglutinins	activating
	NKp46	viral hemagglutinins	activating
others	LAIR1	collagens	inhibitory
	Siglec-7	sialic acid	inhibitory
	KLRG1	cadherins	inhibitory
	CEACAM1	CEACAM1	inhibitory
	CD16	IgG	activating
	2B4	CD48	activating

Fig. 10.3 NK cell receptors with well-defined ligands.

Killer immunoglobulin-like receptors recognize MHC class I

The killer immunoglobulin-like receptors, or KIRs, are members of the immunoglobulin superfamily. They are present on the majority of CD56^{low} NK cells, with each individual NK cell expressing a random selection of KIRs. Almost none of the CD56^{hi} NK cells express KIRs.

KIRs fall into two main subsets:

- KIR2D (CD158) have two immunoglobulin domains;
- KIR3D have three immunoglobulin domains.

The KIRs are then further classified by whether they have a long (L) or short (S) cytoplasmic tail. KIRs with long tails are inhibitory and those with short tails are activating (Fig. 10.4). For example, the inhibitory receptor KIR2DL1 has two immunoglobulin domains and a long cytoplasmic tail. It binds alleles of HLA-C that have a lysine residue at position 80 (HLA-C2 alleles). Its activating counterpart, KIR2DS1 also binds HLA-C2 alleles, but with lower affinity. The ligands of most other activating KIRs are not yet known.

Inhibitory KIRs therefore allow NK cells to recognize and respond to cells that have downregulated specific HLA molecules. This is likely to explain genetic associations whereby those individuals who have both a particular KIR and its cognate HLA molecule experience better outcomes in some viral diseases such as hepatitis B and C. The normal functions of the activating KIRs are unknown, although the presence of activating KIR in the donor is associated with better outcomes when hematopoietic stem cell transplantation is used as a treatment for some leukemias.

NK cells in mice do not express KIRs. Instead, they use Ly49 receptors, which are members of the lectin-like

Killer immunologloblulin-like receptors

inhibitory receptors	non-inhibitory receptors

Fig. 10.4 KIRs consist of either two or three extracellular immunoglobulin superfamily domains. The inhibitory forms have long cytoplasmic tails that contain ITIMs (immunoreceptor tyrosine inhibitory motifs). The activating forms have short cytoplasmic tails and a charged lysine residue (K) in their transmembrane domains, which allows them to associate with an ITAM–containing adaptor molecule.

receptor family. Like KIRs, Ly49 receptors come in inhibitory and activating forms, bind to specific MHC class I molecules, and are expressed stochastically. Unlike KIRs, which recognize the top of the peptide binding groove of MHC class I, Ly49 receptors recognize the underside of the

Lectin-like receptors of NK cells

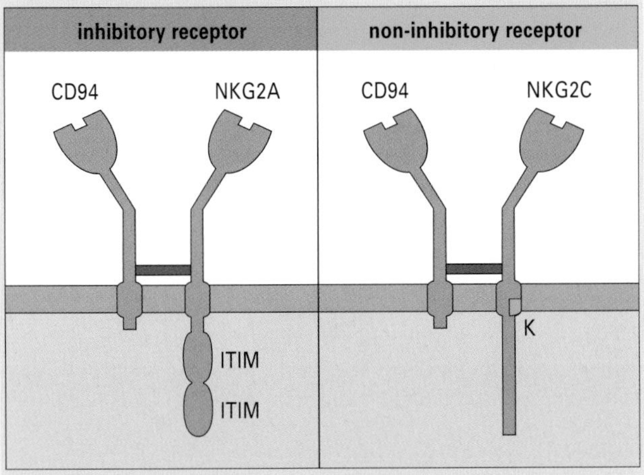

inhibitory receptor	non-inhibitory receptor

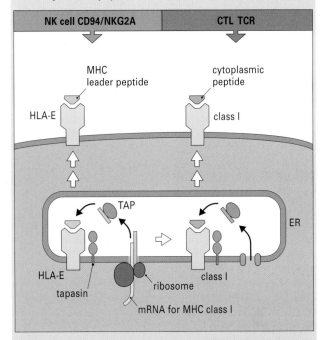

Fig. 10.5 CD94 associates with members of the NKG2 family via a disulphide bond. NKG2A contains intracellular ITIMs (immunoreceptor tyrosine inhibitory motifs) and so forms an inhibitory receptor. NKG2C lacks ITIMs but has a charged lysine residue (K) in its transmembrane segment, which allows it to interact with ITAM (immunoreceptor tyrosine activatory motif) – containing adaptor molecules.

HLA-E presents peptides of other MHC class I molecules

Fig. 10.6 Leader peptides from MHC class I molecules are loaded onto HLA-E molecules in the endoplasmic reticulum, a process that requires TAP transporters and tapasin to assemble functional HLA-E molecules. These are presented at the cell surface for review by CD94 receptors on NK cells. The MHC class I molecules meanwhile present antigenic peptides from cytoplasmic proteins that have been transported into the endoplasmic reticulum. These complexes are presented to the TCR on CD8$^+$ CTLs.

molecule. Ly49 and KIRs are unrelated molecules that perform the same function in different species, providing an interesting illustration of convergent evolution.

The lectin-like receptor CD94 recognizes HLA-E

The lectin-like receptor CD94 is present on the majority of CD56^{hi} NK cells, a large subset of CD56^{low} NK cells and is also found on a small subset of CTLs. It covalently associates with different members of another group of lectin-like receptors called NKG2, and the dimers are expressed at the cell membrane.

There are at least six members of the NKG2 family (NKG2A-F), of which all except NKG2D associate with CD94. NKG2A-CD94 is an inhibitory receptor that blocks NK cell activation. By contrast, CD94-NKG2C is an activating receptor (Fig. 10.5). The ligand for both CD94-NKG2A and CD94-NKG2C is HLA-E, although the inhibitory CD94-NKG2A has greater affinity for HLA-E than its activating counterpart. The function of CD94-NKG2A is to allow NK cells to recognize and respond to cells, such as those that are virally infected or cancerous, that are expressing low levels of MHC class I molecules

The *HLA-E* gene locus encodes an MHC class I-like molecule. These are sometimes called non-classical class I molecules, or class Ib molecules, to distinguish them from the classical MHC molecules that present antigen to CTLs. The function of HLA-E is to present peptides from other MHC class I molecules. The leader peptides from other MHC molecules are transported to the endoplasmic reticulum and are loaded into the peptide binding groove of HLA-E molecules, stabilizing them and allowing them to be transported to the plasma membrane (Fig. 10.6). Cells lacking classical MHC class I molecules do not express HLA-E at the cell surface. Thus, surface HLA-E levels provide

a sensitive mechanism for monitoring global MHC class I expression by the cell.

Q. Unlike the classical MHC class I molecules, HLA-E is not highly polymorphic. Additionally, the leader peptides of classical MHC class I molecules are very similar, regardless of the haplotype of the molecules. From these observations, what can you infer about immune regulation mediated by CD94-NKG2A?

A. The combination of HLA-E plus leader peptide is similar regardless of the haplotype, therefore the CD94-NKG2A receptor does not need to be able to recombine to recognize MHC molecules of different haplotypes. Compare this with antigen presentation by classical MHC class I molecules, and their recognition by the TCR.

LILRB1 recognizes all MHC class I molecules including HLA-G

LILRB1 belongs to the LILR family of type I transmembrane proteins with multiple extracellular immunoglobulin domains (previously called the ILT family, or CD85). Of this family, only two inhibitory receptors, LILRB1 and LILRB2 have well-defined ligands, and these interact with a broad spectrum of MHC class I molecules. LILRB1 is expressed by a proportion of NK cells, as well as some T cells, B cells and all monocytes, whereas LILRB2 is only expressed by monocytes and dendritic cells. Thus LILRB1, like CD94-NKG2A, allows NK cells to detect target cells that are expressing low levels of any MHC class I molecule.

LILRB1 recognizes both classical and non-classical MHC class I molecules, but it has a particularly high affinity for the non-classical molecule HLA-G, whose expression is restricted to extravillous trophoblast cells in the placenta. Interaction of LILRB1 with HLA-G inhibits NK cell cytotoxicity more strongly than that with other class I molecules. The significance of this observation is not yet clear.

NK cells are self-tolerant

The MHC and NK receptor loci are polygenic, polymorphic and unlinked. Furthermore, NK cells are highly heterogenous with respect to their receptor repertoire, with some NK cells failing to express any inhibitory receptors that recognize self MHC class I molecules. Since they cannot be inhibited by self MHC class I molecules, these NK cells might be expected to be activated in response to autologous cells and so are potentially autoreactive. Therefore, similar to the cells of the adaptive immune system, there must be some mechanism by which NK cell tolerance to self is established and maintained. This process has been called 'education' or 'licensing'.

The mechanisms that maintain NK tolerance to self have not yet been defined, but some simple rules are clear:

- an NK cell lacking an inhibitory receptor that recognizes a self MHC class I molecule cannot carry out cytotoxicity or cytokine production in response to target cells;
- an NK receptor that has an activating receptor that recognizes a self MHC class I molecule is also unable to carry out effector functions. Such NK cells are referred to as 'hyporesponsive';
- hyporesponsive NK cells may still be able to carry out effector functions in some situations, such as when activated by IL-2.

Cancerous and virally-infected cells are recognized by NKG2D

Like other NKG2 receptors, NKG2D is a member of the C-type lectin receptor family, but unlike other NKG2 molecules, NKG2D does not associate with CD94, instead forming a disulphide-linked homodimer (Fig. 10.7). It is an activating receptor expressed by all circulating NK cells.

In humans, the ligands for NKG2D are the MHC class I-like molecules ULBP1–3, MICA and MICB. Expression of these molecules is upregulated by a variety of cellular stresses including heat shock, oxidative stress, proliferation and viral infection. Thus, NKG2D allows NK cells to recognize cells that are stressed, including virally infected and cancerous cells. For this reason, some viruses encode immune evasion proteins that interfere with NKG2D ligand expression, and some cancers produce soluble NKG2D ligands that block NKG2D recognition of its ligands at the cell surface.

The activating NK cell receptor NKp46 is present on all NK cells, and indeed is currently considered to be the best pan-species marker of NK cells. This receptor has been

NKG2D forms disulphide-linked homodimers

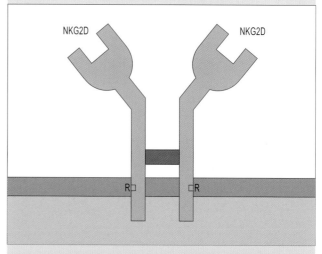

Fig. 10.7 NKG2D forms disulphide-linked homodimers. Its transmembrane domain contains an arginine residue (R), which allows it to recruit the adaptor protein DAP10.

Fluorescence micrograph of two NK cells attacking a tumor cell

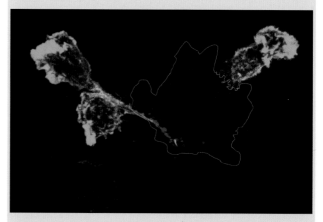

Fig. 10.8 Fluorescence micrograph of two NK cells attacking a tumor cell. F-actin is stained in red and perforin in green. *(Courtesy of Dr Pedro Roda Navarro and Dr Hugh Reyburn.)*

reported to recognize some viral hemagglutinins, and thus may provide another way for NK cells to recognize virally infected cells directly. Another activating receptor, NKp44, may also be able to recognize viral hemagglutinins.

NK cells can also recognize antibody on target cells using Fc receptors

The Fc receptor CD16 (FcγRIII) is expressed by all CD56^{low} NK cells, but not by CD56^{hi} cells. CD16 binds antibody bound to target cells, activating the NK cell so that it degranulates, mediating antibody dependent cell-mediated cytotoxicity (ADCC) (Fig. 10.8). Historically, this was referred to as K cell activity, but this function may also be

Signaling through activating and inhibitory receptors

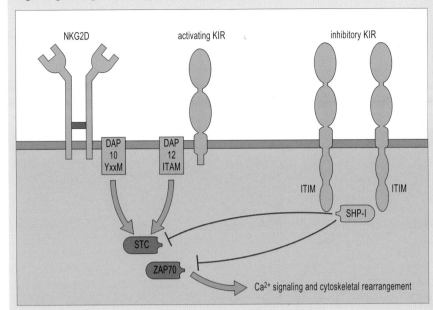

Fig. 10.9 Signaling through activating receptors leads to the recruitment of adaptor molecules that contain either an ITAM or ITAM-like motif. These recruit and phosphorylate intracellular signaling molecules, leading to NK cell activation. Signaling through inhibitory receptors recruits inhibitory phosphatases, which inhibit the phosphorylation of activating signaling molecules.

performed by other cell types with Fc receptors, including T cells. NK cell-mediated ADCC requires both an adaptive immune stimulus (cells coated with antibody) and an innate immune effector mechanism (NK cells) and is thus an example of cross-talk between the innate and adaptive immune systems.

The balance of inhibitory and activating signals determines whether an NK is activated

During an interaction with a target cell, an NK cell must decide between cytotoxic action and inaction. This decision is thought to depend on the coordination of intracellular signaling pathways, and may involve the balance between activating and inhibitory signals.

Both the KIRs and CD94-associated lectin-like receptors occur as inhibitory or activating receptors.

- Inhibitory receptors contain an immunoreceptor tyrosine inhibitory motif (ITIM) in their cytoplasmic tails. These recruit inhibitory phosphatases, which disrupt phosphorylation of activating receptors and intracellular signaling molecules, and prevent NK cell activation. All NK cell inhibitory receptors contain an ITIM.
- CD94-NKG2C and activating KIR associate with intracellular proteins that have an immunoreceptor tyrosine activation motif (ITAM). This allows them to phosphorylate and recruit tyrosine kinases including ZAP-70, which lead to cellular activation. CD16, NKp46, NKp44 and NKp30 also associate with ITAM-bearing intracellular molecules.
- Some other activating receptors recruit an intracellular adaptor that does not bear an ITAM. For example, NKG2D recruits the adaptor molecule DAP10, which bears an ITAM-like YXXM motif.

As well as inhibitory receptors that recognize MHC class I, NK cells express inhibitory receptors for collagens (LAIR1, CD305) and sialic acid (siglecs). These may affect the balance of activation and inhibition at locations where these are present in large amounts, such as in tissues.

It is not yet known precisely how the balance of activation and inhibition is resolved. To degranulate, NK cells require a longer contact period with their targets than CTLs do. This is thought to reflect more complex processing that must occur to integrate activating and inhibitory signals at the NK cell immunological synapse (Fig. 10.9).

Cytoxicity

Cytotoxicity is effected by direct cellular interactions, granule exocytosis, and cytokines

CTLs and NK cells use a variety of different mechanisms to kill their targets. These include:

- direct cell–cell signaling via TNF family molecules;
- pore formation, which allows apoptosis-inducing proteins to access the target cell cytoplasm;
- indirect signaling via cytokines.

All of these mechanisms culminate in target cell death by apoptosis. Apoptosis is a form of programmed cell death in which the nucleus fragments and the cytoplasm, plasma membranes and organelles condense into apoptotic bodies and are digested. Any remnants are phagocytosed by tissue macrophages.

Apoptosis is usually mediated by a family of proteases called the caspases. There are two caspase-dependent pathways of apoptosis:

- the extrinsic pathway begins outside the cell. Recognition of pro-apoptotic proteins by specific receptors initiates the caspase cascade;

CTLs and NK cells can trigger apoptosis

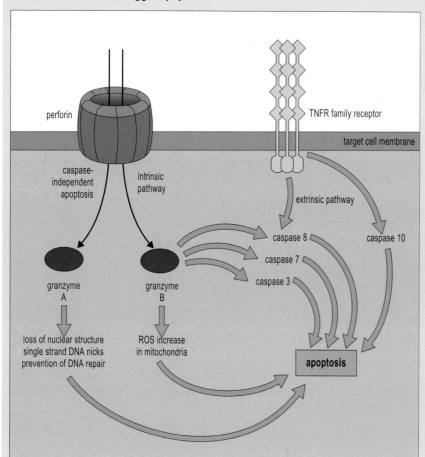

Fig. 10.10 CTLs and NK cells can trigger apoptosis in their targets by signaling through TNF receptor family of molecules. These activate caspases 8 and 10, initiating apoptosis via the extrinsic pathway. CTLs and NK cells also trigger apoptosis in their targets by releasing cytotoxic granules. Perforin forms a pore in the target cell membrane, allowing granzymes access to the cytoplasm. Granzyme B activates caspases 3, 7, and 8, triggering apoptosis via the intrinsic pathway. Granzyme A initiates a caspase-independent pathway of apoptosis.

- the intrinsic pathway is initiated from within the cell. In response to DNA damage or other types of severe cell stress, pro-apoptotic proteins are released from the mitochondria and initiate the caspase cascade.

There are also caspase-independent pathways of apoptosis. All of these may be triggered by CTLs and NK cells. The target cell remains in control of its internal processes throughout apoptosis. Thus CTLs and NK cells effectively instruct their targets to commit suicide (Fig. 10.10).

Cytotoxicity may be signaled via TNF receptor family molecules on the target cell

CTLs and NK cells can initiate apoptosis in their targets via the extrinsic pathway using members of the tumor necrosis factor (TNF) receptor group of molecules. These include:

- Fas (CD95);
- TNF receptors.

$CD4^+$ and $CD8^+$ T cells and NK cells can initiate cell death via expression of Fas ligand, a member of the TNF family. Fas ligand recognizes the widely expressed cell surface protein Fas. Cross-linking leads to trimerization of Fas and recruitment of FADD to the death domain in the cytoplasmic tail of Fas. FADD recruits caspase 8 or 10, leading to apoptosis.

Other members of the TNF receptor family can also trigger caspase-dependent cell death upon engagement with their ligand by a similar mechanism. TNFα is primarily produced by macrophages, but is also produced by CTLs and NK cells. TNFR1, one of the receptors for TNFα, recruits caspases 8 and 10 via TRADD. The ability to induce cell death is dependent on the presence of the death domain in the cytoplasmic tail. TNF receptor family members that lack the death domain do not mediate caspase-dependent cell death. Apoptotic signals delivered by members of the TNF family are Ca^{2+} independent.

CTL and NK cell granules contain perforin and granzymes

Activated CTLs and resting $CD56^{low}$ NK cells contain numerous cytoplasmic granules called lytic granules. Upon recognition of a target cell, these granules polarize to the site of contact, the immunological synapse, releasing their contents into a small cleft between the two cells (Fig. 10.11). The lytic granules contain the pore-forming protein perforin, as well as a series of granule-associated enzymes, called granzymes.

Perforin is a monomeric pore-forming protein that is related both structurally and functionally to the complement component C9.

Intracellular reorganizations during effector-target cell interaction

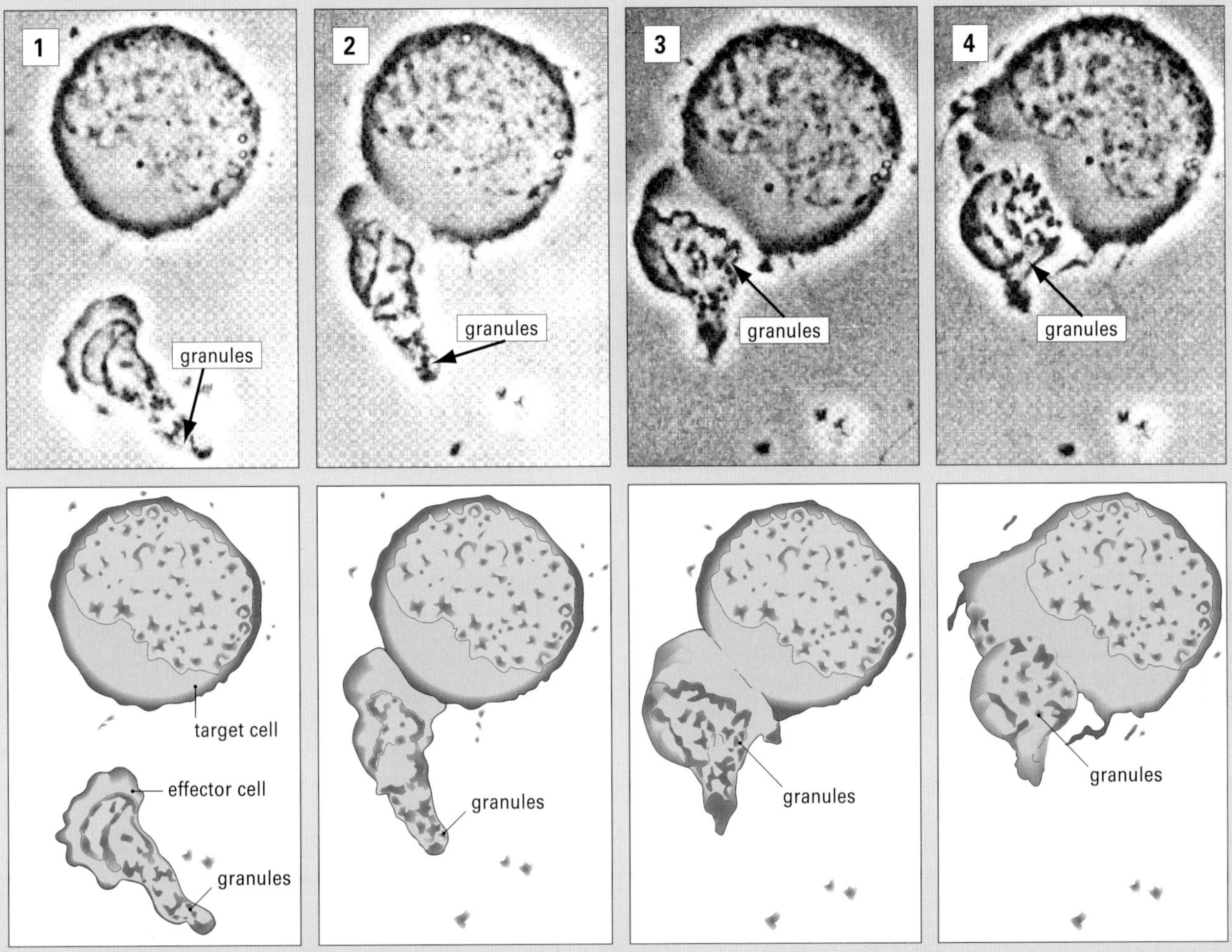

Fig. 10.11 Early events in the interaction of CTLs with specific targets were studied with high-resolution cinematographic techniques. The figure shows four frames (together with interpretative drawings), taken at different times, of a CTL interacting with its target. The location of the granules within the effector cell is indicated in each case. Before contact with the target (**1**), the effector has granules located in a uropod at the rear, and is seen to move randomly by extending pseudopods from the organelle-free, broad, leading edge of the cell. Within 2 minutes of contacting the target (**2**), the CTL has begun to round up and initiate granule reorientation (**3**). After 10 minutes (**4**) the granules occupy a position in the zone of contact with the target, where they appear to be in the process of emptying their contents into the intercellular space between the two cells. *(Courtesy of Dr VH Engelhard.)*

Q. What function does C9 perform?

A. It polymerizes to form channels across membranes, as the final step in the formation of the membrane attack complex (MAC).

Perforin is inactive when located within the granules, but undergoes a conformational activation, which is Ca^{2+} dependent. Like C9, perforin is able to form homopolymers, inserting into the membrane to form a circular pore of approximately 16 nm diameter. Unlike C9, perforin is able to bind membrane phospholipids directly in the presence of Ca^{2+} (Fig. 10.12).

Perforin-deficient mice show greatly reduced cytotoxicity. The fact that some cytotoxicity remains demonstrates that other mechanisms contribute to CTL- and NK cell-mediated death. Some of the residual killing is likely to come from the Fas ligand and TNF pathways.

Granzymes are serine proteases that are released from the lytic granules alongside perforin. Once perforin has formed a pore in the cell membrane, granzymes may enter the target cell cytoplasm and cleave a number of substrates, leading to apoptosis via the intrinsic pathway:

- granzyme B cleaves pro-caspases 3, 7, and 8, triggering apoptosis in the target cell. Granzyme B-deficient mice show delayed but not ablated cytotoxicity, illustrating the importance of other pathways;
- granzyme A triggers apoptosis via a caspase-independent pathway. It targets the ER-associated protein complex SET, activating DNAse, which nicks the target cell DNA. It also cleaves nuclear laminins, leading to loss of nuclear structure, and acts in the mitochondria to increase ROI production.

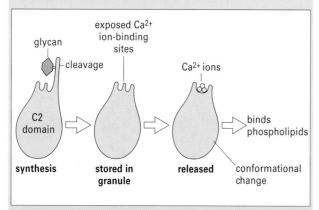

Perforin undergoes a conformational activation

Fig. 10.12 Perforin is synthesized with a tailpiece of 20 amino acid residues with a large glycan residue attached. In this form, it is inactive. Cleavage of the tailpiece within the granules allows Ca^{2+} ions to access a site associated with the C2 domain of the molecule, but the molecule is thought to be maintained in an inactive state by the low Ca^{2+} concentration in the granules. Following secretion, the increased Ca^{2+} concentration permits a conformational change, which exposes a phospholipid-binding site, allowing the perforin to bind to the target membrane as a precursor to polymerization.

Granzymes other than A and B have been identified, although mice with these genes knocked out are less severely affected than granzyme A and B knockout mice, suggesting that A and B are the most important death-inducing granzymes. Some of these minor granzymes, such as granzyme C, contribute to apoptosis via a caspase dependent pathway whereas others, such as granzyme K, seem to act in a manner similar to that of granzyme A. The large number of granzymes is likely to provide multiple pathways to trigger apoptosis, ensuring that cell death ensues.

Some cell types are resistant to cell-mediated cytotoxicity

A number of cell types display some resistance to cell-mediated cytotoxicity, including: the CTLs and NK cells themselves. CTLs and NK cells can be killed by other cytotoxic effector cells, but do not destroy themselves when they kill a target cell. A number of mechanisms contribute to this protection:

- both perforin and granzymes are synthesized as inactive precursors that need to be activated by cleavage;
- activation takes place only after perforin and granzymes have been released from the granules. Inside granules, pH, Ca^{2+} levels and the presence of proteoglycans that bind perforin and granzymes are thought to keep them inactive;
- during degranulation, a membrane-bound form of cathepsin B lines the granule membrane and cleaves perforin on the CTL or NK side of the synapse;

- CTL and NK express cFLIP, a protein that inhibits the cleavage of caspase 8 and prevents apoptosis via the caspase 8 pathway;
- they also express protease inhibitor 8 (PI-8), a serpin that can inhibit granzyme B activity.

Neurons, hepatocytes and some placental cell populations are resistant to CTL and NK cell attack under normal circumstances. These cells express little or no MHC class I and for this reason, they are largely resistant to CTL-mediated cytotoxicity. They would, however, be expected to be susceptible to killing by NK cells. They evade NK cell killing in a number of ways:

- neurons, as well as cells in other immune privileged sites, such as the cornea and testes, express FasL. This induces apoptosis in Fas-expressing T and NK cells as they enter the tissue;
- tissue-resident NK cells are generally not efficient killers. In non-pathological situations, neurons, hepatocytes and most placental extravillous trophoblast cells are only exposed to tissue-resident, and not blood NK cells;
- placental villous trophoblast cells express no MHC class I molecules, and are in direct contact with peripheral blood NK cells. They form a syncytium, and this may confer some resistance to killing, but other mechanisms, as yet undefined, are also likely to be important;
- some placental extravillous trophoblast cells are exposed to peripheral blood NK cells. These express the classical MHC class I molecule HLA-C, and the non-classical class I molecules HLA-E and -G, which effectively inhibit NK cell activation.

Cytokine stimulated CTL and NK cells are able to kill these cell types *in vitro*, and under inflammatory conditions, CTL and NK cells can kill neurons and hepatocytes *in vivo*. Therefore, these cell types are only resistant to cell-mediated cytotoxicity in the absence of inflammation or infection.

Non-lymphoid cytotoxic cells

A number of non-lymphoid cells may be cytotoxic to other cells or to invading microorganisms, such as bacteria or parasites. Macrophages and neutrophils may phagocytose cells and debris in a non-specific way, but also express FcγRI and FcγRII, which allow them to recognize antibody-coated target cells. Eosinophils also recognize antibody-coated targets via Fc receptors, triggering degranulation.

Macrophages and neutrophils primarily kill target cells by phagocytosis

In general, macrophages and neutrophils destroy pathogens by internalizing them and barraging them with toxic molecules and enzymes within the phagolysosome. These include:

- the production of reactive oxygen species, toxic oxidants, and nitric oxide;
- the secretion of molecules such as neutrophil defensins, lysosomal enzymes and cytostatic proteins (Fig. 10.13).

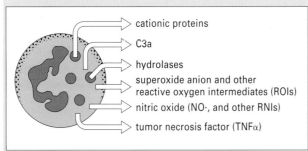

Mechanisms that may contribute to the cytotoxicity of myeloid cells

- cationic proteins
- C3a
- hydrolases
- superoxide anion and other reactive oxygen intermediates (ROIs)
- nitric oxide (NO·, and other RNIs)
- tumor necrosis factor (TNFα)

Fig. 10.13 Reactive oxygen intermediates (ROIs) and reactive nitrogen intermediates (RNIs), cationic proteins, hydrolytic enzymes, and complement proteins released from myeloid cells may damage the target cell, in addition to cytokine-mediated attack.

If the target is engaged by surface receptors but is too large to phagocytose, the phagosome may fail to internalize its target. In this case, molecules from the phagolysosome may be released into the extracellular environment and contribute to localized cell damage. This is called 'frustrated phagocytosis'. Frustrated phagocytosis can be considered a type of ADCC, but unlike ADCC mediated by NK cells, the mediators produced by the phagocyte damage the target cell, inducing necrosis rather than apoptosis.

Activated macrophages also secrete TNFα, which can induce apoptosis in a similar way to CTLs and NK cells. Macrophages can therefore induce necrosis, apoptosis or a combination of both, depending on the state of activation of the macrophages and the target cell involved.

Eosinophils kill target cells by ADCC

Mature eosinophils contain two types of granules: 'specific' granules are unique to eosinophils and have a crystalloid core that binds the dye eosin, whereas 'primary' granules are similar to those found in other cells of the granulocyte lineage. Eosinophils are only weakly phagocytic. They are capable of ingesting some bacteria following activation, but are less efficient than neutrophils at intracellular killing.

The major function of eosinophils appears to be the secretion of various toxic granule constituents following activation. They are therefore effective at extracellular killing of microorganisms, particularly of large parasites such as schistosomes.

Eosinophil degranulation can be triggered in a number of ways:

- binding to IgG-coated targets via FcγRII;
- binding to IgE-coated targets via FcεRII;
- by exposure to cytokines, including IL-3, IL-5, granulocyte-macrophage colony stimulating factor (GM-CSF), TNF, IFNβ and platelet-activating factor (PAF). The cytokines also enhance ADCC-mediated degranulation.

Different modes of activation can alter the balance of toxic proteins released during degranulation, although the details of this are not yet understood.

The components of the eosinophil specific granule include:

- major basic protein (MBP), which is the major component of the granules, forming the crystalloid core. It increases membrane permeability, causing damage to, and sometimes killing, parasites. It can also damage host cells;
- eosinophil peroxidase (EPO), a highly cationic heterodimeric hemoprotein distinct from the myeloperoxidase of neutrophils and macrophages. In the presence of H_2O_2, which is also produced by eosinophils, EPO will oxidize a variety of substrates, including halide ions and nitric oxide to produce highly toxic oxidant species. These may represent the eosinophil's most potent killing mechanism for some parasites, but are also toxic to host cells;
- eosinophil cationic protein (ECP), an eosinophil-specific protein that is toxic to many parasites, particularly *Schistosoma mansoni* schistosomulae. It is a ribonuclease that binds avidly to negatively charged surfaces. It is possible that it forms membrane channels, which allow other mediators access to the target cell cytoplasm. Eosinophils also produce eosinophil-derived neurotoxin (EDN), another ribonuclease but with strong neurotoxic activity. The ribonuclease activity of these proteins is not required for their toxicity.

Eosinophils are prominent in the inflammatory lesions of a number of diseases, particularly atopic disorders of the gut, skin and respiratory tract, where they are often closely associated with fibrotic reactions. Examples are atopic eczema, asthma, and inflammatory bowel disease. Although eosinophils may play some regulatory role in these conditions, such as inactivating histamine, their toxic products and cytotoxic mechanisms are a major cause of the tissue damage. For example, in asthma, MBP can kill some pneumocytes and tracheal epithelial cells while EPO kills type II pneumocytes. MBP can also induce mast cells to secrete histamine, so exacerbating allergic inflammation.

CRITICAL THINKING: MECHANISMS OF CYTOTOXICITY (SEE P. 436 FOR EXPLANATIONS)

Lymphocytes from a normal individual were stimulated *in vitro* by co-culture with irradiated T lymphoma cells. (Irradiation of these stimulator cells prevents them from dividing in culture.) After 7 days, the lymphocytes were harvested and sorted to obtain a population of CTLs (CD3$^+$CD8$^+$) and a population of

NK cells (CD56^{low}CD16$^+$). These effector cells were set up in a cytotoxicity assay with two tumor cell lines as targets: Tumor line 1 and Tumor line 1 S, which is derived from Tumor line 1. The percentage of cells displaying DNA fragmentation in each condition is shown in the table.

Treatment	Tumor line 1	Tumor line 1 S
no effector cells	1%	2%
CTLs	84%	2%
NK cells	15%	88%
anti-class I antibody	2%	1%
CTLs + anti-class I antibody	6%	1%
NK cells + anti-class I antibody	46%	85%

1 Why is target cell DNA fragmentation a good indication of CTL and NK cell activity?

2 From the cultures with CTLs or NK cells alone, what can you deduce about Tumor lines 1 and 1 S?

3 How can you account for the observation that NK cells do cause some DNA fragmentation in Tumor line 1? How would you test your hypothesis?

4 The cultures were repeated including an antibody that recognizes MHC class I molecules, and blocks their interactions. How can you account for the effects on DNA fragmentation observed in Tumor line 1?

CASE STUDY: GRISCELLI SYNDROME

A number of genetic diseases have been identified that result from loss of function of one of the proteins involved in CTL- and NK-mediated killing. One of these is Griscelli syndrome type II, which is associated with a mutation in the GTPase Rab27.

Rab27 is present on mature secretory vesicles, and is required for their recruitment to the plasma membrane. Thus, it is critical for CTL and NK cell degranulation. Griscelli syndrome patients have CTLs and NK cells that are unable to kill target cells, and they suffer from frequent infections. These patients go on to develop hemophagocytic

lymphohistiocytosis, a syndrome in which leukocytes proliferate out of control, and tissue macrophages are inappropriately activated. This demonstrates the importance of cytotoxic lymphoid effector cells in controlling other cells of the immune system, as well as in defense against pathogenic microorganisms.

Rab27 is also required for secretion of melanin by melanocytes, so these patients present with partial albinism. Some patients may have neurological disorders as a result of defective neurotransmitter secretion.

Further reading

Cheent K, Khakoo SI. Natural killer cells: integrating diversity with function. Immunology 2009;126:449–457.

Colonna M. Interleukin-22-producing natural killer cell and lymphoid tissue inducer-like cells in mucosal immunity. Immunity 2009;31:15–23.

Colucci F, Caligiuri MA, Di Santo JP. What does it take to make a natural killer? Nat Rev Immunol 2003;3:413–425.

Cullen SP, Martin SJ. Mechanisms of granule-dependent killing. Cell Death Differ 2008;15:251–262.

Di Santo JP. A defining factor for natural killer cell development. Nat Immunol 2009;10:1051–1052.

Dustin ML, Long EO. Cytotoxic immunological synapses. Immunol Rev 2010;235:24–34.

Joncker NT, Raulet DH. 2010. Regulation of NK cell responsiveness to achieve self-tolerance and maximal

responses to diseased target cells. Immunol Rev 2008;224:85–97.

Kärre K. Natural killer cell recognition of missing self. Nat Immunol 2008;9:477–480.

Lanier LL. Up on the tightrope: natural killer cell activation and inhibition. Nat Immunol 2008;9:495–502.

López-Larrea C, Suárez-Alvarez B, López-Soto A, et al. The NKG2D receptor: sensing stressed cells. Trends Mol Med 2008;14:179–189.

Rothenberg ME, Hogan SP. The Eosinophil. Annu Rev Immunol 2006;24:147–174.

Vivier E, Tomasello E, Baratin M, et al. Functions of natural killer cells. Nat Immunol 2008;9:503–510.

Weninger W, Manjunath N, von Adrian UH. Migration and differentiation of CD8$^+$ T cells. Immunol Rev 2002;186:221–233.

CHAPTER 11

Regulation of the Immune Response

SUMMARY

- **Many factors govern the outcome of any immune response.** These include the antigen itself, its dose and route of administration, and the genetic background of the individual responding to antigenic challenge. A variety of control mechanisms serve to restore the immune system to a resting state when the response to a given antigen is no longer required.

- **The APC has an important effect on the immune response** through its ability to provide co-stimulation to T cells and by the production of cytokines and chemokines that influence both the nature and make-up of the ensuing reponse. In addition, APC heterogeneity aids in the promotion of different modes of immune response.

- **T cells regulate the immune response.** Cytokine production by T cells influences the type of immune response elicited by antigen. CD4$^+$ T cells can differentiate into several effector phenotypes such as TH1, TH2 or TH17. These subsets play important roles in the protection of the host against a diversity of pathogen challenges. Regulatory T cells may belong to the CD4 or CD8 subpopulations. They may inhibit responses via a variety of mechanisms such as via

cell-to-cell contact or by the production of the anti-inflammatory cytokines IL-10 and TGFβ.

- **Immunoglobulins can influence the immune response.** They may act positively, through the formation of immune complexes, or negatively, by reducing antigenic challenge or by feedback inhibition of B cells.

- **Selective migration of lymphocyte subsets to different sites can modulate the local type of immune response** because different TH subsets respond to different sets of chemokines.

- **The neuroendocrine system influences immune responses.** Cells from both systems share similar ligands and receptors, which permit cross-interactions between them. Corticosteroids in particular downregulate TH1 responses and macrophage activation.

- **Genetic factors influence the immune system and include both MHC-linked and non-MHC-linked genes.** They affect the level of immune response and susceptibility to infection.

Ideally, an immune response is mounted quickly to clear away a pathogenic challenge with the minimum of collateral damage and then the system is returned to a resting state once the antigen is eliminated. The immune response, like many other biological systems, is therefore subject to a variety of control mechanisms. Additional mechanisms help regulate the levels of immunopathology that are often a necessary sacrifice for pathogen elimination. An insufficient immune response can result in an individual being overwhelmed by infection. An inappropriate, or over vigorous immune response can lead to high levels of immunopathology or even autoimmunity (see Chapter 20). The balance between these two is therefore critical.

At its most basic, an effective immune response is an outcome of the interplay between antigen and a network of immunologically competent cells. The nature of the immune response, both qualitatively and quantitatively, is determined by many factors, including:

- the form, dose, and route of administration of the antigen;
- the antigen-presenting cell (APC);
- the genetic background of the individual;
- any history of previous exposure to the cognate antigen; and
- any concurrent infections that the individual may have.

Specific antibodies may also modulate the immune response to an antigen.

Regulation by antigen

T cells and B cells are activated by antigen after effective engagement of their antigen-specific receptors together with appropriate co-stimulation. Repeated antigen exposure is required to maintain T and B cell proliferation, and during an effective immune response there is often a dramatic expansion of specifically reactive effector cells.

At the end of an immune response, reduced antigen exposure results in a reduced expression of IL-2 and its receptor, leading to **apoptosis** of the antigen-specific T cells. The majority of antigen-specific cells therefore die at the end of an immune response leaving a minor population of long-lived T and B cells to survive and give rise to the memory population.

> **Q. What process leads to the inactivation of T cells and loss of the IL-2 receptor?**
> A. Ligation of CTLA-4, the alternative receptor for the co-stimulatory molecule B7 (see Fig. 8.17).

Different antigens elicit different kinds of immune response

Intracellular organisms such as some bacteria, parasites, or viruses induce a cell-mediated immune response. Cell-mediated immune responses are also induced by agents such as silica. In contrast, extracellular organisms and soluble antigens induce a humoral response, with the polysaccharide capsule antigens of bacteria generally inducing IgM responses.

In some situations, antigens (e.g. those of intracellular microorganisms) may not be cleared effectively leading to a sustained immune response. Chronic immune responses have several possible pathological consequences and can lead to autoimmunity and hypersensitivity (see Chapters 20 and 23–26).

Large doses of antigen can induce tolerance

Very large doses of antigen often result in specific T – and sometimes B – cell tolerance.

Administration of antigen to neonatal mice often results in tolerance to the antigen. It was once speculated that this might be the result of immaturity of the immune system. However, neonatal mice can develop efficient immune responses (Fig. 11.1) and their non-responsiveness may in some cases be attributable, not to the immaturity of T cells, but to immune deviation. In this case a non-protective TH2-type cytokine response would dominate a protective TH1-type cytokine response.

T-independent polysaccharide antigens have been shown to generate tolerance in B cells after administration in high doses. Tolerance and its underlying mechanisms are discussed in Chapter 19.

Antigen route of administration can determine whether an immune response occurs

The route of administration of antigen has been shown to influence the immune response:

- antigens administered subcutaneously or intradermally evoke an active immune response; whereas
- antigens given intravenously, orally, or as an aerosol may cause tolerance or an immune deviation from one type of CD4⁺ T cell response to another.

For example, rodents that have been fed ovalbumin do not respond effectively to a subsequent challenge with the corresponding antigen. This phenomenon may have some therapeutic value in allergy. Studies have shown that oral administration of a T cell epitope of the Der p1 allergen of house dust mite (*Dermatophagoides pteronyssimus*) could tolerize to the whole antigen. The potential mechanisms of such tolerance induction include anergy, immune deviation, and the generation of regulatory T cells that act through the production of cytokines such as TGFβ and IL-10.

Similar observations have been made when antigen is given as an aerosol. Studies in mice have shown that aerosol administration of an encephalitogenic peptide of myelin basic protein (MBP) inhibits the development of experimental allergic encephalomyelitis (EAE) that would normally be induced by a conventional (subcutaneous) administration of the peptide (Fig. 11.2).

Effect of antigen dose on the outcome of the immune response to murine leukemia virus

virus (pfu)	antiviral cytotoxicity	TH1 response (IFNγ)	TH2 response (IL-4)
0.3	+ + +		
1000	+		

80 60 40 20 0 20 40 60 80

Fig. 11.1 Newborn mice were infected with either 0.3 or 1000 plaque-forming units (pfu) of virus and the CTL response against virally infected targets was assessed together with the production of interferon-γ (IFNγ – a TH cell type 1 [TH1] cytokine) or interleukin-4 (IL-4 – a TH2 cytokine) in response to viral challenge. Mice infected with a low dose of virus make a TH1-type response and are protected. The results are presented as arbitrary units.

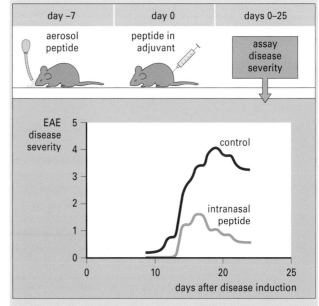

Aerosol administration of antigen modifies the immune response

day –7	day 0	days 0–25
aerosol peptide	peptide in adjuvant	assay disease severity

Fig. 11.2 Mice were treated with a single aerosol dose of either 100 µg peptide (residues 1–11 of MBP) or just the carrier. Seven days later the same peptide, this time in adjuvant, was administered subcutaneously. The subsequent development of experimental allergic encephalomyelitis (EAE) was significantly modified in pretreated animals.

A clear example of how different routes of administration affect the outcome of the immune response is provided by studies of infection with lymphocytic choriomeningitis virus (LCMV). Mice primed subcutaneously with peptide in incomplete Freund's adjuvant develop immunity to LCMV. However, if the same peptide is repeatedly injected intraperitoneally the animal becomes tolerized and cannot clear the virus (Fig. 11.3).

Regulation by the antigen presenting cell

The nature of the APC initially presenting the antigen may determine whether immune responsiveness or tolerance ensues. Effective activation of T cells requires the expression of co-stimulatory molecules on the surface of the APC. Therefore, presentation by dendritic cells or activated macrophages that express high levels of MHC class II molecules, in addition to co-stimulatory molecules, results in highly effective T cell activation. Furthermore, the interaction of CD40L on activated T cells with CD40 on dendritic cells is important for the high-level production of IL-12 necessary for the generation of an effective TH1 response.

If antigen is presented to T cells by a 'non-professional' APC that is unable to provide co-stimulation, unresponsiveness, or immune deviation results. For example, when naive T cells are exposed to antigen by resting B cells they fail to

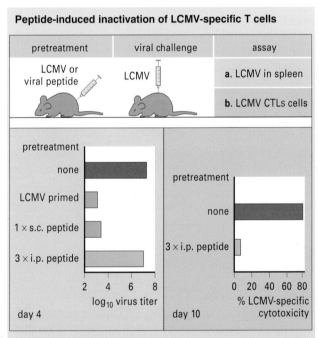

Peptide-induced inactivation of LCMV-specific T cells

Fig. 11.3 Mice were either primed with LCMV or injected with 100 mg LCMV peptide. The peptide was given either subcutaneously (s.c.) or three times intraperitoneally (i.p.) with incomplete Freund's adjuvant. The animals were later infected with LCMV (day 0). The titer of virus in the spleen was measured on day 4. Animals that had been pretreated with subcutaneous peptide or with LCMV developed neutralizing antibody and protective immunity against the virus; animals pretreated with peptide i.p. did not develop immunity. Cytotoxic T lymphocyte (CTL) activity was assessed in the mice on day 10. Mice that had received no pretreatment demonstrated CTLs specific for the LCMV peptide. Mice pretreated with peptide i.p. failed to show such activity.

respond and become tolerized. Experimental observations illustrate this point.

Neonatal animals are more susceptible to tolerance induction. Therefore mice administered MBP in incomplete Freund's adjuvant during the neonatal period are resistant to the induction of EAE. This is due to the development of a dominant TH2 response (see Fig. 11.1). The prior TH2 response to MBP prevents the development of the TH1/TH17 pathological response, which mediates EAE. This effect is not restricted to neonatal animals. Indeed, adult Lewis rats can be tolerized to the induction of EAE by similar administration of MBP in incomplete Freund's adjuvant.

Adjuvants may facilitate immune responses by inducing the expression of high levels of MHC and co-stimulatory molecules on APCs. Furthermore, their ability to activate Langerhans' cells leads to the migration of these skin dendritic cells to the local draining lymph nodes where effective T cell activation can occur.

The importance of dendritic cells in initiating a cytotoxic T lymphocyte (CTL) response is illustrated by experiments showing that newborn female mice injected with male spleen cells fail to develop a CTL response to the male antigen, H-Y. However, if male dendritic cells are injected into female newborn mice, a good H-Y-specific CTL response develops.

Cytokine production by APCs influences T cell responses

Cytokines are part of an extracellular signaling network that controls every function of the innate and adaptive immune system and have:

- numerous effects on cell phenotypes; and
- the ability to regulate the type of immune response generated and its extent.

Activation of APCs by pathogen stimulation can lead to the production of cytokines and the expression of costimulatory molecules. The local cytokine milieu is heavily influenced by cytokines derived from innate immune cells in the early stages of an immune response. For instance the production of type one interferons and IL-12 in response to viral challenge will evoke cell-mediated immunity by the polarization of naive CD4$^+$ T cells to the TH1 phenotype. Conversely early production of IL-4 by innate immune cells will cultivate a humoral TH2 response and act to inhibit any TH1 response.

Q. Aside from driving effector T cell responses, how else may APCs affect T cell responses?
A. Dendritic cells or macrophages may produce cytokines such as TGFβ and IL-10 in response to some antigens. These cytokines can drive the conversion of naive CD4$^+$ T cells into regulatory T cells (see Fig. 11.8), which can act as suppressors.

T cell regulation of the immune response

Differentiation into CD4$^+$ TH subsets is an important step in selecting effector functions

A single TH cell precursor is able to differentiate into a variety of phenotypes, the best characterized and understood being the TH1 and TH2 phenotypes. A recently-described subset, TH17 (producing IL-17A and IL-17F), is proposed to have important roles in mucosal immunity to certain bacteria and fungi. The differentiation fates of TH cells are crucial to the generation of effective immunity; factors that may influence the differentiation of TH cells include:

- the sites of antigen presentation;
- co-stimulatory molecules involved in cognate cellular interactions;
- peptide density and binding affinity – high MHC class II peptide density favors TH1 or TH17, low densities favor TH2;
- APCs and the cytokines they produce;
- the cytokine profile and balance of cytokines evoked by antigen;
- receptors expressed on the T cell;
- activity of co-stimulatory molecules and hormones present in the local environment;
- host genetic background.

The cytokine balance controls T cell differentiation

IL-12 is a potent initial stimulus for IFNγ production by T cells and natural killer (NK) cells and therefore promotes TH1 differentiation. IFNα, a cytokine produced early during viral infection, induces IL-12 and can also switch cells from a TH2 to a TH1 profile.

By contrast, early production of IL-4 favors the generation of TH2 cells. NKT cells, specialized macrophages (called alternatively activated macrophages) and basophils have all been suggested to be early producers of IL-4.

Very recent studies have suggested the existence of a novel TH2 promoting innate cell population present in gut associated lymphoid tissues (GALT). These cells respond rapidly to the cytokines IL-25 and IL-33, which can be produced by epithelial cells, in response to antigens derived from helminths or allergens. These cells have been reported to produce large amounts of IL-5 and IL-13, with lesser amounts of IL-4.

TH17 cells in mice develop in the presence of TGFβ with IL-6 or IL-21 and share an interesting reciprocal developmental relationship with inducible Tregs, which is discussed in more detail below.

Cytokines from the various TH subsets can cross-regulate each other's development. Thus, cross-regulation of TH subsets has been demonstrated whereby IFNγ secreted by TH1 cells can inhibit the responsiveness of TH2 cells; also IL-17A can inhibit the development of TH1 responses (Fig. 11.4) whereas IL-10 produced by TH2 cells downregulates B7 and IL-12 expression by APCs, which in turn inhibits TH1 activation.

The TH subset balance is modulated not only by the level of expression of cytokines such as IL-12 or IL-4, but also by expression of cytokine receptors. For instance, the high-affinity IL-12R is composed of two chains, β1 and β2, with both chains being constitutively expressed on TH1 cells. TH1, TH2, and TH17 cells express the β1 chain, but expression of the β2 chain is induced by IFNγ and inhibited by IL-4 (Fig. 11.5). Therefore cytokines reinforce the lineage decisions of the various TH subsets at least in part by controlling the expression of lineage specific receptors.

An immune response therefore tends to settle into a TH1, TH2 or TH17 type of response, but immune responses are not always strongly polarized in this way particularly

Differentiation of murine TH cells

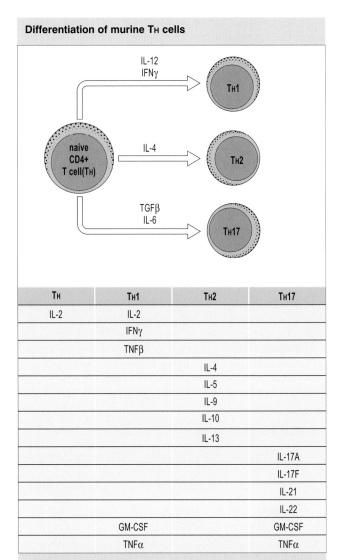

TH	TH1	TH2	TH17
IL-2	IL-2		
	IFNγ		
	TNFβ		
		IL-4	
		IL-5	
		IL-9	
		IL-10	
		IL-13	
			IL-17A
			IL-17F
			IL-21
			IL-22
	GM-CSF		GM-CSF
	TNFα		TNFα

Fig. 11.4 IL-12 and IFNγ favor differentiation of TH1 cells, and IL-4 favors differentiation of TH2 cells. TGFβ and IL-6 will drive TH17 cell development. (GM-CSF, granulocyte–macrophage colony stimulating factor; TNF, tumor necrosis factor.)

in humans. It is conceptually useful to consider TH1 and TH2 as extremes on a scale, and TH1 and TH2 responses do play different roles both in immune defence and immunopathology. However it is important to appreciate that other TH subsets such as TH17 do exist and that the well-established TH1/TH2 paradigm is an oversimplification. It should also be noted that some recent studies have suggested that many TH subsets are in fact not terminally differentiated; and when given the right signals; some TH cells can undergo conversion to another phenotype.

Q. Apart from the cross-regulation by cytokines described above, in what other ways can a TH1- or TH2-type immune response reinforce itself?

A. The chemokines induced by TH1 and TH2 cells tend to induce the accumulation of the same sets of lymphocytes and their associated effector cells (see Chapter 6).

Regulation of the Th1 response by IL-12

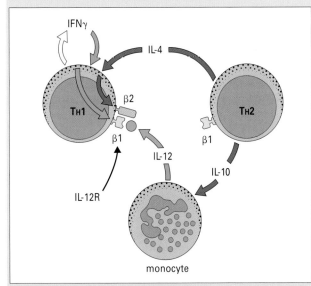

Fig. 11.5 The high-affinity IL-12R consisting of the β1 and β2 chains is constitutively expressed on Th1 cells. IL-12 released by mononuclear phagocytes promotes the development and activation of Th1 cells, but IL-12 production is inhibited by IL-10 released by Th2 cells. IFNγ from Th1 cells promotes production of the β2 chain and therefore production of the high-affinity IL-12R. However, this is inhibited by IL-4.

TH cell subsets determine the type of immune response

It is clear that:

- local patterns of cytokine and hormone expression help to select lymphocyte effector mechanism; and
- the polarized responses of CD4+ TH cells are based on their profile of cytokine secretion (Fig. 11.6).

Q. In what way do cytokines that are normally associated with Th1 responses (IFNγ, IL-2) affect B cell differentiation?
A. IL-2 promotes B cell division. IFNγ promotes affinity maturation and class switching to IgG2a, which acts as an opsonin and fixes complement.

Th1 cytokines including IFNγ, TNFβ, and IL-2 also promote:

- macrophage activation;
- antibody-dependent cell-mediated cytotoxicity; and
- delayed-type hypersensitivity.

Th2 clones are typified by production of IL-4, IL-5, IL-9, IL-10 and IL-13 (see Fig. 11.4). These cells provide optimal help for humoral immune responses biased towards:

- IgG1 and IgE isotype switching;
- mucosal immunity;
- stimulation of mast cells, eosinophil growth and differentiation; and
- IgA synthesis.

Th17 cell cytokines include IL-17A, IL-17F, TNFα, and IL-22. Since many stromal cells express receptors for these cytokines the effects of Th17 cells can promote inflammation. In addition:

Selection of effector mechanisms by Th1 and Th2 cells

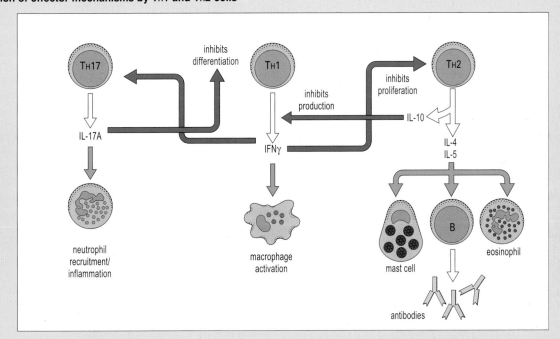

Fig. 11.6 The cytokine patterns of Th1, Th2 and Th17 cells drive different effector pathways. Th1 cells activate macrophages and are involved in antiviral and inflammatory responses. Th2 cells are involved in humoral responses and allergy. Th17 cells are an important defense at mucosal barriers recruiting neutrophils to sites of infection and tightening epithelial barriers.

- IL-17A has been proposed to be important for the recruitment of neutrophils and induction of anti-microbial peptides from resident cells.
- IL-17A is important for host defence against *Klebsiella pneumonia* and *Candida albicans*.

Therefore, in essence, TH1 cells are associated with cell-mediated inflammatory reactions and TH2 cells are associated with strong antibody and allergic responses. TH17 cells appear important in defense against certain infections, particularly at mucosal surfaces.

CD8$^+$ T cells can be divided into subsets on the basis of cytokine expression

Many CD8$^+$ CTLs make a spectrum of cytokines similar to TH1 cells and are termed CTL1 cells. CD8$^+$ T cells that make TH2-associated cytokines are associated with regulatory functions and CD8$^+$ T cells that make IL-17A have also been observed. The differentiation of these cells may be affected by the CD4$^+$ cell cytokine profile, with CTLs commonly associated with TH1 responses and less commonly found when TH2 cells are present. Thus:

- IFNγ and IL-12 may encourage CTL1 generation; and
- IL-4 may encourage CTL2 generation.

However, both CTL1 and CTL2 cells can be cytotoxic and kill mainly by a Ca^{2+}/perforin-dependent mechanism (see Fig. 10.10).

Regulatory T cells exert important suppressive functions

Although T cells modulate the immune response in a positive sense by providing T cell help as discussed above, T cells are also capable of downregulating immune responses, and both CD4$^+$ and CD8$^+$ T cell subsets can induce this inhibition.

A naturally occurring population of CD4$^+$CD25$^+$ regulatory T cells (Tregs) is generated in the thymus. Additionally, CD4$^+$ Tregs can be induced from non-regulatory T cells in the periphery.

Tregs function to maintain peripheral tolerance and have important roles in the prevention of autoimmune diseases such as type 1 diabetes. They are also thought to play critical roles in limiting the levels of immunopathology during an active immune response.

Treg differentiation is induced by Foxp3

The immunosuppressive functions of CD4$^+$ cells were initially observed by adoptively transferring T cells depleted of CD25$^+$ cells into immunodeficient mice. This resulted in multiorgan autoimmunity suggesting that CD25$^+$ cells play an important role in preventing self-reactivity. When the CD25$^+$ T cells were replaced, autoimmune disease was prevented.

Comparison of CD4$^+$CD25$^+$ Tregs with naive and activated CD4$^+$ T cells shows that regulatory cells selectively express **Foxp3**, a member of the forkhead/winged helix transcription factors (Fig. 11.7) essential for the development and function of CD4$^+$CD25$^+$ Tregs. Mutations in the *Foxp3* gene cause immune dysregulation, poly-endocrinopathy enteropathy, X-linked syndrome (IPEX).

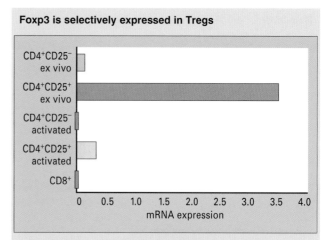

Foxp3 is selectively expressed in Tregs

Fig. 11.7 Cell populations were collected and real-time polymerase chain reaction (PCR) was performed to assess levels of Foxp3. Foxp3 mRNA is expressed selectively in CD4$^+$CD25$^+$ cells *ex vivo*. It was expressed at low levels in activated CD4$^+$CD25$^+$ cells and was not present in CD25$^-$ cells or CD8$^+$ cells. *(Adapted from Fontenot JD, Gavin MA, Rudensky AY. Nat Immunol 2003;4:330–336.)*

Individuals with this disease have increased autoimmune and inflammatory diseases.

The importance of Foxp3 in the development of CD4$^+$CD25$^+$ Tregs was underlined following transfection of Foxp3 into naive T cells (which do not express Foxp3). This increased expression of CD25 and induced suppressor function.

Evidence for the origin of these naturally occurring Tregs came from the finding that mice thymectomized at three days old developed multi-organ autoimmune disease. Further analysis revealed that CD4$^+$ CD8$^-$ thymocytes begin expressing Foxp3 at day 2 after birth and after that CD4$^+$ Foxp3$^+$ cells accumulate in the periphery. Therefore naturally occurring Tregs are educated in the thymus during thymic selection. CD4$^+$CD25$^+$ Foxp3$^+$ Tregs constitute 5–10% of peripheral CD4$^+$ T cells in both mice and humans, and whilst athymic mice have severely reduced levels of Tregs, it is clear that Foxp3$^+$ Tregs can arise in the periphery. These so called induced Tregs have been extensively studied *in vitro*. If naive CD4$^+$ T cells are stimulated in the presence of TGFβ then many cells start expressing Foxp3. The additional presence of retinoic acid is thought to accentuate the conversion of naive CD4$^+$ T cells into Foxp3$^+$ Tregs.

Interestingly, it is thought that induced Treg populations and inflammatory TH17 cells share a reciprocal developmental pathway.

Tr1 regulatory cells

CD4$^+$ regulatory T cells can also be generated from naive TH cells in the presence of certain cytokines (Fig. 11.8) such as IL-10. These cells do not express CD25 or Foxp3 and they mediate suppression through the secretion of IL-10.

Mechanisms of Treg suppression

Many mechanisms of Treg suppression have been proposed. For instance, initial studies suggested that natural Tregs require cell contact to suppress, whilst induced Treg

Regulatory T cells can be generated in the periphery

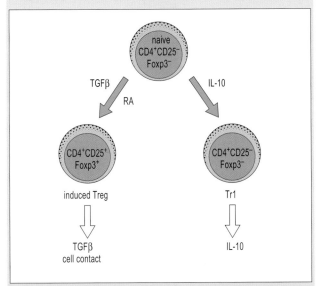

Fig. 11.8 Naive CD4⁺CD25⁻ cells in the periphery can be stimulated to become suppressive. If TGFβ is present, cells upregulate Foxp3 and CD25. In the presence of IL-10 cells can become suppressive, but they do not express Foxp3 or CD25. (RA, retinoic acid.)

populations may suppress by the release of soluble factors. The vast majority of these studies have examined the behaviour of Tregs with *in vitro* culture systems. These highly controlled environments do not take into account the need for regulatory T cell populations to home to different locations in order to interact with target cells. Therefore, our knowledge of the exact functions of Tregs *in vivo* is less clear. This is further confounded by the different types of regulatory T cell, and the exact contribution of natural and induced regulatory populations may differ depending on the antigenic challenges encountered.

In spite of this at least four mechanisms of Treg suppression have been proposed (Fig. 11.9).

Role of Tregs in infection

Although CD4⁺ Tregs play a vital role in the prevention of autoimmune diseases (see Chapter 20), their role in infections is less clear. CD4⁺ Tregs have a protective role against immune-mediated pathology and their ability to suppress is important in reducing inflammation. For example, lesions in the eye in stromal keratitis are less severe in the presence of CD4⁺CD25⁺ Tregs.

CD4⁺ Tregs can also suppress virus-specific responses. Many pathogens induce high levels of IL-10 and TGFβ, which promote the induction of CD4⁺CD25⁺ Tregs. In chronic viral infections, including HIV, cytomegalovirus (CMV), and herpes simplex virus (HSV) infections, increased numbers of Tregs are responsible for decreased antigen-specific responses by CD4⁺ and CD8⁺ T cells. This can lead to disease development.

CD8⁺ T cells suppress secondary immune responses

CD8⁺ suppressive Tregs can be generated *in vitro* by stimulating highly differentiated CD8⁺ cells with antigen and IL-10. Many CD8⁺ Tregs work in a cell contact-dependent manner. They cause a reduction of co-stimulatory molecules on dendritic cells and endothelial cells. This induces tolerance because upon the interaction with the TCR and peptide there is insufficient co-stimulation to generate a functional immune response.

In mice the non-classical MHC class Ib molecule, Qa-1, is crucial for suppression. Mice lacking Qa-1 are unable to suppress responses. However when Qa-1 is replaced into these cells their ability to suppress immune responses is restored (Fig. 11.10).

CD8⁺ Tregs:

- need to be primed by CD4⁺ cells during a primary response; they then suppress secondary immune responses;

Mechanisms of Treg suppression

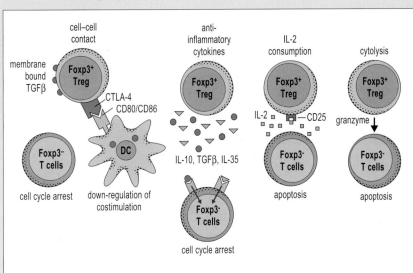

Fig. 11.9 Tregs may suppress by a variety of mechanisms. (**1**) Via cell-to-cell contact (secreted or cell surface molecules such as CTLA-4 expression, or membrane bound TGFβ). (**2**) Release of suppressor cytokines such as IL-10, TGFβ and IL-35. (**3**) IL-2 consumption (Tregs can express high levels of CD25, the IL-2 receptor). (**4**) Cytolysis, akin to CD8⁺ T cell killing. (*Adapted from Shevach EM, Immunity 2009:30:636–645.*)

CD4 Qa-1 is essential for CD8⁺ T suppressor function

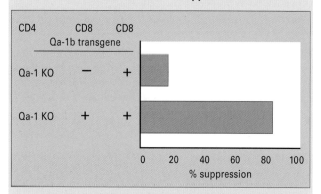

Fig. 11.10 Qa-1 knockout (KO) mice were generated. Qa-1 KO CD4⁺ cells were mixed with CD8⁺ cells and the level of suppression was assessed. CD8⁺ cells could not suppress CD4 cells lacking Qa-1 expression. Insertion of the Qa-1b allele into CD4⁺ cells resulted in effective suppression of responses. *(Adapted from Hu D, Ikizawa K, Lu L, et al. Nat Immunol 2004;5:516–523.)*

- can target activated effector T cells;
- can kill by direct lysis of target cells;
- can suppress immune responses through the secretion of cytokines such as IL-10.

NK and NKT cells produce immunoregulatory cytokines and chemokines

NK cells make cytokines and chemokines and therefore play an important role in the innate immune response to infections and tumors.

The production of immunoregulatory cytokines and chemokines at early stages in the immune response influences the characteristics of the subsequent adaptive immune reaction and can, therefore, affect the overall outcome of the immune response.

NK cells play a key role in the early immune response to intracellular pathogens, largely through their production of IFNγ, which activates macrophages and facilitates differentiation of TH1 cells.

NK cell activity itself is induced by a variety of cytokines including:

- IFNα/β;
- IL-15;
- IL-18; and
- IL-12.

NK cells in turn are negatively regulated by cytokines such as IL-10 and TGFβ.

Q. Which cells will tend to promote the development of NK cells?

A. The TH1 population and macrophages through the production of IL-12, IL-15, and IL-18, whereas the TH2 population will tend to inhibit their development through the production of IL-10.

NK T cells produce cytokines when their TCR engages glycolipids in association with CD1d. It has been suggested that these cells play an immunoregulatory role in the control of autoimmunity, parasite infection, and tumor cell growth.

NK T cells produce both TH1- and TH2-type cytokines

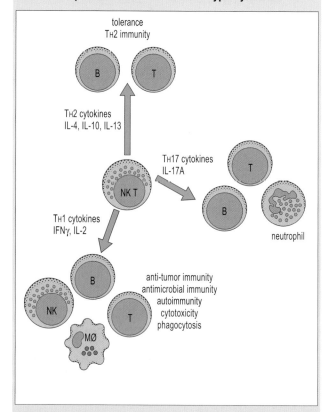

Fig. 11.11 NK T cells exert effects on many cell types. They can produce TH1, TH2, and TH17 cytokines and are involved in all aspects of the immune response.

T cells secreting IFNγ are able to induce NK cell activation, increasing both NK proliferation and cytotoxicity. They are capable of making both TH1-type (IFNγ), TH2-type (IL-4), and TH17 (IL-17A) cytokines depending on the cytokines present in the microenvironment when they are activated (Fig. 11.11). These early sources of cytokine are important in influencing the nature of the T cell response.

Deficiencies of NK T cells have also been reported in animal and human autoimmune diseases, highlighting their regulatory roles. For example, non obese diabetic (NOD) mice have a deficit in NK T cells and injection of NK T cells into these mice prevents the spontaneous development of autoimmune diabetes. Human examples where NK T deficiencies may play a role include:

- rheumatoid arthritis;
- psoriasis;
- ulcerative colitis; and
- multiple sclerosis.

Regulation of the immune response by immunoglobulins

Antibody has been shown to exert feedback control on the immune response.

Passive administration of IgM antibody together with an antigen specifically enhances the immune response to that

Feedback control by antibody

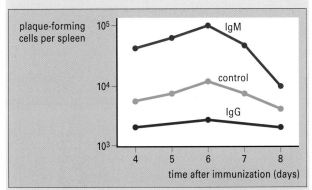

Fig. 11.12 Mice received a monoclonal IgM anti-SRBC (sheep red blood cells), a IgG anti-SRBC, or a medium alone (control). Two hours later all groups were immunized with SRBC. The antibody response measured over the following 8 days was enhanced by IgM and suppressed by IgG.

Antibody-dependent B cell suppression

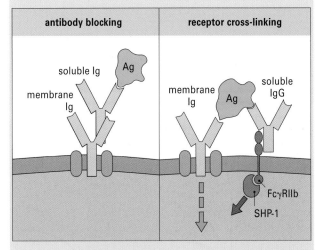

Fig. 11.13 Antibody blocking – high doses of soluble immunoglobulin (Ig) block the interaction between an antigenic determinant (epitope) and membrane immunoglobulin on B cells. The B cell is then effectively unable to recognize the antigen. This receptor-blocking mechanism also prevents B cell priming, but only antibodies that bind to the same epitope to which the B cell's receptors bind can do this. Receptor cross-linking – low doses of antibody allow cross-linking by antigen of a B cell's Fc receptors and its antigen receptors. The FcγRIIb receptor associates with a tyrosine phosphatase (SHP-1), which interferes with cell activation by tyrosine kinases associated with the antigen receptor. This allows B cell priming, but inhibits antibody synthesis. Antibodies against different epitopes on the antigen can all act by this mechanism.

antigen, whereas IgG antibody suppresses the response. This was originally shown with polyclonal antibodies, but has since been confirmed using monoclonal antibodies (Fig. 11.12).

The ability of passively administered antibody to enhance or suppress the immune response has certain clinical consequences and applications:

- certain vaccines (e.g. mumps and measles) are not generally given to infants before 1 year of age because levels of maternally derived IgG remain high for at least 6 months after birth and the presence of such passively acquired IgG at the time of vaccination would result in the development of an inadequate immune response in the baby;
- in cases of Rhesus (Rh) incompatibility, the administration of anti-RhD antibody to Rh⁻ mothers prevents primary sensitization by fetally derived Rh⁺ blood cells, presumably by removing the foreign antigen (fetal erythrocytes) from the maternal circulation (see Chapters 24 and 25).

The mechanisms by which antibody modulates the immune response are not completely defined. In the case of IgM-enhancing plaque-forming cells, there are thought to be two possible interpretations:

- IgM-containing immune complexes are taken up by Fc or C3 receptors on APCs and are processed more efficiently than antigen alone;
- IgM-containing immune complexes stimulate an anti-idiotypic response to the IgM, which amplifies the immune response.

IgG antibody can regulate specific IgG synthesis

IgG can suppress antibody responses in a number of ways.

- Passively administered antibody binds antigen in competition with B cells (antibody blocking) (Fig. 11.13). In this case suppression is highly dependent on the concentration of the antibody, and on its affinity for the antigen compared with the affinity of the B cell

receptors. Only high-affinity B cells compete successfully for the antigen. This mechanism is independent of the Fc portion of the antibody.

- Immunoglobulin can inhibit B cell differentiation by cross-linking (receptor cross-linking) the antigen receptor with the Fc receptor (FcγRIIb) on the same cell (see Fig. 11.13). In this case, the suppressive antibody and the B cell's receptor antibody may recognize different epitopes.
- Doses of IgG that are insufficient to inhibit the production of antibodies completely have the effect of increasing the average antibody affinity because only those B cells with high-affinity receptors can successfully compete with the passively acquired antibody for antigen. For this reason, antibody feedback is believed to be an important factor driving the process of affinity maturation (Fig. 11.14).

Immune complexes may enhance or suppress immune responses

One of the ways in which antibody (either IgM or IgG) might act to modulate the immune response involves an Fc-dependent mechanism and immune complex formation with antigen.

Immune complexes can inhibit or augment the immune response (Fig. 11.15). By activating complement, immune complexes may become localized via interactions with CR2 on follicular dendritic cells (FDCs). This could

Antibody feedback on affinity maturation

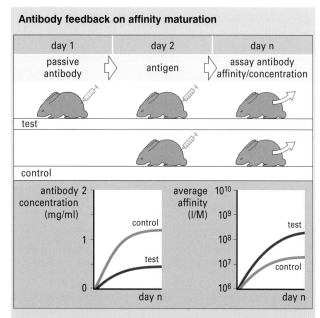

Fig. 11.14 The effect of passive antibody on the affinity and concentration of secreted antibody. One of two rabbits was injected with antibody (passive antibody) on day 1. Both rabbits were immunized with antigen on day 2 and the affinity and concentration of antibody raised to this antigen were assayed at a later time (day n). The antibody assay results show that passive antibody reduces the concentration, but increases the affinity of antibody produced.

Regulatory effects of immune complexes

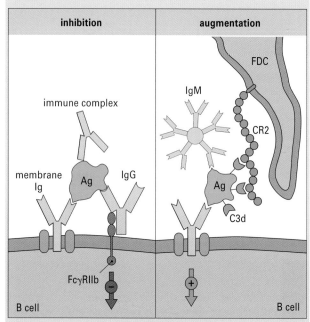

Fig. 11.15 Immune complexes can act either to inhibit or to augment an immune response. Inhibition – when the Fc receptor of the B cell is cross-linked to its antigen receptor by an antigen–antibody complex, a signal is delivered to the B cell, inhibiting it from entering the antibody production phase. Passive IgG may have this effect. Augmentation – antibody encourages presentation of antigen to B cells when it is present on an APC, bound via Fc receptors or, in this case, complement receptors (CR2) on a follicular dendritic cell (FDC). Passive IgM may have this effect.

facilitate the immune response by maintaining a source of antigen.

Q. How does the presence of antigen on FDCs facilitate the immune response?
A. The antigen is available for uptake by B cells and presentation to T cells within the follicle, a process required for class switching and affinity maturation (see Fig. 9.15).

CR2 is also expressed on B cells and, as co-ligation of CR2 with membrane IgM has been shown to activate B cells, immune complex interaction with CR2 of the B cell–co-receptor complex and membrane Ig might lead to an enhanced specific immune response.

Apoptosis in the immune system

Apoptosis is a cellular clearance mechanism through which homeostasis is maintained.

Unlike cell damage-induced death (i.e. **necrosis**), which can trigger immune responses, apoptosis maintains intracellular structures within the cell. Apoptopic cells undergo nuclear fragmentation and the condensation of cytoplasm, plasma membranes, and organelles into apoptopic bodies. Apoptopic cells are rapidly phagocytosed by macrophages, which prevents the release of toxic cellular components into tissues, so avoiding immune responses to the dead cells.

Apoptosis is:

- involved in clearing cells with a high avidity for antigen in the thymus and is an important mechanism of immunological tolerance (see Chapter 19);
- an important mechanism in maintaining homeostasis in the immune system.

Following resolution of an immune response the majority of antigen-specific cells die by apoptosis. This ensures that no unwanted effector cells remain and also maintains a constant number of cells in the immune system.

A small number of cells are prevented from undergoing apoptosis and enter the memory T cell pool.

Apoptosis is controlled by a number of factors in the cell and depends on expression of the death trigger molecule **CD95 (Fas)**. Deficiencies in the FAS/ FASL pathway can give rise to lymphoproliferative disorders with autoimmune manifestations.

Q. How does ligation of Fas lead to apoptosis?
A. It causes activation of a series of inducer and effector caspases.

Expression of the anti-apoptotic molecule **Bcl-2** makes cells more resistant to cell death. Memory T cells generally express high levels of Bcl-2, which may contribute to the rescue of memory populations from apoptosis.

Different cell populations can express both pro- and anti-apoptotic molecules with the balance of these molecules determining whether a cell survives to participate in immune responses. Interestingly, at least *in vitro*, TH1 cells appear more susceptible to Fas induced apoptosis than TH2 or TH17 cells. The exact significance of this finding, however, remains to be determined.

Mechanisms for local reinforcement of different modes of immune response

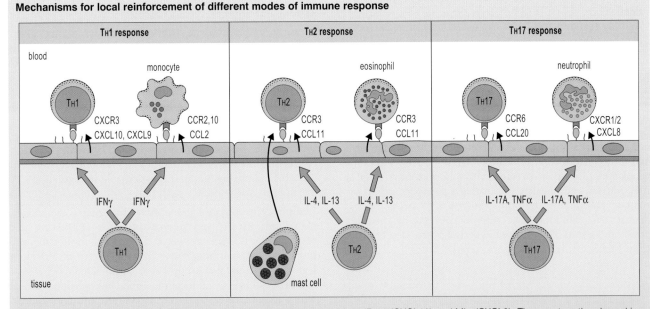

Fig. 11.16 Activated TH1 cells release IFNγ, which induces the chemokines IP-10 (CXCL10) and Mig (CXCL9). These act on the chemokine receptors CXCR3, which are selectively expressed on TH1 cells, thereby reinforcing this type of response. Macrophage chemotactic protein-1 (MCP-1, CCL2), which attracts macrophages and monocytes, is also induced by IFNγ. Mast cells release eotaxin (CCL11) when activated, and endothelial cells and bronchial epithelium can also synthesize this chemokine in response to IL-4 and IL-13 from TH2 cells. Eotaxin acts on CCR3, which is selectively expressed on TH2 cells, thereby reinforcing the TH2 response. Eosinophils and basophils, which mediate allergic responses in airways, also express CCR3. TH17 cells express the chemokine receptor CCR6. IL-17A production by TH17 cells induces expression of CCL20 which acts on CCR6 thus recruiting TH17 cells to the site of infection. Chemokines can therefore potentiate both the initiation and effector phases of a specific type of immune response.

Immune regulation by selective cell migration

The spatial and temporal production of chemokines by different cell types is an important mechanism of immune regulation. There is good evidence to suggest that the recruitment of TH1, TH2 and TH17 cells is differentially controlled, thereby ensuring the maintenance of locally polarized immune responses.

The expression of different chemokine receptors on TH1 cells (CXCR3 and CCR5), TH2 cells (CCR3, CCR4, CCR8), and TH17 (CCR6) allows chemotactic signals to produce the differential localization of T cell subsets to sites of inflammation (see Fig. 6.10).

Chemokines can be induced by cytokines released at sites of inflammation, so providing a mechanism for local reinforcement of particular types of response (Fig. 11.16). Once a response is established the T cells can induce further migration of appropriate effector cells. This is clearly illustrated in TH1 responses where the secondary production of CCL2, CCL3, CXCL10, and CCL5 serves to attract mononuclear phagocytes to the area of inflammation. Production of IL-17A can drive the expression of CCL20, the ligand for CCR6, recruiting more TH17 cells to the site of inflammation. The ability of cytokines such as TGFβ, IL-12, and IL-4 to influence chemokine or chemokine receptor expression provides a further level of control on cell migration or recruitment.

Immune responses do not normally occur at certain sites in the body such as the anterior chamber of the eye and the testes. These sites are called **immune privileged**.

The failure to evoke immune responses in these sites is partly due to the presence of inhibitory cytokines such as TGFβ and IL-10, which inhibit inflammatory responses. The presence of migration inhibition factor (MIF) in the anterior chamber of the eye also inhibits NK cell activity.

T cell expression of different molecules can mediate tissue localization

Most studies on the human immune system are performed on blood due to the ethical issues in obtaining tissues. However, only a small proportion of the lymphocyte pool is circulating in the blood, most being resident in lymphoid or effector tissues.

The expression of molecules on T cells can mediate circulation through different tissues. Loss of the lymph node homing molecules CCR7 and CD62L on the surface of T cells prevents cells from circulating through lymphoid tissue – in this way a population of highly differentiated memory cells migrate to non-lymphoid sites where they can exert effector functions.

It has recently been suggested that there are two types of memory cell:

- **central memory cells** express CCR7, home to lymphoid tissues, and do not have immediate effector function;
- **effector memory cells** do not express CCR7, migrate to non-lymphoid tissues, and produce effector cytokines – effector cells in non-lymphoid tissues, such as the skin, can proliferate and senesce and this has a direct effect on the level of local immune responses.

Q. Why do cells that express CCR7 migrate to lymphoid tissues?

A. They respond to CCL21 expressed only in secondary lymphoid tissues (see Fig. 6.14).

Neuroendocrine regulation of immune responses

It is now widely accepted that there is extensive cross-talk between the neuroendocrine and immune systems. Both systems share similar ligands and receptors that permit intra and inter-system communication. These networks of communication are deemed essential for normal physiological function and good health. For instance they play important roles in modulating the body's response to stress, injury, disease and infection. The interconnections of the nervous, endocrine, and immune systems are depicted in (Fig. 11.17).

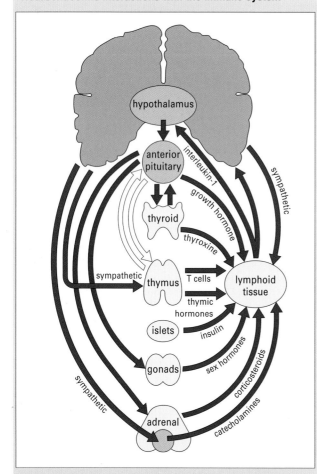

Neuroendocrine interactions with the immune system

Fig. 11.17 The diagram indicates some of the potential connections between the endocrine, nervous, and immune systems. Blue arrows indicate nervous connections, red arrows indicate hormonal interactions, and white arrows indicate postulated connections for which the effector molecules have not been established.

There are several routes by which the central nervous system and immune system can interact:

- most lymphoid tissues (e.g. spleen and lymph nodes) receive direct sympathetic innervation to the blood vessels passing through the tissues and directly to lymphocytes;
- the nervous system directly and indirectly controls the output of various hormones, in particular corticosteroids, growth hormone, prolactin, α-melanocyte-stimulating hormone, thyroxine, and epinephrine (adrenaline);
- immune derived growth factors and cytokines can in turn feed back on the neural and endocrine systems, which probably has an important role in regulating the use of the body's resources.

Lymphocytes express receptors for many hormones, neurotransmitters, and neuropeptides – expression and responsiveness vary between different lymphocyte and monocyte populations, such that the effect of different transmitters may vary in different circumstances.

Corticosteroids, endorphins, and enkephalins, all of which may be released during stress, are immunosuppressive in vivo. Such hormones can have strong effects on lymphocyte proliferation. In particular stress hormones can bring about the reactivation of latent viral infections. The precise *in vitro* effects of endorphins vary depending on the system and on the doses used – some levels are suppressive and others enhance immune functions.

It is certain, however, that corticosteroids act as a major feedback control on immune responses. It has been found that lymphocytes themselves can respond to corticotrophin releasing factor to generate their own adrenocorticotrophic hormone (ACTH), which in turn induces corticosteroid release. Corticosteroids:

- inhibit TH1 cytokine production while sparing TH2 responses; and
- induce the production of TGFβ, which in turn may inhibit the immune response.

For example, the low levels of plasma corticosteroids found in Lewis rats are believed to contribute to their susceptibility to a variety of induced TH1-type autoimmune conditions.

This interplay between the neuroendocrine system and the immune system is bidirectional. Cytokines, in particular IL-1 and IL-6 produced by T cells, neurons, glial cells and cells in the pituitary and adrenal glands, are potent stimulators of ACTH production through their effect on corticotrophin releasing hormone (CRH).

Q. In what other ways does IL-1 mediate interactions between the immune and nervous systems?

A. It causes an increase in body temperature, suppresses appetite, and enhances the duration of slow-wave sleep (see Chapter 6).

Gender based differences in immune responses also occur. Immune cells have been shown to express receptors for estrogens and androgens, so it is likely that circulating levels of these hormones can affect their function. It is noted that, during reproductive years, females demonstrate more pronounced humoral and cellular immunity than males.

Some autoimmune diseases also show a gender bias. The systemic autoimmune disease systemic lupus erythematosus (SLE) is ten times more common in females than males.

Additionally, in animal models of autoimmunity, female NOD mice develop a much higher incidence of diabetes than males (though interestingly this sex bias is not observed in humans) and male BXSB mice have a spontaneously higher incidence of an-SLE like syndrome when compared to females. This provides some evidence for the effects of sex hormones on immune function.

Genetic influences on the immune response

Familial patterns of susceptibility to infectious agents suggest that resistance or susceptibility might be an inherited characteristic. Such patterns of resistance and susceptibility also occur in autoimmune diseases.

Many genes are involved in governing susceptibility or resistance to disease and the disease is said to be under polygenic control. Considerable advances have been made in mapping and identifying the genes governing the response to some diseases as a result of:

- the development of techniques such as microsatellite mapping;
- increased availability of DNA samples; and
- sequencing of the human genome.

In most cases these studies have led to the identification of potential candidate genes, but their real role in disease susceptibility remains to be clarified. In other cases single mutations in genes of known function have been found and the mechanism by which they contribute to disease identified.

MHC haplotypes influence the ability to respond to an antigen

The development of inbred mouse strains conclusively demonstrated that genetic factors have a role in determining immune responsiveness. For example, strains of mice with different MHC haplotypes vary in their ability to mount an antibody response to specific antigens (Fig. 11.18). This function depends on MHC class II molecules (see Chapter 5) and is specific for each antigen – a high responder strain for some antigens may be a low responder strain for others.

MHC-linked genes control the response to infections

MHC-linked genes (see Chapter 5) are involved in the immune response to infectious agents. In some cases the gene involved is the MHC gene itself, but in others it can be a gene linked to the MHC.

Susceptibility to infection by Trichinella spiralis is affected by the I-E locus in mice

The first observation that genes within the MHC could influence the response to parasites involved the susceptibility to *Trichinella spiralis* infection. The response of different recombinant mouse strains to infection with *T. spiralis* is affected by the I-E locus. Mouse strains that express I-E (B10.BR, B10.P) appear to be susceptible whereas those that do not (B10.S, B10.M) are resistant to infection (Fig. 11.19). The response to *T. spiralis* is also influenced by the MHC-linked gene *Ts-2*, which maps close to the *TNF* genes.

The I-E locus also influences susceptibility to Leishmania donovani

Using H-2 congenic mice, it was shown that mice expressing the I-E locus were susceptible to visceral leishmaniasis. Parasite clearance was enhanced by anti-I-E antibody, but not by anti-I-A antibody, showing direct involvement of the I-E product. Furthermore, insertion of an I-E transgene into mice lacking the locus prevented effective clearance of parasites from the liver and spleen when compared to the original strain.

Strain differences in the antibody response

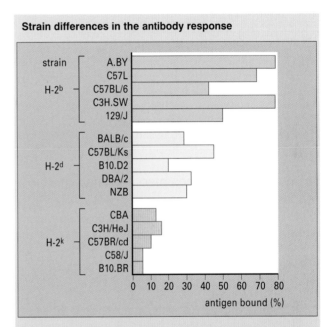

Fig. 11.18 Fifteen strains of mice were given a standard dose of the synthetic antigen (TG)-A-L. Antibody responses are expressed as the antigen-binding capacity of the sera. Animals of the H-2^b haplotype are high responders, whereas those of the H-2^d and H-2^k haplotypes are intermediate and low responders, respectively. However, there is some overlap between the levels of response in different haplotypes, indicating that H-2-linked genes are not the only ones controlling the antibody response.

Susceptibility to *Trichinella spiralis*

mouse strain	H-2 haplotype	I-E expression	resistance index	resistance phenotype
B10.BR	k	+	0	sus
B10.P	p	+	−22	sus
B10.RIII	r	+	33	sus
B10	b	−	63	res/int
B10.S	s	−	100	res
B10.M	f	−	104	res
B10.Q	q	−	105	res

Fig. 11.19 Association of H-2 haplotype, expression of cell surface I-E molecules, and susceptibility to infection with *T. spiralis*. The resistance index is measured as the number of parasites present after a constant challenge relative to strains B10.BR (susceptible = 0% resistance) and B10.S (resistant = 100% resistance). B10 shows intermediate resistance.

Certain HLA haplotypes confer protection from infection

Comparison of HLA haplotypes in humans revealed that certain MHC class I and class II alleles (HLA-B*5301 and DRB1*1302, respectively) are associated with a reduced risk of severe malaria. DRB1*1302 binds different peptides from those bound by DRB1*1301 as a result of a single amino acid difference in the β chain. This change is sufficient to influence the response to the malaria parasite.

HLA-DRB1*1302 has also been associated with an increased clearance of the hepatitis B virus and consequently a decreased risk of chronic liver disease.

The MHC class I type, HLA-A*02, is associated with a reduced risk of disease development following human T-lymphotropic virus-1 (HTLV-1) infection. The viral load was lower in HLA-A*02-positive healthy carriers of HTLV-1 correlating with the presence of high levels of virus-specific CTLs.

In HIV-1 infection a selective advantage against disease has been noted in individuals expressing maximal HLA heterozygosity of class I loci (A, B, and C) and lacking expression of HLA-B*35 and HLA-Cw*04.

Many non-MHC genes also modulate immune responses

Some genes outside the MHC region also govern the immune response. However, these genes are generally less polymorphic than MHC genes and contribute less to variations in disease susceptibility. Nevertheless, their effects are found in autoimmune diseases, allergy, and infection. For example:

- individuals with defects in the complement components C1q, C1r, and C1s (see Chapter 4) are predisposed to develop systemic lupus erythematosus (SLE) and lupus nephritis – the development of SLE-like symptoms in C1q knockout mice parallels the human situation;
- deficiency in C3 leads to an increased susceptibility to bacterial infections and a predisposition to immune complex disease – this is also seen with a deficiency in C2 and C4, both of which are located within the MHC region;
- high IgE production in some allergy-prone families associates with the presence of an 'atopy gene' on human chromosome 11q;
- Biozzi generated two lines of mice based on their responsiveness to erythrocyte antigens. The high responder and low responder Biozzi mice make quantitatively different amounts of antibody in response to antigenic challenge and the basis for these differences has in part been attributed to genetic differences in macrophage activity; the high and low responder strains also differ in their ability to respond to parasitic infections, but this does not correlate with the level of antibody produced.

Q. Why would deficiency in the components of the classical pathway lead to immune complex disease?
A. C3b deposition is required to transport complexes on erythrocytes and their ultimate phagocytosis by macrophages in the liver and spleen (see Chapter 4).

Polymorphisms in cytokine and chemokine genes affect susceptibility to infections

Polymorphisms in the genes encoding cytokine receptors have been shown to correlate with an increased susceptibility to:

- infection;
- severe combined immune deficiency (SCID); and
- inflammatory conditions.

The outcome of the mutation is dependent on which cytokine gene is affected.

Q. What effect would you expect a deficiency in the IL-7 receptor (IL-7R) to produce?
A. It causes a reduction in T cell numbers because IL-7 is required for early thymocyte development.

For example, humans with:

- mutations in the IL-7R α chain have a reduced number of T cells;
- whereas those with deficiency in the common cytokine receptor γ chain (γc), a component of IL-2, IL-4, IL-7, IL-9, and IL-15 receptors, have reduced numbers of T and NK cells and impaired B cell function, in part attributable to the lack of T cell help (Fig. 11.20).

Further examples are the mutations in the IFNγ receptor (IFNγR) or IL-12 receptor (IL-12R), which increase

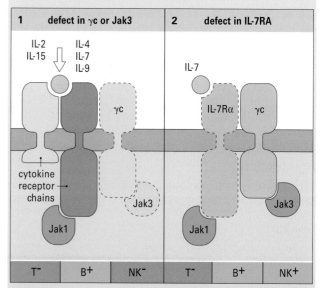

Role of mutations in cytokine receptor genes in severe combined immune deficiency (SCID)

Fig. 11.20 (**1**) A defect in the common chain (γc) of the cytokine receptors IL-2, IL-15, IL-4, IL-7, and IL-9 leads to a SCID, with loss of both T and NK cells. A similar deficiency results from mutation in the janus kinase (Jak3), which transduces signals from the γc chain. Note that IL-2 and IL-15 have three chains in their high-affinity receptor, whereas IL-4, IL-7, and IL-9 have only two chains. (**2**) Absence of the specific IL-7R chain also produces a severe immunodeficiency, but this primarily affects T cell development.

susceptibility to mycobacterial infection. A list of genetic defects that contribute to impaired immune responses is given in Figure 11.21.

Mutations in the cytokine promoters influence the levels of expression of cytokines. Polymorphisms such as these have been linked to certain autoimmune conditions and also to susceptibility to infections. For example, polymorphisms in the promoter region of the *TNFα* gene, which lies within the MHC, influence its level of expression through altered binding of the transcription factor OCT-1. One of these polymorphisms, commonly associated with cerebral malaria, results in high levels of TNF expression. This may lead to upregulation of intercellular adhesion molecule-1 (ICAM-1) on vascular endothelium, increased adherence of infected erythrocytes, and subsequent blockage of blood flow.

This polymorphism in the TNFα promoter has also been associated with:

- lepromatous leprosy;
- mucocutaneous leishmaniasis; and
- death from meningococcal disease.

Some genes involved in immune responses affect disease susceptibility, but do not affect immune responsiveness. For example, disease progression to AIDS has been shown to be associated with polymorphisms in the chemokine receptor gene-5 (CCR5).

CCR5 is a co-receptor used in the entry of macrophage-tropic strains of HIV-1 into cells. A mutation that inactivates this receptor is found in some individuals of European origin, but is rare in populations of Asian or sub-Saharan African descent. Individuals homozygous for this CCR5 mutation are very resistant to HIV-1 infection. In this case resistance is related to the reduced primary spread of the virus rather than an enhanced immune response against it.

Genetic defects associated with immune deficiency or abnormalities

condition	defective gene	result
SCID	γc	failure of signal transduction by cytokines
	IL-2Rα	failure of IL-2 signal in activation and development
	IL-7Rα	failure of IL-7 signal in lymphocyte development
	Jak3	lack of signal transduction by cytokines
	CD3γ	no signal transduced from TCR
	CD3ε	no signal transduced from TCR
	ZAP70	no signal transduced from TCR
	ADA	T cell toxicity
	RAG1/2	failure in TCR and BCR gene recombination
T cell deficiency	PNP	T cell development failure
class II deficiency	CIIT	failure to express MHC class II molecules
class I deficiency	TAP1/2	failure to load MHC class I molecules
X-linked hyper-IgM	CD40L	no maturation of antibody response
X-linked-agamma-globulinemia	Btk	failure of B cell development
X-linked lymphoproliferative syndrome	SH2DIA/SAP	impaired negative signals to B cells
Autoimmune lymphoproliferative syndrome	Fas(CD95) or FasL	extended lymphocyte life span due to reduced apoptosis
mycobacterial infection	IFNγR1/2, IL-12R	impaired TH1 responses

ADA, adenosine deaminase gene; BCR, B cell receptor; *Btk,* Bruton's tyrosine kinase gene; TCR, T cell receptor; *PNP*, purine nucleoside phosphorylase gene; *RAG*, recombination activating gene

Fig. 11.21 Genetic defects associated with immune deficiency or abnormalities. See also Chapter 16. (*Based on a review by Leonard, Curr Opin Immunol 2000;12:465–467.*)

CRITICAL THINKING: REGULATION OF THE IMMUNE RESPONSE (SEE P. 436 FOR EXPLANATIONS)

1. Why is there a need to regulate the extent of immune activation and lymphocyte proliferation?

2. In what ways can antibody regulate the immune response?

3. How could regulatory T cells be used to modulate aberrant immune responses?

Further reading

Agnello D, Lankford CS, Bream J, et al. Cytokines and transcription factors that regulate T helper cell differentiation: new players and new insights. J Clin Immunol 2003;23:147–161.

Bettelli E, Carrier Y, Gao W, et al. Reciprocal developmental pathways for the generation of pathogenic effector TH17 and regulatory T cells. Nature 2006;441:235–238.

Blalock JE. Shared ligands and receptors as a molecular mechanism for communication between immune and neuroendocrine systems. Ann N Y Acad Sci 1994;741:292–298.

Chess L, Jiang H. Resurrecting CD8+ suppressor cells. Nat Immunol 2004;5:569–571.

Cua DJ, Tato DM. Innate IL-17-producing cells: the sentinels of the immune system. Nat Rev Immunol 2010;10:479–489.

Ferwerda B, McCall MB, Alonso S, et al. TLR4 polymorphisms, infectious diseases, and evolutionary pressure during migration of modern humans. Proc Nat Acad Sci U S A 2007;104:16645–16650.

Heymann B. Regulation of antibody responses via antibodies, complement, and Fc receptors. Annu Rev Immunol 2000;18:709–738.

Korn T, Bettelli E, Oukka M, Kuchroo VK. IL-17 and Th17 cells. Annu Rev Immunol 2009;27:485–517.

Leonard WJ. Genetic effects on immunity. Curr Opin Immunol 2000;12:465–467.

Metzler B, Wraith DC. Inhibition of experimental autoimmune encephalomyelitis by inhalation but not oral administration of the encephalitogenic peptide: influence of MHC binding affinity. Int Immunol 1993;5:1159–1165.

Mills KHG, McGuirk P. Antigen-specific regulatory T cells – their induction and role in infection. Semin Immunol 2004;16:107–117.

Murphy KM, Stockinger B. Effector T cell plasticity: flexibility in the face of changing circumstances. Nat Immunol 2010;11:674–690.

Romagnani S. Th1/Th2 cells. Inflamm Bowel Dis 1999;5:285–294.

Shevach EM. Mechanisms of Foxp3+ T regulatory cell-mediated suppression. Immunity 2009;30:636–645.

Taub DD. Neuroendocrine Interactions in the Immune System. Cell Immunol 2008;252:1–10.

Van der Vliet HJJ, Molling JW, von Blomberg BM, et al. The immunoregulatory role of CD1d-restricted natural killer T cells in disease. Clin Immunol 2004;112:8–23.

Zlotnik A, Yoshie O. Chemokines: a new classification system and their role in immunity. Immunity 2000;12:121–127.

CHAPTER 12

Immune Responses in Tissues

SUMMARY

- **A tissue can influence local immune responses**, promoting some classes of immunity and suppressing others. Vascular endothelium in each tissue expresses chemokines and adhesion molecules that attract specific subsets of leukocytes.

- **Certain sites in the body are immunologically privileged** and fully allogeneic tissue can be transplanted into them without risk of rejection. These sites, which include the anterior chamber of the eye and the CNS, promote beneficial classes of immune responses while suppressing classes that can do irreparable local damage.

- **The endothelium in the CNS has barrier properties, which exclude most serum proteins from the tissue.** Acute inflammation in the CNS is characterized by TH1 cells, TH17 cells and mononuclear phagocytes.

- **Immune responses in gut and lung distinguish between pathogens and innocuous organisms and antigens.** The immune response in mucosal tissues tends to promote TH2-type responses with IgA production. Gut enterocytes influence the local immune response. Intraepithelial lymphocytes (IELs) respond to stress-induced class Ib molecules and produce many immunomodulatory cytokines. Regulatory T cells normally limit the level of inflammatory reactions.

- **T cells are present in normal skin and immune responses are characterized by T-cell infiltration.** The endothelium of the dermis attracts TH1 cells, which express cutaneous lymphocyte antigen (CLA) and receptors for IFNγ-induced chemokines.

Tissue-specific immune responses

What determines whether an immune response should be comprised of, for example, activated cytotoxic T lymphocytes (CTLs) or a particular class of antibodies? Although immune responses are primarily tailored to the pathogen, there is also a strong influence from the local tissue, where the immune response occurs (Fig. 12.1).

This chapter focuses on:

- the features of immune responses that are unique to individual tissues; and
- the mechanisms by which the tissues influence local and systemic characteristics.

There are several reasons why a particular organ may need to modify local immunity.

Q. Herpes simplex virus infects sensory neurons and causes cold sores. Why might a CTL response be inappropriate for controlling such an infection?

A. An effective cytotoxic response would kill the infected neuron, which cannot be replaced. This would be worse for the host than the moderate inconvenience caused by the sporadically reactivating viral infection.

This is an example of how an immune response summoned to clear an infection can interfere with a tissue's physiology as seriously as the infection itself. A similar outcome can occur in both the eye and the gut, which may be damaged by cytokines such as tumor necrosis factor-α (TNFα) and interferon-γ (IFNγ) produced locally during cell-mediated immune reactions.

Indeed, when TNFα and IFNγ reach high systemic levels, they can result in shock and rapid death. An example is seen in Dengue shock syndrome. Individuals who are immune to the Dengue virus or infants with maternal antibodies may develop rapid circulatory collapse. It is thought that interaction between activated T cells and macrophages causes the release of TNFα, which acts on endothelium leading to an increase in capillary permeability and consequent fall in blood pressure.

Moreover, some types of immune response are only appropriate in specific tissues.

Q. What type of immune response is suited to the gut and mucosal surfaces?

A. The production of IgA antibodies, promoted by a TH2-type immune response. Accumulation and recirculation

Factors controlling the characteristic immune response of a tissue

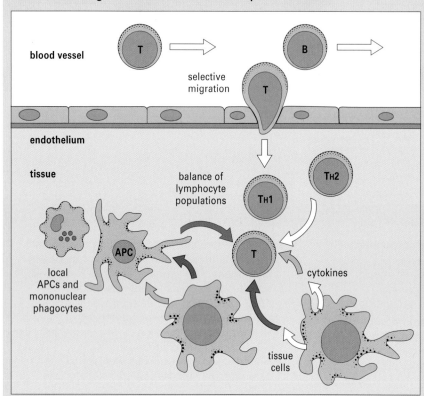

Fig. 12.1 The characteristic immune response of a tissue is controlled both by the leukocyte populations present and by the direct and indirect signals from the endogenous cells of the tissue. The population of lymphocytes that enter a particular tissue is controlled by the vascular endothelium in that tissue. Antigen presentation within the tissue depends on the populations of antigen-presenting cells (APCs), which include resident mononuclear phagocytes. APCs and T cells are influenced directly by endogenous cells of the tissue, and indirectly via cytokines.

of IgA-producing B cells within submucosal tissues means that IgA antibodies are produced near the point of secretion.

These observations suggest that the immune responses in tissues are modulated in order to be appropriate for and effective at that site. Consequently, tissues have evolved regulatory mechanisms that influence the immune response that occurs within them.

Locally produced cytokine and chemokines influence tissue-specific immune responses

Knowledge of the distinctive immunological characteristics of each tissue is only just emerging. Nevertheless a number of principles can be discerned:

* a tissue can promote some classes of immunity and suppress others;
* the vascular endothelium plays a major role in determining which leukocytes will enter the tissue by secretion of distinct blends of chemokines, and expression of site specific adhesion molecules;
* cells in the tissue can exert their effects via cytokines or by direct cell–cell interactions. In effect, cells of the tissue can signal infection, damage or distress;
* a tissue can have several microenvironments, each of which has its own physiology and preferred immune response;
* the local immune response can produce systemic changes.

Endothelium controls which leukocytes enter a tissue

Migration of leukocytes into different tissues of the body is dependent on the vascular endothelium in each tissue. For many years, it was thought that the endothelium in different tissues was essentially similar, with the possible exception of tissues such as the brain and retina, which have barrier properties (see below). Despite this common belief, it was well known that inflammation in different tissues had different characteristics, even when the inducing agents were similar.

It is now clear that a major element controlling inflammation and the immune response is the vascular endothelium in each tissue, which has its own characteristics; different endothelia produce distinctive blends of chemokines (Fig. 12.2). In addition the endothelium can transport chemokines produced by cells in the tissue from the basal to the lumenal surface by transcytosis, or by surface diffusion in tissues that lack barrier properties (Fig. 12.3).

The surface (glycocalyx) of vascular endothelium also varies considerably between tissues, and this affects which chemokines are retained on the lumenal surface, to signal to circulating leukocytes.

Q. Why would the glycocalyx of endothelium affect the chemokines presented?
A. Chemokines have two binding sites, one for the chemokine receptor and another that binds to sites in extracellular matrix and cell-surface molecules, particularly negatively charged proteoglycans. The binding affinity varies depending on the proteoglycan and the chemokine.

Production of chemokines by endothelium derived from different human tissues

	endothelium		
	lung	dermis	brain
CXCL8	++	++	+++
CXCL10	+	+	+++
CCL2	+++	++	+
CCL5	+	++	+

Fig. 12.2 Brain endothelium produces high levels of CXCL8 and CXCL10 associated with a TH1-type immune response. Dermal endothelium produces high levels of CCL5 associated with T cell migration, whereas lung endothelium produces high levels of CCL2, a chemokine that causes macrophage migration.

Histological section of an airway from a case of fatal asthma

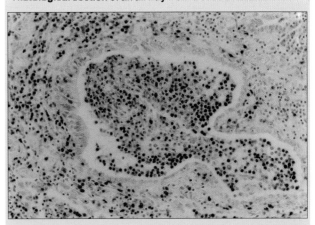

Fig. 12.4 The lumen of an alveolus of the lung is heavily infiltrated with inflammatory exudates, fibrin, and cellular debris. Immunohistochemical staining with monoclonal antibody against EG2 indicates that the majority of cells are eosinophils. *(Courtesy of Arshad SH. Allergy: An Illustrated Colour Text. Philadelphia: Churchill Livingstone, 2002. With permission from Elsevier.)*

Transport of chemokines

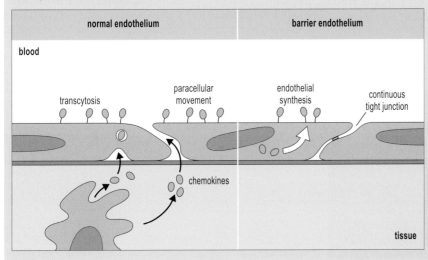

Fig. 12.3 In most tissues, chemokines produced by cells in the tissue can move to the lumenal surface of the endothelium by transcytosis or by movement through the paracellular junctions, to be held on the endothelial glycocalyx. In tissues such as the brain, which have a barrier endothelium, there is limited transcytosis, and almost no paracellular movement of proteins such as chemokines. In these tissues, chemokine production by the endothelium is particularly important in controlling leukocyte migration.

Hence the different sets of leukocytes present in each tissue can be partly related to the chemokines synthesized by the cells present, particularly the endothelium. For example, in normal lung there is a high level of macrophage migration, which relates to the high expression of CCL2 (macrophage chemotactic protein-1) by lung endothelium. In allergic asthma, the proportion of eosinophils increases, due to the production of IL-5 and CCL3 (eotaxin), which are characteristic of the TH2 response that tends to predominate in mucosal tissues (Fig. 12.4). By contrast, in the CNS lymphocytes and mononuclear phagocytes predominate in most immune reactions.

Q. How would you expect the high production of CXCL10 to affect immune reactions in the CNS?

A. CXCL10 is induced in response to IFNγ and acts on CXCR3, which is selectively expressed on TH1 cells (see Fig. 6.11). Therefore brain endothelium produces chemokines that promote a TH1-type reaction.

Some tissues are immunologically privileged

There are certain sites in the body where fully allogeneic tissue can be transplanted without risk of rejection. These include the anterior chamber of the eye, the brain, and testes. Several factors may contribute to the **immunological privilege** of these sites, some of which affect the initiation of the immune response and some affect the effector phase.

The 'privileged sites' were long thought to be locations where adaptive immune responses are so dangerous that the immune system is either not allowed entry, is destroyed upon arrival, or is prevented from functioning. Recent evidence suggests that the concept of privileged sites may have been a misconception based on the limitations of the experimental assay systems. Once the experiments were expanded to include a wider variety of assays it became apparent that privileged sites are not immunologically impaired. They are simply sites that are able to promote certain kinds of beneficial classes of immune responses while suppressing classes that can do irreparable local damage. The mechanisms controlling immune reactions in the CNS are explored below.

Immune reactions in the CNS

The CNS, including the brain, spinal cord, and retina of the eye is substantially shielded from immune reactions. The peripheral nervous system is also partially protected. The low levels of immune reactivity in the brain are ascribed to a number of factors:

- the blood–brain barrier (endothelium plus astrocytes) prevents the movement of over 99% of large serum proteins into the brain tissue (IgG, complement, etc.); there are similar barriers in the eye (blood–retinal barrier);
- low levels of MHC molecule expression, and co-stimulatory molecules result in inefficient antigen presentation;
- there is no conventional lymphatic drainage system from brain tissue to local lymph nodes;
- there are low levels of leukocyte traffic into the CNS in comparison with other tissues;
- neurons have direct immunosuppressive actions on glial cells;
- astrocytes, neurons and some glial cells produce immunosuppressive cytokines.

The blood–brain barrier excludes most antibodies from the CNS

The blood–brain barrier is a composite structure formed by the specialized brain endothelium and the foot processes of astrocytes. Astrocytes are required to induce the special properties of brain endothelial cells, which have continuous belts of tight junctions connecting them to other endothelial cells (Fig. 12.5). An estimate of the tightness of the barrier is given by its trans-endothelial resistance, which is up to 2000 Ω/cm^2 in the CNS by comparison with values $<10\,\Omega/cm^2$ in most other tissues. In addition the brain endothelial cells have an array of transporters that allow nutrients into the CNS and a set of multi-drug resistance pumps that prevent many toxic molecules and therapeutic drugs from entering the brain. However, it is the very low permeability of the endothelium to serum proteins which is of particular interest for immunologists (see Fig. 12.5). For example, the level of IgG found in the CNS is normally approximately 0.2% of the level found in serum. The level may rise during an immune reaction as the endothelial barrier becomes more permeable in response to inflammatory cytokines. In some conditions, such as multiple sclerosis, there is often local synthesis of antibody within the CNS, which is reflected in abnormally high antibody levels in cerebrospinal fluid, even accounting for the increased leakage into the CNS. This finding demonstrates that some B cells have migrated into the CNS, and plasma cells have been identified in the spaces surrounding the larger blood vessels. Macrophages also contribute to immune reactions in CNS and they can synthesize some complement components locally (e.g. C3). However the overall level of serum proteins

The blood–brain barrier

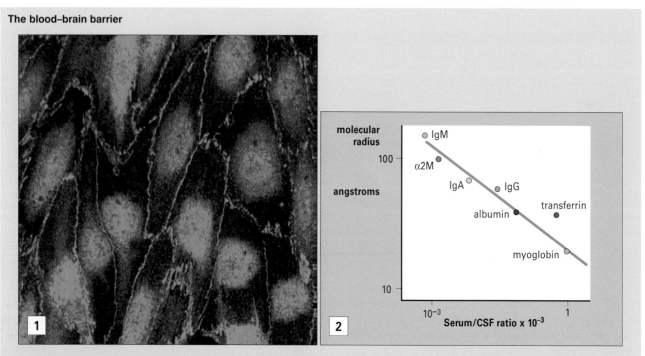

Fig. 12.5   (1) Brain endothelial cells have a continuous ring of tight junctions, identified in this micrograph by the junctional marker ZO-1. The resulting permeability barrier excludes serum proteins from the brain tissue. (2) The graph shows the serum/cerebrospinal fluid (CSF) ratio for different proteins. There is an inverse relationship between molecular size and the level in CSF. Molecules such as transferrin, which are transported into the brain, are present at higher levels than would be expected from their size. Immunoglobulins are not transported.

including antibodies and complement rarely exceeds 2% of the levels in serum even in the most severe inflammatory reactions.

Neurons suppress immune reactivity in neighboring glial cells

Researchers first examined single populations of cells from the CNS in vitro. For example, they found that astrocytes would respond to IFNγ by increasing their expression of MHC class I molecules and IFNγ would also induce the normally-absent MHC class II molecules. However, in vivo, astrocytes rarely respond in this way. It appeared that the local environment of the CNS could in some way suppress the ability of astrocytes to respond to IFNγ.

Subsequently it was found that when neurons are co-cultured in contact with astrocytes, then the ability to induce MHC molecules was suppressed, but if the cells were not in contact, they were not repressed (Fig. 12.6).

Q. How do you interpret the repression of MHC induction described in Figure 12.6?
A. Because repression of MHC induction requires contact between the cells it implies that the effect is not caused by a cytokine.

Subsequently it became clear that electrically active neurons are required. This means that neurons that are functioning normally can suppress their neighboring glial cells (and downregulate their own MHC molecules) whereas

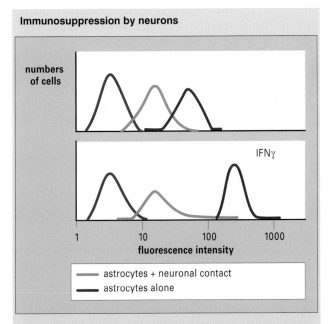

Immunosuppression by neurons

numbers of cells

IFNγ

fluorescence intensity

— astrocytes + neuronal contact
— astrocytes alone

Fig. 12.6 The top graph is a FACS histogram which shows the expression of MHC class I molecules on astrocytes cultured in contact with (*green*) or separate from neurons (*purple*). Note that when neurons are in contact with astrocytes, the astrocytes have lower MHC class I expression. Staining of the negative control antibody is shown in blue. If IFNγ is added to the cultures (*lower graph*), astrocytes cultured alone (*purple*) increase their expression of MHC class I molecules, but those cocultured with neurons are still suppressed (*green*). *(Based on data from Tonsch U, Rott O. Immunology 1993;80:507.)*

damaged neurons will lift the local immunosuppression to allow an immune response to develop.

Neurons can also act on microglia, which are resident mononuclear phagocytes of the CNS. The molecular mechanisms that underlie the suppressive activity of neurons include:

- expression of CD200 and fractalkine (a cell surface chemokine CX3CL1) on the surface of neurons inhibits the activation of microglia, by binding to CD200L and the chemokine receptor CX3CR1 respectively, on the microglia;
- neuronal CD47 binds to a microglial signal regulatory protein (SIRP-1α) which inhibits phagocytosis and TNFα production by the microglia.

Immunosuppressive cytokines regulate immunity in the normal CNS

Observations of immune reactions in the CNS have led to the view that TH1-type immune responses with macrophage activation are generally most damaging, as are responses mediated by IL-17-secreting T cells (TH17 cells). By comparison TH2-type immune responses are generally less damaging, and strains of animals that make strong autoantibody responses against CNS antigens, are often less susceptible to CNS pathology than strains that make weaker antibody responses. Certainly, the production of IL-12, IL-23, and TNFα are associated with damaging responses in CNS. Interestingly IFNγ appears to have a dual role, involved in the acute-phase of CNS inflammation, but also necessary for the recovery phase (Fig. 12.7). Such observations have led to the view that **immune deviation** (the switching of an immune response from TH1 towards a TH2 type) can be protective in the CNS (see Fig. 11.2).

This view is supported by findings that cells of the normal CNS can produce cytokines associated with TH2 responses. For example, astrocytes produce TGF-β, while microglia can produce IL-10 when cocultured with T cells, and both astrocytes and neurons secrete prostaglandins, which inhibit lymphocyte activation. Additionally, several neuropeptides and transmitters (e.g. vaso-active intestinal peptide, VIP) are suppressive. Acute immune responses can develop in the CNS, particularly in susceptible strains, but the normal immunosuppresive controls usually reassert themselves within 1–2 weeks, causing remission. Such a relapsing-remitting pattern of disease occurs in multiple sclerosis and the animal model of CNS inflammation, CREAE (chronic relapsing experimental allergic encephalomyelitis) (Fig. 12.8).

Immune reactions in CNS damage oligodendrocytes

Oligodendrocytes are glial cells that produce the myelin sheaths which act as electrical insulation around nerve axons. When immune reactions occur in the CNS these cells appear to be particularly vulnerable (Fig. 12.9). For example, multiple sclerosis is characterized by focal areas of myelin loss called plaques, typically a few millimeters in diameter. Nerve transmission through these demyelinated areas is seriously impaired, which may cause disease symptoms – weakness and loss of sensation. But it is only in the

Immune regulation in the CNS

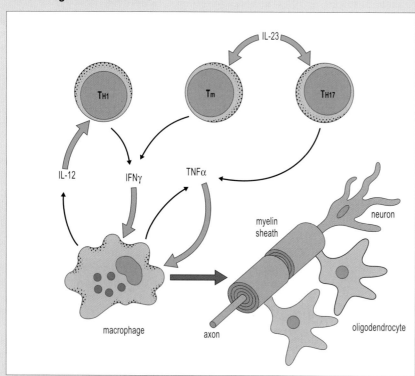

Fig. 12.7 In immune reactions in the CNS the myelin sheath formed by oligodendrocytes around nerve axons is particularly susceptible to damage by activated macrophages. Macrophages are activated by IFNγ produced by TH1 cells and memory T cells (Tm), and IL-12 is important in promoting this type of immune response. Alternatively TH17 cells induced by IL-23 and mononuclear phagocytes (macrophages and microglia) can also produce TNFα, which enhances macrophage activation and contributes to myelin damage. (Black arrows = production, green arrows = activation.)

Chronic relapsing experimental allergic encephalomyelitis

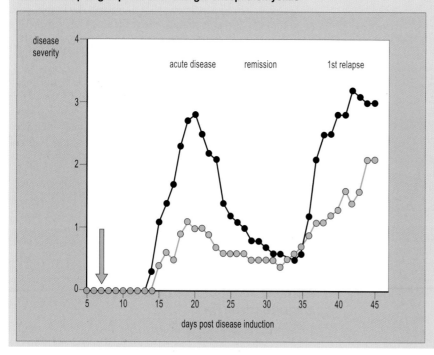

Fig 12.8 The relapsing remitting disease course of CREAE in Biozzi Ab/H mice is shown in the days following immunization with myelin components on day 0 (*black*). Animals that were treated at day 7 with a cell line expressing a soluble TNF-receptor (to mop up TNFα in the brain) had a less serious acute disease and relapse. *(Based on data of Croxford et al. The Journal of Immunology 2000;164: 2776–2781.)*

later stages of the disease that the neurons themselves are damaged.

The reason that oligodendrocytes are vulnerable in multiple sclerosis is less clear. It is possible that they are most readily damaged, because they normally maintain very large amounts of plasma-membrane forming the myelin sheath. Another theory suggests that they are particularly susceptible to damage by serum molecules (e.g. complement), which leak into the CNS as a result of blood–brain barrier breakdown. Many researchers consider that they are

Type IV hypersensitivity in CNS

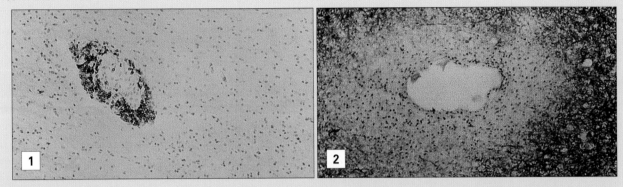

Fig. 12.9 (1) The perivenous infiltrations of lymphocytes in parainfectious encephalomyelitis are confined to the area around the venule. There is little disruption of the tissue, but a stain for myelin shows that demyelination (2) extends out beyond the initial area of infiltration. *(Courtesy of Dr N Woodroofe and Dr H Okazaki.)*

IgA synthesis in the lamina propria

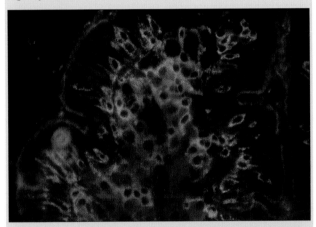

Fig. 12.10 Lymphoid cells in the epithelium and lamina propria fluoresce green using antibody to leukocyte common antigen (CD45). Red cytoplasmic staining is obtained with anti-IgA antibody, which detects plasma cells in the lamina propria and IgA in the mucus. *(Courtesy of Professor G Janossy.)*

targeted by autoantibodies which allow macrophages and activated microglia to recognize them, and that release of reactive oxygen and nitrogen intermediates from the phagocytes then damage the myelin.

Immune responses in the gut and lung

In contrast to the CNS, the gut and lung are examples of tissues that are continuously in contact with high levels of harmless commensal organisms and innocuous antigens as well as potential pathogens. Mucosal tissues contain a high proportion of the body's lymphoid tissues, but the responses in these tissues are concerned not just with whether an immune response takes place, but also on the quality of that response. Antigens introduced orally tend to invoke an immune response that is appropriate for the gut and other mucosal surfaces, namely the production of local IgA, and some systemic IgG (Fig. 12.10). There is generally little production of TH1 cells or CTLs, and no cell-mediated immune response.

It is essential that the immune system in the gut does not make strong immune responses against the enormous load of antigens in food, or harmless commensal bacteria. Similarly, many airborne antigens (e.g. pollen) are harmless, and a strong immune response in the lung is inappropriate i.e., it would be considered hypersensitivity.

Q. What factors allow the immune system to distinguish between pathogens and innocuous organisms and antigens?
A. Many pathogenic organisms have components that are recognized by pattern recognition receptors (PRRs) including Toll-like receptors (see Fig. 6.20), which when ligated can lead to efficient antigen presentation.

The gut immune system tolerates many antigens but reacts to pathogens

There are many examples, where an individual encounters an antigen in food, and subsequently becomes tolerant to it – they do not make an immune response when the antigen is subsequently given in an immunogenic form. This phenomenon is called **oral tolerance** and it is related to **nasal tolerance** where antigen delivered to nasal mucosa as an aerosol inhibits subsequent immunization.

Q. Can you give an example of tolerance induced by administration of antigen across mucosal tissues?
A. Tolerance in mice administered myelin basic protein (MBP) by aerosol can suppress the induction of experimental allergic encephalomyelitis (EAE) in response to the same antigen given intradermally in adjuvant (see Fig. 11.2).

Oral tolerance, and the related phenomenon of nasal tolerance, illustrate two points:

- it is systemic in that it can influence responses at non-mucosal sites;
- it is dominant in that it is transferable to naive individuals by CD4 (or occasionally CD8) T cells.

Tolerance is not the only form of immunity that arises from ingestion of antigens. **Oral vaccination** has been recognized since 1919 when Besredka noticed that rabbits were protected from fatal dysentery by oral immunization with killed shigellae. The attenuated polio vaccine that was

2 Immune responses in tissues

Structure of the villi and crypts of the small intestine

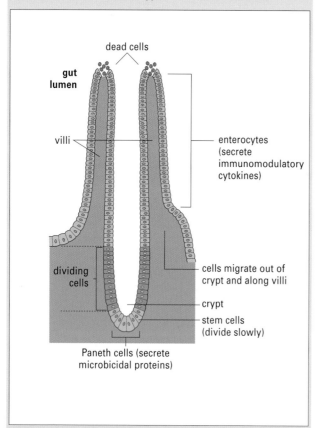

Fig. 12.11 Stem cells give rise to Paneth cells at the base of the crypt, which secrete antimicrobial peptides. The enterocytes are derived from the rapidly dividing transit-amplifying population and will eventually be shed from the tips of the villi. These cells secrete immunomodulatory cytokines.

developed in the 1950s was also given as an oral vaccination. In both cases these vaccines are not viewed as harmless antigens by the immune system:

- shigellae contain antigens that activate the intracellular PRR, NOD-1 (see Fig. 7.w6);
- the polio genome is ssRNA (recognized by TLR7 and TLR8) and it replicates using a dsRNA intermediate, which is recognized by TLR3. Also, the attenuated polio vaccine proliferates in the gut and lymphoid tissue, and therefore induces tissue damage.

Gut enterocytes influence the local immune response

Intestinal epithelial cells (enterocytes) are the major cell-type forming the epithelium of the gut. These cells have continuous tight junctions and thus form a barrier to prevent antigens from entering the body. The enterocytes of the gut considerably influence the local immune response by secreting a variety of immunomodulatory factors such as TGFβ, VIP, IL-1, IL-6, IL-7, CXCL8, and CCL3. The Paneth cells at the bottoms of the crypts meanwhile produce several natural antibiotic peptides (Fig. 12.11), which help prevent

bacterial overgrowth in these sensitive sites of cellular differentiation.

Intra-epithelial cells (IEL) and some dendritic cells are located in the epithelial layer and enterocytes may promote their migration. More lymphocytes and phagocytes are found in the lamina propria, which lies beneath the epithelium.

Q. What are the characteristics of IELs?
A. IELs have a dendritic morphology and express the γδ form of the T cell receptor (TCR) and often CD8.

By expressing E-cadherin, a ligand for αEβ7-integrin, and by secreting TGFβ, which upregulates the expression of αEβ7, enterocytes may provide a signal for the selective accumulation of IELs that express this integrin. In this way, the tissue cells invite the residency of cells that promote certain types of immunity and aid in repair.

The major areas of gut-associated lymphoid tissue (GALT) include the Peyer's patches in the small intestine, the lymphoid follicles throughout the gut, and the mesenteric lymph nodes which receive lymph draining from the intestinal villi and the other lymphoid tissues (see Fig. 2.53). It is worth noting that food antigens are primarily present in the small intestine, whereas bacterial antigens are more prevalent in the large intestine.

IELs produce many immunomodulatory cytokines

Tolerance to food antigens depends on a variety of overlapping mechanisms, but the production of TGFβ and IL-10 are particularly important. For example, IL-10 knockout mice develop colitis, if they contact appropriate triggering micro-organisms and in humans, IL-10 is a susceptibility locus for ulcerative colitis. TGFβ is an important element in the TH2 spectrum of cytokines and also induces FoxP3 in naive T cells, thus promoting development of regulatory T cells. Tregs, which are abundant in the lamina propria also produce IL-10 and TGFβ, which further limit inflammatory reactions in the gut (Fig. 12.12). It is not clear exactly how Tregs are stimulated within the gut; they express high levels of TLRs, particularly TLR2, 4, and 8, so they can respond to the high potential load of MAMPs, but they clearly respond differently to APCs and effector CD4$^+$ T cells.

When immune responses develop in the gut, IELs can produce IL-1, lymphotoxin (LT), IFNγ, and TNFα, so a switch in the balance of pro-inflammatory cytokines and regulatory cytokines in the epithelium and lamina propria occurs when damaging immune reactions develop in the gut.

Many IELs have an activated or memory phenotype and recognize the ancient conserved MHC class I-like molecules, **MICA** and **MICB**, which are upregulated by cellular stress. When activated by MICA and MICB some of the mucosa-associated lymphocytes secrete epidermal cell growth factor (ECGF) and may therefore function to repair and renew damaged intestinal epithelial cells.

Hence, by expressing molecules, the tissue cells can activate their local resident lymphocytes regardless of the specific antigen that is the target of the immune response. In this way the tissue can influence local immunity against many different antigens.

206

Immune cells in the intestine

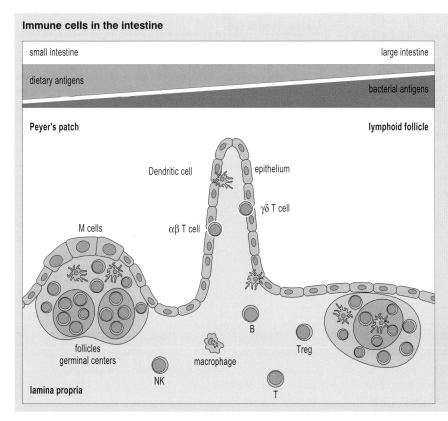

small intestine   large intestine

dietary antigens

bacterial antigens

Peyer's patch   lymphoid follicle

Dendritic cell   epithelium

γδ T cell

M cells   αβ T cell

B

follicles
germinal centers   macrophage   Treg

NK

lamina propria   T

Fig 12.12 Immune cells in the intestine include the intra-epithelial γδ T cells, effector αβ T cells and dendritic cells found in the epithelial layer. The lamina propria includes populations of macrophages, effector T cells and regulatory T cells (Tregs). IgA-producing B cells and associated T cells are found in the encapsulated lymphoid organs, including the Peyer's patches and the lymphoid follicles. Tregs are also found in T cell areas of the lymphoid tissues.

Chronic inflammation in the gut

The most common types of chronic inflammatory disease of the gut are inflammatory bowel disease (IBD) including Crohn's disease, which may affect the entire intestinal tract, and ulcerative colitis affecting the large intestine. Both of these conditions are thought to occur because of an over-reaction to intestinal bacteria; both have a strong genetic component and pattern recognition receptors (e.g. NOD2) are disease susceptibility loci.

In celiac disease, the subject is sensitive to gluten in the food, and susceptibility is strongly related to HLA haplo-type and to loci for inflammatory cytokines and chemo-kines. In all three conditions, ulcerative colitis, celiac disease and Crohn's disease, there is production of TNFα and IFNγ, dysregulation of the normal mucosal immune response and damage to tissue, including the epithelium responsible for absorbing nutrients.

The chronic inflammatory diseases all appear to be due to a reduction of the normal tolerogenic mechanisms in the gut, so that the immune response is tipped towards inflammation.

Immune reactions in the skin

The skin is the largest organ of the body, and in humans there may be up to 10^6 T cells/cm^2, in the dermis, tissue macrophages and at least two major populations of dendritic cells, the Langerhans' cells in the epidermis and the plasmacytoid dendritic cells, mostly in the dermis. T cells constitute the major cell type present both in normal skin and in immune reactions (Fig. 12.13). They are characterized by a skin-homing marker CLA (cutaneous lympho-cyte antigen) and the chemokine receptors CCR4 and

Tregs in the skin

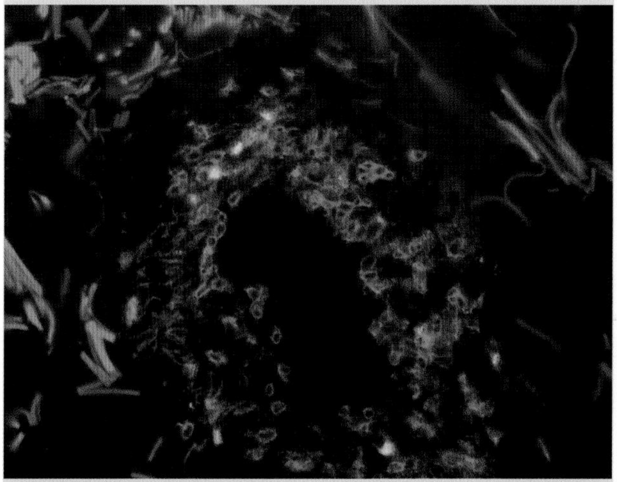

Fig 12.13 A section of normal human skin (dermis) costained with antibody to CD3 (*red*) and FOXP3 (*green*) to identify regulatory T cells. T cell infiltrates, including Tregs, are seen around a vessel. *(Courtesy of Dr Rachael Clark, Clark and Kupper, 2007, Blood 109:194–202.)*

CCR6; CCR4 recognizes CCL5 (RANTES) which is strongly expressed by dermal endothelium (see Fig. 12.2). CLA is a sialylated molecule that binds to ELAM-1 (endothelial leukocyte adhesion molecule-1), a lectin-like molecule that is strongly expressed on endothelium in the skin. CLA$^+$ lymphocytes also express high levels of receptors for IL-12 and IL-2 and the chemokine receptor CXCR3, which recognizes IFNγ-induced chemokines. This can explain why active immune responses in skin are characterized by a TH1-type immune response, with high expression of IFNγ and low IL-4. However, as inflammation subsides, there is an increase in IL-4 production and a shift towards a TH2-type response. An outline of the intiation and effector phases of immune responses in the skin (type-IV hypersensitivity) are shown in Figures 26.4–26.7. Immune reactions in skin are also seen in psoriasis and mycosis fungoides, both with strong T cell infiltration.

The cells of the tissue also contribute to the development of the immune response. Keratinocytes, which form the epidermis, express high levels of IL-1, which may be released when the skin is damaged, to promote inflammation and repair. Fibroblasts in the dermis respond to TNFα by releasing IL-15, which activates effector T cells as an immune response develops, and induces Tregs during the resolution phase.

Conclusions

The immune responses and inflammatory reactions that occur in each tissue are distinctive, and are directed by interactions between the endothelial chemokines and adhesion molecules and the circulating leukocytes. The endothelium in each tissue synthesizes distinct sets of chemokines, and expresses specific adhesion molecules, which attracts distinct leukocyte subsets. In the CNS and the skin, TH1-type immune responses are favored, whereas TH2-type responses predominate in mucosal tissues. The type of immune response may switch within individual tissues as the reaction resolves, although this is very much dependent on the inducing antigen, and the immune status of the individual. In tissues with barrier properties, the endothelium also limits entrance of immunoglobulins and serum molecules and the movement of cytokines from cells in the tissue to the blood. Consequently vascular endothelium and the resident cells of the tissue play a central role in determining the characteristics of the inflammatory response in each tissue.

CRITICAL THINKING: IMMUNE REACTIONS IN THE GUT (SEE P. 436 FOR EXPLANATIONS)

Oyster poisoning occurs when an individual eats an oyster that has concentrated bacteria or Protoctista in itself from sea water. Often an individual who has eaten an infected oyster will then be unable to eat oysters again – even good oysters make them ill. Construct a logical explanation for this observation, based on your understanding of immune reactions in the gut.

Further reading

Galea I, Bechmann I, Perry VH. What is immune privilege? Trends Immunol 2007;28:12–18.

Brandtzaeg P. History of oral tolerance and mucosal immunity. Ann N Y Acad Sci 1996;778:1–27.

Cheroutre H. Starting at the beginning: new perspectives on the biology of mucosal T cells. Annu Rev Immunol 2004;22:217–246.

Debendictis C, Joubeh S, Zhang G, et al. Immune functions of the skin. Clin Dermatol 2001;19:573–585.

Engelhardt B, Ransohoff RM. The ins and outs of T-lymphocyte trafficking to the CNS: anatomical sites and molecular mechanisms. Trends Immunol 2005;26:485–495.

Fagarasan S, Kawamoto S, Kanagawa O. Adaptive immune regulation in the gut: T cell dependent and T cell independent IgA synthesis. Ann Rev Immunol 2010;28:243–273.

Greenwood J, Begley DJ, Segal MB, eds. New concepts of a blood brain barrier. New York: Plenum Press; 1995.

Izcue A, Coombes JL. Regulatory lymphocytes and intestinal inflammation. Ann Rev Immunol 2009;27:313–318.

Spellberg B. The cutaneous citadel: a holistic view of skin and immunity. Life Sci 2002;67:477–502.

Wayne Streilein J. Regional immunology of the eye. In: Pepose JS, Holland GN, Wilhelmus KR, eds. Ocular infection and immunity. Oxford: Elsevier;1996:19–33.

Defense Against Infectious Agents

CHAPTER 13

Immunity to Viruses

SUMMARY

- Innate immune responses (mediated by anti-microbial peptides, type I interferons (IFNs), dendritic cells (DCs), natural killer (NK) cells, and macrophages) restrict the early stages of infection, delay spread of virus and promote the activation of adaptive responses. Innate defences are triggered following recognition of molecular 'patterns' characteristic of viral but not host components. Type I IFNs exert direct antiviral activity and also activate other innate and adaptive responses. NK cells are cytotoxic for virally infected cells. Macrophages act at three levels to destroy virus and virus-infected cells.

- As a viral infection proceeds, the adaptive (specific) immune response unfolds. Antibodies and complement can limit viral spread or reinfection. T cells mediate viral immunity in several ways – CD8$^+$ T cells destroy virus-infected cells or cure them of infection; CD4$^+$ T cells promote antibody and CD8$^+$ T cell responses and are a major effector cell population in the response to some virus infections.

- Viruses have evolved strategies to evade the immune response. They may impair the host immune response at the induction and/or effector stages; avoid recognition by the immune response, e.g. via latency or antigenic variation; or resist control by immune effector mechanisms. Many viruses employ multiple strategies to prolong their replication in the host.

- Responses induced during viral infections can have pathological consequences. Damage can be mediated by antiviral responses (e.g. via the formation of immune complexes or T cell-induced damage to host tissues) or by autoimmune responses triggered during the course of infection.

Innate immune defenses against viruses

The early stage of a viral infection is often a race between the virus and the host's defense system, in which the virus tries to overcome host defenses in order to establish an infection and then spread to other tissues.

The initial defense against virus invasion is the integrity of the body surface – for a virus to infect its host it needs to overcome anatomical barriers such as acid pH, proteolytic enzymes, bile and mucous layers. Once these outer defenses are breached, the presence of infection triggers activation of an inflammatory response with activation of local DCs and macrophages and production of a variety of cytokines, chemokines and antimicrobial peptides that establish a local anti-viral state and guide immune system cells to the site of infection.

The innate response plays a critical role in control of early virus replication and spread. Key innate antiviral effectors include type I IFNs, TNFα, defensins, NK cells, neutrophils, and macrophages. A second important role of the innate response is to promote the activation of adaptive responses to eliminate the infection and provide protection against re-infection.

Microbicidal peptides have broad-spectrum antiviral effects

The innate immune response to viruses involves complex interactions between soluble factors and cells. For example during influenza virus infection mucins, gp-340 and pentraxins compete with the virus for its receptor, sialic acid, and cause aggregation of virus particles. Respiratory secretions are also rich in the collectin surfactant proteins (SP)-A and SP-D. These molecules bind to carbohydrates on a range of pathogens, including influenza virus where they adhere to the hemagglutinin protein (HA) resulting in virus neutralization. Some strains of influenza virus fail to be recognized by collectins due to reduced levels of glycosylation of HA. An example of this was the H1N1 virus that caused the 1918 pandemic.

Other families of antimicrobial peptides with antiviral activity include the defensins and the related cathelicidins. Alpha-defensin and the cathelicidin LL37 are produced by epithelial cells and neutrophils in reponse to infection. They have broad-spectrum direct antiviral activity, and also modulate the inflammatory response at sites of infection.

Type I interferons have critical antiviral and immunostimulatory roles

The activation of the IFN system is arguably the most important defence for containing the initial stages of virus infection. There are three major families of IFNs:

- type I (multiple subtypes of IFNα and one subtype of IFNβ);
- type II (IFNγ); and
- type III (IFNλ1, IFNλ2, and IFNλ3, also known as IL-29, IL-28a, and IL-28b).

Other types of IFN exist, including IFN-ω, -τ, -δ, and -κ, some of which play a role during pregnancy. Here we will focus on the IFNs with antiviral activity. Of these, it is the type I and type III IFNs that are induced directly following virus infection, whereas IFNγ is produced by activated T cells and NK cells. Type III IFNs are much less well characterized than type I IFNs, but their functions are thought to be similar.

Type I IFN production typically starts to be induced within the first few hours after virus infection. Type I IFNs can be produced by almost any cell type in the body if it becomes infected with a virus. There are also specialized interferon-producing cells, plasmacytoid DCs, which can be triggered to produce high levels of type I IFN following exposure to virus without themselves becoming infected. This is important because, as discussed below, many viruses have evolved strategies for impairing type I IFN production in the cells they infect. Plasmacytoid DCs typically make at least half of the type I IFN produced during a virus infection.

Type I IFN production is triggered following recognition of molecular patterns characteristic of viral but not host components (Fig. 13.1). Host pattern-recognition receptors involved in detecting the presence of virus infections include:

- cytoplasmic pattern-recognition receptors expressed by almost all cells (e.g. the retinoic acid-inducible gene I (RIG-I)-like receptors, which recognize viral 5'-triphosphorylated ssRNA and dsRNA, and cytoplasmic DNA sensors);
- members of the Toll-like family of receptors (TLRs), which are expressed on the cell membrane or within endosomes/lysosomes of immune system cells and certain non-immune cells located at common sites of pathogen entry, e.g. epithelial cells (TLR3, TLR7, and TLR9, which recognize viral dsRNA, viral ssRNA, and DNA containing CpG motifs, respectively).

Q. What role does dsRNA play in the normal metabolism of a mammalian cell?
A. dsRNA is formed as part of the replication/transcription of RNA viruses. However, because mammals have a DNA genome, dsRNA is not produced during transcription of mRNA; consequently dsRNA is a signature of viral replication. At least, this was the view until recently. It is now known that dsRNA is formed in eukaryotic cells as part of the process that controls mRNA activity by small inhibitory RNAs (siRNA). Mammalian cells therefore have an intrinsic normal mechanism that leads to the recognition and degradation of dsRNA.

Pathways by which type I IFN production can be triggered following virus infection

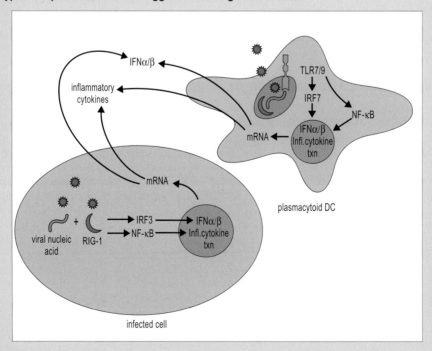

Fig. 13.1 Most cells in the body express cytoplasmic pattern-recognition receptors such as RIG-I. If the cell becomes infected, these detect the presence of viral nucleic acids in the cytoplasm and stimulate IRF3 and NF-κB activation, leading to transcription (txn) of type I IFN and inflammatory cytokine genes and production of these factors. Plasmacytoid DCs can detect the presence of virus and up-regulate type I IFN production without becoming infected. Following virion uptake, viral nucleic acids are detected by TLRs 7 and 9 in endosomal compartments. This stimulates IRF7 and NF-κB activation, leading to production of type I IFNs and inflammatory cytokines.

Triggering of pattern-recognition receptors initiates signaling along pathways that culminate in the activation of transcription factors including IFN regulatory factor (IRF)3 and NFκB, which translocate into the nucleus and activate the transcription of type I IFNs and inflammatory cytokines, respectively (see Fig. 13.1). Plasmacytoid DCs also have a unique signaling pathway for induction of type I IFN production in response to TLR7 or TLR9 ligation that involves the transcription factor IRF7.

The IFN released acts on both the cell producing it and also neighboring cells where it establishes an antiviral state, enabling them to resist virus infection (Fig. 13.2).

IFNs mediate their activity by up-regulating the expression of a large number of genes known as IFN-stimulated genes (ISGs), some of which encode proteins that mediate an antiviral response. These include the key dsRNA-dependent enzymes protein kinase R (PKR) and 2′,5′-oligoadenylate synthetase.

- PKR disrupts virus infection by phosphorylating and inhibiting eukaryotic initiation factor (eIF)-2α, hence blocking the translation of viral mRNA and by initiating apoptosis via Bcl-2 and caspase-dependent mechanisms, killing the cell before virus can be released.
- 2′,5′-oligoadenylate synthetase specifically activates a latent endonuclease (RNaseL) that targets the degradation of viral RNA.

Another inhibitor of transcriptional activation is the Mx protein, which is active against variety of RNA viruses, most notably influenza virus. Although some ISGs have broad activity against multiple viruses there are also other ISGs that mediate antiviral activity against selected classes of viruses, e.g. apolipoprotein B mRNA editing enzyme, catalytic polypeptide-like (APOBEC)s, which combat infection with retroviruses including HIV-1.

In addition to the direct inhibition of virus replication, IFNs also activate macrophages and NK cells and enhance their antiviral activity (see Fig. 13.2). In addition, they help to promote the activation of adaptive responses. They act on antigen presenting cells including conventional DCs to stimulate increased expression of MHC class I and II, along with components of the antigen processing machinery; and they also act directly on T and B cells to promote an antiviral response (see Fig. 13.2).

The importance of type I IFNs *in vivo* is underlined by the increased susceptibility of mice lacking the IFNα/β receptor to virus infection. Similarly, depletion of IFNs by specific antibody treatment also augments virus infection.

NK cells are cytotoxic for virally-infected cells

Activated NK cells can typically be detected within 2 days of virus infection. Since viruses require the replicative machinery of live cells to reproduce, NK cells act to combat virus replication directly by recognizing and killing infected cells; they also produce cytokines such as IFNγ and TNFα and mediate important immunomodulatory effects, stimulating the activation of macrophages via IFNγ and regulating DC responses.

NK cells are non-specifically activated by innate cytokines including type I IFNs, IL-12, IL-15, and IL-18, but their

---

Type I IFNs mediate direct antiviral effects and play an important role in activating other antiviral defenses

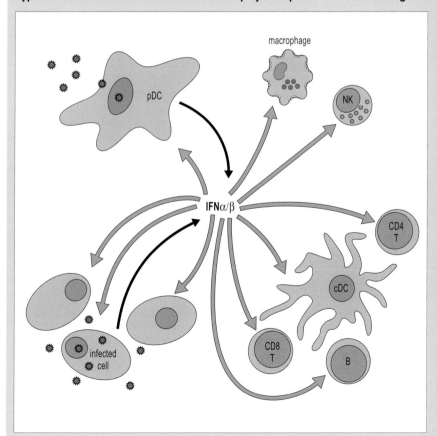

Fig. 13.2 Type I IFNs produced by infected cells and plasmacytoid DCs (pDCs) detecting virion components up-regulate the expression of antiviral genes in both infected and uninfected cells, thereby helping to eradicate infection and block its spread. Type I IFNs also activate cells participating in the innate response, including pDCs, conventional DCs (cDCs), NK cells and macrophages (mØs) and promote the activation of adaptive responses not only via DC activation but also by acting directly on T and B cells.

activation state and effector activity are also regulated by signaling through multiple activating and inhibitory receptors.

- Inhibitory NK receptors typically recognize ligands expressed on 'normal' host cells, such as MHC class I molecules. As discussed below, many viruses downregulate MHC class I expression on the cells they infect to limit recognition by CD8$^+$ T cells, but this helps to trigger NK cell activation.
- Activating NK receptors typically recognize host cell proteins that are up-regulated in response to stress or viral proteins, e.g. the natural cytotoxicity receptors NKp44 and NKp46 recognize certain viral glycoproteins including the influenza virus HA. Mice deficient in NKp46 are highly susceptible to influenza virus infection.
- NK cells can also be activated via antibody coating of the target cell which mediates crosslinking of the NK surface receptor FcγRIII. As discussed below, NK cells are one of the principal mediators of antibody-dependent cell-mediated cytotoxicity (ADCC).

Macrophages act at three levels to destroy virus and virus-infected cells

Macrophages are ever present in the tissues of the body and act as a first line of defense against many pathogens. In virus infection they act at three levels to destroy virus and virus-infected cells:

- phagocytosis of virus and virus-infected cells;
- killing of virus-infected cells; and
- production of antiviral molecules such as TNFα, nitric oxide, and IFNα.

Phagocytosis of infected cells and virus complexes is part of the normal housekeeping role of macrophages at a site of infection.

As with many pathogens the phagolysosome represents a hostile environment for viruses in which oxygen-dependent and oxygen-independent destructive mechanisms prevail. The induction of nitric oxide synthetase and the generation of nitric oxide is a potent inhibitor of herpesvirus and poxvirus infection.

Adaptive immune responses to viral infection

The adaptive immune response typically begins a few days after innate responses are activated (Fig. 13.3). T cells start to appear at sites of infection around 4 days after the initiation of viral expansion. In many virus infections, it is the action of CD8$^+$ T cells that plays a key role in the resolution of infection. Antibodies are frequently induced slightly later, around day 6/7, and contribute to recovery from infection.

A key feature of the adaptive immune response is the establishment of immunological memory which forms the basis of a number of highly successful vaccines against virus infections.

Antibodies and complement can limit viral spread or reinfection

Antibodies can neutralize the infectivity of viruses

Antibodies provide a major barrier to virus spread between cells and tissues and are particularly important in restricting virus spread in the bloodstream. IgA production becomes

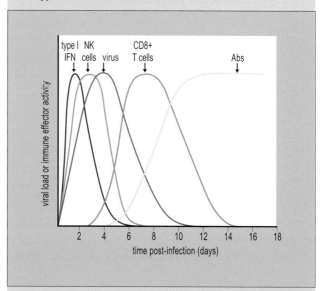

Kinetics of activation of host defenses in response to a typical acute virus infection

Fig. 13.3 During an acute virus infection (e.g. with influenza or lymphocytic choriomeningitis virus), type I IFN production is rapidly initiated in infected tissues and circulating levels of type I IFNs increase. Activated NK cells then start to be detected in the blood and at infection sites. Virus-specific T cell responses are induced in local lymph nodes or the spleen, and effector cells traffic to sites of virus infection. Expansion of virus-specific T cell responses is followed by the appearance of neutralizing antibodies in serum. Virus-specific T cells decline in frequency after virus clearance has been mediated, and activated T cells are no longer present by 2–3 weeks post-infection. However high titres of neutralizing antibodies remain and T cell memory is established and may last for many years.

focused at mucosal surfaces where it serves to prevent reinfection.

An important mechanism of IgA-mediated neutralization occurs intracellularly as IgA passes from the luminal to the apical surface of the cell. During this transcytosis vesicles containing IgA interact with those containing virus, leading to neutralization.

Antibodies may be generated against any viral protein in the infected cell.

Q. Which proteins are likely to be the most important targets of antibody-mediated defenses?
A. Only antibodies directed against glycoproteins that are expressed on the virion envelope or on the infected cell membrane are of importance in controlling infection.

Defense against free virus particles involves neutralization of infectivity, which can occur in various ways (Fig. 13.4). Such mechanisms are likely to operate *in vivo* because injection of neutralizing monoclonal antibodies is highly effective at inhibiting virus replication. The presence of circulating virus-neutralizing antibodies is an important factor in the prevention of reinfection. Passively-administered monoclonal antibodies have been used therapeutically to inhibit respiratory syncytial virus and influenza virus infections.

Antiviral effects of antibody

target	agent	mechanism
free virus	antibody alone	blocks binding to cell blocks entry into cell blocks uncoating of virus
	antibody + complement	damage to virus envelope blockade of virus receptor
virus-infected cells	antibody + complement	damage of infected cell opsonization of coated virus or infected cells for phagocytosis
	antibody bound to infected cells	ADCVI by NK cells, macrophage and neutrophils

ADCVI – antibody-dependent cell-mediated virus inhibition

Fig. 13.4 Mechanisms by which antibody acts to neutralize virus or kill virally infected cells.

Complement is involved in the neutralization of some free viruses

Complement can also damage the virion envelope, a process known as virolysis, and some viruses can directly activate the classical and alternative complement pathways. However, complement is not considered to be a major factor in the defense against viruses because individuals with complement deficiencies are not predisposed to severe viral infection.

This should be contrasted with those herpesviruses and poxviruses that carry viral homologues of complement regulatory proteins (CD46, CD55) that regulate complement activation. Presumably these viruses are susceptible to control by complement-dependent mechanisms.

Antibodies mobilize complement and/or effector cells to destroy virus-infected cells

Antibodies are also effective in mediating the destruction of virus-infected cells. This can occur by antibody-mediated activation of the complement system, leading to the assembly of the membrane attack complex and lysis of the infected cell (see Chapter 4). This process requires a high density of viral antigens on the membrane (about 5×10^6/cell) to be effective. In contrast, ADCC mediated by NK cells requires as few as 10^3 IgG molecules in order to activate NK cell binding to and lysis of the infected cell.

Q. How can NK cells use antibody to recognize and destroy virus-infected cells?
A. The IgG-coated target cells are bound using the NK cell's FcγRIII (CD16; see Chapter 3), and are rapidly destroyed by a perforin-dependent killing mechanism (see Fig. 10.12).

Just how important these mechanisms are for destroying virus-infected cells *in vivo* is difficult to resolve. The best evidence in favor of ADCC comes from studying the protective effect of non-neutralizing monoclonal antibodies in mice. Although these antibodies fail to neutralize virus *in vivo*, they can protect C5-deficient mice from a high-dose virus challenge. (C5-deficient mice are used in this study to eliminate the role of the late complement components.)

T cells mediate viral immunity in several ways

T cells exhibit a variety of functions in antiviral immunity:
*   CD8⁺ T cells are important effector cells that play a key role in the control of established virus infections;
*   most of the antibody response is T-dependent, requiring the presence of helper CD4⁺ T cells for class switching and affinity maturation;
*   CD4⁺ T cells also help in the induction of CD8⁺ T cell responses and in the recruitment and activation of macrophages at sites of virus infection;
*   memory CD8⁺ T cells are effective in combating reinfection with viruses such as influenza virus and respiratory syncytial virus – however, even memory T cells need time to develop a response when infection is re-encountered, so antibodies typically assume a more dominant role in protection against *reinfection* by neutralizing incoming virus, containing the infection and preventing spread to other tissues.

An absence of T cells renders the host highly susceptible to virus attack. For example, cutaneous infection of congenitally athymic 'nude' mice (which lack mature T cells) with herpes simplex virus (HSV) results in a spreading lesion and the virus eventually travels to the central nervous system, resulting in death of the animal. The transfer of HSV-specific T cells shortly after infection is sufficient to protect the mice.

Q. How do CD4⁺ T cells help to induce and recruit CD8⁺ T cells?
A. CD4⁺ T cells interact with dendritic cells and help to activate them to stimulate an effective CD8⁺ T cell response. Cytokines, including IL-2, released by CD4⁺ T cells are also required for division of CD8⁺ T cells. CD4⁺ T cells can recruit CD8⁺ T cells to sites of infection by the release of chemokines and induction of chemokine synthesis by endothelium.

CD8⁺ T cells target virus-infected cells

The principal T cell surveillance system operating against viruses is highly efficient and selective. CD8⁺ T cells identify virus-infected cells by recognizing MHC class I molecules presenting virus-derived peptides on the cell surface, and are triggered to mediate effector functions that clear the infection.
CD8⁺ T cells:
*   kill infected cells through the release of perforin, granzymes, and other cytolytic proteins;
*   trigger the death of infected cells through binding of soluble factors (e.g. TNFα) or ligands they express (e.g. FasL) to cell-surface receptors (such as Fas) that signal the cell to undergo apoptosis, i.e. effectively 'commit suicide'; and
*   produce soluble factors such as IFNγ and/or TNFα that can 'cure' infection with some viruses (e.g. hepatitis B virus) without death of the cell. This can result in eradication of virus from not only the target cell with which the CD8⁺ T cell is interacting, but also from neighboring cells.

'Curative' mechanisms are particularly important when infection is very widespread and it would be neither feasible for CD8$^+$ T cells to interact with and kill every infected cell, nor desirable for so many host cells to be destroyed.

Virtually all cells in the body express MHC class I molecules, making this an important mechanism for identifying and eliminating or curing virus-infected cells.

Because of the central role played by MHC class I in targeting CD8$^+$ T cells to infected cells, some viruses have evolved elaborate strategies to disrupt MHC class I expression, thereby interfering with T cell recognition and favoring virus persistence (see below).

Almost any viral protein can be processed in the cytoplasm to generate peptides that are transported to the endoplasmic reticulum where they interact with MHC class I molecules.

Q. Why might it be advantageous to the host to present viral peptides that are produced early in the replication cycle, and which may not be part of the assembled virus?

A. Viral proteins expressed early in the replication cycle can be presented on infected cells relatively soon after they have been infected, enabling T cell recognition to occur long before new viral progeny are produced. For example, CD8$^+$ T cell-mediated immunity against murine cytomegalovirus (MCMV) is mediated predominantly by T cells recognizing an epitope in the immediate early protein pp89 (80–90% of the T cell response is directed against pp89). Immunization of mice with a recombinant vaccinia virus containing pp89 is sufficient to confer complete protection from MCMV-induced disease.

The importance of T cells in *in vivo* control of virus infections has been identified using various techniques.

In animals:

- the adoptive transfer of specific T cell subpopulations or T cell clones to infected animals;
- depletion of T cell populations *in vivo* using monoclonal antibodies to CD4 or CD8; and
- creation of 'gene knockout' mice, in which genes encoding cell surface receptors (e.g. CD8, CD4), signal transduction molecules (e.g. signal transducer and activator of transcription (STAT)) or transcription factors (e.g. T-bet) are removed from the germline.

In humans:

- correlative studies addressing the relationship between the magnitude or functional efficacy of antigen-specific T cell responses and the efficiency of control of virus replication in different infected individuals;
- assessment of control of virus replication in patients with defects in selected immune functions (e.g. DiGeorge syndrome patients lacking a thymus); and
- finding of evidence that viruses have evolved strategies to escape recognition by host T cells (this would not happen unless T cells were exerting selective pressure on virus replication).

The ability of knockout mice that lack particular lymphocyte populations to mediate control of some virus infections illustrates the redundancy that can occur in the immune system. For example, in the absence of CD8$^+$ T cells, CD4$^+$ T cells, antibodies or other mechanisms, individuals are sometimes able to compensate and still bring the infection under control.

Experiment demonstrating that CD4$^+$ T cells, macrophages, and IFNγ all have a protective role in cutaneous infections with HSV-1

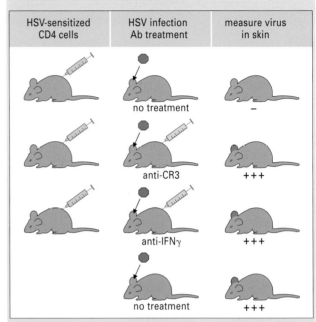

Fig. 13.5 CD4$^+$ T cells were obtained from mice infected with HSV-1 8 days previously. The cells were transferred to syngeneic mice infected with HSV-1 in the skin. These mice were treated with anti-CR3 (to block macrophage migration to the site of infection), or anti-IFNγ (to block the activation of macrophages), or were untreated. An additional control group was infected, but did not receive CD4$^+$ T cells. The amount of infectious virus remaining after 5 days was then determined. The results demonstrate that the protective effects of CD4$^+$ T cells are mediated by macrophages and IFNγ.

CD4$^+$ T cells are a major effector cell population in the response to some virus infections

CD4$^+$ T cells have also been identified as a major effector cell population in the immune response to some virus infections. A good example is in HSV-1 infection of epithelial surfaces. Here, CD4$^+$ T cells participate in a delayed-type hypersensitivity response (see Chapter 26) that results in accelerated clearance of virus. They produce cytokines such as IFNγ and TNFα, which mediate direct antiviral effects and also help to activate macrophages at the site of infection. Macrophages play an important role in inhibiting virus infection, probably through the generation and action of nitric oxide (Fig. 13.5).

In measles virus and Epstein–Barr virus (EBV) infections, CD4$^+$ CTLs are generated that recognize and kill MHC class II-positive cells infected with the virus using the cytolytic mechanisms also employed by CD8$^+$ CTLs. This suggests that measles virus and EBV peptides are generated by normal pathways of antigen presentation (i.e. following phagocytosis and degradation, see Chapter 8). However, other pathways have been implicated in which some measles proteins/peptides enter class II vesicles from the cytosol.

A summary of antiviral defense mechanisms is illustrated in Figure 13.6.

Effector mechanisms by which adaptive responses combat virus replication

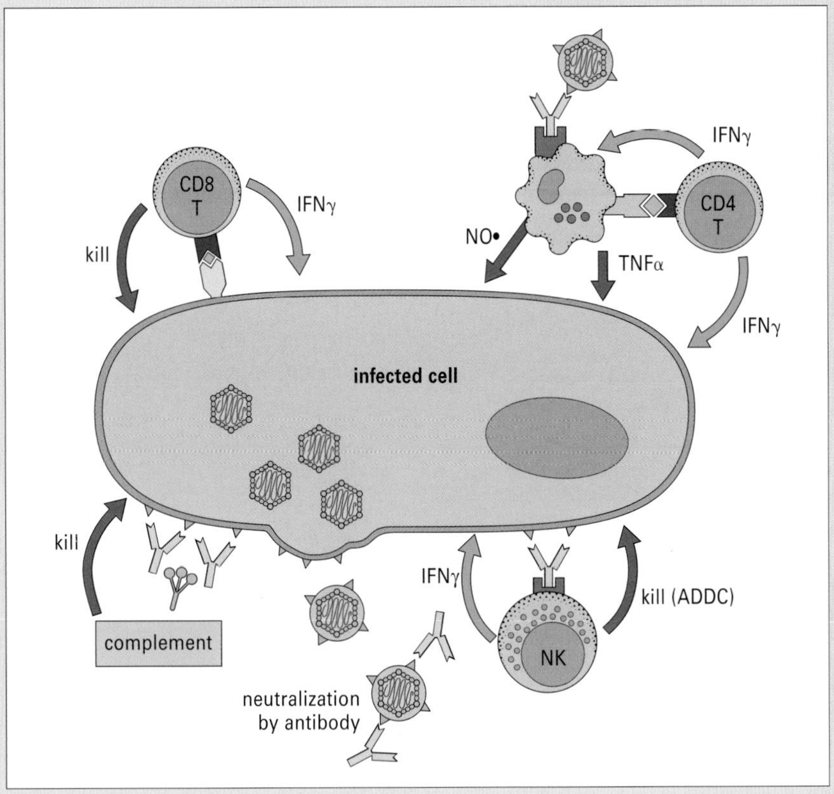

Fig. 13.6 CD8$^+$ T cells typically play a dominant role in control of established virus infections, mediating lysis of virus-infected cells and producing antiviral cytokines. CD4$^+$ T cells are important effectors in the control of certain virus infections, producing cytokines that mediate antiviral effects and activating macrophages to produce cytolytic and antiviral factors. They also help B cells to make antibodies which are important in controlling free virus, and can also target infected cells by activating complement-mediated lysis or triggering antibody-dependent cell-mediated virus inhibition (ADCVI) by effector cells including NK cells and macrophages.

Virus strategies to evade host immune responses

To promote their survival, viruses have evolved multiple strategies for evasion of control by the host immune response. Avoidance of immune clearance is essential for viruses that persist in their hosts for long periods – but even for viruses that cause acute infections, immune evasion strategies are important to prolong infection and increase the opportunities for transmission to new hosts.

Viral immune evasion strategies can be categorized into mechanisms for:

- impairing the host response;
- avoiding recognition by the host immune defences; and
- resisting control by immune effector mechanisms.

Some viruses employ multiple strategies in each category to promote their persistence *in vivo*: human immunodeficiency virus type 1 (HIV-1) provides a particularly good example of this (Fig. 13.7).

Viruses can impair the host immune response

Virus infections can sometimes be associated with a profound widespread impairment of host immune functions, e.g. the generalized immune suppression associated with measles virus infection, or the acquired immunodeficiency syndrome (AIDS) induced in the late stages of HIV-1 infection. Whilst induction of a state of generalized immune dysfunction does impair control of virus replication, it also impacts on host survival – so is not an ideal strategy for promoting virus persistence. Many viruses instead induce impairments in host immunity that are more localized, more limited and/or target virus-specific cellular or humoral responses.

The importance of type I IFNs in innate control of local virus replication and spread is illustrated by the fact that many different families of viruses have evolved strategies for blocking type I IFN production in the cells they infect. Some viruses also impair the recruitment of plasmacytoid DCs to sites of infection, reduce circulating plasmacytoid DC numbers or infect plasmacytoid DCs and impair their functions to reduce type I IFN production by these specialized IFN-producing cells.

Chemokines represent an important traffic-light system for cell migration and viruses have evolved elaborate strategies for disrupting the chemokine network. The herpesviruses encode:

- chemokine homologues (e.g. CCL3);
- chemokine receptor homologues; and
- chemokine-binding proteins, which have powerful effects on delaying or inhibiting cell migration during inflammation.

Viruses may also inhibit the induction of adaptive responses by infecting and interfering with the functions of key antigen presenting cells such as DCs, or by producing cytokine homologues such as vIL-10 (herpesviruses) that modulate the nature of the response induced.

Q. From this observation, what can you infer about an effective immune response to herpesviruses?

A. The vIL-10 will deviate the immune response, inhibiting a T$_H$1-type reaction with macrophage activation. One can

Strategies employed by HIV to evade immune control

host defense mechanism to be evaded	impaired strategies	avoidance strategies	resistance strategies
type I IFN	not impaired in acute infection depletion of pDCs in chronic infection	latency (avoids control by all arms of the immune response)	resistance to antiviral activity of some ISGs e.g. HIV-1 Vif counteracts APOBECs
NK cells	decrease in NK cell number and decline in their functions in chronic infection	expression of MHC I alleles involved in NK inhibition retained on infected cells	inhibition of TNF and Fas-mediated lysis of infected cells by HIV-1 Nef
CD8$^+$ T cells	exhaustion of CD8$^+$ T cell effector functions during chronic infection	down-regulation of MHC I expression aquisition of escape mutations	inhibition of TNF and Fas-mediated lysis of infected cells by HIV-1 Nef
CD4$^+$ T cells	loss of CD4$^+$ T cells due to infection and lysis by HIV	down-regulation of MHC II expression	inhibition of TNF and Fas-mediated lysis of infected cells by HIV-1 Nef
antibodies	delay in neutralizing Ab production – may be due in part to aberrant B cell activ'n	blocks of Ab binding to the virus by glycans acquisition of escape mutations	incorporation of CD59 into the virion envelope to block complement activation

Fig. 13.7 The figure list of the host defense mechanisms affected by the ingenious avoidance mechanisms evolved by the type 1 human immunodeficiency virus.

therefore infer that this type of immune response is the key to anti-herpes immunity and the type of response the viruses aims to deflect.

Given the critical role of T cells, particularly CD8$^+$ CTLs, in elimination of established virus infections, viruses that establish long-term persistent infections in their hosts frequently possess strategies for impairment of the virus-specific CD8$^+$ T cell response.

- Some persistent virus infections are transmitted from mother to offspring *in utero* (e.g. lymphocytic choriomeningitis virus (LCMV) infection of mice and hepatitis B virus infection in humans). This can result in tolerization of virus-specific T cells as self-tolerance is established in the developing host immune system, leading to failure to mount a virus-specific T cell (or an effective antibody) response to the virus.
- Virus-specific CD8$^+$ T cell responses in immunologically-mature hosts may be impaired by processes termed 'exhaustion' or 'stunning' during which virus-specific T cells are rendered increasingly functionally-defective in the face of high-level ongoing virus replication and may eventually be driven to undergo apoptotic death.

Viral strategies for avoidance of recognition by host immune defenses

Strategies viruses use to avoid recognition by host immune defenses include:

- latency;
- infection of 'immune privileged' sites;
- rendering infected cells less visible to host effector cells; and
- antigenic variation.

Some viruses establish a latent infection within certain host cells, during which there is little or no production of viral proteins. Latently-infected cells are thus essentially 'invisible' to the host immune system. Cells such as HSV-infected neurons can thus persist for the life of the host in this form – although if the infection is to be spread to new hosts, latency also needs to be accompanied by continuous or sporadic productive virus replication.

Another strategy that viruses use to avoid recognition by host immune defences is to replicate in 'immune privileged' sites, i.e. parts of the body to which adaptive responses have limited access and where there may also be an 'immune-suppressive' environment, such as in the brain (see Chapter 12). A surprising number of different viruses persist in the brain.

Viruses avoid recognition by T cells by reducing MHC expression on infected cells

Other viruses try to render the cells they infect 'less visible' to host adaptive responses. The critical role played by CD8$^+$ T cells in elimination of virus infections is again underlined by the plethora of strategies that viruses have evolved to reduce the level of MHC class I expression on the surface of infected cells.

MHC class I expression can be disrupted by:

- downregulating MHC class I synthesis (e.g. HIV-1);
- reducing the generation of epitope peptides in the cytoplasm (e.g. EBV);
- blocking peptide uptake into the endoplasmic reticulum (e.g. HSV-1);

Examples of strains of influenza A virus that have caused pandemics since 1933

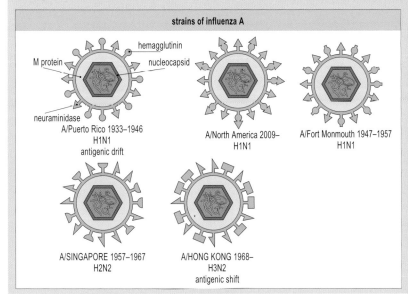

Fig. 13.8 The major surface antigens of influenza virus are the hemagglutinin and neuraminidase. Hemagglutinin is involved in attachment to cells, and antibodies to hemagglutinin are protective. Antibodies to neuraminidase are much less effective. Influenza virus can change its antigenic properties slightly (antigenic drift) or radically (antigenic shift). Alterations in the structure of the hemagglutinin antigen render earlier antibodies ineffective and new virus epidemics therefore break out. The diagram shows strains that have emerged by antigenic shift since 1933. The official influenza antigen nomenclature is based on the type of hemagglutinin (H_1, H_2, etc.) and neuraminidase (N_1, N_2, etc.) expressed on the surface of the virion. Note that, although new strains replace old strains, the internal antigens remain largely unchanged.

- preventing maturation, assembly and migration of the trimolecular MHC complex (e.g. human cytomegalovirus [HCMV]); and/or
- recycling of MHC class I molecules from the cell surface (e.g. HIV-1).

Similar mechanisms apply for MHC class II molecules where some herpesviruses block transcription, whereas other mechanisms involve premature targeting of MHC class II for degradation.

Downregulation of MHC class I may disrupt CD8$^+$ T cell recognition, but NK cells are more efficient killers in the absence of MHC class I. Human and murine CMV have tried to redress the balance by encoding their own MHC class I homologues, which are expressed on infected cells and can inhibit NK cell activation.

Mutation of viral target antigen allows escape from recognition by antibodies or T cells

Antigenic variation involves a virus acquiring sequence changes (mutations) in sites on proteins that are normally targeted by antibody or T cells so that these sites are no longer recognized. Antigenic variation can promote virus persistence within a given host, e.g. during HIV-1 infection mutations are frequently selected for in and around the epitopes recognized by the initial T cell responses and neutralizing antibody responses, which confer escape from recognition by these responses and enable enhanced virus replication. It can also promote virus persistence at the population level, as exemplified by the antigenic shift and drift seen with influenza virus (Fig. 13.8). Humoral immunity to influenza virus provides protection against re-infection only until a new virus strain emerges, making effective long-lasting vaccines difficult to produce.

Viral strategies for resisting control by immune effector mechanisms

Viruses have evolved strategies for resisting control by many different immune effector mechanisms including:

- the antiviral activity of type I IFNs and other cytokines;
- the lytic mechanisms by which NK cells and CD8$^+$ T cells destroy infected cells; and
- antibodies and complement.

In addition to impairing production of type I IFNs, viruses also have many strategies for resisting control by these important antiviral cytokines. This can be achieved via:

- production of soluble IFN receptors (e.g. pox viruses);
- interference with IFN signaling (e.g. paramyxoviruses); and
- disruption of intracellular IFN-induced defences such as PKR or 2′,5′-oligoadenylate synthetase activity (e.g. adenovirus and herpesviruses).

Viruses may also resist control by other antiviral cytokines, e.g. several poxviruses encode soluble receptors to interfere with TNF function.

Other viral proteins produced in infected cells protect the cells from lysis by TNF: adenoviruses, herpesviruses and poxviruses all encode proteins with this function. HIV protects the cells it infects from lysis mediated not only via TNF, but also via Fas.

As noted above some viruses also possess strategies for resisting control by antibodies and complement. Some herpesviruses and poxviruses encode homologues for CD46 and CD55 (complement regulatory proteins that block C3 activation) and also for CD59, which blocks formation of the membrane attack complex. HIV makes use of cellular CD59, which is incorporated into the viral envelope, thereby blocking complement-mediated lysis of the virion.

Examples of virus-encoded homologues or mimics of the host defense system are shown in Figure 13.9.

Examples of homologues or mimics of host proteins encoded by viruses to promote their persistence *in vivo*

host defence affected	virus	host protein that virus encodes a homologue or mimic of	mechanism of action
Type I IFN	HHV-8	IRF homologue	Blocks type I IFN transcription
	Vaccinia	Type I IFN receptor homologue	Secreted and binds to IFNα/β
	Vaccinia	eIF-2α homologue	Prevents eIF-2α phosphorylation and inhibits PKR
Other cytokines	Multiple poxviruses	TNF receptor homologues	Secreted and bind to TNFα
	Vaccinia	IL-1β receptor mimic	Binds IL-1β and blocks the febrile response
	EBV, HCMV	IL-10 mimics	Mimic IL-10 activity and downregulate production of TH1 cytokines e.g. IFNγ
Chemokines	MCMV, HCMV, HHV-6, 7 and 8, MHV-68	Chemokine receptor mimics	Secreted and bind CC and/or CXC chemokines, either enhancing or blocking their activity
	MCMV, HCMV, HHV-6, HHV-8	CC or CXC chemokine mimics	Attract monocytes for viral replication or attract TH2 cells
Complement	Vaccinia, smallpox HSV-1 and 2, HVS HHV-8, MHV-68	Homologues of complement-binding proteins e.g. C4-binding protein, CR1, CD46 and CD55	Inhibit soluble complement factors
	HVS	CD59 homologue	Blocks formation of membrane-attack complex
Antibody	HSV-1 and 2, MCMV, coronavirus	Fc-receptor mimics	Bind IgG and inhibit Fc-dependent effector mechanisms
NK cells	HCMV, MCMV	MHC class I homologues	Inhibit NK recognition of infected cells
Destruction of infected cells	HHV-8, HVS, some poxviruses	FLIP mimics	Inhibit caspase activation, preventing death-receptor-mediated triggering of apoptosis
	HHV-8, HVS, adenovirus	Bcl 2 homologues	Block apoptosis

Fig. 13.9 Many viruses with large DNA genomes encode proteins of this type. (EBV, Epstein–Barr virus; FLIP, FLICE-like inhibitory protein; HCMV, human cytomegalovirus; HHV, human herpesvirus; HHV-8, human herpesvirus-8 (Kaposi's sarcoma-associated herpesvirus); HSV, herpes simplex virus; HVS, herpesvirus saimiri; MCMV, murine cytomegalovirus; MHV-68, murine gammaherpesvirus.)

Pathological consequences of immune responses induced by viral infections

Although the host immune response plays a vital role in combating virus infections, it can also have immunopathological consequences. These can result from inappropriate antiviral immune responses, or from the induction of autoimmune responses during the course of a virus infection.

Excessive cytokine production and immune activation can be pathological

Cytokines and chemokines play a critical role in activation of immune responses following virus infection and recruitment of cells to the site of infection. However excessive cytokine and chemokine production can have pathological consequences. For example:

- Infection with severe acute respiratory syndrome (SARS) virus and the highly pathogenic influenza viruses (H5N1), if not rapidly controlled by the early innate response, can be associated with hypercytokinemia (cytokine storms) which drive an aggressive inflammatory response that can result in massive tissue damage (pneumonia) leading to death.
- Activated CD4$^+$ T cells constitute the main cellular sites for HIV replication. The virus triggers an intense cytokine storm associated with extensive immune activation during acute infection, which helps to fuel virus replication by providing a large pool of activated CD4$^+$ target cells. A key difference between non-pathogenic simian immunodeficiency virus (SIV) infections of non-human primates and pathogenic SIV infection or HIV infection is that in non-pathogenic infections immune activation is rapidly down-modulated after the acute phase of infection, whilst a constant state of immune activation is maintained in pathogenic infections. This helps to drive ongoing virus replication and CD4$^+$ T cell loss, ultimately leading to the development of AIDS.

Pathological consequences of antiviral antibody production

Poorly-neutralizing antibodies can enhance viral infectivity

An unusual pathological consequence of some virus interactions, where weakly-neutralizing antibodies are produced, is antibody-dependent enhancement of virus infection (ADE). This involves Fc receptor-mediated uptake of antibody–virus complexes by macrophages and subsequent enhancement of virus infectivity. This is seen in many persistent or viremic virus infections where the common target for replication is the macrophage. An example is dengue virus infection where weakly cross-reactive antibodies induced during prior infections with different dengue virus subtypes can result in ADE with the initiation of:

- dengue hemorrhagic fever; and
- dengue shock syndrome, which results in excessive procoagulant release by monocytes.

Antiviral antibodies can form immune complexes that cause tissue damage

Immune complexes may arise in body fluids or on cell surfaces and are most common during persistent or chronic infections (e.g. with hepatitis B virus). Antibody is ineffective (non-neutralizing) in the presence of large amounts of the viral antigen; instead, immune complexes form and are deposited in the kidney or in blood vessels, where they evoke inflammatory responses leading to tissue damage (e.g. glomerulonephritis, see Chapter 25).

Virus-specific T cell responses can cause severe tissue damage

In any virus infection some tissue damage is likely to arise from the activity of infiltrating T cells. However, in some situations this damage may be considerable, resulting in the death of the host. A classic illustration of this is the CD8$^+$ T cell response to LCMV in the central nervous system (Fig. 13.10). Removal of T cells protects LCMV-infected mice from death, indicating that they, rather than the virus, are mediating damage to the brain.

The different outcomes of lymphocytic choriomeningitis virus (LCMV) infection of mice are related to differences in immune status

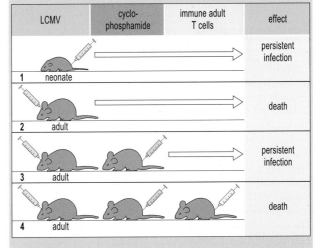

Fig. 13.10 Infection of neonatal mice (**1**) results in virus persistence, because virus-specific T cells are clonally-deleted as self tolerance is established in the newborn animal. In the absence of T cell help, non-neutralizing antibodies are produced, and virus persistence is associated with immune complex disease, manifesting itself as glomerulonephritis and vasculitis. Intracerebral infection of adult mice (**2**) results in death from lymphocytic choriomeningitis. This is due to the recruitment of virus-specific T cells to sites of virus replication in the brain. Suppression of immunity with cyclophosphamide (**3**) prevents death, but leads to the establishment of a persistent infection. The 'protective' effect produced by cyclophosphamide can be reversed by adoptive transfer of T cells from an LCMV-immune animal (**4**).

Viral infection may provoke autoimmunity

Viruses may trigger autoimmune disease in a number of ways, including:

- Virus-induced damage – during the course of some virus infections, tissues become damaged, provoking an inflammatory response during which 'hidden' antigens become exposed and can be processed and presented to the immune system. Examples of this include Theiler's virus (a murine picornavirus) and murine hepatitis virus infection of the nervous system, in which the constituents of myelin (the insulating material of axons) become targets for antibody and T cells.

- Molecular mimicry – a sequence in a viral protein that is homologous to a 'self' protein can become recognized, leading to a breakdown in immunological tolerance to cryptic self antigens in the consequent attack on host tissues by the immune system (see Chapter 19). A good example is coxsackie B virus-induced myocarditis. Patients with inflammatory cardiomyopathy have antibodies that cross-react with peptides derived from coxsackie B3 protein and with peptides derived from cellular adenine nucleotide translocator.

CRITICAL THINKING: VIRUS–IMMUNE SYSTEM INTERACTIONS (SEE P. 436 FOR EXPLANATIONS)

A series of IgG monoclonal antibodies were developed against glycoprotein D of herpes simplex virus. When tested *in vitro* for virus neutralizing activity the antibodies could be divided into two groups: those capable of neutralizing virus infectivity and non-neutralizing antibodies. However, when individual neutralizing or non-neutralizing antibodies were injected into mice infected with herpes simplex virus, both sets of antibodies protected the animals from an overwhelming infection.

1 How do you explain the protection achieved by the non-neutralizing monoclonal antibodies?

2 What experiments would you propose to support some of your conclusions?

3 Why might memory CD8$^+$ T cells be unable to prevent the establishment of HIV infection?

4 Would T cell responses directed against epitopes in any of the HIV proteins be likely to control viral replication equally well?

5 How could viral escape from vaccine-elicited T cell responses be minimized?

Further reading

Alcami A. Viral mimicry of cytokines, chemokines and their receptors. Nat Rev Immunol 2003;3:36–50.

Goulder PJ, Watkins DI. HIV and SIV CTL escape: implications for vaccine design. Nat Rev Immunol 2004;4:630–640.

Guidotti LG, Chisari FV. Noncytolytic control of viral infections by the innate and adaptive immune response. Annu Rev Immunol 2001;19:65–91.

Hansen TH, Bouvier M. MHC class I antigen presentation: learning from viral evasion strategies. Nat Rev Immunol 2009;9:503–513.

Kawai T, Akira S. Innate immune recognition of viral infection. Nat Immunol 2006;7:131–137.

Klenerman P, Hill A. T cells and viral persistence: lessons from diverse infections. Nat Immunol 2005;6:873–879.

Klotman ME, Chang TL. Defensins in antiviral immunity. Nat Rev Immun. 2006;6:247–256.

Koelle DM, Corey L. Herpes simplex: insights on pathogenesis and possible vaccines. Annu Rev Med 2008;59:381–395.

Kohlmeier JE, Woodland DL. Immunity to respiratory viruses. Annu Rev Immunol 2009;27:61–82.

Lanier L. Evolutionary struggles between NK cells and viruses. Nat Rev Immunol 2008;8:259–268.

McMichael AJ, Borrow P, Tomaras GD, et al. The immune response during acute HIV-1 infection: clues for vaccine development. Nat Rev Immunol 2010;10:11–23.

Paiardini M, Pandrea I, Apetrei C, Silvestri G. Lessons learned from the natural hosts of HIV-related viruses. Annu Rev Med 2009;60:485–495.

Peiris JS, Hui KP, Yen HL. Host response to influenza virus: protection versus immunopathology. Curr Opin Immunol 2010;22:475–481.

Powers C, DeFilippis V, Malouli D, Früh K. Cytomegalovirus immune evasion. Curr Top Microbiol Immunol 2008;325:333–359.

Randall RE, Goodbourn S. Interferons and viruses: An interplay between induction, signalling, antiviral responses and virus countermeasures. J Gen Virol 2008;89:1–47.

Reading SA, Dimmock NJ. Neutralization of animal virus infectivity by antibody. Arch Virol 2007;152:1047–1059.

Rehermann B, Hepatitis C. virus versus innate and adaptive immune responses: a tale of coevolution and coexistence. J Clin Invest 2009;119:1745–1754.

Sadler AJ, Williams BRG. Interferon-inducible antiviral effectors. Nat Rev Immunol 2008;8:559–568.

Tirado SM, Yoon KJ. Antibody-dependent enhancement of virus infection and disease. Viral Immunol 2003;16:69–86.

Tortorella D, Gewurz BE, Furman MH, et al. Viral subversion of the immune system. Annu Rev Immunol 2000;18:861–926.

CHAPTER 14

Immunity to Bacteria and Fungi

SUMMARY

- **Mechanisms of protection from bacteria can be deduced from their structure and pathogenicity.** There are four main types of bacterial cell wall and pathogenicity varies between two extreme patterns. Non-specific, phylogenetically ancient recognition pathways for conserved bacterial structures trigger protective innate immune responses and guide the development of adaptive immunity.

- **Lymphocyte-independent bacterial recognition pathways have several consequences.** Complement is activated via the alternative pathway. Release of proinflammatory cytokines and chemokines increases the adhesive properties of the vascular endothelium and promotes neutrophil and macrophage recruitment. Pathogen recognition generates signals then regulate the lymphocyte-mediated response.

- **Antibody provides an antigen-specific protective mechanism.** Neutralizing antibody may be all that is needed for protection if the organism is pathogenic only because of a single toxin or adhesion molecule. Opsonizing antibody responses are particularly important for resistance to extracellular bacterial pathogens. Complement can kill some bacteria, particularly those with an exposed outer lipid bilayer, such as Gram-negative bacteria.

- **Ultimately most bacteria are killed by phagocytes** following a multistage process of chemotaxis, attachment, uptake, and killing. Macrophage killing can be enhanced on activation. Optimal activation of macrophages is dependent on T_H1 CD4 T cells, whereas neutrophil responses are promoted by T_H17 CD4 T cells. Persistent macrophage recruitment and activation can result in granuloma formation, which is a hallmark of cell-mediated immunity to intracellular bacteria.

- **Successful pathogens have evolved mechanisms to avoid phagocyte-mediated killing** and have evolved a startling diversity of mechanisms for avoiding other aspects of innate and adaptive immunity.

- **Infected cells can be killed by CTLs.** Other T cell populations and some tissue cells can contribute to antibacterial immunity.

- **The response to bacteria can result in immunological tissue damage.** Excessive release of cytokines caused by microorganisms can result in immunopathological syndromes, such as endotoxin shock and the Schwartzman reaction.

- **Fungi can cause life-threatening infections.** Immunity to fungi is predominantly cell mediated and shares many similarities with immunity to bacteria.

Innate recognition of bacterial components

Bacterial infections have had an enormous impact on human society and despite the discovery of antibiotics continue to be a major threat to public health.

Plague caused by *Yersinia pestis* is estimated to have killed one-quarter of the European population in the Middle Ages, whereas infection with *Mycobacterium tuberculosis* is currently a global health emergency.

The immune defense mechanisms elicited against pathogenic bacteria are determined by their:

- surface chemistry;
- mechanism(s) of pathogenicity; and
- whether they are predominantly extracellular or also have the ability to survive inside mammalian cells.

There are four main types of bacterial cell wall

The four main types of bacterial cell wall (Fig. 14.1) belong to the following groups.

- Gram-positive bacteria;
- Gram-negative bacteria;
- mycobacteria;
- spirochetes.

The outer lipid bilayer of Gram-negative organisms is of particular importance because it is often susceptible to lysis by complement. However, killing of most bacteria usually

Bacterial cell walls

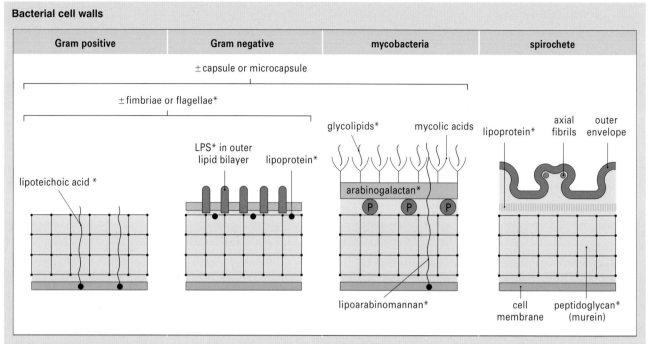

Fig. 14.1 Different immunological mechanisms have evolved to destroy the cell wall structure of the different groups of bacteria. All types have an inner cell membrane and a peptidoglycan wall. Gram-negative bacteria also have an outer lipid bilayer in which lipopolysaccharide (LPS) is embedded. Lysosomal enzymes and lysozyme are active against the peptidoglycan layer, whereas cationic proteins and complement are effective against the outer lipid bilayer of the Gram-negative bacteria. The compound cell wall of mycobacteria is extremely resistant to breakdown, and it is likely that this can be achieved only with the assistance of the bacterial enzymes working from within. Some bacteria also have fimbriae or flagellae, which can provide targets for the antibody response. Others have an outer capsule, which renders the organisms more resistant to phagocytosis or to complement. The components indicated with an asterisk (*) are recognized by the innate immune system as a non-specific 'danger' signal that selectively boosts some aspects of immune activity. (Gram staining is a method that exploits the fact that crystal violet and iodine form a complex that is more abundant on Gram-positive bacteria. The complex easily elutes from Gram-negative bacteria.)

requires uptake by phagocytes. The outer surface of the bacterium may also contain fimbriae or flagellae, or it may be covered by a protective capsule. These can impede the functions of phagocytes or complement, but they also act as targets for the antibody response, the role of which is discussed later.

Pathogenicity varies between two extreme patterns

The two extreme patterns of pathogenicity are:

- toxicity without invasiveness;
- invasiveness without toxicity (Fig. 14.2).

However, most bacteria are intermediate between these extremes, having some invasiveness assisted by some locally acting toxins and spreading factors (tissue-degrading enzymes).

Corynebacterium diphtheriae and *Vibrio cholerae* are examples of organisms that are toxic, but not invasive. Because their pathogenicity depends almost entirely on toxin production, neutralizing antibody to the toxin is probably sufficient for immunity, though antibody binding to the bacteria and so blocking their adhesion to the epithelium could also be important.

In contrast, the pathogenicity of most invasive organisms does not rely so heavily on a single toxin, so immunity requires killing of the organisms themselves.

The first lines of defense do not depend on antigen recognition

The body's first line of defense against pathogenic bacteria consists of simple barriers to the entry or establishment of the infection. Thus, the skin and exposed epithelial surfaces have non-specific or innate protective systems, which limit the entry of potentially invasive organisms.

Intact skin is impenetrable to most bacteria. Additionally, fatty acids produced by the skin are toxic to many organisms. Indeed, the pathogenicity of some strains correlates with their ability to survive on the skin. Epithelial surfaces are cleansed, for example, by ciliary action in the trachea or by flushing of the urinary tract.

Many bacteria are destroyed by pH changes in the stomach and vagina, both of which provide an acidic environment. In the vagina, the epithelium secretes glycogen, which is metabolized by particular species of commensal bacteria, producing lactic acid.

Commensals can limit pathogen invasion

Commensal bacteria have co-evolved with us over millions of years, providing an essential protective function against more pathogenic species by occupying an ecological niche that would otherwise be occupied by something more unpleasant. In fact it has been estimated that the human body contains approximately 10 times more bacterial cells than human cells. This is mostly because of the gut microbiota,

Mechanisms of immunopathogenicity

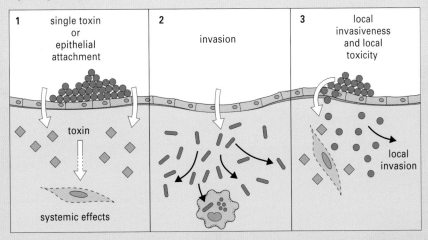

Fig. 14.2 (**1**) Some bacteria cause disease as a result of only a single toxin (e.g. *Corynebacterium diphtheriae*, *Clostridium tetani*) or because of an ability to attach to epithelial surfaces (e.g. in group A streptococcal sore throat). Immunity to such organisms may require only antibody to neutralize this critical function. (**2**) At the other extreme there are organisms that are not toxic, and cause disease by invasion of tissues and sometimes cells, where damage results mostly from the bulk of organisms or from immunopathology (e.g. lepromatous leprosy). Where organisms invade cells, they must be destroyed and degraded by the cell-mediated immune response. (**3**) Most organisms fall between the two extremes, with some local invasiveness assisted by local toxicity and enzymes that degrade extracellular matrix (e.g. *Staphylococcus aureus*, *Clostridium perfringens*). Antibody and cell-mediated responses are both involved in resistance and the latter is a major cause of antibiotic-induced colitis and diarrhea.

made up of perhaps thousands of different bacterial species many of which have not been cultured but identified more recently by high throughput sequencing technology of 16S ribosomal RNA sequences. The precise makeup of this microbiota is different between individuals, with a core of common species together with an additional set that is determined in part by the genetics of the host. The normal flora protect against pathogens by competing more efficiently for nutrients, by producing antibacterial proteins termed colicins and by stimulating immune responses which act to limit pathogen entry.

Maintaining this protective flora without eliciting inflammatory reactions is a delicate and immunologically complicated process as even these bacteria are not immunologically inert. The host attempts to minimize contact between the bacteria and the epithelial cells of the gut lumen by production of mucins, and by effector molecules including antimicrobial peptides and secretory IgA. Nevertheless, some commensal bacteria do penetrate these barriers and are sampled by intestinal dendritic cells, inducing local (but not systemic) immune responses involving CD4 T cells and regulatory T cells.

When the normal flora are disturbed by antibiotics, infections by *Candida* spp. or *Clostridium difficile* can occur. Several studies suggest that the reintroduction of non-pathogenic 'probiotic' organisms such as lactobacilli into the intestinal tract (or in extreme circumstances even the normal flora from an otherwise healthy person) can alleviate the symptoms, presumably by replacing those killed by the antibiotics.

In practice, only a minute proportion of the potentially pathogenic organisms around us ever succeed in gaining access to the tissues.

The second line of defense is mediated by recognition of bacterial components

If organisms do enter the tissues, they can be combated initially by further elements of the innate immune system. Numerous bacterial components are recognized in ways that do not rely on the antigen-specific receptors of either B cells or T cells. These types of recognition are phylogenetically ancient 'broad-spectrum' mechanisms that evolved before antigen-specific T cells and immunoglobulins, allowing protective responses to be triggered by common microbial components bearing so-called '**pathogen-associated molecular patterns**' (**PAMPs**), recognized by '**pattern recognition molecules**' of the innate immune system (see Chapter 6).

Q. List some examples of soluble molecules, cell surface receptors, and intracellular molecules that recognize PAMPs.
A. Collectins and ficolins (see Fig. 6.w3), the Toll-like receptors (see Fig. 6.21), the mannose receptor (see Fig. 7.11), and the NOD-like receptor proteins (see Fig. 7.13) all recognize PAMPs.

Many organisms, such as non-pathogenic cocci, are probably removed from the tissues as a consequence of these pathways, without the need for a specific adaptive immune reaction. Figure 14.3 shows some of the microbial components involved and the host responses that are triggered.

The immune system has selected these structures for recognition because they are not only characteristic of microbes, but are essential for their growth and cannot be easily mutated to evade discovery (though, as might be

Protective mechanisms not involving antigen-specific B or T cells

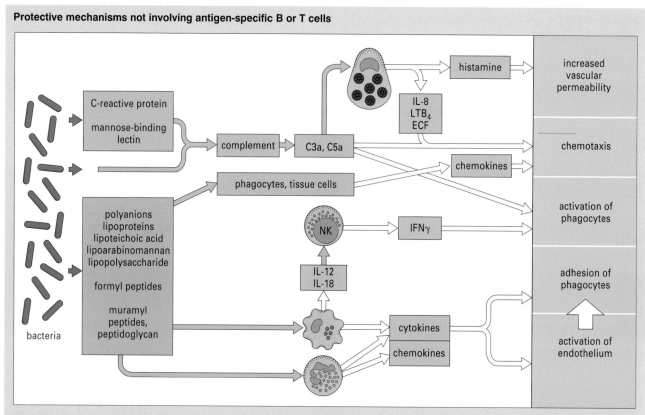

Fig. 14.3 Several common bacterial PAMPs are recognized by molecules present in serum and by receptors on cells. These recognition pathways result in activation of the alternative complement pathway (factors C3, B, D, P), with consequent release of C3a and C5a; activation of neutrophils, macrophages, and NK cells; triggering of cytokine and chemokine release; mast cell degranulation, leading to increased blood flow in the local capillary network; and increased adhesion of cells and fibrin to endothelial cells. These mechanisms, plus tissue injury caused by the bacteria, may activate the clotting system and fibrin formation, which limit bacterial spread.

predicted, there are increasing examples of pathogen strategies that attempt to subvert this process).

It is interesting to note that the 'Limulus assay', which is used to detect contaminating lipopolysaccharide (LPS) in preparations for use in humans, is based on one such recognition pathway found in an invertebrate species. In *Limulus polyphemus* (the horseshoe crab), tiny quantities of LPS trigger fibrin formation, which walls off the LPS-bearing infectious agent.

LPS is the dominant activator of innate immunity in Gram-negative bacterial infection

Injection of pure LPS into mice or even humans is sufficient to mimic most of the features of acute Gram-negative infection, including massive production of proinflammatory cytokines, such as IL-1, IL-6, and tumor necrosis factor (TNF), leading to severe shock.

Q. How does release of proinflammatory cytokines cause shock?

A. These proinflammatory cytokines act directly on endothelium to increase vascular adhesiveness, and indirectly activate other plasma enzyme systems to release vasoactive peptides and amines leading to a drop in blood pressure.

Recognition of LPS is a complex process involving molecules that bind LPS and pass it on to cell membrane-associated receptors on leukocytes, and endothelial and other cells, which initiate this proinflammatory cascade (Fig. 14.4).

Binding of LPS to TLR4 is a critical event in immune activation. TLR4 knockout mice are resistant to LPS-induced shock and there is some evidence that polymorphisms in human TLR4 may influence the course of infection with these bacteria.

The LBP and CD14, which bind LPS, are also involved in recognition of lipid-containing bacterial components from mycoplasmas, mycobacteria, and spirochetes.

Other bacterial components are also potent immune activators

Gram-positive bacteria do not possess LPS yet still induce intense inflammatory responses and severe infection via the actions of other chemical structures such as peptidoglycans and lipotechoic acids of their cell wall, which can be recognized by TLR2, often in cooperation with TLR1 or TLR6.

Most capsular polysaccharides are not potent activators of inflammation (though some can activate macrophages) but they shield the bacterium from host immune defenses.

Effects of lipopolysaccharide

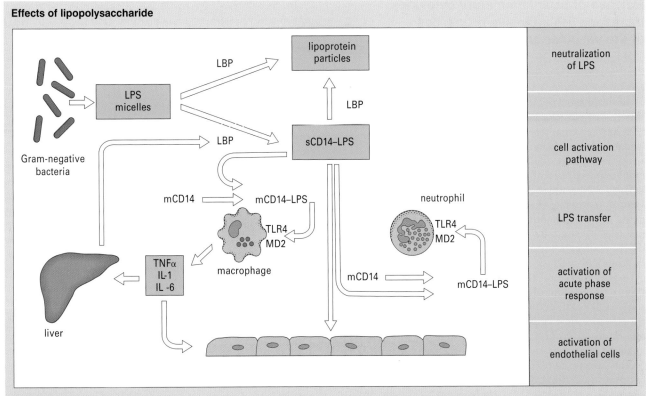

Fig. 14.4   LPS released from Gram-negative bacteria becomes bound to LPS-binding protein (LBP) which promotes transfer of LPS to either soluble CD14 (sCD14) or to a GPI-linked membrane form of the protein (mCD14) expressed on neutrophils and macrophages and to a lesser extent on epithelial and endothelial cells. LBP then dissociates and transfers LPS to the TLR4/MD2 complex, allowing TLR4 to transduce intracellular signals that increase release of many proinflammatory cytokines including TNFα and IL-6, as well as type I IFN and IL-1. These in turn activate endothelial cells, increasing adhesion molecule expression and also drive the acute phase response in the liver. One product of the acute phase response is further production of LBP and sCD14.

Other bacterial molecules that trigger innate immunity include lipoproteins (via TLR 2/6), flagellin (via TLR5), and DNA (due to its distinct **CpG motifs**) via TLR9.

Most pattern recognition receptors are expressed on the plasma membrane of cells, making contact with microbes during the process of binding and/or phagocytosis.

However, others are designed to detect intracellular pathogens and their products inside phagosomes (such as TLR9) or in the cytosol.

Q. Which proteins can recognize pathogens in the cytosol, and which pathogen components?
A. NOD-1 and NOD-2 proteins are members of the larger family of NOD-like receptors (NLRs) and recognize peptidoglycans of both Gram-positive and Gram-negative bacteria (see Fig. 7.w6).

Epithelial cells of the gut and lung can have few TLRs on their luminal surface, but can be triggered by pathogens that:

- actively invade the cell (such as *Listeria* spp.);
- inject their components (such as *Helicobacter pylori*); or
- actively reach the basolateral surface (e.g. *Salmonella* spp.).

This helps to explain why constant exposure to non-pathogenic microbes in the intestine and airways does not induce a chronic state of inflammation – the host waits until they move beyond the lumen, signifying the presence of a real pathogenic threat.

Lymphocyte-independent effector systems

Complement is activated via the alternative pathway

Complement activation can result in the killing of some bacteria, particularly those with an outer lipid bilayer susceptible to the **lytic complex (C5b–9)**.

Q. To which strains of bacteria are individuals with C9 deficiency more susceptible?
A. *Neisseria* spp. (see Fig. 4.16).

Perhaps more importantly, complement activation releases C5a, which attracts and activates neutrophils and causes degranulation of mast cells (see Chapter 3). The consequent release of **histamine** and **leukotriene (LTB₄)** contributes to further increases in vascular permeability (see Fig. 14.3).

Opsonization of the bacteria, by attachment of **cleaved derivatives of C3**, is also critically important in subsequent interactions with phagocytes.

Release of proinflammatory cytokines increases the adhesive properties of the vascular endothelium

The rapid release of cytokines such as TNF and IL-1 (see Fig. 14.4) from macrophages increases the adhesive properties of the vascular endothelium and facilitates the passage of more phagocytes into inflamed tissue. Combined with the release of chemokines such as CCL2, CCL3, and CXCL8 (see Chapter 6), this directs the recruitment of different leukocyte populations.

Epithelial cells, neutrophils, and mast cells are also important sources of proinflammatory cytokines.

IL-1, TNF, and IL-6 also initiate the **acute phase response**, increasing the production of complement components as well as other proteins involved in scavenging material released by tissue damage and, in the case of CRP, an opsonin for improving phagocytosis of bacteria.

When NK cells are stimulated by the phagocyte-derived cytokines **IL-12** and **IL-18** they rapidly release large quantities of interferon-γ (IFNγ). This response happens within the first day of infection, well before the clonal expansion of antigen-specific T cells, and provides a rapid source of IFNγ to activate macrophages. This T cell-independent pathway helps to explain the considerable resistance of mice with SCID (severe combined immune deficiency, a defect in lymphocyte maturation) to infections such as with *Listeria monocytogenes*. In mice, CD1d-restricted NK T cells also secrete IFNγ in response to IL-12 and IL-18 and other ligands, and help to further activate both NK cells and macrophages.

Pathogen recognition generates signals that regulate the lymphocyte-mediated response

The signals generated following the recognition of pathogens not only generate a cascade of innate immune events, but also regulate the development of the appropriate lymphocyte-mediated response.

Dendritic cells (DCs) are crucial for the initial priming of naive T cells specific for bacterial antigens. Contact with bacteria in the periphery induces immature DCs to migrate to the draining lymph nodes and augments their antigen-presenting ability by increasing their:

- display of MHC molecule–peptide complexes;
- expression of co-stimulatory molecules (such as CD40, CD80, and CD86); and
- secretion of T cell differentiating cytokines.

Some of this DC activation occurs secondary to their production of cytokines such as type I IFN.

Activated macrophages also act as antigen-presenting cells (APCs), but probably function more at the site of infection, providing further activation of effector rather than naive T cells. Following initial T cell activation by dendritic cells, B cells are also able to act as APCs during B cell–T cell cooperation and are essential for the protective action of polysaccharide-conjugate vaccines in children against encapsulated bacteria such as *S. pneumoniae* and *H. influenzae*.

Binding of bacterial components to pattern recognition receptors such as TLRs induces a local environment rich in cytokines such as IFNγ, IL-12, and IL-18, which promote T cell differentiation down the TH1 rather than TH2 pathway.

Immunologists have made use of these effects for many decades (even without knowing their true molecular basis) in the use of **adjuvants** in vaccination. 'Adjuvant' is derived from the Latin *adjuvare*, to help. When given experimentally, soluble antigens evoke stronger T and B cell-mediated responses if they are mixed with bacterial components that act as adjuvants. Components with this property are indicated in Figure 14.1. This effect probably reflects that the antigen-specific immune response evolved in a tissue environment that already contained these pharmacologically active bacterial components.

With the exception of proteins such as **flagellin**, which itself stimulates TLR5 and is also a strong T cell immunogen, the response to pure bacterial antigens, injected without adjuvant-active bacterial components, is essentially an artificial situation that does not occur in nature.

The best known adjuvant in laboratory use, **complete Freund's adjuvant**, consists of killed mycobacteria suspended in oil, which is then emulsified with the aqueous antigen solution.

New-generation adjuvants based on bacterial components (and safe to use in humans, unlike Freund's adjuvant) include synthetic TLR activators such as CpG motifs and monophosphoryl lipid A (MPL) as well as recombinant cytokines such as IL-12, IL-1, and IFNγ. Identifying the best adjuvant for inclusion in a vaccine is arguably as important as the choice of antigens and is dramatically illustrated in the RTS,S malaria vaccine – a product which was not effective until reformulated with a new MPL based adjuvant.

Antibody dependent anti-bacterial defenses

The relevance to protection of interactions of bacteria with antibody depends on the mechanism of pathogenicity. Antibody clearly plays a crucial role in dealing with bacterial toxins:

- it neutralizes diphtheria toxin by blocking the attachment of the binding portion of the molecule to its target cells;
- similarly it may block locally acting toxins or extracellular matrix-degrading enzymes, which act as spreading factors.

Antibody can also interfere with motility by binding to flagellae.

An important function on external and mucosal surfaces, often performed by secretory IgA (sIgA, see Chapter 3), is to stop bacteria binding to epithelial cells – for instance, antibody to the M proteins of group A streptococci gives type-specific immunity to streptococcal sore throats.

It is likely that some antibodies to the bacterial surface can block functional requirements of the organism such as binding of iron-chelating compounds or intake of nutrients (Fig. 14.5).

An important role of antibody in immunity to non-toxigenic bacteria is the more efficient targeting of complement.

Naturally occurring IgM antibodies, which bind to common bacterial structures such as phosphorylcholine, are important for protection against some bacteria (particularly streptococci) via their complement fixing activity.

The antibacterial roles of antibody

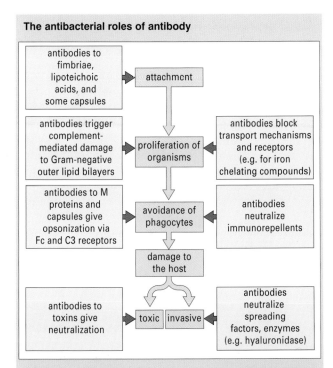

Fig. 14.5 This diagram lists the stages of bacterial invasion (blue) and indicates the antibacterial effects of antibody (yellow) that operate at the different stages. Antibodies to fimbriae, lipoteichoic acid, and some capsules block attachment of the bacterium to the host cell membrane. Antibody triggers complement-mediated damage to Gram-negative outer lipid bilayers. Antibody directly blocks bacterial surface proteins that pick up useful molecules from the environment and transport them across the membrane. Antibody to M proteins and capsules opsonizes the bacteria via Fc and C3 receptors for phagocytosis. Bacterial factors that interfere with normal chemotaxis or phagocytosis are neutralized. Bacterial toxins may be neutralized by antibody, as may bacterial spreading factors that facilitate invasion (e.g. by the destruction of connective tissue or fibrin).

Specific, high-affinity IgG antibodies elicited in response to infection are most important. This is particularly true for anti-toxin responses where the antibody must compete against the affinity of the toxin receptor on host cells *in vivo*. Children with primary immune deficiencies in B cell development or in T cell help have increased susceptibility to extracellular rather than intracellular bacteria.

With the aid of antibodies, even organisms that resist the alternative (i.e. innate) complement pathway (see below) are damaged by complement or become coated with C3 products, which then enhance the binding and uptake by phagocytes (Figs 14.6 and 14.7).

Q. How do C3 products attach to pathogens?
A. Following activation by cleavage the larger fragment, C3b, attaches covalently to hydroxyl and amine groups on the target (see Fig. 4.6).

The most efficient **complement-fixing antibodies** in humans are IgM, then IgG3 and to a lesser extent IgG1, whereas IgG1 and IgG3 are the subclasses with the highest affinity for Fc receptors.

Effect of antibody and complement on rate or clearance of virulent bacteria from the blood

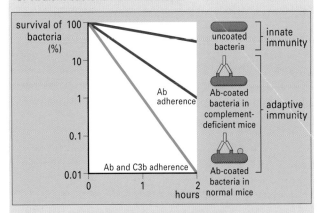

Fig. 14.6 Uncoated bacteria are phagocytosed rather slowly (unless the alternative complement pathway is activated by the strain of bacterium); on coating with antibody (Ab), adherence to phagocytes is greatly increased. The adherence is somewhat less effective in animals temporarily depleted of complement.

The interaction between bacteria and phagocytic cells

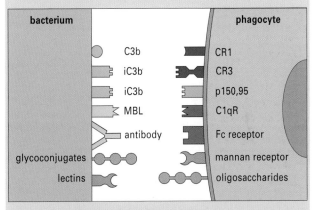

Fig. 14.7 A variety of molecules facilitate the binding of the organisms to the phagocyte membrane. These are in addition to the TLR system (e.g. TLR4 for LPS, TLR5 for flagellin, and TLR2 [plus TLR1/TLR6] for bacterial lipoproteins and peptidoglycans). The precise nature of the interaction will determine whether uptake occurs and whether cytokine secretion and appropriate killing mechanisms are triggered. Recognition invariably involves combinations of different receptor families. Note that apart from complement, antibody, and mannose-binding lectin (MBL), which bind to the bacterial surface, the other components are constitutive bacterial molecules.

Pathogenic bacteria may avoid the effects of antibody

Neisseria gonorrhoeae is an example of a pathogenic bacterium that uses several immune evasion strategies (Fig. 14.8) and humans can be repeatedly infected with *N. gonorrhoeae* with no evidence of protective immunity.

Antibodies may also be important for effective immunity against some intracellular bacteria such as *Legionella* and *Salmonella* spp.

Mechanisms used by *Neisseria gonorrhoeae* to avoid the effects of antibody

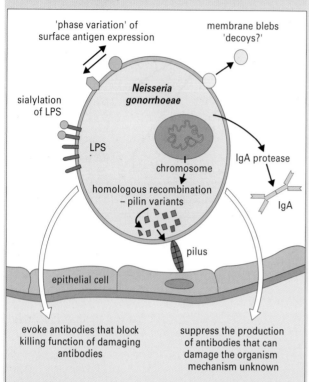

Fig. 14.8 *N. gonorrhoeae* is an example of a bacterium that uses several strategies to avoid the damaging effects of antibody. First, it fails to evoke a large antibody response, and the antibody that does form tends to block the function of damaging antibodies. Second, the organism secretes an IgA protease to destroy antibody. Third, blebs of membrane are released, and these appear to adsorb and so deplete local antibody levels. Finally, the organism uses three strategies to alter its antigenic composition: (i) the LPS may be sialylated, so that it more closely resembles mammalian oligosaccharides and promotes rapid removal of complement; (ii) the organism can undergo phase variation, so that it expresses an alternative set of surface molecules; (iii) the gene encoding pilin, the subunits of the pilus, undergoes homologous recombination to generate variants. *N. gonorrhoeae* also impairs T cell activation by engaging a co-inhibitory receptor CEACAM-1 on the lymphocyte surface by one of its OPA proteins.

Pathogenic bacteria can avoid the detrimental effects of complement

Some bacterial capsules are very poor activators of the alternative pathway (Fig. 14.9).

For other bacteria, long side chains (O antigens) on their LPS may fix C3b at a distance from the otherwise vulnerable lipid bilayer. Similarly, smooth-surfaced Gram-negative organisms (*Escherichia coli*, *Salmonella* spp., *Pseudomonas* spp.) may fix but then rapidly shed the C5b–C9 membrane lytic complex.

Other organisms exploit the physiological mechanisms that block destruction of host cells by complement. When C3b has attached to a surface it can interact with factor B leading to further C3b amplification or it can become inactivated by factors H and I. Capsules rich in sialic acid

Avoidance of complement-mediated damage

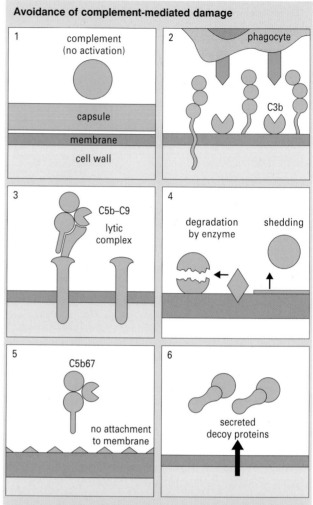

Fig. 14.9 Bacteria avoid complement-mediated damage by a variety of strategies. (**1**) An outer capsule or coat prevents complement activation. (**2**) An outer surface can be configured so that complement receptors on phagocytes cannot obtain access to fixed C3b. (**3**) Surface structures can be expressed that divert attachment of the lytic complex (MAC) from the cell membrane. (**4**) Membrane-bound enzyme can degrade fixed complement or cause it to be shed. (**5**) The outer membrane can resist the insertion of the lytic complex. (**6**) Secreted decoy proteins can cause complement to be deposited on them and not on the bacterium itself.

(as host cell membranes are) seem to promote the interaction with factors H and I.

Neisseria meningitidis, *E. coli* K1, and group B streptococci all resist complement attachment in this way.

The M protein of group A streptococci acts as an acceptor for factor H, thus potentiating C3bB dissociation. These bacteria also have a gene for a C5a protease.

Q. What value is a C5a protease to bacteria?
A. C5a is a major chemotactic molecule generated by complement activation that acts on specific receptors on macrophages, neutrophils, and mast cells (see Fig. 4.13).

Bactericidal killing by phagocytes

A few, mostly Gram-negative, bacteria are directly killed by complement. However, immunity to most bacteria, whether considered as extracellular or intracellular pathogens, ultimately needs the killing activity of neutrophils and macrophages. This process involves several steps.

Bacterial components attract phagocytes by chemotaxis

Unlike neutrophils, which in the uninfected host are found almost entirely in the blood, resident macrophages are constitutively present in tissues where exposure to pathogens first occurs (such as alveolar macrophages in the lung and Kupffer cells in the liver). These macrophages have some killing activity, but invariably need to be supplemented by recruitment of neutrophils and/or monocytes across the blood vessel wall. Phagocytes are attracted by:

- bacterial components such as **f-Met-Leu-Phe** (which is chemotactic for leukocytes);
- complement products such as C5a; and
- locally released chemokines and cytokines derived from resident macrophages and epithelial cells (see Chapter 6).

The cellular composition of this inflammatory response varies according to the pathogen and the time since infection. For instance:

- acute infection with encapsulated bacteria such as *Streptococcus pyogenes* give rise to tissue lesions rich in neutrophils (typical of so-called pyogenic or pus-forming infections);
- at the other extreme, chronic infections with *M. tuberculosis* result in granulomas rich in macrophages, macrophage-derived multinucleated giant cells, and T cells;
- other organisms, such as *Listeria* and *Salmonella* spp., result in lesions of more mixed composition.

The choice of receptors is critical

The choice of receptors used for attachment of the phagocyte to the organism is critical and will determine:

- the efficiency of uptake;
- whether killing mechanisms are triggered;
- whether the process favors the pathogen by subverting immunity.

The binding can be mediated by lectins on the organism (e.g. on the fimbriae *of E. coli*), but receptors on the phagocyte are the most important. These either bind directly to the bacterium or indirectly via host complement and antibody deposited on the bacterial surface (**opsonization**).

- direct binding is mediated by pattern recognition molecules including Toll-like receptors and scavenger receptors (such as SRA, MARCO), mannose receptor, and dectin-1;
- opsonization is mediated through complement receptors such as CR1, CR3, and CR4, which recognize complement fragments deposited on the organism via the alternative or classic complement pathways.

Complement can also be fixed by MBL present in serum, which can itself bind to **C1q receptors** and CR1.

Additionally, Fc receptors on the phagocyte (**FcγRI, FcγRII, and FcγRIII**, see Chapter 3) bind antibody that has coated bacteria (see Fig. 14.7), whereas various integrins can bind **fibronectin** and **vitronectin** opsonized particles.

Uptake can be enhanced by macrophage-activating cytokines

The binding of an organism to a receptor on the macrophage membrane does not always lead to its uptake. For example, zymosan particles (derived from yeast) bind via the glucan-recognizing lectin-like site on the CR3 of the macrophage and are taken up, whereas erythrocytes coated with iC3b are not, even though the iC3b also binds to CR3. This can, however, be enhanced by macrophage-activating cytokines such as granulocyte–macrophage colony stimulating factor (GM-CSF).

Different membrane receptors vary in their efficiency at inducing a microbicidal response

Just as the binding of an organism to membrane receptors does not guarantee uptake, so different membrane receptors vary in their efficiency at inducing a microbicidal response – for example, mannose receptors and Fc receptors are particularly efficient at inducing the respiratory burst, but complement receptors are not, providing an evasion strategy for some organisms.

Phagocytic cells have many killing methods

Killing of bacteria and fungi occurs most efficiently when the organisms have been internalized by the phagocyte and are now within a host membrane bound phagosome. This confinement helps to deliver antimicrobial molecules to the organism at high concentrations and reduces collateral damage to the host. Maturation of the phagosome into a killing zone occurs by acquisition of microbicidal mediators following fusion with other intracellular vesicles such as lysosomes.

The killing pathways of phagocytic cells can be oxygen dependent, with the generation of reactive oxygen intermediates, or oxygen independent (see Chapter 7). In neutrophils, the oxidative burst may also act indirectly, by promoting the flux of K^+ ions into the phagosome and activating microbicidal proteases.

A second oxygen-dependent pathway involves the creation of nitric oxide ($NO^{\bullet}$) from the guanidino nitrogen of L-arginine. This in turn leads to further toxic substances such as the peroxynitrites, which result from interactions of $NO^{\bullet}$ with the products of the oxygen reduction pathway.

Q. What pathway leads to the production of NO by macrophages?
A. Cytokine activation by IFNγ and TNFα leads to production of inducible NO synthase, which generates NO from L-arginine (see Fig. 7.19).

Oxygen-independent killing mechanisms may be more important than previously thought. Many organisms can be killed by cells from patients with chronic granulomatous disease (CGD), which cannot produce reactive oxygen intermediates, and from patients with myeloperoxidase (MPO) deficiency, which cannot produce hypohalous acids. Some of this killing may be due to $NO^{\bullet}$, but many organisms can be killed anaerobically, so other mechanisms must exist. Some have been identified and are discussed below. Indeed, many innate immune factors have actually evolved to work optimally in the hypoxic environment of infected tissues. Under conditions of low oxygen tension and pH, phagocytes specifically upregulate genes which contain hypoxic-response elements, resulting in increased phago-cytic activity, a longer life span and the production of antimicrobial molecules and inflammatory cytokines.

Some cationic proteins have antibiotic-like properties

The **defensins** (Fig. 14.10) are cysteine- and arginine-rich cationic peptides of 30–33 amino acids found in phagocytes such as neutrophils, where they comprise 30–50% of the granule proteins.

Q. Which other cells secrete antimicrobial peptides?
A. Paneth cells of the intestine (see Fig. 12.11) and airway epithelial cells (i.e. sites of primary contact with pathogens).

Defensins evolved early in evolution and similar molecules are found in insects. They act by integrating into microbial lipid membranes (in some cases forming ion-permeable channels) and disrupting membrane function and structure, resulting in lysis of the pathogen. Defensins can act both in-side and outside of host cells and kill organisms as diverse as *Staphylococcus aureus*, *Pseudomonas aeruginosa*, *E. coli*, as well as fungi such as *Cryptococcus neoformans*.

Defensins also have important immunostimulatory prop-erties including:

- promoting chemotaxis and phagocytosis;
- regulating cytokine production; and

Cationic host defense peptides in immunity to fungi and bacteria

cell sources	mediators	actions
neutrophils	α-defensins (e.g. HNPs)	**directly antimicrobial**
		Gram +ve
epithelia	β-defensins (e.g. HBDI-4)	Gram –ve
		fungi
	cathelicidins (e.g. LL-37)	**inflammation**
e.g. epidermis, lung, genitourinary tract, gut (Paneth cells)	bacterial permeability inducing protein (BPI)	cytokine/chemokine secretion mast cell degranulation wound repair monocyte/neutrophil chemotaxis
mast cells	protegrins	anti-endotoxic activity
		adaptive immunity
	histatins	dendritic cell chemotaxis T cell recruitment

Fig. 14.10 Numerous cationic host defense peptides are produced by neutrophils, monocytes, epithelia, and mast cells. Their synthesis is usually constitutive but is also enhanced by proinflammatory cytokines such as TNF, IL-1, IL-22, and IFNγ generated following infection. Originally defined by their direct killing activity against pathogens, they are now known also to act on immune cells, having multiple immunomodulatory effects on inflammation and adaptive immunity.

- acting as adjuvants for adaptive immunity by promoting multiple facets of dendritic cell function including antigen uptake, processing and presentation as well as their migration and maturation.

Other antibacterial peptides include the **cathelicidins** (which can kill *Mycobacterium tuberculosis* under the regu-lation of Vitamin D) and **protegrins**, which can bind LPS and also form membrane pores.

There are also cationic proteins with different pH optima, including **cathepsin G** and **azurocidin**, both of which are re-lated to elastase, but have activity against Gram-negative bacteria – this is unrelated to their enzyme activity.

Neutrophils (and possibly mast cells and eosinophils) possess an extracellular mechanism of microbicidal activity by release of so called neutrophil extracellular traps (NETs). This involves the release of chromatin, histones, and antimi-crobial proteins which bind and kill bacteria and fungi as well as generating a barrier against the spread of infection.

Other antimicrobial mechanisms also play a role

Following lysosome fusion there is a transient rise in pH before acidification of the phagolysosome takes place. This occurs within 10–15 minutes.

The acidification of phagosomes containing bacteria fol-lowing their fusion with lysosomes is an important step in the killing process and is related to the low pH optima of lysosomal enzymes.

Certain Gram-positive organisms may be killed by **lyso-zyme**, which is active against their exposed peptidoglycan layer.

Restricting the access of intracellular bacteria to essential nutrients is a microbistatic strategy of host defense. Induc-tion of indoleamine 2-3 dioxygenase (IDO) in macrophages by IFNγ depletes tryptophan which is an essential amino acid for growth of *Chlamydia* and mycobacteria. NRAMP 1 (also known as SLC11A1) performs its microbistatic func-tion by removing divalent cations from the phagosome; these are needed for bacterial metabolism and their evasion of the respiratory burst. (The tryptophan starvation path-way also functions in endothelial cells and fibroblasts.)

The availability of intracellular iron is another important factor in the interplay between host and pathogen. Iron is essential for the growth of many bacteria and also influences their expression of key virulence genes. Sequestration of iron can therefore be an effective antimicrobial strategy, particularly for intracellular bacteria.

Lactoferrin is a mammalian iron-binding protein released by degranulating neutrophils that sequesters iron from pathogens, inhibiting their growth, and in the case of *P. aeruginosa* also reducing biofilm formation, a key event in the pathogenesis of infection in cystic fibrosis patients. **Lactoferricin**, an antimicrobial peptide derived from lacto-ferrin, kills other bacteria.

Iron is also required for many host immune functions in-cluding the respiratory burst, the generation of NO•, and the development of pathogen-specific T cells.

Both iron excess and iron deficiency can therefore have complex effects on the outcome of infection. For example, individuals with iron overload syndromes resulting from genetic defects (such as thalassemia or hemochromato-sis), nutritional excess, or following iron or red cell supplementation (such as in the treatment of anemias) have increased susceptibility to infection with *Yersinia* and *Salmonella* spp., and *M. tuberculosis*.

Macrophage killing can be enhanced on activation

Unlike neutrophils, which have a short life span but are efficient killers even in their normal state, macrophages are long-lived cells that without appropriate activation can actually provide a haven for microbial growth.

Macrophage activation occurs most effectively by the combination of exposure to:

- microbial products (through the receptors described above); and
- cytokines (particularly IFNγ) derived from cells of the innate and adaptive immune system.

Optimal activation of macrophages is dependent on TH1 CD4 T cells

Microbial products can directly activate monocytes and resident macrophages to secrete proinflammatory cytokines and thus initiate the immune process. However, complete activation, including the ability to kill intracellular microbes, requires the action of IFNγ. IFNγ knockout mice are extremely susceptible to infection and children with deficiencies in either the IFNγ receptor or the cytokines necessary for its production (such as IL-12, IL-18, and IL-23) have increased susceptibility to intracellular bacteria such as *Salmonella* spp., and mycobacteria including bacille Calmette–Guérin (BCG).

IFNγ is so potent because it enhances several different microbicidal pathways, including both the respiratory burst and the generation of NO•.

As described above, NK cells, NK T cells, and even macrophages themselves can produce IFNγ during the innate immune response. However, the additional actions of antigen-specific T cells are necessary for optimal cell-mediated immunity.

The most important source of IFNγ during the adaptive immune response to intracellular bacteria is from TH1 CD4$^+$ T cells (Fig. 14.11).

Patients who have AIDS and a reduced CD4 T cell number and function have dramatically increased susceptibility to *M. tuberculosis*, as well as *Mycobacterium avium* and atypical salmonella.

As mentioned above, many bacterial components activate the TLR pattern recognition receptors, ensuring the preferential expression of TH1 rather than TH2 CD4$^+$ T cell responses in most cases.

TH1 T cells provide both IFNγ for macrophage activation and B cell help to produce IgG subclasses for opsonization of bacteria, rather than the eosinophilia and IgE responses typical of helminth infections.

There is mutual antagonism between the TH1 and TH2 pathways at the level of both T cell differentiation and also directly on the macrophage:

- IFNγ upregulates induced NO• synthetase expression; whereas
- IL-4 and -13 promote the expression of arginase, which inhibits NO• production, reducing the macrophage

killing potential and diverting it to a profibrotic phenotype. In some cases these cells are called alternatively activated macrophages.

Other cytokines such as GM-CSF and TNF can also contribute to macrophage activation.

Macrophage activation is also promoted by direct contact with CD4 T cells via **CD40–CD40L interactions**.

Thus T cell-mediated help for macrophages and B cells shares the common themes of soluble and cell-contact mediated activation by CD4 TH1 cells.

While this functional link between CD4 TH1 cells and macrophages has been known for many years, only recently have we discovered that a different T cell subset (CD4 TH17 cells) mediate a link to neutrophils, the other major phagocyte group in the body. TH17 cells preferentially produce IL-17 and IL-22 and were originally discovered for their role in autoimmune diseases. TH17 cells appear to be particularly important in resistance to extracellular (rather than intracellular) fungi and bacteria at mucosal surfaces. The major biological activity of IL-17 is to increase neutrophil recruitment and differentiation in an indirect manner by acting on epithelial cells to produce CXC chemokines, TNF, IL-6 and G-CSF, whilst IL-22 induces the production of anti-microbial peptides. Since neutrophil responses can also cause pathology if excessive, in different animal models TH17 cells can either be protective or contribute to immune pathology. These cells are also found in humans but to date their importance is not clear.

Persistent macrophage recruitment and activation can result in granuloma formation

If intracellular pathogens are not quickly eliminated, the persistent recruitment and activation of macrophages and T cells to an infected tissue can result in the formation of **granulomas**. These are generally associated with chronic bacterial infections such as tuberculosis and syphilis, but similar (although not identical) structures are also induced in parasitic diseases such as schistosomiasis and in response to non-infectious materials such as asbestos.

In the classical example of tuberculosis, granulomas are composed of a core of infected (and uninfected) macrophages, epithelioid cells, and multinucleated giant cells (derived from the fusion of activated macrophages), and a peripheral accumulation of T cells. Neutrophils and dendritic cells can also be found in granulomas, along with extracellular matrix components such as collagen. In human tuberculosis, the center of granulomas undergoes caseating necrosis. The presence of activated macrophages and the fibrosis that ensues is believed to control bacterial growth and prevent dissemination to other organs but may also provide a niche for bacterial persistence and can be an obstacle to penetration of antibiotics. There is also experimental evidence that at least initially, the TB bacillus actively induces the granulomatous response in order to have a source of naive macrophages in which to grow. Generating these new immunological structures is a highly complex event involving multiple adhesion molecules, chemokines, and cytokines. Once formed, their continued existence also requires active immunological input. New intra-vital imaging techniques where the movement of host cells in and out of the granuloma can be measured in real time are

Overview of CD4⁺ T cell-mediated immunity to bacteria and fungi

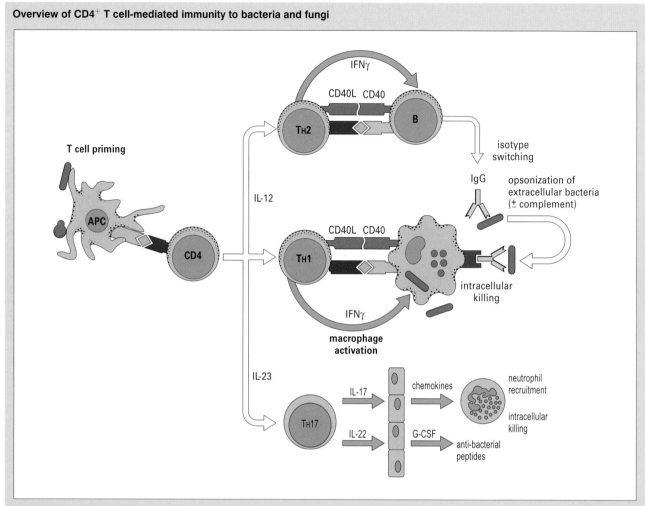

Fig. 14.11 Naive CD4⁺ T cells are stimulated by class II MHC positive antigen-bearing dendritic cells (DCs) via the TCR, in conjunction with co-stimulatory molecules such as CD80/86 and CD28, which induce T cell activation and proliferation. Differentiation into T$_H$1, T$_H$17, or T$_H$2 effector cells is strongly influenced by the cytokine environment during this interaction – microbial pattern recognition events that favor production of IL-12 promote T$_H$1 development, low IL-12 favors T$_H$2 responses, whereas combinations of IL-6, IL-1 TGFβ, IL-21, and IL-23 are required for development and maintenance of T$_H$17 responses. T$_H$17 cells mediate their biological activities via secretion of IL-17 which induces G-CSF and CXC family chemokines to enhance neutrophil differentiation and recruitment, and of IL-22 which induces antimicrobial peptides such as defensins and mucins. Although not shown here, conditions with high levels of IL-10 or TGFβ can induce regulatory T cells, rather than effector (i.e. T$_H$1, T$_H$2, or T$_H$17) subsets. Optimal T cell help for either B cells or macrophage responses involves T cell-derived cytokines and direct cell contact. T$_H$1 cells also promote opsonizing antibody production of high affinity (Fig. 9.8), which complements their activation of phagocytes by IFNγ, but the main activators of antibody synthesis are T$_H$2 cells, themselves induced by IL-4, producing IL-4, 5, 6, 10 and 13 (Fig. 9.7).

now providing insights into just how dynamic these structures are *in vivo*.

AIDS and diabetes mellitus are important risk factors for loss of control of *M. tuberculosis*. TNF is also critical for granuloma maintenance – some patients given TNF-blocking antibodies to alleviate the symptoms of rheumatoid arthritis rapidly reactivate tuberculosis that had otherwise been controlled for many years.

Successful pathogens have evolved mechanisms to avoid phagocyte-mediated killing

Because most organisms are ultimately killed by phagocytes, it is not surprising that successful pathogens have evolved an array of mechanisms to counteract this risk (Fig. 14.12).

Intracellular pathogens may 'hide' in cells

Some organisms may thrive inside metabolically damaged host phagocytes, or escape killing by moving out of phagosomes into the cytoplasm.

Listeria monocytogenes, *Shigella* spp., and *Burkholderia pseudomallei* achieve this by releasing enzymes that lyse the phagosome membrane and allow entry into the cytoplasm. However all is not lost, as the host can still capture cytosolic bacteria into the lysosome system for destruction, a process termed autophagy, which these pathogens also actively attempt to evade. These organisms clearly illustrate the concept that bacteria are not just inert particles, but have evolved multiple strategies for taking control of functions of the host cell.

Other organisms, such as *M. leprae* and salmonellae, cause themselves to be taken up by cells that are not

Evasion mechanisms of bacteria (and some fungi)

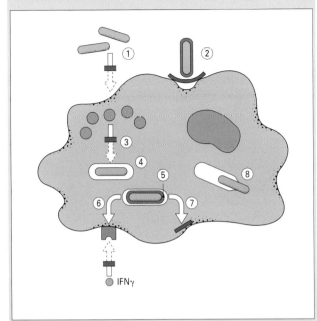

IFNγ

Fig. 14.12 Evasion mechanisms of bacteria (and some fungi), particularly those that are successful intracellular parasites, have evolved the ability to evade different aspects of phagocyte-mediated killing. (**1**) Some can secrete repellents or toxins that inhibit chemotaxis. (**2**) Others have capsules or outer coats that inhibit attachment by the phagocyte (e.g. *Streptococcus pneumoniae* or the yeast *C. neoformans*). (**3**) Others permit uptake, but release factors that block subsequent triggering of killing mechanisms. Once ingested, some, such as *M. tuberculosis*, inhibit lysosome fusion with the phagosome. They also inhibit the proton pump that acidifies the phagosome, so the pH does not fall. (**4**) They may also secrete catalase (e.g. staphylococci), which breaks down hydrogen peroxide. (**5**) Organisms such as *M. leprae* have highly resistant outer coats. *M. leprae* surrounds itself with a phenolic glycolipid, which scavenges free radicals. (**6**) Mycobacteria also release a lipoarabinomannan, which blocks the ability of macrophages to respond to the activating effects of IFNγ. (**7**) Cells infected with *Salmonella enterica*, *M. tuberculosis*, or *Chlamydia trachomatis* have impaired antigen-presenting function. (**8**) Several organisms (e.g. *Listeria* and *Shigella* spp.) can escape from the phagosome to multiply in the cytoplasm. Finally, the organism may kill the phagocyte via either necrosis (e.g. staphylococci) or induction of apoptosis (e.g. *Yersinia* spp.).

normally considered phagocytic and have little antibacterial potential such as Schwann cells, hepatocytes, and epithelial cells.

Before they can be taken up by activated phagocytes or exposed to other killing mechanisms, the organisms may need to be released from such cells.

Direct anti-bacterial actions of T cells

Infected cells can be killed by CTLs

CD8$^+$ cytotoxic T lymphocytes (CTLs) can release intracellular organisms by killing the infected cell. For example, mice become strikingly susceptible to *M. tuberculosis* if

class I MHC genes are knocked out so that antigen-specific CD8$^+$ T cells do not develop, and kill infected macrophages.

This is consistent with an essential role for CTLs in resistance to intracellular bacteria, and inducing these responses is now a primary goal of new vaccines against bacteria such as *M. tuberculosis* as well as other pathogens.

Tissue cells that are not components of the immune system can also harbor bacteria such as *M. leprae*, invasive *Shigella* and *Salmonella* spp., and *Rickettsia* and *Chlamydia* spp. These infected cells may also be sacrificed by CTLs.

Dendritic cells appear to be particularly important in the generation of strong CD8 T cell responses to bacteria such as *L. monocytogenes* and *Salmonella* spp.

Although antigen processing and presentation via the class I MHC pathway (see Chapter 8) is most efficient for microbial antigens derived from the cytosol, nevertheless, CTLs are also clearly induced by bacteria that never escape the phagosome such as *M. tuberculosis*, salmonellae, and chlamydiae. This occurs either by **cross-presentation** of antigens within the same cell or by **cross-priming** where antigens are released from infected cells undergoing apoptosis and then transferred to nearby DCs for efficient presentation via the MHC I pathway. In some cases, lysis of infected host cells by CTLs can result in killing of the organism inside. This can be due to the action of **granulysin** – an antibacterial peptide stored in the cytotoxic granules and released during the cytotoxic process.

CTLs can also secrete IFNγ when they recognize infected targets, providing an additional pathway of macrophage activation and protective immunity (Fig. 14.13).

Other T cell populations can contribute to antibacterial immunity

In addition to the classical MHC class I- and MHC class II-mediated recognition of bacterial proteins by αβ CD4 and CD8 T cells, other 'non-conventional' T cell populations allow the host to respond rapidly to other microbial chemistries.

T cells bearing γδ (rather than αβ) receptors (see Chapter 5) proliferate in response to bacterial infection.

Q. Where in the body are γδ T cells located?
A. They preferentially home to epithelial surfaces (see Chapter 2).

Some γδ T cells recognize small phospholigands derived from *M. tuberculosis* and possibly other bacteria, whereas others are triggered in an antigen-independent manner by the presence of pathogen-activated dendritic cells expressing high levels of co-stimulatory molecules and IL-12.

NK T cells are a diverse group of T cells, some of which have an invariant T cell antigen receptor. They recognize not proteins, but hydrophobic antigens, particularly microbial glycolipids such as the **lipoarabinomannan** from *M. tuberculosis*, presented via CD1 molecules (see Fig. 5.w3).

Such γδ and NKT cells can have cytotoxic activity and also secrete multiple cytokines including IFNγ and IL-17 (depending on how they are stimulated) giving a potential role in host defense. In animal models of infection these non-conventional T cells can be protective or

Pathways of CD8 T cell activation and function

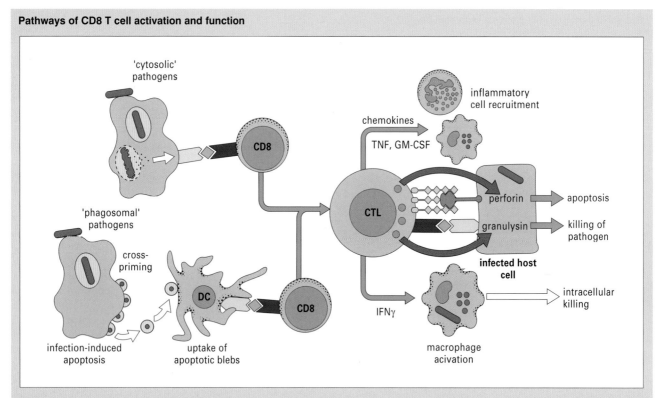

Fig. 14.13 Naive CD8 T cells are activated by peptides presented via MHC class I molecules, primarily derived from microorganisms that reside in the cytoplasm, such as viruses and some intracellular bacteria that escape the phagosome such as *Listeria* spp. Other pathogens that do not escape the phagosome (such as *M. tuberculosis*) can still induce CD8 T cell responses via cross-priming, in which infected and apoptotic host cells release antigenic fragments that are taken up by dendritic cells (DCs). Effector CD8 T cells (CTLs) provide protection by releasing proinflammatory and macrophage-activating cytokines and killing infected host cells via perforin release and Fas. In some cases, the release of granulysin from the CTL can also result in killing of the pathogen.

Immunity in some important bacterial infections

infection	pathogenesis	major defense mechanisms
Corynebacterium diphtheriae	non-invasive pharyngitis – toxin	neutralizing antibody
Vibrio cholerae	non-invasive enteritis – toxin	neutralizing and adhesion-blocking antibodies
Neisseria meningitidis (Gram-negative)	nasopharynx →bacteremia →meningitis →endotoxemia	killed by antibody and lytic complement; opsonized and phagocytosed
Staphylococcus aureus (Gram-positive)	locally invasive and toxic in skin, etc.	osponized by antibody and complement; killed by phagocytes
Mycobacterium tuberculosis	invasive, evokes immunopathology	macrophage activation by cytokines from T cells, CTLs
Mycobacterium leprae	invasive, space-occupying and/or immunopathology	

Fig. 14.14 This table provides examples of how a knowledge of the organism, and the mechanism of disease, can lead to a prediction of the relevant protective mechanism.

immunoregulatory, but their relative importance in human immunity is not resolved.

Examples to illustrate the relationship between the nature of an organism, the disease, and immunopathology caused, and the mechanism of immune response that leads to protection, are given in Figure 14.14.

Immunopathological reactions induced by bacteria

The events described so far are generally beneficial to the host and critical for resistance against pathogenic bacteria. However, all immune responses designed to kill invading pathogens have the potential for causing collateral damage to the host.

Excessive cytokine release can lead to endotoxin shock

If cytokine release is sudden and massive, several acute tissue-damaging syndromes can result and are potentially fatal.

One of the most severe examples of this is **endotoxin (septicemic) shock**, when there is massive production of cytokines, usually caused by bacterial products released during septicemic episodes. Endotoxin (LPS) from Gram-negative bacteria is usually responsible, though Gram-positive septicemia can cause a similar syndrome. There can be life-threatening fever, circulatory collapse, diffuse intravascular coagulation, and hemorrhagic necrosis, leading eventually to multiple organ failure (Fig. 14.15).

Paradoxically, individuals who recover from the initial life-threatening phase often overcompensate and switch from a hyper- to a hyporesponsive phase, in which excessive production of endogenous immune regulators such as IL-10 and TGFβ (and possibly other mechanisms) results in immune paralysis, making them susceptible to secondary infection.

The toxicity of superantigens results from massive cytokine release

Certain bacterial components called **superantigens** bind directly to the variable regions of β chains (Vβ) of antigen receptors on subsets of T cells, and cross-link them to the MHC molecules of APCs, usually outside the normal antigen-binding groove (Fig. 14.16). Between them staphylococci

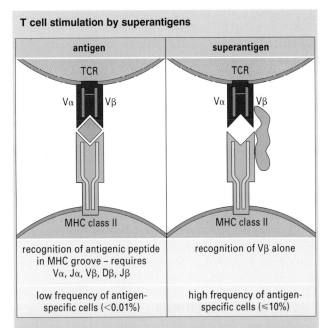

T cell stimulation by superantigens

antigen	superantigen
TCR Vα Vβ	TCR Vα Vβ
MHC class II	MHC class II
recognition of antigenic peptide in MHC groove – requires Vα, Jα, Vβ, Dβ, Jβ	recognition of Vβ alone
low frequency of antigen-specific cells (<0.01%)	high frequency of antigen-specific cells (≤10%)

Fig 14.16 Normally antigenic peptides are processed and presented on MHC molecules (left). Superantigens, such as staphylococcal enterotoxins, are not processed but bind directly to MHC class II molecules and Vβ of the TCR (right). Each superantigen activates a distinct set of Vβ-expressing T cells.

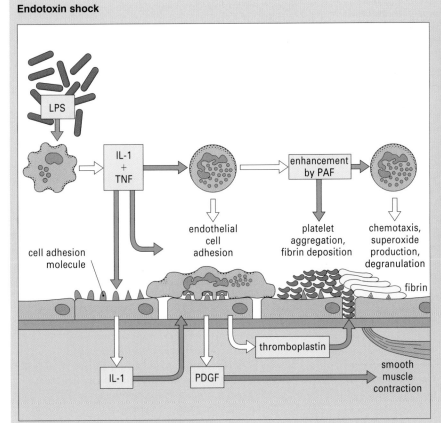

Endotoxin shock

LPS

IL-1 + TNF

enhancement by PAF

endothelial cell adhesion

platelet aggregation, fibrin deposition

chemotaxis, superoxide production, degranulation

cell adhesion molecule

fibrin

thromboplastin

IL-1

PDGF

smooth muscle contraction

Fig. 14.15 Excessive release of cytokines, often triggered by the endotoxin (LPS) of Gram-negative bacteria, can lead to diffuse intravascular coagulation with consequent defective clotting, changes in vascular permeability, loss of fluid into the tissues, a fall in blood pressure, circulatory collapse, and hemorrhagic necrosis, particularly in the gut. This figure illustrates some important parts of this pathway at the cellular level. The cytokines TNF and IL-1 cause endothelial cells to express cell adhesion molecules and tissue thromboplastin. These promote adhesion of circulating cells and deposition of fibrin, respectively. Platelet activating factor (PAF) enhances these effects. In experimental models, shock can be blocked by neutralizing antibodies to TNF, and greatly diminished by antibodies to tissue thromboplastin, or by inhibitors of PAF or of nitric oxide production, but these have not been successful clinically. Gram-positive bacteria can induce shock, for example by massive release of cytokines mediated by superantigens. (PDGF, platelet-derived growth factor, produced by both platelets and endothelium.)

and streptococci have some 21 different superantigens and these molecules can also be found in other bacteria such as mycoplasmas. The full biological significance of this bacterial adaptation is not yet clear – it could be to the organism's advantage to exhaust or deplete T cells that would otherwise be protective.

One certain effect is the toxicity of the massive release of cytokines (including IL-2, TNFα, and TNFβ, together with IL-1β from activated macrophages) due to the simultaneous stimulation of up to 20% of the entire T cell pool.

The staphylococcal toxins responsible for the **toxic shock syndrome** (toxic shock syndrome toxin-1 [TSST-1], etc.) operate in this way, though not all shock syndromes caused by staphylococci are the result of T cell activation.

Recent evidence suggests that streptococcal M protein, a known virulence factor of *S. pyogenes*, forms a complex with fibrinogen, which then binds to β-integrins on neutrophils, causing the release of inflammatory mediators, which also result in massive vascular leakage and shock.

The 'hygiene hypothesis'

Several groups of diseases, all characterized by defects in the regulation of the immune system, are becoming more common, particularly in developed countries. These diseases include:

* allergies;
* inflammatory bowel diseases (Crohn's disease and ulcerative colitis); and
* autoimmune conditions such as multiple sclerosis.

This may have many causes but the 'hygiene hypothesis' suggests that increasing immunological dysregulation correlates with decreasing exposure to environmental microorganisms. Decreased exposure could be due to hygiene, vaccines, and antibiotic use. This was mostly thought to act on infants as they develop in the first few years of life but there are now indications that this can be preceded by immune programming *in utero*, where infection and inflammatory stresses acting on the mother (such as aerosol exposure to microbe containing dust) during pregnancy directly influence the immune response of the newborn. If proved correct, the solution would clearly not be the abandonment of the most important achievements of medicine (hygiene, vaccines, antibiotics), but rather the improvement of maternal health and identification of other environmental factors that are lacking from the modern lifestyle so that they can be replaced as vaccines or probiotics.

However, recent data suggest that the correlation does not always hold true – some viral infections (such as respiratory syncytial virus) seem to promote rather than decrease allergy and asthma in animal models and in humans.

Whatever their cause, prevention or treatment of these diseases will need to address:

* the balance of TH1/TH2 responses; and
* manipulation of the regulatory T cell circuits that normally control allergy and autoimmunity.

Fungal infections

Fungi are eukaryotes with a rigid cell wall enriched in complex polysaccharides such as chitin, glucans, and mannan.

Among the 70 000 or so species of fungi, only a small number are pathogenic for humans. However, because there are no approved vaccines and antifungal drugs often have severe side effects, fungi can cause serious and sometimes life-threatening infections.

Q. Why has it been more difficult to identify antifungal antibiotics than antibacterial antibiotics?
A. Fungi are eukaryotic organisms and therefore have similar protein synthesis machinery and mechanisms to organize and replicate the genome as mammalian cells.

Fungi can exist as:

* single cells (yeasts) small enough to be ingested by host phagocytes; or
* long slender, branching hyphae, which may require extracellular killing processes.

Some pathogenic fungi are dimorphic, in that they switch from a hyphal form in the environment to a yeast form as they adapt to life in the host. Both phases possess important virulence determinants and pose different problems to the immune system.

There are four categories of fungal infection

Although some fungi can cause disease in otherwise healthy individuals, severe fungal infections are a growing problem because of the markedly increased numbers of immunologically compromised hosts. Fungal infections are therefore regularly seen in:

* patients with untreated AIDS;
* patients with cancer and undergoing chemotherapy;
* patients with transplants on immunosuppressive agents; and
* some patients taking long-term corticosteroids.

These clinical findings point to the key roles of neutrophils and macrophages and the CD4 T cell subsets that regulate their activity (i.e. TH1 and TH17) in antifungal immunity.

Human fungal infections fall into the following four major categories:

* **superficial mycoses** caused by fungi known as dermatophytes, usually restricted to the non-living keratinized components of skin, hair, and nails, and including infection by *Trichophyton* and *Microsporum* spp. (which cause ringworm and athlete's foot) and *Malassezia* spp. (which causes pityriasis);
* **subcutaneous mycoses** in which saprophytic fungi cause chronic nodules or ulcers in subcutaneous tissues following trauma (e.g. chromomycosis, sporotrichosis, and mycetoma);
* **systemic mycoses** caused by soil saprophytes, which are inhaled from the environment and produce subclinical or acute lung infections that can disseminate to almost any tissue in the immunocompromised host – *Histoplasma, Blastomyces, Coccidioides,* and *Paracoccidioides* spp. can all cause primary disease in otherwise immunocompetent individuals, whereas *Aspergillus* spp., *Pneumocystis jiroveci,* and C. *neoformans* act more as opportunists;

- candidiasis caused by *Candida albicans*, a ubiquitous commensal and the most common opportunistic fungal pathogen – disturbance of normal physiology by immunosuppressive drugs, of normal flora by antibiotics, or T cell function (as in severe combined immune deficiency, thymic aplasia, and AIDS), results in superficial infections of the skin and mucous membranes, and systemic disease can occur in intravenous drug users and patients with lymphoma or leukemia.

Innate immune responses to fungi include defensins and phagocytes

The basic protective features of the skin and normal commensal flora described against bacterial infections above are also important in resistance to fungi.

Defensins have antifungal as well as antibacterial properties, and collectins such as MBL and the surfactant proteins A and D can bind, aggregate, and opsonize fungi for phagocytosis.

Phagocytes, particularly neutrophils (Fig. 14.17) and macrophages, are essential for killing fungi, either by:

- degranulation and release of toxic materials onto large indigestible hyphae; or
- ingestion of yeast or conidia.

The oxidative burst plays a crucial role in some antifungal responses, as seen in the susceptibility to severe aspergillosis by patients with CGD who have defects in the NADPH oxidase system. However, phagocytes from such patients with defective oxygen reduction pathways nevertheless kill other yeast and hyphae with near normal efficiency, so demonstrating the role of other killing mechanisms (Fig. 14.18). For instance, NO• and its derivatives are important for resistance to *C. neoformans*.

These responses rely on the recognition of PAMPs in the fungal cell wall by either soluble or cell-bound pattern recognition molecules. The TLR family again plays an important role in this process, along with the mannose receptor and complement receptors:

Evidence for neutrophil-mediated immunity to mucormycosis

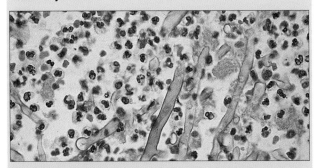

Fig. 14.17 This is a section from the lung of a patient suffering from mucormycosis – an opportunistic infection in an immunosuppressed subject. The inflammatory reaction consists almost entirely of neutrophil polymorphs around the fungal hyphae. The disease is particularly associated with neutropenia (lack of neutrophils). Silver stain. × 400. *(Courtesy of Professor RJ Hay.)*

- TLR2 (which can cooperate with the β-glucan receptor dectin-1) recognizes fungal phospholipomannans, *C. albicans* yeasts, and *A. fumigatus* hyphae and conidia;
- TLR4/CD14 recognizes *C. albicans*, *Aspergillus fumigatus*, and the glucuronoxylomannan capsule of *C. neoformans*.

Dectin-1, a C type lectin receptor is widely expressed on myeloid cells of the gut and airway mucosa. Recognition of fungi via this receptor promotes phagocytosis, triggers the respiratory burst and elicits inflammatory cytokine, chemokine and prostaglandin responses. TNF is one of these important cytokines in humans, since individuals given anti-TNF therapy have increased susceptibility to multiple fungal pathogens. Not all of these recognition events are to the host's advantage, for example binding of *Candida albicans* mannan via TLR4 induces proinflammatory chemokine responses, whereas ligation of candidal phospholipomannan and glucans with TLR2/dectin-1 generates a strong IL-10 response, which may inhibit the relevant immune response.

Monocyte/macrophage killing of fungi

organism	source of monocytes/macrophages		
	normal	CGD	MPO deficiency
Candida albicans	killed	sometimes killed	sometimes killed
Candida parapsilosis	killed	not killed	unknown
Cryptococcus neoformans	killed	unknown	killed
Aspergillus fumigatus conidia	killed	sometimes killed	killed
Aspergillus fumigatus hyphae	killed	killed	killed

Fig. 14.18 Many fungi are killed by monocytes or macrophages. Individuals with chronic granulomatous disease (CGD) are highly susceptible to *Aspergillus* spp. infections whereas myeloperoxidase (MPO) deficiency does not usually lead to opportunistic infection, suggesting that non-oxygen-dependent mechanisms are also important in host defense.

T cell-mediated immunity is critical for resistance to fungi

Most fungi are highly immunogenic and induce strong antibody and T cell-mediated immune responses, which can be detected by serology and delayed-type (type IV) hypersensitivity skin reactions (see Chapter 26).

Considerable evidence points to the dominant protective role of TH1 (and perhaps also TH17 T cells) and phagocyte activation, rather than antibody-mediated responses.

Patients with T cell deficiencies, rather than defects in antibody production, are more at risk of disseminated fungal disease, and antibody titers, though useful as an epidemiological tool to determine exposure, do not necessarily correlate with prognosis. Nevertheless, fungi can elicit both protective and non-protective antibodies and the protection afforded by some experimental vaccines can be adoptively transferred by immune sera.

Resistance to most pathogenic fungi (including dermatophytes and most systemic mycoses including C. neoformans, Histoplasma capsulatum, etc., but not Aspergillus spp.) is clearly dependent upon T cell-mediated immunity, particularly CD4$^+$ TH1 cells secreting IFNγ and to a lesser extent CD8 T cells (Fig. 14.19). As in the case of bacteria, dendritic cells are necessary for this response and produce IL-12 after engulfing fungi.

The clinical relevance of TH1 versus TH2 responses is also clear for some human mycoses, for example:

- individuals with mild paracoccidioidomycosis have TH1-biased immune responses; whereas
- individuals with severe, disseminated infection have high levels of TH2 cytokines such as IL-4 and IL-10, and eosinophilia.

Children with the primary immunodeficiency hyper IgE syndrome have defects in the production of IFNγ, fail to develop TH17 cells and have increased susceptibility to fungal infections.

An increased level of IL-10 (with concomitant reductions in IFNγ) is also a marker of impaired immunity to systemic mycoses, C. albicans, and in neutropenia-associated aspergillosis.

Fungi possess many evasion strategies to promote their survival

Evasion strategies used by fungi to promote their survival include the following:

- Cryptococcus neoformans produces a polysaccharide capsule, which inhibits phagocytosis (similar in principle to that of encapsulated bacteria), though this can be overcome by the opsonic effects of complement and antibodies;
- similarly, Candida conceal the β glucans of their cell wall which would otherwise be efficiently recognized by host dectin-1, underneath an external coat of mannan, a molecule which is considerably less immune-reactive. β glucans are also differentially expressed in the yeast versus filamentous forms of some fungi, contributing to the differences in immune response to these two distinct phases of infection;
- Histoplasma capsulatum is an obligate intracellular pathogen that evades macrophage killing by entering the cell via CR3 and then altering the normal pathways of phagosome maturation, in parallel to the strategies of intracellular bacteria such as M. tuberculosis;
- dermatophytes suppress host T cell responses to delay cell-mediated destruction.

Immune responses to fungi are therefore as complex and interesting as those against bacteria and for many infections (such as the subcutaneous mycoses) these responses remain poorly understood.

New immunological approaches are being developed to prevent and treat fungal infections

Unlike many antibiotics, which are directly microbicidal, antifungal drugs need significant assistance from the immune system to be most effective.

Reducing the underlying immunosuppression that leads to susceptibility to fungi is an important goal and generic immunotherapies such as cytokine administration (using IFNγ in patients with CGD and granulocyte colony stimulating factor [G-CSF] therapy to reduce neutropenia in patients with cancer) have had some success. Human antibodies specific for fungal antigens are being tested for their protective effects by passive transfer. In a clinical trial, administration of Aspergillus specific donor CD4 T cells reduced the incidence of invasive aspergillosis in patients undergoing allogeneic bone marrow transplantation. There is also considerable interest in dendritic cell-based vaccine strategies to promote TH1-mediated immunity.

Evidence for T cell immunity in chromomycosis

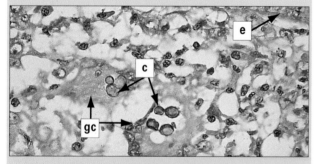

Fig. 14.19 The pigmented fungal cells of chromomycosis (a subcutaneous mycosis) (c) are visible inside giant cells (gc) in the dermis of a patient. The area is surrounded by a predominantly mononuclear cell infiltrate. The basal layer of epidermis (e) is visible at the top of the frame. H & E stain. × 400. (Courtesy of Professor RJ Hay.)

CRITICAL THINKING: IMMUNOENDOCRINE INTERACTIONS IN THE RESPONSE TO INFECTION (SEE P. 437 FOR EXPLANATIONS)

Humans subclinically infected with tuberculosis (about one-third of the world's population) may harbor live organisms for the rest of their lives. Similarly tuberculosis can establish a latent non-progressive infection in mice. If animals with such latent infection are subjected to a period of restraint stress (placed in a tube that limits movement) each day for several days, the infection may reactivate. This also happens if cattle with latent disease are transported in trucks. Similarly tuberculosis increases in human populations in war zones, probably due to reactivation of latent disease.

1 What is the physiology of this reactivation? When American military trainees were subjected to an extremely stressful training schedule their serum IgE levels rose and they lost their previously positive delayed hypersensitivity skin-test responses. The levels of mRNA encoding IFNγ in the peripheral blood mononuclear cells of medical students were lower during the examination period than at other times of the year.

2 Do these observations suggest changes in cytokine profile? If so, why did it happen?

Further reading

Anas A, van der Poll T, de Vos AF. Role of CD14 in lung inflammation and infection. Crit Care 2010;14:209.

Andrea M. Cooper cell-mediated immune responses in tuberculosis. Annu Rev Immunol 2009;27:393–422.

Borghetti P, Saleri R, Mocchegiani E, et al. Infection, immunity and the neuroendocrine response. Vet Immunol Immunopathol 2009;130:141–162.

Cerf-Bensussan N, Gaboriau-Routhiau V. The immune system and the gut microbiota: friends or foes? Nat Rev Immunol 2010;10:735–744.

Cunha C, Romani L, Carvalho A. Cracking the Toll-like receptor code in fungal infections. Expert Rev Anti Infect Ther 2010;8:112.

Curtis MM, Way SS. Interleukin 17 in host defence against bacterial, mycobacterial and fungal pathogens. Immunology 2009;126:177–185.

Davis M, Ramakrishnan L. The role of the granuloma in expansion and dissemination of early tuberculous infection. Cell 2009;136:37–49.

Deretic V. Autophagy in infection. Curr Opin Cell Biol 2010;22:252–262.

Dietrrich J, Doherty TM. Interaction of mycobacterium tuberculosis with the host: consequence for vaccine development. APMIS 2010;117:440–457.

Flannagan RS, Cosio G, Grinstein S. Antimicrobial mechanisms of phagocytes and bacterial evasion strategies. Nat Rev Microbiol 2009;7:355–366.

van de Veerdonk FL, Mihai G. Netea T-cell subsets and antifungal host defenses. Curr Fungal Infect Rep 2010;4:238–243.

Harty JT, Tvinnereim AR, White DW. CD8 + T cell effector mechanisms in resistance to infection. Annu Rev Immunol 2000;18:275–308.

Hazlett L, Wu M. Defensins in innate immunity. Cell Tissue Res 2011;343:175–188.

Hooper LV, Macpherson AJ. Immune adaptations that maintain homeostasis with the intestinal microbiota. Nat Rev Immunol 2010;10:159–169.

Hohl TM, Pamer EG. Cracking the fungal armor. Nat Med 2006;12:730–732.

Hohl TM, Rivera A, Pamer EG. Immunity to fungi. Curr Opin Immunol 2006;18:465–472.

Holt PG, Strickland DH. Soothing signals: transplacental transmission of resistance to asthma and allergy. J Exp Med 2010;206:2861–2864.

Jo EK. Innate immunity to mycobacteria: vitamin D and autophagy. Cell Microbiol 2010;12:1026–1035.

Kaufmann SH, Hussey G, Lambert PH. New vaccines for tuberculosis. Lancet 2010;375:2110–2119.

Kaufmann SH, Schaible UE. Antigen presentation and recognition in bacterial infections. Curr Opin Immunol 2005;17:79–87.

Kronenberg M, Kinjo Y. Innate-like recognition of microbes by invariant natural killer T cells. Curr Opin Immunol 2009;21:391–396.

Kumar V, Sharma A. Neutrophils: Cinderella of innate immune system. Int Immunopharmacol 2010;10:1325–1334.

Lambris JD, Ricklin D, Geisbrecht BV. Complement evasion by human pathogens. Nat Rev Microbiol 2008;6:132–142.

Mackenzie CR, Heselar K, Muller A, Daubener W. Role of indole 2,3-dioxygenase in antimicrobial defence and immune regulation: tryptophan depletion versus production of toxic kynurenes. Curr Drug Metab 2007;8:237–244.

MacLennan C, Fieschi C, Lammas DA, et al. Interleukin (IL)-12 and IL-23 are key cytokines for immunity against Salmonella in humans. J Infect Dis 2004;190:1755–1757.

Monack DM, Mueller A, Falkow S. Persistent bacterial infections: the interface of the pathogen and the host immune system. Nat Rev Microbiol 2004;2:747–765.

Papayannopoulos V, Zychlinsky A. NETs: a new strategy for using old weapons. Trends Immunol 2009;30:513–521.

Park SJ, Mehrad B. Innate immunity to Aspergillus species. Clin Microbiol Rev 2009;22:535–551.

Philpott DJ, Girardin SE. NOD like receptors: sentinels at host membranes. Curr Opin Immunol 2010;22:428–434.

Puel A, Picard C, Cypowyj S, et al. Inborn errors of mucocutaneous immunity to Candida albicans in humans: a role for IL-17 cytokines? Curr Opin Immunol 2010;22:467–474.

Sansonetti PJ. To be or not to be a pathogen: that is the mucosally relevant question. Mucosal Immunol 2011;4:8–14.

Schaible UE, Kaufmann SH. Iron and microbial infection. Nat Rev Microbiol 2004;2:946–953.

Stewart GR, Young DB. Heat-shock proteins and the host–pathogen interaction during bacterial infection. Curr Opin Immunol 2004;16:506–510.

Thornton CA, Macfarlane TV, Holt PG. The hygiene hypothesis revisited: role of maternal–fetal interactions. Curr Allergy Asthma Rep 2010;10:444–452.

Umetsu DT. Revising the immunological theories of asthma and allergy. Lancet 2005;365:98–100.

van de Vosse E, Hoeve MA, Ottenhoff TH. Human genetics of intracellular infectious diseases: molecular and cellular immunity against mycobacteria and salmonellae. Lancet Infect Dis 2004;4:739–749.

Voyich JM, Musser JM, DeLeo FR. *Streptococcus pyogenes* and human neutrophils: a paradigm for evasion of innate host defense by bacterial pathogens. Microbes Infect 2004;6:1117–1123.

Wills-Karp M, Santeliz J, Karp CL. The germless theory of allergic disease: revisiting the hygiene hypothesis. Nat Rev Immunol 2001;1:69–75.

Zelante T, DeLuca A, D'Angelo C, et al. IL-17/T$_H$17 in antifungal immunity: what's new. Eur J Immunol 2009;39:645.

CHAPTER 15

Immunity to Protozoa and Worms

SUMMARY

- **Parasites stimulate a variety of immune defense mechanisms.**

- **Parasitic infections are often chronic and affect many people.** They are generally host specific and most cause chronic infections. Many are spread by invertebrate vectors and have complicated life cycles. Their antigens are often stage specific.

- **Innate immune responses are the first line of immune defense.**

- **T and B cells are pivotal in the development of immunity.** Both CD4 and CD8 T cells are needed for protection from some parasites, and cytokines, chemokines, and their receptors have important roles.

- **Effector cells such as macrophages, neutrophils, eosinophils, and platelets can kill both protozoa and worms.** They secrete cytotoxic molecules such as reactive oxygen radicals and nitric oxide (NO•). All are more effective when activated by cytokines.

- Worm infections are usually associated with an increase in eosinophil number and circulating IgE, which are characteristic of TH2 responses. TH2 cells are necessary for the elimination of intestinal worms.

- **Parasites have many different escape mechanisms to avoid being eliminated by the immune system.** Some exploit the host response for their own development.

- **Inflammatory responses can be a consequence of eliminating parasitic infections.**

- **Parasitic infections have immunopathological consequences.** Parasitic infections are associated with pathology, which can include autoimmunity, splenomegaly, and hepatomegaly. Much immunopathology may be mediated by the adaptive immune response.

- **Vaccines against human parasites are not yet routinely available.**

Parasite infections

Parasitic infections typically stimulate a number of immune defense mechanisms, both antibody and cell mediated, and the responses that are most effective depend upon the particular parasite and the stage of infection. Some of the more important parasitic infections of humans (Fig. 15.1) affect the host in diverse ways. Parasitic protozoa may live:

- in the gut (e.g. amoebae);
- in the blood (e.g. African trypanosomes);
- within erythrocytes (e.g. *Plasmodium* spp.);
- in macrophages (e.g. *Leishmania* spp., *Toxoplasma gondii*);
- in liver and spleen (e.g. *Leishmania* spp.); or
- in muscle (e.g. *Trypanosoma cruzi*).

Parasitic worms that infect humans include trematodes or flukes (e.g. schistosomes), cestodes (e.g. tapeworms), and nematodes or roundworms (e.g. *Trichinella spiralis*, hookworms, pinworms, *Ascaris* spp., and the filarial worms).

Tapeworms and adult hookworms inhabit the gut, adult schistosomes live in blood vessels, and some filarial worms live in the lymphatics (Fig. 15.2). It is clear that there is widespread potential for damaging pathological reactions.

Many parasitic worms pass through complicated life cycles, including migration through various parts of the host's body:

- hookworms and schistosome larvae invade their hosts directly by penetrating the skin;
- tapeworms, pinworms, and roundworms are ingested; and
- filarial worms depend upon an intermediate insect host or vector to transmit them from person to person.

Most protozoa rely upon an insect vector, apart from *Toxoplasma* and *Giardia* spp. and amoebae, which are transmitted by ingestion. Thus:

- malarial parasites are spread by mosquitoes;
- trypanosomes by tsetse flies;
- *T. cruzi* by triatomine bugs; and
- *Leishmania* by sandflies.

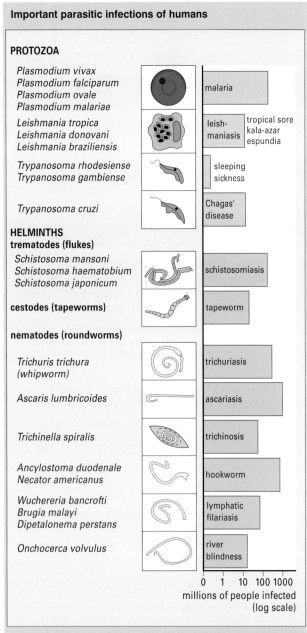

Important parasitic infections of humans

PROTOZOA

Plasmodium vivax
Plasmodium falciparum
Plasmodium ovale
Plasmodium malariae — malaria

Leishmania tropica
Leishmania donovani
Leishmania braziliensis — leish-maniasis / tropical sore / kala-azar / espundia

Trypanosoma rhodesiense
Trypanosoma gambiense — sleeping sickness

Trypanosoma cruzi — Chagas' disease

HELMINTHS
trematodes (flukes)

Schistosoma mansoni
Schistosoma haematobium
Schistosoma japonicum — schistosomiasis

cestodes (tapeworms) — tapeworm

nematodes (roundworms)

Trichuris trichura (whipworm) — trichuriasis

Ascaris lumbricoides — ascariasis

Trichinella spiralis — trichinosis

Ancylostoma duodenale
Necator americanus — hookworm

Wuchereria bancrofti
Brugia malayi
Dipetalonema perstans — lymphatic filariasis

Onchocerca volvulus — river blindness

0   1   10   100 1000
millions of people infected
(log scale)

Fig. 15.1 Important parasitic infections, including data from the World Health Organization (1993). Their sizes range from 1 m for the tapeworm to around 10^{-5} m for *Plasmodium* spp. (cf. Fig. 15.w1).

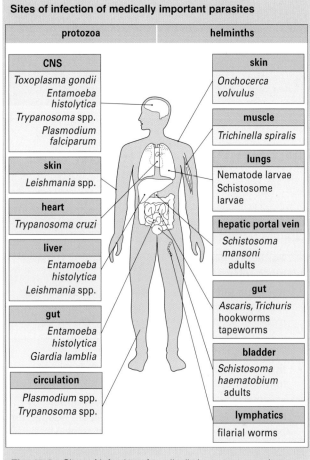

Sites of infection of medically important parasites

protozoa	helminths

protozoa

CNS
Toxoplasma gondii
Entamoeba histolytica
Trypanosoma spp.
Plasmodium falciparum

skin
Leishmania spp.

heart
Trypanosoma cruzi

liver
Entamoeba histolytica
Leishmania spp.

gut
Entamoeba histolytica
Giardia lamblia

circulation
Plasmodium spp.
Trypanosoma spp.

helminths

skin
Onchocerca volvulus

muscle
Trichinella spiralis

lungs
Nematode larvae
Schistosome larvae

hepatic portal vein
Schistosoma mansoni adults

gut
Ascaris, Trichuris hookworms
tapeworms

bladder
Schistosoma haematobium adults

lymphatics
filarial worms

Fig. 15.2 Sites of infection of medically important parasites.

shown that human behavior can account for large variation in exposure between families.

Many parasitic infections are long-lived

It is not in the interest of a parasite to kill its host, at least not until transmission to another host has been ensured. During the course of a chronic infection the type of immune response may change and immunosuppression and immunopathological effects are common.

Host defense depends upon a number of immunological mechanisms

The development of immunity is a complex process arising from the activation of both adaptive and innate immune responses and the switching on of many different kinds of cell over a period of time. Effects are often local and many cell types secreting different mediators may be present at sites of immune rejection. Moreover, the processes involved in controlling the multiplication of a parasite within an infected individual may differ from those responsible for the ultimate development of resistance to further infection.

In some helminth infections a process of 'concomitant immunity' occurs, whereby an initial infection is not eliminated, but becomes established, and the host then acquires resistance to invasion by new parasites, mostly worms, of the same species.

Immune defenses against parasites

Host resistance to parasite infection may be genetic

The resistance of individual hosts to infection varies, and may be controlled by a number of genes. These may be MHC, non-MHC, or other genes (Fig. 15.3).

One should not assume that host genetic background is the only reason determining the outcome of infection. There may be many factors involved. In most helminth infections, for example, a heavy worm burden occurs in comparatively few individuals, but may cluster in families, implying a genetic basis. On the other hand, studies have

Human gene polymorphisms that affect the outcome of parasite infection

parasite	genetic trait
Plasmodium spp.	sickle cell hemoglobin (HbS) protects from malaria certain MHC genes common in West Africans, but rare in Caucasians, protect from malaria (e.g. HLA-B53) Duffy blood group antigen (Fy/Fy)-negative erythrocytes protect from *Plasmodium vivax*
Leishmania spp.	polymorphisms in *Nramp1* govern susceptibility to macrophage invasion
Schistosoma spp.	candidate polymorphic genes on chromosome 5q31-q33, a region that includes key cytokines IL-4 and IL-5
Ascaris spp.	candidate polymorphic genes on chromosomes 1 and 13, a region that includes the TNF family of cytokines

Fig. 15.3 Human gene polymorphisms that affect the outcome of parasite infection.

Adult schistosome worm pairs in mesenteric blood vessels

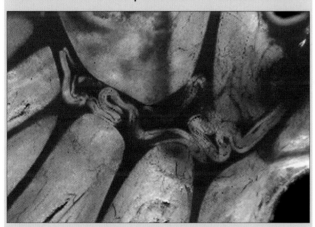

Fig. 15.4 Although very exposed to immune effectors, adult schistosomes are highly resistant and can persist for an average of 3–5 years. *(Courtesy of Dr Alison Agnew.)*

In very general terms, humoral responses are important to eliminate extracellular parasites such as those that live in blood (Fig. 15.4), body fluids, or the gut.

However, the type of response conferring most protection varies with the parasite. For example, antibody, alone or with complement, can damage some extracellular parasites, but is better when acting with an effector cell.

As emphasized above, within a single infection different effector mechanisms act against different developmental stages of parasites. Thus in malaria:

• antibody against extracellular forms blocks their capacity to invade new cells;
• cell-mediated responses prevent the development of the liver stage within hepatocytes.

Innate immune responses

The innate and adaptive immune responses are co-evolving to allow mammals to identify and eliminate parasites.

The innate immune system provides the first line of immune defense by detecting the immediate presence and nature of infection.

Many different cells are involved in generating innate responses including phagocytic cells and NK cells. It is also becoming clear that early recognition of parasites by antigen-presenting cells (APCs), for example dendritic cells, determines the phenotype of the adaptive response (Fig. 15.5).

Innate immune recognition relies on **pattern recognition receptors (PRRs)** that have evolved to recognize pathogen-associated molecular patterns (PAMPs).

Q. Which groups of receptors and soluble molecules recognize PAMPs?
A. Toll-like receptors (see Fig. 6.20), the mannose receptor (see Fig. 7.11) and scavenger receptors (see Fig. 7.10) allow phagocytes to directly recognize pathogens. Ficolins, collectins, and pentraxins act as soluble opsonins by binding to pathogen surfaces (see Fig. 6.w3).

A unifying feature of these targets is their highly conserved structures, which are invariant between parasites of a given class.

Although many parasites are known to activate the immune system in a non-specific manner shortly after infection, it is only recently that attention has been given to the mechanisms involved.

While major advances are being achieved in the area of microbial recognition by PRRs, a small but growing number of studies show that parasites also possess specific molecular patterns capable of engaging PRRs. Examples of some parasite PAMPs along with their receptors are given in Figure 15.6.

Toll-like receptors recognize parasite molecules

The discovery of the TLR family, an evolutionarily conserved group of mammalian PRRs involved in antimicrobial immunity, has enriched our understanding of how innate and adaptive immunity are mutually dependent.

Cytokines secreted by the different subsets of T cells

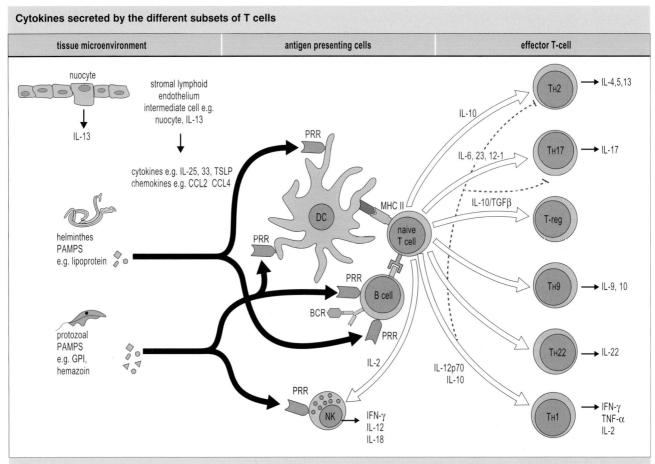

Fig. 15.5 The cytokines secreted by the different subsets of T cells are shown. Note the importance of antigen presenting cells, e.g. DCs and B cells in driving maturation of different TH cell subsets.

A few studies have examined the role of TLRs in immunity to parasites. For example:

- *T. gondii* binds TLR11 via profilin and associates with TLR3, TLR7, and TLR9 via the endoplasmic reticulum protein UNC93B1;
- TLR9 mediates innate immune activation by the malaria pigment hemozoin;
- lyso-phosphatidylserine (lyso-PS) from *S. mansoni*, glycophosphatidylinositol (GPI) anchors, and Tc52 from *T. cruzi* are capable of signaling through TLR2.

Interestingly, TLR2 triggering by these diverse parasite patterns leads to different immune outcomes: for *S. mansoni*, triggering leads to the development of fully mature dendritic cells capable of inducing a Treg response (see Chapter 11), characterized by elevated IL-10 levels; for *T. cruzi*, mature dendritic cells induce a TH1 response (see Chapter 7) with raised levels of IL-12. This dichotomous response could, in part, be explained by the cooperation between TLR2 and other TLRs. However, there has been difficulty in assigning definitive contributions of TLRs to activation by specific parasite proteins since samples are easily contaminated, e.g. with bacterial PAMPs.

Classical human PRRs also contribute to recognition of parasites

Classical PRRs also play important roles in the innate response to parasite infection (see Fig. 15.6) and include collectins (e.g. MBL), pentraxins (e.g. CRP), C-type lectins (e.g. macrophage mannose receptor, and scavenger receptors (e.g. CD36) – see Chapters 6 and 7. For example, MBL binds mannose-rich LPG from *Leishmania*, *Plasmodium*, trypanosomes, and schistosomes; and polymorphisms in the *MBL* gene are associated with increased susceptibility to severe malaria.

Complement receptors are archetypal PRRs

Complement receptors, in particular CR3, are archetypal PRRs involved in innate immune responses (see Fig. 15.6). They are truly multifunctional, being involved in phagocyte adhesion, recognition, migration, activation, and microbe elimination.

Why then is CR3, a linchpin of phagocyte responses, the favored portal of entry for diverse intracellular parasites, including *Leishmania* via LPG?

Innate immune receptors involved in parasite recognition

family	member	parasite ligand(s)
collectins (see Fig. 6.w3)	MBL	mannose-rich sugars from numerous protozoans and helminths
pentraxins	CRP	phospholipids and phosphosugars
		Leishmania spp. LPG
C-type lectins (see Fig. 7.11)	macrophage mannose receptor, DC-SIGN	*Trypanosoma cruzi, Schistosoma* spp. (Lewis X and/or Omega-1)
scavenger receptors (see Fig. 7.10)	SR-B (CD36)	*Plasmodium falciparum* (PfEMP1)
complement receptors	CR1/CR3	*Leishmania* spp. LPG
		Necator NIF
		Plasmodium PfEMP1
Toll-like receptors (see Fig. 6.21)	TLR2 (with TLR1/ TLR6)	GPI anchors from many protozoa
		lyso-PS from *Schistosoma* spp.
	TLR3	double-stranded RNA from *Schistosoma* spp.
	TLR2/6	Diacetylated lipoprotein from the filarial endosymbiont *Wolbachia* spp.
	TLR9	protozoal DNA
		malarial pigment hemozoin

CRP, C-reactive protein; GPI, glycosylphosphatidylinositol; LPG, lipophosphoglycan; lyso-PS, lyso-phosphatidylserine; MBL, mannose-binding lectin; NIF, neutrophil inhibition factor (NIF); PfEMP1, *P. falciparum* erythrocyte membrane protein-1

Fig. 15.6 Innate immune receptors involved in parasite recognition.

- CR3 offers a multiplicity of binding sites, enabling opsonic or non-opsonic binding;
- phagocytosis by CR3 alone does not generate an oxidative burst in phagocytic cells;
- binding of CR3 suppresses the secretion of IL-12.

Q. What effect would suppression of IL-12 secretion have on the immune response?
A. Because IL-12 promotes the development of the TH1 response, reduced expression will tend to reduce macrophage-mediated immunity.

In isolation, CR3 is not an activating receptor. It requires cooperation from other receptors, most notably Fc receptors, for pathogen killing. Helminths have also exploited this chink in the immune armory. Hookworm NIF has been shown to bind a domain in the α subunit of CR3, presumably to downregulate cell-mediated immunity.

Adaptive immune responses to parasites

T and B cells are pivotal in the development of immunity

In most parasitic infections, protection can be conferred experimentally on normal animals by the transfer of spleen cells, especially T cells, from immune animals.

The T cell requirement is also demonstrable because nude (athymic) or T-deprived mice fail to clear otherwise non-lethal infections of protozoa such as *T. cruzi* or *Plasmodium yoelii*, and T cell-deprived rats fail to expel the intestinal worm *Nippostrongylus brasiliensis* (Fig. 15.7).

Counterintuitively, many parasites require signals from immune cells to thrive – for example, schistosomes fail to develop in the absence of hepatic CD4+ lymphocytes.

Parasitic infections in T cell-deprived mice

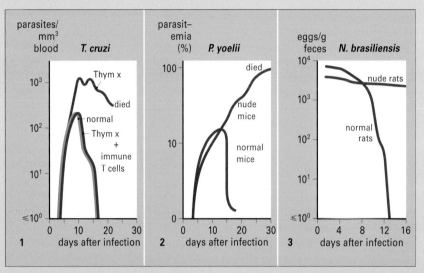

Fig. 15.7   The first two graphs plot the increase in number of blood-borne protozoa (parasitemia) following infection. (**1**) *T. cruzi* multiplies faster (and gives fatal parasitemia) in mice that have been thymectomized and irradiated to destroy T cells (Thym x). In normal mice, parasites are cleared from the blood by day 16. Reconstitution of T cell-deprived mice with T cells from immune mice restores their ability to control the parasitemia. In these experiments both thymectomized groups were given fetal liver cells to restore vital hematopoietic function. (**2**) *P. yoelii* causes a self-limiting infection in normal mice and the parasites are cleared from the blood by day 20. In nude mice the parasites continue to multiply, killing the mice after about 30 days. (**3**) This graph illustrates the time course of the elimination of the intestinal nematode *N. brasiliensis* from the gut of rats. In normal rats the worms are all expelled by day 13, as determined by the number of worm eggs present in the rats' feces. T cells are necessary for this expulsion to occur, as shown by the establishment of a chronic infection in the gut of nude rats.

B cells also play key roles in regulating and controlling immunity to parasites. For example:

- B cells and antibodies are required for resistance to the parasitic gastrointestinal nematode *Trichuris muris*; and
- passive transfer of IgG can protect people from malaria.

Both CD4 and CD8 T cells are needed for protection from some parasites

The type of T cell responsible for controlling an infection varies with the parasite and the stage of infection, and depends upon the kinds of cytokine they produce. For example, $CD4^+$ and $CD8^+$ T cells protect against different phases of *Plasmodium* infection:

- $CD4^+$ T cells mediate immunity against blood-stage *P. yoelii*;
- $CD8^+$ T cells protect against the liver stage of *Plasmodium berghei*.

The action of $CD8^+$ T cells is twofold:

- they secrete IFNγ, which inhibits the multiplication of parasites within hepatocytes;
- they are able to kill infected hepatocytes, but not infected erythrocytes.

Q. By what mechanism are the hepatocytes killed, and why do the $CD8^+$ cells not recognize infected erythrocytes?

A. The $CD8^+$ T cells recognize parasite antigens presented by MHC class I molecules and induce apoptosis in the target, via Fas ligand, tumor necrosis factor (TNFα), lymphotoxin, and granzymes. Erythrocytes do not express MHC molecules.

The immune response against *T. cruzi* depends not only upon $CD4^+$ and $CD8^+$ T cells, but also on NK cells and

antibody production; the same is true for the immune response against *T. gondii*.

$CD8^+$ T cells confer protection in mice depleted of $CD4^+$ T cells, both through their production of IFNγ and because they are cytotoxic for infected macrophages.

NK cells, stimulated by IL-12 secreted by the macrophages, are another source of IFNγ – chronic infections are associated with reduced production of IFNγ.

These observations probably underlie the high incidence of toxoplasmosis in patients with AIDS, who are deficient in $CD4^+$ T cells.

$CD4^+$ T cells are critical for the expulsion of intestinal nematodes and as immunity to *T. muris* can be transferred to a SCID (severe combined immune deficiency) mouse by the transfer of $CD4^+$ T cells alone there is no evidence for a role of $CD8^+$ T cells.

The cytokines produced by $CD4^+$ T cells can be important in determining the outcome of infection. As TH1 and TH2 cells have contrasting and cross-regulating cytokine profiles, the roles of TH1 or TH2 cells in determining the outcome of parasitic infections have been extensively investigated.

As a result of early studies, predominantly in mouse infections, certain dogmas have arisen suggesting that:

- TH1 responses mediate killing of intracellular pathogens; and
- TH2 responses eliminate extracellular ones.

However, this is very much an oversimplification of the true picture, and based on work in animal models that may not fully recapitulate the human immune system.

Although the TH1/TH2 paradigm may be a useful tool in some situations, it is probably more realistic in humans to consider that TH1 and TH2 phenotypes represent the extremes of a continuum of cytokine profiles, and that perhaps it may be more accurate to look at the role of the cytokines themselves in the resolution of infectious disease, particularly as new TH subsets are being discovered, e.g. TH17, TH22, and TH9, and their roles in immunity to parasites investigated.

Regulatory T cells are able to modulate the extremes of both TH2 and TH1 responses.

Cytokines, chemokines, and their receptors have important roles

Q. What experimental methods can be used to elucidate whether a particular cytokine is needed to clear a parasite infection?
A. Experiments with cytokine-knockout animals or cytokine blocking with specific antibody can determine whether a particular cytokine is required. This can be confirmed by observing whether exogenously administered cytokine speeds recovery.

Cytokines not only act on effector cells to enhance their cytotoxic or cytostatic capabilities, but also act as growth factors to increase cell numbers, while chemokines attract cells to the sites of infection. Thus in malaria, the characteristic enlargement of the spleen is caused by an enormous increase in cell numbers.

Other examples include:

• the accumulation of macrophages in the granulomas that develop in the liver in schistosomiasis;
• the eosinophilia characteristic of helminth infections; and
• the recruitment of eosinophils and mast cells into the gut mucosa that occurs in worm infections of the gastrointestinal tract.

Mucosal mast cells and eosinophils are both important in determining the outcome of some helminth infections

and proliferate in response to the products of T cells – IL-3, granulocyte–macrophage colony stimulating factor (GM-CSF), and IL-5 respectively.

However, an increase in cell number can itself harm the host. Thus administration of IL-3 to mice infected with *Leishmania major* can exacerbate the local infection and increase the dissemination of the parasites, probably through the proliferation of bone marrow precursors of the cells the parasites inhabit.

IL-10 and transforming growth factor-β (TGFβ), the regulatory cytokines (see Chapter 11), downregulate the proinflammatory response and thus minimize pathological damage.

Chemokines are key molecules in recruiting immune cells by chemotaxis, but also act in leukocyte activation, hematopoiesis, inflammation, and antiparasite immunity.

Protozoan parasites have been most studied in the context of chemokines and their diverse roles in the parasite–host relationship. For example, *T. gondii* possesses cyclophilin-18, which binds to the chemokine receptor CCR5 and induces IL-12 production by dendritic cells.

T cell responses to protozoa depend on the species

T cell-mediated immunity operating to control protozoan parasites depends on the species of animal infected and the location and complexity of the parasite life cycle within the host.

For example, in mouse models, the induction of TH1 cells with concomitant upregulation of IFNγ and nitric oxide (NO•) is crucial for protection of mice from *Leishmania*. Strains of mice driving TH2 responses on infection, manifested by high levels of IL-4, IL-13, IL-10, and antibody, develop progressive and ultimately lethal disease (Fig. 15.8).

Development of the immune response to *Leishmania major* and *Trichuris muris* infection

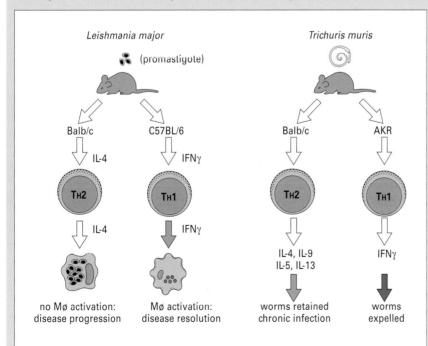

Fig. 15.8 The cytokines secreted by the different subsets of T cells and their effect on the resolution of the disease are shown. Note that resolution of infection is dependent on mouse strain. (Mø, macrophage.)

The polarization of TH cell responses in murine models does not conveniently translate to humans, where both TH1 and TH2 responses appear to be involved in protection

The importance of TH1 cells for protection from toxoplasmosis is also evident in murine models.

For malaria, the TH1/TH2 paradigm is less helpful in understanding immunity, because the type of immune response mounted and the ensuing risk of pathology depends on whether the first exposure to the parasite occurs during infancy or adulthood. As a consequence, immunity to malaria is best thought of in the context of regulated TH1 responses. Thus, in endemic populations, primary malaria infections in infants induce low levels of IFNγ and TNFα via an innate pathway (potentially involving NK cells), which leads to T cell priming.

The infection induces minimal pathology and the parasites can be cleared, either immunologically via maternal antibody or because parasites fail to thrive in fetal hemoglobin. On reinfection, the malaria-primed T cells produce massive amounts of IFNγ and TNFα leading to an increased risk of unwanted pathology, including cerebral malaria.

Q. What effects will IFNγ and TNFα have on cerebral blood vessels?

A. These cytokines cause an increase in adhesion molecules (ICAM-1, VCAM-1) and synthesis of inflammatory chemokines (CCL2, CXCL10) producing leukocyte migration into the brain (see Chapter 6). They also cause an increase in the permeability of the vessels so that large serum molecules enter the CNS, and ionic equilibria are disturbed. This is referred to as a breakdown in the blood–brain barrier.

Further infections induce effective anti-parasite immunity principally through the development of an individual's own repertoire of high-affinity antibodies, which inhibit parasite development. This change in immune environment ultimately leads to a switch in T cell phenotype from TH1 to a regulatory T cell phenotype in which raised levels of IL-10 and TGFβ can be detected.

By contrast, non-immune individuals who contract malaria for the first time in adulthood are unable to control their infections and are more likely to develop severe pathology. This is believed to arise from cross-reactively primed T cells generated against other microbes that appear to contribute to the development of severe disease.

The immune response to worms depends upon TH2-secreted cytokines

IgE and eosinophilia are the hallmarks of the immune response to worm infections, and depend upon cytokines secreted by TH2 cells (see Fig. 15.8).

In humans schistosomiasis and infection with gastrointestinal nematodes, resistance to reinfection after drug treatment is correlated with the production of IgE and high pre-treatment levels of TH2 cytokines such as IL-4, IL-5, and IL-13.

The primary stimuli for TH2 development in schistosomiasis are egg antigens. Similarly the excretory and secretory products of nematodes have been shown to polarize cells towards TH2 responses. Again the control of T cell phenotype

seems to be exerted by the dendritic cell after exposure to these substances.

The mechanisms of induction of TH2 responses are less well understood than TH1 responses.

* one hypothesis, the default hypothesis, suggests that unless the triggers for TH1 responses are received (including high IL-12), TH2 responses occur;
* more recent evidence, however, suggests that specific signals induce the T cell to make TH2 cytokines, probably including cell–cell interactions.

The pattern of cytokine production in infected hosts may be different from that in vaccinated hosts. For example:

* in mice infected with *S. mansoni*, IL-5-producing TH2 cells predominate;
* in mice that have been immunized, IgE levels and eosinophil numbers are low and TH1 cells predominate.

IFNγ activates effector cells that destroy lung stage larvae, via the production of NO•.

Q. How does IFNγ lead to the production of NO•?

A. It causes the production of inducible NO• synthase in macrophages (see Fig. 7.19).

However, when adult worms start to produce eggs, a soluble egg antigen is released that has an effect only in susceptible mice. The antigen reduces levels of IFNγ and increases production of IL-5.

TH2 cytokines control effector mechanisms important in controlling intestinal worm infections. Perhaps the example that demonstrates this most clearly is *T. muris* infection in mice.

* animals normally resistant to infection develop persistent infections in IL-4 and/or IL-13 knockout mice;
* conversely, susceptible mice expel the worms if IL-4 activity is promoted by administration of neutralizing antibody against IFNγ.

IL-9 is another TH2 cytokine that seems to be important in resistance to intestinal nematode infection and is involved in the production of mucosal mast cell responses and the production of IgE. IL-9 transgenic mice that produce higher levels of this cytokine have enhanced expulsion of *T. muris*.

What is clear from a number of studies is that there is no single mechanism by which a TH2 response mediates expulsion of all intestinal worms. The species of worm, its anatomical position within the gut, and the immune status of the host are all factors likely to influence whether a particular immune mechanism will be effective at promoting worm loss.

Some worm infections deviate the immune response

The role of IFNγ in promoting chronic infection is again shown by the administration of IL-12 to mice soon after infection with the intestinal worm *Nippostrongylus braziliensis* (Fig. 15.w2).

N. braziliensis stimulates IFNγ production, which delays expulsion of the worms.

IL-12 acts by inhibiting the production of TH2 cytokines – in particular IL-4 and IL-5, thereby preventing the production of IgE, eosinophilia, and mast cell hypertrophy.

The host may isolate the parasite with inflammatory cells

In some parasitic infections, the immune system cannot completely eliminate the parasite, but reacts by isolating the organism with inflammatory cells. The host reacts to locally released antigen, which stimulates the production of cytokines that recruit cells to the region. An example of this has been shown in mice vaccinated with radiation-attenuated schistosome cercariae. Infiltrating cells, which are mostly TH1-type lymphocytes, surround the lung-stage larvae as early as 24 hours after intravenous challenge infection. This prevents subsequent migration to the site necessary for development into the adult parasite.

The schistosome egg granuloma in the liver is another example of the host reacting by 'walling off' the parasite. This reaction is a chronic cell-mediated response to soluble antigens released by eggs that have become trapped in the liver. Macrophages accumulate and release fibrogenic factors, which stimulate the formation of granulomatous tissue and, ultimately, fibrosis. Although this reaction may benefit the host, in that it insulates the liver cells from toxins secreted by the worm eggs, it is also the major source of pathology, causing irreversible changes in the liver and the loss of liver function. In the absence of T cells, there is no granuloma formation and no subsequent fibrous encapsulation. Different mechanisms may affect:

- worms that inhabit different anatomical sites, such as the gut (e.g. *T. trichura*) or the tissues (e.g. *Onchocerca volvulus*); and
- different stages of the life cycle (e.g. schistosome larvae in the lungs and adult worms in the veins).

Parasites induce non-specific and specific antibody production

Many parasitic infections provoke a non-specific hyper-gammaglobulinemia, much of which is probably due to substances released from the parasites acting as B cell mitogens.

Levels of total immunoglobulins are raised:

- IgM in trypanosomiasis and malaria;
- IgG in malaria and visceral leishmaniasis.

The relative importance of antibody-dependent and antibody-independent responses varies with the infection and host (Fig. 15.9).

The mechanisms by which specific antibody can control parasitic infections and its effects are summarized in Figure 15.10. Antibody:

- can act directly on protozoa to damage them, either by itself or by activating the complement system (Fig. 15.11);
- can neutralize a parasite directly by blocking its attachment to a new host cell, as with *Plasmodium* spp., whose merozoites enter red blood cells through a special receptor – their entry is inhibited by specific antibody (Fig. 15.w3);
- may prevent spread (e.g. in the acute phase of infection by *T. cruzi*);
- can enhance phagocytosis by macrophages – phagocytosis is increased even more by the addition of complement; these effects are mediated by Fc and C3 receptors on macrophages, which may increase in number as a result of macrophage activation;
- is involved in antibody-dependent cell-mediated cytotoxicity (ADCC), for example in infections caused

Relative importance of antibody-dependent and antibody-independent responses in protozoal infections

parasite and habitat		antibody-dependent			antibody-independent	
		importance	mechanism	means of evasion	importance	mechanism
T. brucei free in blood		+ + + +	lysis with complement, which also opsonizes for phagocytosis	antigenic variation	–	
Plasmodium spp. inside red cell		+ + +	blocks invasion, opsonizes for phagocytosis	intracellular; antigenic variation	liver stage + + + blood stage + + +	cytokines macrophage activation
T. cruzi inside macrophage		+ +	limits spread in acute infection, sensitizes for ADCC	intracellular	+ + + (chronic phase)	macrophage activation by IFNγ and TNFα, and killing by NO• and metabolites of O₂
Leishmania spp. inside macrophage		+	limits spread	intracellular	+ + + +	

Fig. 15.9 This table summarizes the relative importance of the two immune responses, the mechanisms involved, and, for antibody, the means by which the protozoon can evade damage by antibody. Antibody is the most important part of the immune response against those parasites that live in the blood stream, such as African trypanosomes and malarial parasites, whereas cell-mediated immunity is active against those like *Leishmania* that live in the tissues. Antibody can damage parasites directly, enhance their clearance by phagocytosis, activate complement, or block their entry into their host cell and so limit the spread of infection. Once inside the cell the parasite is safe from the effects of antibody. *Trypanosoma cruzi* and *Leishmania* spp. are both susceptible to the action of oxygen metabolites released by the respiratory burst of macrophages, and to NO•. Treating macrophages with cytokines enhances release of these products and diminishes the entry and survival of the parasites. (ADCC, antibody-dependent cell-mediated cytotoxicity.)

Mechanisms by which specific antibody controls some parasitic infections

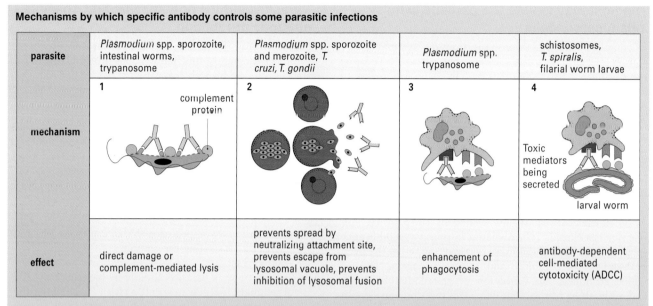

parasite	*Plasmodium* spp. sporozoite, intestinal worms, trypanosome	*Plasmodium* spp. sporozoite and merozoite, *T. cruzi, T. gondii*	*Plasmodium* spp. trypanosome	schistosomes, *T. spiralis*, filarial worm larvae
mechanism	1	2	3	4
effect	direct damage or complement-mediated lysis	prevents spread by neutralizing attachment site, prevents escape from lysosomal vacuole, prevents inhibition of lysosomal fusion	enhancement of phagocytosis	antibody-dependent cell-mediated cytotoxicity (ADCC)

Fig. 15.10 (1) Direct damage. Antibody activates the classical complement pathway, causing damage to the parasite membrane and increasing susceptibility to other mediators. (2) Neutralization. Parasites such as *Plasmodium* spp. spread to new cells by specific receptor attachment; blocking the merozoite binding site with antibody prevents attachment to the receptors on the erythrocyte surface and prevents further multiplication. (3) Enhancement of phagocytosis. Complement C3b deposited on the parasite membrane opsonizes it for phagocytosis by cells with C3b receptors (e.g. macrophages). Macrophages also have Fc receptors. (4) Eosinophils, neutrophils, platelets, and macrophages may be cytotoxic for some parasites when they recognize the parasite via specific antibody (ADCC). The reaction is enhanced by complement.

Direct effect of specific antibody on sporozoites of malaria parasites

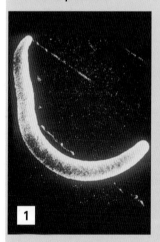
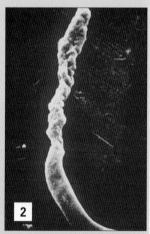

Fig. 15.11 These scanning electron micrographs show a sporozoite of *P. berghei*, which causes malaria in rodents, before (1) and after (2) incubation in immune serum. The surface of the sporozoite is damaged by the antibody, which perturbs the outer membrane, causing leakage of fluid. Specific antibody protects against infection with *Plasmodium* spp. at several of the extracellular stages of the life cycle. The antibody is stage specific in each case. (Courtesy of Dr R Nussenzweig.)

Different antibody isotypes may have different effects. In individuals infected with schistosomes, parasite-specific IgE and IgA are associated with resistance to infection and there is an inverse relationship between the amount of IgE in the blood and reinfection.

Q. What roles does IgE have in immune defense?
A. IgE mediates inflammation by binding to mast cells and basophils, sensitizing them to parasite antigens. Additionally it can act as an opsonin for eosinophils (see Chapter 3). Polyclonal activation of IgE production can inhibit cross-linking of specific IgE on mast cells by 'crowding out'.

IgG4 appears to block the action of IgE; reinfection is more likely in children who have high levels of IgG4 and infection rates are highest in 10–14-year-olds when IgG4 levels are also at their highest. Class switching to IgG4 appears to occur in the context of a modified TH2 response involving the induction of Tregs.

In many infections it is difficult to distinguish between cell-mediated and antibody-mediated responses because both can act in concert against the parasite. This is illustrated in Figure 15.12, which summarizes the immune reaction that can be mounted against schistosome larvae.

Immune effector cells

Macrophages, neutrophils, eosinophils, mast cells and platelets can all damage parasites. Antibody and cytokines produced specifically in response to parasite antigens enhance the antiparasitic activities of all these effector cells, though tissue macrophages, monocytes, and granulocytes have some intrinsic activity before enhancement. The point of entry of the parasite is obviously important, for example:

by *T. cruzi, T. spiralis, S. mansoni*, and filarial worms – cytotoxic cells such as macrophages, neutrophils, and eosinophils adhere to antibody-coated worms by means of their Fc and C3 receptors and degranulate, spilling their toxic contents onto the worm (see Fig. 15.13).

Possible effector responses to schistosomules

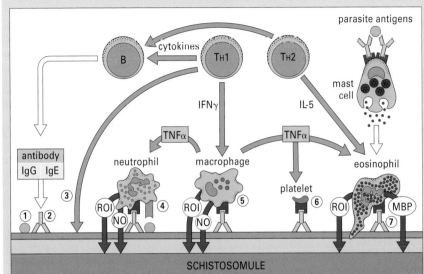

Fig. 15.12 The various effector mechanisms damaging schistosomes *in vitro* are shown. Complement alone damages worms (**1**) and also does so in combination with antibody (**2**). TH1 cells may act directly, reducing the number of larvae in the lungs (**3**). Antibody sensitizes neutrophils (**4**), macrophages (**5**), platelets (**6**), and eosinophils (**7**) for ADCC. Neutrophils and macrophages probably act by releasing toxic oxygen and nitrogen metabolites, whereas eosinophils damage the worm tegument by the release of major basic protein (MBP) plus reactive oxygen intermediates (ROI). The response is potentiated by cytokines (e.g. TNFα). IgE antibody is important in sensitizing both eosinophils and local mast cells, which release a variety of mediators, including those that activate the eosinophils.

- the cercariae of *S. mansoni* enter through the skin – experimental depletion of macrophages, neutrophils, and eosinophils from the skin of mice increases their susceptibility to infection;
- trypanosomes and malarial parasites entering the blood are removed from the circulation by phagocytic cells in the skin, spleen and liver;
- comparison of strains of mice with various immunological defects for their resistance to infection by *Trypanosoma rhodesiense* shows that the African trypanosomes are destroyed by macrophages, and later in infection, when opsonized with antibodies and complement C3b, they are taken up by macrophages in the liver more quickly still.

Before acting as APCs initiating an immune response, macrophages act as effector cells to inhibit the multiplication of parasites or even to destroy them. They also secrete molecules that regulate the inflammatory response:

- some of these molecules – IL-1, IL-12, TNFα, and the colony stimulating factors (CSFs) – enhance immunity by activating other cells or stimulating their proliferation;
- others, like IL-10, prostaglandins, and TGFβ, may be anti-inflammatory and immunosuppressive.

Macrophages can kill extracellular parasites

Phagocytosis by macrophages provides an important defense against the smaller parasites. Macrophages also secrete many cytotoxic factors, enabling them to kill parasites without ingesting them.

When activated by cytokines, macrophages can kill both relatively small extracellular parasites, such as the erythrocytic stages of malaria, and also larger parasites, such as the larval stages of the schistosome. Macrophages also:

- act as killer cells through ADCC – specific IgG and IgE, for instance, enhance their ability to kill schistosomules;

- secrete cytokines, such as TNFα and IL-1, which interact with other types of cell, for example rendering hepatocytes resistant to malarial parasites.

Reactive oxygen intermediates (ROIs) are generated by macrophages and granulocytes following phagocytosis of *T. cruzi*, *T. gondii*, *Leishmania* spp., and malarial parasites, for instance. Filarial worms and schistosomes also stimulate the respiratory burst.

When activated by cytokines, macrophages release more superoxide and hydrogen peroxide than normal resident macrophages, and their oxygen-independent killing mechanisms are similarly enhanced.

Nitric oxide, a product of L-arginine metabolism, is another potent toxin. Its synthesis by macrophages in mouse experimental systems is induced by the cytokines IFNγ and TNFα and is greatly increased when they act synergistically. NO• can also be produced by endothelial cells. It contributes to host resistance in leishmaniasis, schistosomiasis, and malaria, and is probably important in the control of most parasitic infections (see Fig. 15.13). For instance, the innate resistance to infection by *T. gondii* that is lost in immunocompromised individuals appears to be due to the inhibition of parasite multiplication by such an oxygen-independent mechanism.

Activation of macrophages is a feature of early infection

All macrophage effector functions are enhanced soon after infection. Although their specific activation is by cytokines secreted by T cells (e.g. IFNγ, GM-CSF, IL-3, and IL-4), they can also be activated by T cell-independent mechanisms, for example:

- NK cells secrete IFNγ when stimulated by IL-12 produced by macrophages;
- macrophages secrete TNFα in response to some parasite products (e.g. phospholipid-containing antigens of malarial parasites and some *T. brucei* antigens) – this TNFα then activates other macrophages.

Although TNFα may be secreted by several other cell types, activated macrophages are the most important source of TNFα, which is necessary for protective responses to several species of protozoa (e.g. *Leishmania* spp.) and helminths. Thus TNFα activates macrophages, eosinophils, and platelets to kill the larval form of *S. mansoni*, its effects being enhanced by IFNγ.

TNFα may be harmful as well as beneficial to the infected host, depending upon the amount produced and whether it is free in the circulation or locally confined. Serum concentrations of TNFα in falciparum malaria correlate with the severity of the disease. Administration of TNFα cures a susceptible strain of mice infected with the rodent malarial parasite *Plasmodium chabaudi*, but kills a genetically resistant strain. Presumably the latter can already make enough TNFα to control parasite replication, and any more has toxic effects.

Neutrophils can kill large and small parasites

The effector properties displayed by macrophages are also seen in neutrophils. Neutrophils are phagocytic and can kill by both oxygen-dependent and oxygen-independent mechanisms, including NO•. They produce a more intense respiratory burst than macrophages and their secretory granules contain highly cytotoxic proteins.

> **Q. Which groups of cytotoxic protein are found in neutrophil granules?**
> A. Defensins, seprocidins, and cathelicidins (see Chapter 2).

Neutrophils can be activated by cytokines, such as IL-8, IFNγ, TNFα, and GM-CSF.

Extracellular destruction by neutrophils is mediated by hydrogen peroxide, whereas granular components are involved in the intracellular destruction of ingested organisms.

Neutrophils are present in parasite-infected inflammatory lesions and probably act to clear parasites from bursting cells.

Like macrophages, neutrophils bear Fc and complement receptors and can participate in antibody-dependent cytotoxic reactions to kill the larvae of *S. mansoni*, for example. In this mode, they can be more destructive than eosinophils against several species of nematode, including *T. spiralis*, though the relative effectiveness of the two types of cell may depend upon the isotype and specificity of antibody present.

Eosinophils are characteristically associated with worm infections

It has been suggested that:

- the eosinophil evolved specifically as a defense against the tissue stages of parasites that are too large to be phagocytosed;
- the IgE-dependent mast cell reaction has evolved primarily to localize eosinophils near the parasite and enhance their antiparasitic functions.

The importance of eosinophils *in vivo* has been shown by experiments using antiserum against eosinophils. Mice infected with *T. spiralis* and treated with the antiserum develop more cysts in their muscles than the controls – without the protection offered by eosinophils, the mice

cannot eliminate the worms and so encyst the parasites to minimize damage.

However, recent work has shown that although eosinophils can help the host to control a worm infection, particularly by limiting migration through the tissues, they do not always do so. For instance, their removal does not abolish the immunity of mice infected with *S. mansoni*, nor does this increase the parasite load in a tapeworm infection.

Removal of IL-5, which is important in the generation and activation of eosinophils, did not change the outcome of *T. spiralis* or *T. muris* infection. In contrast the infectivity of *Strongyloides venezuelensis* is enhanced in IL-5-deficient mice. Although *T. spiralis* worm burdens were not affected in a primary infection of IL-5 deleted mice, the worm numbers were significantly higher after challenge infection.

The role of IL-5 and therefore eosinophils has also been suggested from human epidemiological studies on gastrointestinal nematode infections where, after drug treatment, low reinfection worm burdens were associated with high pre-treatment levels of IL-5.

Elevated eosinophilia is often associated with high levels of IgE, both of which are hallmarks of infection with parasites. Although eosinophils express FcεRI, most of the protein is confined to the cytoplasm, and there is little evidence for IgE-dependent function.

Eosinophils can kill helminths by oxygen-dependent and independent mechanisms

Eosinophils are less phagocytic than neutrophils. They degranulate in response to perturbation of their surface membrane and their activities are enhanced by cytokines such as TNFα and GM-CSF. Most of their activities, however, are controlled by antigen-specific mechanisms. Thus their binding *in vitro* to the larvae of worms (e.g. *S. mansoni* and *T. spiralis*) increases the release of their granular contents onto the surface of the worms (Fig. 15.13).

Damage to schistosomules can be caused by the major basic protein (MBP) of the eosinophil crystalloid core. MBP is not specific for any particular target, but because it is

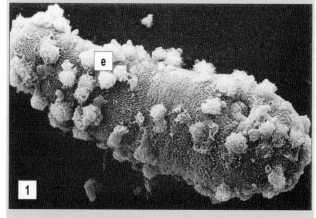

Eosinophil adhesion and degranulation

Fig. 15.13   A schistosomule being killed by eosinophils from mouse bone marrow, cultured in the presence of IL-5. The larval helminth has been first treated with IgG and the eosinophils adhere by means of their Fcγ receptors. *(Courtesy of Dr C Sanderson.)*

confined to a small space between the eosinophil and the schistosome, there is little damage to nearby host cells.

Eosinophils and mast cells can act together

The killing of *S. mansoni* larvae by eosinophils is enhanced by mast cell products, and when studied *in vitro* eosinophils from patients with schistosomiasis are found to be more effective than those from normal subjects. The antigens released cause local IgE-dependent degranulation of mast cells and the release of mediators. These selectively attract eosinophils to the site and further enhance their activity. Other products of eosinophils later block the mast cell reactions. These effector mechanisms may function *in vivo*, as has been shown in monkeys, where schistosome killing is associated with eosinophil accumulation.

Mast cells control gastrointestinal helminths

In the case of *T. spiralis* and *Heligmosomoides polygyrus* there is good evidence to suggest the involvement of mucosal mast cells (Fig. 15.14)

Following mast cell activation, the mast cell contents are released resulting in changes to the permeability of the intestinal epithelium and ultimately an environment that appears hostile for continued *T. spiralis* survival. By contrast, expulsion of *N. braziliensis* and *T. muris* still proceeds normally following depression of mastocytosis, suggesting that the mast cell is not the major effector cell type.

Therefore, although TH2 cytokines are critical for the elimination of worms from the gut, the exact effector mechanism may vary.

Platelets can kill many types of parasite

Potential targets for platelets include the larval stage of flukes, *T. gondii*, and *T. cruzi*.

Like other effector cells, the cytotoxic activity of platelets is enhanced by treatment with cytokines (e.g. IFNγ and TNFα). In rats infected with *S. mansoni*, platelets become larvicidal when acute phase reactants appear in the serum but before antibody can be detected. Incubation of normal platelets in such serum can cause their activation.

Platelets, like macrophages and the other effector cells, also bear Fcε and Fcγ receptors, by which they mediate antibody-dependent cytotoxicity associated with IgE.

Parasite escape mechanisms

It is a necessary characteristic of all successful parasitic infections that they can evade the full effects of their host's immune responses. Parasites have developed many different ways of doing this. Some even exploit cells and molecules of the immune system to their own advantage – *Leishmania* parasites, by using complement receptors to gain entry into macrophages, avoid triggering the oxidative burst and thus destruction by its toxic products.

Despite their protective role in the immune response to many different parasites:

- host TNFα actually stimulates egg production by adult worms of *S. mansoni*;
- IFN is used as a growth factor by *T. brucei*.

Parasites can resist destruction by complement

In the case of *Leishmania*, resistance correlates with virulence:

- *L. tropica*, which is easily killed by complement, causes a localized self-healing infection in the skin; whereas
- *L. donovani*, which is ten times more resistant to complement, becomes disseminated throughout the viscera, causing a disease that is often fatal.

The mechanisms whereby parasites can resist the effect of complement differ:

- the lipophosphoglycan (LPG) surface coat of *L. major* activates complement, but the complex is then shed so the parasite avoids lysis;
- the trypomastigotes of *T. cruzi* bear a surface glycoprotein that has activity resembling the decay accelerating factor (DAF) that limits the complement reaction. The resistance that schistosomules acquire as they mature is also correlated with the appearance of a surface molecule similar to DAF.

Section through the gut of a mouse infected with *Heligmosomoides polygyrus*

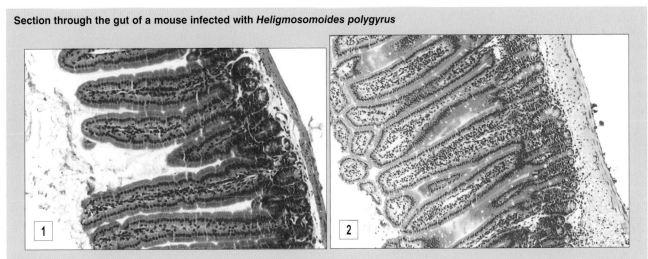

Fig. 15.14 (**1**) Gut of an uninfected mouse. (**2**) Gut of an infected mouse. The crypts have shortened and a large influx of mast cells can be clearly seen.

Intracellular parasites can avoid being killed by oxygen metabolites and lysosomal enzymes

Intracellular parasites that live inside macrophages have evolved different ways of avoiding being killed by oxygen metabolites and lysosomal enzymes (Fig. 15.15):

- *T. gondii* penetrates the macrophage by a non-phagocytic pathway and so avoids triggering the oxidative burst;
- *Leishmania* spp. can enter by binding to complement receptors – another way of avoiding the respiratory burst.

Leishmania organisms also possess enzymes such as super-oxide dismutase, which protects them against the action of oxygen radicals.

It can be demonstrated that the vacuole in which *Leishmania* organisms survive is lyosomal in nature (Fig. 15.16), but the parasites have evolved mechanisms that protect it against enzymatic attack. The LPG surface coat acts as a scavenger of oxygen metabolites and affords protection against enzymatic attack, but a glycoprotein, Gp63 (Fig 15.w4) inhibits the action of the macrophage's lysosomal enzymes.

Leishmania spp. can also downregulate the expression of MHC class II molecules on the macrophages they inhabit, thus reducing their capacity to stimulate TH cells.

These escape mechanisms, however, are less efficient in the immune host.

Q. Why would reduction in MHC molecule expression be less effective in an immune host?

A. In immune hosts, the release of IFNγ enhances MHC molecule expression by APCs. In addition the level of stimulation required by a primed T cell is less than for a naive T cell, due in part to its enhanced level of receptors for co-stimulatory signals (see Chapter 8).

Parasites can disguise themselves

Parasites that are vulnerable to specific antibody have evolved different methods of evading its effects.

African trypanosomes and malaria undergo antigenic variation

The molecule that forms the surface coat of the African trypanosome, the variable surface glycoprotein (VSG), changes to protect the underlying surface membrane from the host's

The leishmanial vacuole is lysosomal in nature

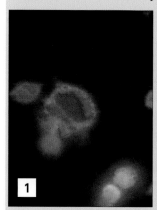
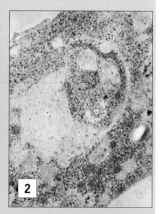

Fig. 15.16 (**1**) Immunofluorescence of *Leishmania mexicana*-infected murine macrophages probed with a rhodamine-conjugated anti-tubulin antibody to illustrate the parasite (stained yellow/red) and a fluorescein-conjugated monoclonal antibody, which reacts with the late endosomal/lysosomal marker LAMP-1 (stained green). (**2**) Immunoelectron micrograph of *L. mexicana*-infected murine macrophage probed with gold-labeled anti-cathepsin D demonstrating the lysosomal aspartic proteinase in the leishmanial vacuole. *(Courtesy of Dr David Russell.)*

The different ways by which protozoa that multiply within macrophages escape digestion by lysosomal enzymes

Toxoplasma gondii	*Trypanosoma cruzi*	*Leishmania* spp.
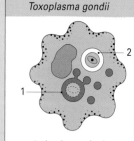	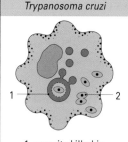	
1. dead parasite in phagosome – fusion with lysosome	1. parasite killed in phagosome following lysosomal fusion	1. parasites resist lysosomal enzyme and divide inside phagosome
2. live parasite in endosome – no fusion with lysosome	2. parasites escape phagosome and divide free in cytoplasm	

Fig. 15.15 *T. gondii* – live parasites enter the cell actively into a membrane-bound vacuole. They are not attacked by enzymes because lysosomes do not fuse with this vacuole. Dead parasites, however, are taken up by normal phagocytosis into a phagosome (by interaction with the Fc receptors on the macrophage if they are coated with antibody) and are then destroyed by the enzymes of the lysosomes that fuse with it. *T. cruzi* – survival of these parasites depends upon their stage of development; trypomastigotes escape from the phagosome and divide in the cytoplasm whereas epimastigotes do not escape and are killed. The proportion of parasites found in the cytoplasm is decreased if the macrophages are activated. *Leishmania* spp. – These parasites multiply within the phagosome and the presence of a surface protease helps them resist digestion. If the macrophages are first activated by cytokines, the number of parasites entering the cell and the number that replicate diminish.

Antigenic variation in trypanosomes

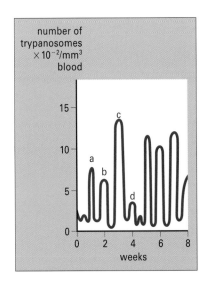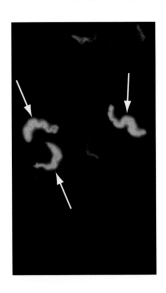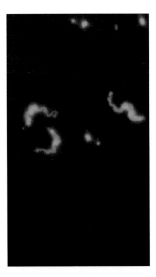

Fig. 15.17 Trypanosome infections may run for several months giving rise to successive waves of parasitemia. The graph shows a chart of the fluctuation in parasitemia in a patient with sleeping sickness. Although infection was initiated by a single parasite, each wave is caused by an immunologically distinct population of parasites (a, b, c, d); protection is not afforded by antibody against any of the preceding variants. There is a strong tendency for new variants to appear in the same order in different hosts. The micrographs show immunofluorescent labeling of trypanosomes with a variant antigen-type specific monoclonal antibody (left). The panel on the right shows the same field but with the nuclei and kinetoplasts of all the parasites stained with a dye that binds to DNA. Only some of the parasites express a given antigen variant. *(Courtesy of Dr Mike Turner.)*

defense mechanisms. New populations of parasites are antigenically distinct from previous ones (Fig. 15.17).

Several antigens of malarial parasites also undergo antigenic variation.

For example, the *P. falciparum* erythrocyte membrane protein-1 (PfEMP1) is extremely polymorphic and variable between different strains of the parasite because it is perpetually exposed to the immune system by its location on the red cell membrane. PfEMP1 can bind numerous host immune proteins, but particularly scavenger receptors, e.g. CD36 and scavenging antibodies that eliminate apoptotic, or damaged cells, e.g. natural IgM (see Fig. 15.20).

Other parasites acquire a surface layer of host antigens

Schistosomes acquire a surface layer of host antigens so that the host does not distinguish them from 'self'. Schistosomules cultured in medium containing human serum and red blood cells can acquire surface molecules containing A, B, and H blood group determinants. They can also acquire MHC molecules and immunoglobulins. However, schistosomules maintained in a medium devoid of host molecules also become resistant to attack by antibody and complement, as mentioned above.

Some extracellular parasites hide from or resist immune attack

Some species of protozoa (e.g. *Entamoeba histolytica*) and helminths (e.g. *T. spiralis*) form protective cysts, while adult worms of *Onchocerca volvulus* in the skin induce the host to surround them with collagenous nodules.

Intestinal nematodes and tapeworms are preserved from many host responses simply because they live in the gut.

There are numerous examples of simple, physical, protective strategies in parasites:

- nematodes have a thick extracellular cuticle, which protects them from the toxic effects of an immune response;
- the tegument of schistosomes thickens during maturation to offer similar protection;
- the loose surface coat of many nematodes may slough off under immune attack;
- tapeworms actually prevent attack by secreting an elastase inhibitor, which stops them attracting neutrophils.

Many parasitic worms have evolved methods of resisting the oxidative burst. For instance, schistosomes have surface-associated glutathione S-transferases, and *Onchocerca* spp. can secrete superoxide dismutase.

Some nematodes and trematodes have evolved an elegant method of disabling antibodies by secreting proteases, which cleave immunoglobulins, removing the Fc portion, and preventing their interaction with Fc receptors on phagocytic cells; for example, schistosomes can cleave IgE.

Most parasites interfere with immune responses for their benefit

Parasites produce molecules that interfere with host immune function

Parasites produce molecules that can affect the phenotype of the adaptive response, which may be to their own advantage (Figs 15.18 and 15.19).

Some mechanisms by which parasites avoid host immunity

parasite	habitat	main host effector mechanism	method of avoidance
Trypanosoma brucei	blood stream	antibody + complement	antigenic variation
Plasmodium spp.	hepatocyte blood stream	T cells, antibody	antigenic variation, sequestration
Toxoplasma gondii	macrophage	ROI, NO•, lysosomal enzymes	suppresses IL-12, inhibits fusion of lysozymes
Trypanosoma cruzi	many cells	ROI, NO•, lysosomal enzymes	escapes to cytoplasm so avoiding digestion
Leishmania spp.	macrophage	ROI, NO•, lysosomal enzymes	induction of Tregs, resists digestion by phagolysosome
Schistosoma spp.	skin, blood, lungs, portal veins	myeloid cells antibody + complement	acquisition of host antigens (e.g. IgG), proteolytic cleavage of immune proteins, inhibition of dendritic cell maturation
filariasis	lymphatics	myeloid cells	induction of Tregs, secretion of cytokine mimics, interference with antigen processing

NO•, nitric oxide; ROI, reactive oxygen intermediates

Fig. 15.18 A summary of the various methods that parasites have evolved to avoid host defense mechanisms.

In leishmaniasis, T cells from patients infected with *L. donovani* when cultured with specific antigen do not secrete IL-2 or IFNγ. Their production of IL-1 and expression of MHC class II molecules is also decreased, whereas secretion of prostaglandins is increased. IL-2, characteristic of TH1 responses, is also deficient in other protozoal infections including malaria, African trypanosomiasis, and Chagas' disease. In mice infected with *T. cruzi*, a parasite product appears to interfere with expression of the IL-2 receptor.

Filarial worms secrete a protease inhibitor that has been shown to affect the proteases critical in the processing of antigens to peptides resulting in the reduction of class II molecule presentation in filariasis. Onchocystatin – one such protease inhibitor – is also able to modulate T cell proliferation and elicit the upregulation of IL-10 expression and is therefore able to modulate the T cell phenotype. Prostaglandins (PGs) produced by helminth parasites may also perform a similar role by modulating APC function. PGE2 is produced by filarial parasites and tapeworms and blocks the production of IL-12 by dendritic cells and thus may direct responses towards TH2.

Phosphorylcholine (PC)-containing molecules are commonly found in infectious organisms and experiments using a nematode PC-bearing glycoconjugate, ES-62, have been shown to desensitize APCs to subsequent exposure to LPS and may therefore also skew against a TH1 response (LPS is a classical inducer of TH1 responses). ES-62 is able to inhibit proliferation of T cells and B cells and inhibit IgE-mediated mast cell responses.

Parasites also produce cytokine-like molecules mimicking TGFβ, migration inhibitory factor (MIF), and a histamine-releasing factor.

Genes encoding possible cytokine homologs are being found as part of the genome sequencing projects that are under way for many parasites. Although the sequences are related to cytokines or cytokine receptors, their functions remain to be established.

Soluble parasite antigens released in huge quantities may impair the host's response by a process termed immune distraction. Thus the soluble antigens (S or heat-stable antigens) of *P. falciparum* are thought to mop up circulating antibody, providing a 'smokescreen' and diverting the antibody from the body of the parasite.

Many of the surface antigens that are shed are soluble forms of molecules inserted into the parasite membrane by a GPI anchor, including the VSG of *T. brucei*, the LPG or 'excreted factor' of *Leishmania* (see Fig. 15.w4) and several surface antigens of schistosomules. These are released by endogenous phosphatidylinositol-specific phospholipases.

The hypergammaglobulinemic immunoglobulins induced by malaria parasites can bind to FcγRIIB, which may benefit the parasite.

Q. Which cells express FcγRIIB and what effect does ligation of this receptor have on them?
A. B cells express the receptor and ligation inhibits B cell function.

Some immunomodulatory effects of parasites

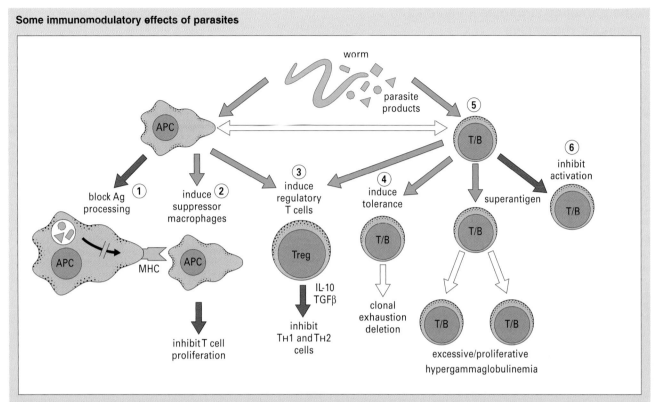

Fig. 15.19 Interference with the host's immune response by molecules released by protozoa or worms. Parasite products act via the APC to (**1**) interfere with antigen processing or presentation (e.g. protease inhibitors from filarial parasites interfere with proteases in the MHC signaling pathway and block antigen presentation); (**2**) induce suppressor macrophages, which can inhibit T cell proliferation; (**3**) induce regulatory T cells (e.g. lyso-PS from schistosomes acts via TLR2 on dendritic cells to induce T cells that secrete IL-10, which inhibits the inflammatory response). Parasite products may also affect lymphocytes to (**3**) make them become regulatory; (**4**) induce T or B cell tolerance by clonal exhaustion or by the induction of anergy; (**5**) cause polyclonal activation (many parasite products are mitogenic to T or B cells, and the high serum concentrations of non-specific IgM [and IgG] commonly found in parasitic infections probably result from this polyclonal stimulation – its continuation is believed to lead to impairment of B cell function, the progressive depletion of antigen-reactive B cells, and thus immunosuppression); (**6**) directly inhibit the activation of T or B cells (e.g. ES-62, a secreted product of a filarial parasite, is able to inhibit the proliferation of both T and B cells).

Malarial pathology resulting from interactions with PfEMP1

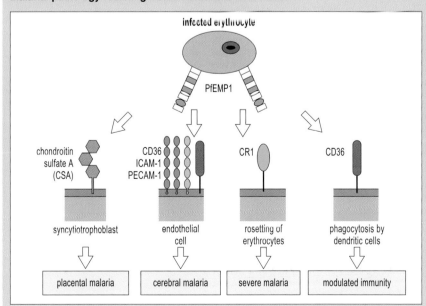

Fig. 15.20 Malaria-infected erythrocytes cause disease through many mechanisms involving the interaction between *P. falciparum* erythrocyte membrane protein-1 (PfEMP1) and diverse host receptors.

Some parasites suppress inflammation or immune responses

Immunosuppression is a common feature of chronic helminth infections, both parasite-specific and generalized. For example, patients with schistosomiasis and filariasis have diminished responsiveness to antigens from the infecting parasite. Studies have also shown diminished responses to bystander infections and vaccinations. This spillover suppression may in fact be beneficial to the host in some situations. For example, reduced inflammatory responses have been observed in *Helicobacter pylori* infection with malaria.

Parasites have co-evolved with humans over millions of years and until recently it was normal for people to carry worms, a fact that argues for their importance in the 'hygiene hypothesis', which proposes that the rise in immune disorders, including allergies and autoimmune illness, is due to cleaner living conditions and the almost complete elimination of parasitic infections in westernized societies.

The ability of parasites to suppress hyperactive immune responses is believed to be due to the induction of regulatory T cells (see Fig. 15.19). Understanding how regulatory T cells, also known as suppressor T cells, are induced and how they dampen immune responses is the focus of intensive research. It seems to be the dendritic cell that polarizes the T cell towards a regulator phenotype after exposure to parasite extracts.

Immunopathological consequences of parasite infections

Apart from the directly destructive effects of some parasites and their products on host tissues, many immune responses themselves have pathological effects.

In malaria, African trypanosomiasis, and visceral leishmaniasis, the increased number and heightened activity of macrophages and lymphocytes in the liver and spleen lead to enlargement of those organs. In schistosomiasis much of the pathology results from the T cell-dependent granulomas forming around eggs in the liver. The gross changes in individuals with elephantiasis are probably caused by immunopathological responses to adult filariae in the lymphatics.

The formation of immune complexes is common – they may be deposited in the kidney, as in the nephrotic syndrome of quartan malaria, and may give rise to many other pathological changes. For example, tissue bound immunoglobulins have been found in the muscles of mice infected with African trypanosomes and in the choroid plexus of mice with malaria.

The IgE of worm infections can have severe effects on the host due to release of mast cell mediators. Anaphylactic shock may occur when a hydatid cyst ruptures. Asthma-like reactions occur in *T. canis* infections and in tropical pulmonary eosinophilia when filarial worms migrate through the lungs.

Autoantibodies, which probably arise as a result of polyclonal activation, have been detected against red blood cells, lymphocytes, and DNA (e.g. in trypanosomiasis and in malaria).

Antibodies against the parasite may cross-react with host tissues. For example, the chronic cardiomyopathy, enlarged esophagus, and megacolon that occur in Chagas' disease are thought to result from the autoimmune effects on nerve ganglia of antibody and Tc cells that cross-react with *T. cruzi*. Similarly *O. volvulus*, the cause of river blindness, possesses an antigen that cross-reacts with a protein in the retina.

Excessive production of cytokines may contribute to some of the manifestations of disease. Thus the fever, anemia, diarrhea, and pulmonary changes of acute malaria closely resemble the symptoms of endotoxemia and are probably caused by TNFα. The severe wasting of cattle with trypanosomiasis may also be mediated by TNFα.

A single parasite protein may produce multiple pathological effects, as seen with PfEMP1, coded by the *var* genes, and expressed on the surface of infected erythrocytes (Fig. 15.20).

Lastly, the non-specific immunosuppression that is so widespread probably explains why people with parasitic infections are especially susceptible to bacterial and viral infections (e.g. measles). It may also account for the association of Burkitt's lymphoma with malaria because malaria-infected individuals are less able to control infection with the Epstein–Barr virus that causes Burkitt's lymphoma.

CRITICAL THINKING: IMMUNITY TO PROTOZOA AND HELMINTHS (SEE P. 437 FOR EXPLANATIONS)

1 In general, protozoa and helminths adopt different strategies for survival and for transmission to the subsequent host. How do they differ?

2 Many parasites have evolved to live in host cells. Consider the advantages and disadvantages to this mode of existence. Consider the different cell types and how parasites have to adapt this environment to their advantage. In particular *Toxoplasma gondii*,

Trypanosoma cruzi, and *Leishmania* spp. have adapted to live in the macrophage and can escape destruction by lysosomal enzymes, but the way in which they do this differs. How have these adaptations helped parasite survival?

3 Extracellular parasites have evolved sophisticated mechanisms to avoid the immune response. Consider examples of how they do this.

Further reading

Anthony RM, Rutitzky LI, Urban JF Jr, et al. Protective immune mechanisms in helminth infection. Nat Rev Immunol 2007;7:975–987.

Couper KN, Blount DG, Riley EM. IL-10: the master regulator of immunity to infection. J Immunol 2008;180:5771–5777.

Czajkowsky DM, Salanti A, Ditlev SB, et al. IgM, Fc mu Rs, and malarial immune evasion. J Immunol 2010;184:4597–4603.

Erb KJ. Helminths, allergic disorders and IgE-mediated immune responses: where do we stand? Eur J Immunol 2007;37:1170–1173.

Langhorne J, Ndungu FM, Sponaas AM, Marsh K. Immunity to malaria: more questions than answers. Nat Immunol 2008;9:725–732.

Martinez FO, Helming L, Gordon S. Alternative activation of macrophages: an immunologic functional perspective. Annu Rev Immunol 2009;27:451–483.

Paul WE, Zhu J. How are T(H)2-type immune responses initiated and amplified? Nat Rev Immunol 2010;10:225–235.

Pleass RJ, Behnke JM. B-cells get the T-cells but antibodies get the worms. Trends Parasitol 2009;25:443–446.

Soong L. Modulation of dendritic cell function by Leishmania parasites. J Immunol 2008;180:4355–4360.

Voehringer D. The role of basophils in helminth infection. Trends Parasitol 2009;25:551–556.

Websites

Various news groups on the www (though not all dedicated to immunology) can be accessed by exploring keywords

Several discussion groups operate through the bionet, for example http://www.bio.net/archives.html (a parasitology mail newsgroup) and http://www.parasitology.org.uk (British Society for Parasitology)

CHAPTER 16

Primary Immunodeficiencies

SUMMARY

- **Primary immunodeficiency diseases** result from intrinsic defects in cells and mediators of the innate and adaptive immune system.

- **Defects in B cell function** result in recurrent pyogenic infections. Defective antibody responses are due to failure of B cell function, as occurs in X-linked agammaglobulinemia, or failure of proper T cell signals to B cells, as occurs in hyper-IgM (HIgM) syndrome and common variable immunodeficiency (CVID).

- **Defects in T cell function** due to ineffective antigen presentation or immune recognition result in susceptibility to opportunistic infections. Other abnormalities of T cells may also lead to immune dysregulation with autoimmunity or overactive immune responses.

- **Hereditary complement component defects** cause a number of clinical syndromes; the most common affects C1 inhibitor, which results in hereditary angioedema (HAE). Deficiencies of the terminal complement components (C5, C6, C7, and C8) and the alternative pathway proteins (factor H, factor I, and properdin) lead to increased susceptibility to infections with *N. gonorrheae* and *N. meningitidis*.

- **Phagocyte defects**, due to reduced numbers or impaired function, can result in overwhelming bacterial and fungal infections. Failure to kill bacteria and persistence of bacterial products in phagocytes leads to abscesses or granulomas, depending on the pathogen.

- **Leukocyte adhesion deficiency (LAD)** is associated with a persistent leukocytosis because phagocytic cells cannot migrate into the tissues.

Primary immunodeficiency diseases (PIDs) comprise a heterogeneous group of disorders characterized by defects in development and/or function of the immune system. The classification of PIDs is based on the nature of the underlying immunological defect.

- **Antibody deficiencies** reflect impaired function of B lymphocytes as a result of intrinsic B cell abnormalities or of defects in T lymphocytes that affect activation and terminal maturation of B lymphocytes
- **Combined immunodeficiencies** are characterized by impaired development and/or function of T lymphocytes, and functional B cell abnormalities
- **Phagocytic cell disorders** include defects in development and/or function of myeloid cells (granulocytes, macrophages)
- **Complement deficiencies** are represented by genetically-determined defects of functional or regulatory components of the complement system
- **Disorders of immune regulation** include diseases characterized by abnormalities in the mechanisms that control autoimmunity, apoptosis, or extinction of immune responses

- **Immunodeficiency syndromes** represent a heterogeneous group of PIDs in which defects of one or more components of the immune system are associated with extra-immune manifestations.

PIDs cause increased susceptibility to infections, consistent with the role played by the immune system in surveillance against pathogens. However, several forms of PID are also characterized by increased frequency of autoimmunity and malignancies, reflecting disturbances of immune regulation and of tumor surveillance.

Consistent with the role of different elements of the immune responses, PIDs are characterized by a distinct pattern of susceptibility to infections. In particular:

- patients with antibody deficiencies are highly susceptible to recurrent **pyogenic infections** sustained by encapsulated bacteria (*Haemophilus influenzae*, *Streptococcus pneumoniae*, *Staphylococcus aureus*);
- combined immunodeficiencies are characterized by broad susceptibility to infections, that includes not only bacteria, but also viruses and **opportunistic pathogens** (i.e. ubiquitous germs that do not pose significant harm to immunocompetent individuals);

- patients with disorders of neutrophils are prone to bacterial and fungal infections;
- defects of macrophages result in increased susceptibility to mycobacterial disease;
- defects of Toll-like receptors (TLRs), that act as microbial sensors, cause selective susceptibility to specific types of pathogens;
- defects of complement may lead to increased risk of pyogenic infections, but also of autoimmunity, consistent with the role played by complement in removal of immune complexes.

B lymphocyte deficiencies

Defects of B cells result in impaired antibody production. Patients affected with these disorders present with recurrent infections, which involve the upper and lower respiratory tract, particularly pneumonia and sinusitis as well as the ear (otitis media). Recurrent pneumonia may cause irreversible lung damage (bronchiectasis) and obstructive lung disease.

However, infections may also involve other tracts, such as the gut (in particular, infection by *Giardia lamblia*), the skin and, less frequently, other organs.

Congenital agammaglobulinemia results from defects of early B cell development

B lymphocytes develop in the bone marrow from the hematopoietic stem cell (HSC), through various stages of maturation (see Fig. 9.w1) during which time they rearrange their immunogloulin genes to generate the pre-B cell receptor (see Fig. 9.w2). Defects in the expression and/or signaling through the pre-BCR cause congenital agammaglobulinemia with lack of circulating B lymphocytes.

X-linked agammaglobulinemia (XLA) is the prototype of these disorders, and was described by Dr Bruton in 1952. Affected males suffer from recurrent pyogenic infections. They lack serum IgA, IgM, IgD and IgE, and IgG levels are extremely low, usually <100 mg/dL. Circulating B lymphocytes are absent or markedly reduced (<1% of peripheral lymphocytes). Tonsils are absent and lymph nodes are unusually small. XLA is caused by mutations of the Bruton tyrosine kinase (*BTK*) gene, that encodes an enzyme involved in signaling through the pre-BCR and the BCR (Fig. 16.1). *BTK* mutations cause an incomplete, but severe, block at the pre-B cell stage in the bone marrow (Fig. 16.2). The BTK protein is also expressed by other cells (including monocytes and megakaryocytes), but its defect does not affect development of these cell types.

For the first 4–6 months of life, males with XLA are protected by the maternally-derived IgG that has crossed the placenta, but once this supply of IgG is exhausted, they develop recurrent bacterial infections. Patients with XLA are also at risk of enteroviral infections (such as Echovirus) that may cause encephalitis. If immunized with attenuated poliovirus vaccine, they may develop paralytic poliomyelitis. Treatment of XLA is based on regular administration of immunoglobulins (IgG).

More rarely, congenital agammaglobulinemia is inherited as an autosomal recessive trait, due to mutations of other genes that encode for components of the pre-BCR or of the

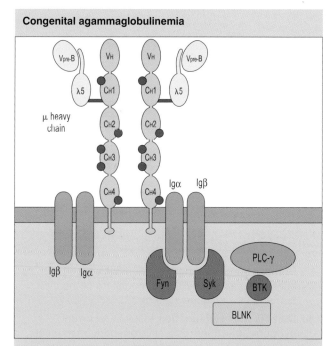

Congenital agammaglobulinemia

Fig. 16.1 Congenital agammaglobulinemia results from defects of proteins that participate at signaling through the pre-B cell receptor (pre-BRC). This is composed of the µ heavy chain, the surrogate light chains V-preB and λ5, and the signal transducing molecules Igα and Igβ. Signaling through the pre-BCR triggers activation of tyrosine kinases such as Fyn, Syk, and BTK, and involves the adaptor molecule BLNK. Ultimately, these signals converge on activation of the phospholipase C-γ (PLC-γ) and induction of calcium flux. The proteins whose mutations result in a known form of congenital agammaglobulinemia in humans are boxed in red.

adaptor molecule BLNK (see Fig. 16.1). In all of these cases, there is a severe block in B-cell development at the pre-B cell stage in the bone marrow. The clinical phenotype is virtually identical to that of XLA.

Defects in terminal differentiation of B cells produces selective antibody deficiencies

Terminal maturation of B lymphocytes is marked by their differentiation into antibody-secreting plasma cells. Generation of plasma cells is markedly reduced in patients with **CVID** (see Fig. 16.2), who typically develop progressive hypogammaglobulinemia in the second and third decades of life. CVID is the most common primary immunodeficiency (1:10 000 affected individuals in the general population), characterized by extensive clinical and immunologic heterogeneity. Some patients have a reduced number of circulating B cells, and especially of CD27[+] memory B lymphocytes; others show impaired function of T lymphocytes. CVID is usually sporadic, and the underlying molecular defect remains unknown in most cases. However, in some families CVID is inherited as an autosomal dominant or an autosomal recessive trait. A minority of CVID patients carry mutations in genes that play a key role in T-B cell interaction and B cell signaling (Fig. 16.3).

B cell maturation in X-linked immunodeficiencies

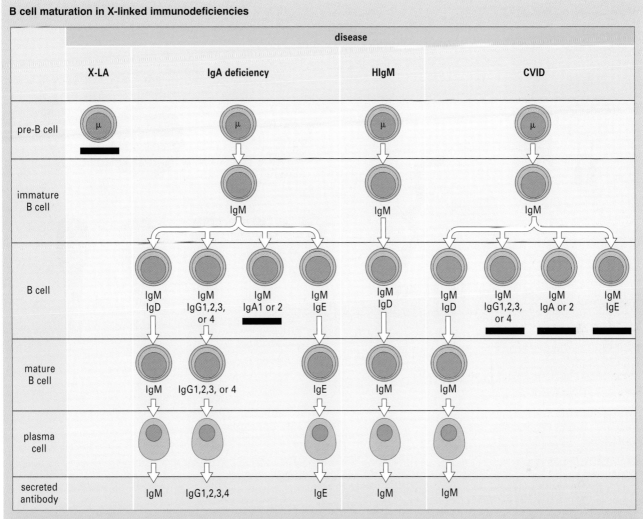

Fig. 16.2 In X-LA, affected male infants have no B cells and no serum immunoglobulins, except for small amounts of maternal IgG. In IgA deficiency, IgA-bearing B cells, and in some cases IgG2- and IgG4-bearing B cells, are unable to differentiate into plasma cells. People with HIgM lack IgG and IgA. In CVID, B cells of most isotypes are unable to differentiate into plasma cells. Black bars denote points of inhibition.

CVID is characterized by reduced levels of specific antibody isotypes

Individuals with CVID have impaired antibody production in response to immunization or to natural infections and there is a virtual absence of plasma cells in lymphoid tissues and in the bone marrow. They suffer from recurrent infections of the respiratory tract (sinusitis, otitis, bronchitis, and pneumonia) sustained by common bacteria (non typeable *H. influenzae*, *S. pneumoniae*, etc.); lack of mucosal antibodies results in increased risk of gastrointestinal infection due to *Giardia lamblia* (Fig. 16.4). They are also highly prone to autoimmune manifestations (cytopenias, inflammatory bowel disease), granulomatous lesions, lymphoid hyperplasia, and tumors (especially lymphomas). Treatment is based on immunoglobulin replacement therapy and antibiotics. Immunosuppressive and anti-inflammatory drugs may be needed in patients with autoimmune or inflammatory complications.

IgA deficiency is relatively common

(IgAD) is common in the general population (1:600 individuals), but remains asymptomatic in the majority of cases. However, recurrent infections, autoimmunity and allergy are possible, especially when IgAD is associated with a defect of IgG2 and IgG4 subclasses. The molecular basis of IgAD remains unknown; occurrence of both CVID and IgAD has been reported in some families.

Defects of class switch recombination (CSR)

Class switch recombination (CSR) is the mechanism by which the μ chain of immunoglobulins is replaced by other heavy chains, resulting in the production of IgG, IgA, and IgE. The process occurs in germinal centres and is accompanied by affinity maturation as described in Chapter 9.

Q. What is the function of CD40 and the CD40 ligand (CD154)?
A. Interaction between the CD40 molecule on the B cell surface and the CD40 ligand on activated T cells is a potent co-stimulatory signal required for class switching and affinity maturation.

Deficiency of CD40L (X-linked) or more rarely of **CD40** (autosomal recessive) results in failure of CSR, with very low or undetectable levels of IgG, IgA, and IgE and normal

Mutations associated with CVID

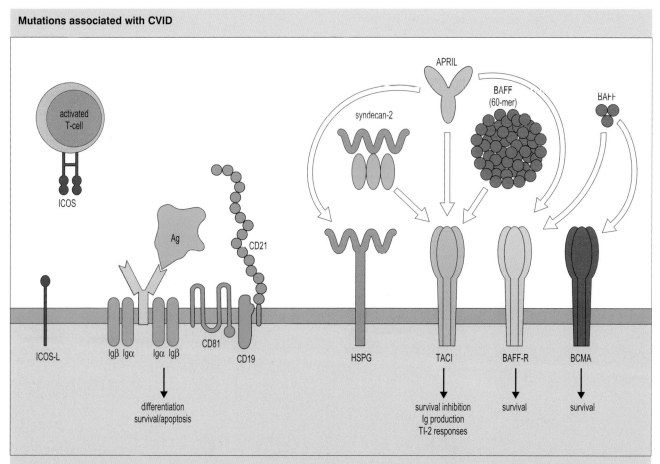

Fig. 16.3 Common variable immunodeficiency may associate with mutations of proteins involved in B cell activation. These include co-stimulatory components of the B cell receptor (CD19, CD81, CD21), ICOS ligand (ICOS-L), transmembrane activator and calcium modulator and cyclophilin ligand interactor (TACI) and the B-cell activating factor receptor (BAFF-R). These molecules deliver survival, activation and differentiation signals in mature B lymphocytes. (APRIL, a proliferation inducing ligand; BCMA, B cell maturation antigen; HSPG, heparan sulfate proteoglycan.)

Giardia lamblia

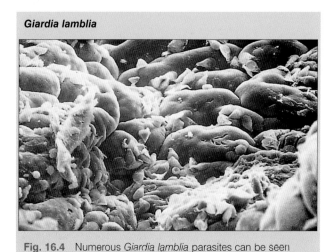

Fig. 16.4 Numerous *Giardia lamblia* parasites can be seen swarming over the mucosa of the jejunum of a patient with CVID.

CD40 ligand deficiency

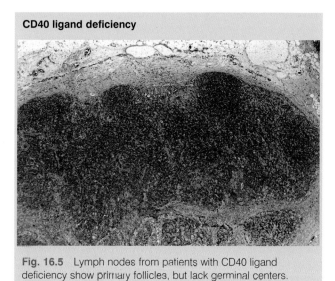

Fig. 16.5 Lymph nodes from patients with CD40 ligand deficiency show primary follicles, but lack germinal centers.

to increased levels of serum IgM (see Fig. 16.2). In the past, this condition was also known as '**hyper-IgM syndrome**'. In the lymph nodes, primary follicles are present, but germinal centers are absent (Fig. 16.5). Binding of CD40L to CD40 is also important to promote interaction between activated

T cells and dendritic cells or monocytes/macrophages. This promotes T cell priming, production of IFNγ and activation of macrophages, that are important in the immune defense against intracellular pathogens. Consistent with this, the clinical phenotype of CD40L and of CD40 deficiency is characterized not only by recurrent bacterial infections, but also by increased risk of early-onset opportunistic infections (*Pneumocystis jiroveci* pneumonia, cytomegalovirus infection, protracted and watery diarrhoea due to *Cryptosporidium*). Neutropenia and severe liver disease are frequent. Therefore, CD40L and CD40 deficiency are not pure antibody deficiency, but rather represent examples of combined immunodeficiency. Treatment of these disorders is based on administration of immunoglobulins and antibiotics, but often requires hematopoietic stem cell transplantation (HSCT).

In B cells, signaling through CD40 promotes transcription of the gene encoding for **activation-induced cytidine deaminase** (AID), a DNA-editing enzyme that replaces deoxycytidine residues with deoxyuracil in the DNA of the immunoglobulin heavy chain switch regions. The resulting mismatch in the DNA is recognized by the enzyme uracil N-glycosylase (UNG) that removes the deoxy-uracil residues, leaving abasic sites that are resolved by means of DNA repair mechanisms. These DNA modifications trigger both CSR and somatic hypermutation. Both AID and UNG mutations cause severe deficiency of IgG, IgA, and IgE production; furthermore, the immunoglobulins (almost entirely IgM) produced by these patients have low affinity for the antigen. Clinically, these immunodeficiency diseases are characterized by recurrent bacterial infections. Dramatic expansion of germinal centers (leading to tonsil and lymph node enlargement), and the lack of susceptibility to opportunistic infections distinguish hyper-IgM syndrome due to AID and UNG mutations from the forms due to defects of CD40L or CD40. Treatment of AID and UNG deficiency is based on administration of immunoglobulins.

T lymphocyte deficiencies

T lymphocytes play a critical role in the defense against intracellular pathogens, such as viruses. In addition, they permit the development of antibody responses to T-dependent antigens. Accordingly, severe defects of T lymphocyte development and/or function cause combined immunodeficiencies, with broad susceptibility to bacterial, viral and opportunistic infections.

Severe combined immunodeficiency (SCID) can be caused by many different genetic defects

SCID includes a heterogeneous group of genetic disorders that affect various stages of T lymphocyte development or function (Fig. 16.6). The main pathophysiology mechanisms of SCID (and the associated diseases) are:

- impaired survival of thymocytes and T lymphocytes (reticular dysgenesis, adenosine deaminase deficiency, purine nucleoside phosphorylase deficiency);
- defective cytokine-mediated expansion of lymphoid progenitors (X-linked SCID, JAK3 deficiency, interleukin-7 receptor deficiency);
- defective expression of the pre-T cell receptor (deficiency of RAG1, RAG2, and of other components of the V(D)J recombination machinery);
- defective signaling through the pre-T cell receptor (deficiency of CD3 chains, CD45 deficiency);

- impaired positive selection of CD4$^+$ or of CD8$^+$ lymphocytes (HLA class II deficiency and ZAP-70 deficiency, respectively);
- defective egress of T lymphocytes from the thymus (coronin 1A deficiency);
- impairment of calcium flux and of T lymphocyte activation (Stim1, Orai1 deficiencies).

While severe T cell abnormalities are a hallmark of all forms of SCID, some of these diseases also involve abnormalities of B and/or NK lymphocytes. In particular, some forms of SCID are characterized by absence of T lymphocytes, but presence of B lymphocytes (T$^-$B$^+$ SCID), whereas others show absence of both T and B lymphocytes (T$^-$B$^-$ SCID). Both of these groups of SCID include forms with or without natural killer (NK) lymphocytes.

SCID has a prevalence of approximately 1:50 000 live births, and is more common in males, reflecting the existence of X-linked SCID (X-SCID), the most common form of SCID in humans. This disease is due to mutation of the gene encoding for the common gamma chain (γc), shared by several cytokine receptors, namely those for IL-2, IL-4, IL-7, IL-9, IL-15, and IL-21.

Q. Which of these cytokines is most critically important in early T cell development?

A. Of these, the binding of IL-7 to the IL-7 receptor is most important for T cell maturation. In humans, IL-7 is critically required for T cell development (but not for B cell development, and this is a major difference as compared to mice), whereas IL-15 is required for the development of NK cells.

Accordingly, patients with X-SCID have a T$^-$B$^+$NK$^-$ phenotype.

Among the autosomal recessive forms of SCID in humans, the most common are represented by defects of RAG1 or RAG2, and by adenosine deaminase (ADA) deficiency. The recombinase activating genes (RAG) 1 and 2 are lymphoid-specific genes that initiate the process of V(D)J recombination, that is required for both T and B lymphocyte development. Therefore, mutations of RAG1 and RAG2 genes cause T$^-$B$^-$NK$^+$ SCID.

ADA is a ubiquitously expressed enzyme involved in purine metabolism. Also purine nucleoside phosphorylase (PNP) is involved in the same metabolic pathway (Fig. 16.7). Lack of ADA results in accumulation of adenosine, deoxyadenosine, and their phosphorylated derivatives. Among them, dATP is particularly toxic; it inhibits the enzyme ribonucleotide reductase, that is required for DNA synthesis and hence for cell replication.

Lymphopenia (typically, less than 3000 lymphocytes/ μL), and marked reduction of the T cell count in particular, is a hallmark of SCID. However, some infants with SCID have circulating T cells, occasionally even in normal numbers. This may reflect the presence of genetic defects that are permissive for T cell development (as in late defects in T cell development, or in patients with hypomorphic mutations in SCID-causing genes), but more often is due to engraftment of maternal T cells. Transplacental passage of maternally-derived T cells is common in pregnancy, but these cells are rejected by the immune system of the fetus. In contrast, maternally-derived T cells persist and expand in infants with SCID, and may cause tissue damage

Gene defects causing SCID

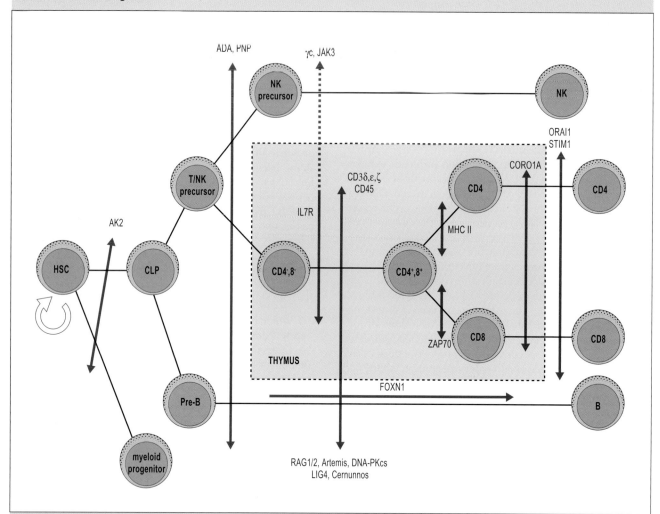

Fig. 16.6 There is a wide range of gene defects that affect T cell development or maturation and cause combined immunodeficiency in humans. Some of these defects also affect B and/or NK cell development. The diagram indicates the main stages that are affected by each deficiency. (γc, common γ chain; ADA, adenosine deaminase; AK2, adenylate kinase 2 (causing reticular dysgenesis); CORO-1A, coronon-1A; DNA-PKcs, DNA-protein kinase catalytic subunit; IL-7R, interleukin 7 receptor; JAK3, janus-associated kinase 3; LIG4, DNA ligase IV; MHC II, major histocompatibility class II antigens (due to mutation of various transcription factors); PNP, purine nucleoside phosphorylase; RAG, recombinase activating gene; STIM1, stromal interaction molecule 1.)

(graft-versus-host disease, GvHD) upon recognition of paternally-derived HLA alloantigens expressed by the patient's cells.

The thymus of SCID infants is very small and typically devoid of lymphoid elements (Fig. 16.8); lymph nodes are often absent or – when present – contain mostly stromal cells. Although B cells are normally present in some forms of SCID, antibody responses are profoundly impaired and immunoglobulin levels are usually reduced.

Clinically, SCID is apparent in the first months of life. Interstitial pneumonia (due to *Pneumocystis jiroveci* or to viral infections: cytomegalovirus, syncytial respiratory virus, adenovirus, parainfluenzae virus type 3), protracted diarrhea leading to failure to grow, and persistent candidiasis (Fig. 16.9) are common clinical findings; however, other infections (meningitis, sepsis) are also possible. Use of live vaccines in SCID infants often leads to severe consequences and should be strictly avoided; in particular, administration

of rotavirus vaccine may cause intractable diarrhea, and immunization with BCG may lead to disseminated infection.

Tн cell deficiency results from HLA class II deficiency

The failure to express class II HLA molecules on antigen-presenting cells is inherited as an autosomal recessive trait, which is not linked to the HLA locus. Affected infants have recurrent infections, particularly of the respiratory and gastrointestinal tracts.

Because the development of CD4+ helper T cells (Tн) depends on positive selection by HLA class II molecules in the thymus (see Chapter 2), HLA class II molecule-deficient infants have a deficiency of CD4+ T cells. This lack of Tн cells leads to a deficiency in antibodies as well. The HLA class II deficiency results from defects in transcription factors that bind to the 5′ untranslated promoter region of the class II HLA genes.

Possible role of adenosine deaminase and purine nucleoside phosphorylase deficiency in SCID

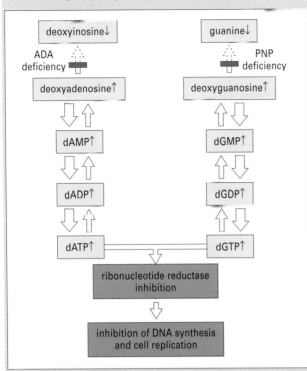

Fig. 16.7 It is thought that deficiencies of ADA and PNP lead to accumulations of dATP and dGTP, respectively. Both of these metabolites are powerful inhibitors of ribonucleotide reductase, which is an essential enzyme for DNA synthesis.

Thymus of SCID

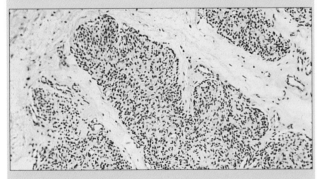

Fig. 16.8 Note that the thymic stroma has not been invaded by lymphoid cells and no Hassall's corpuscles are seen. The gland has a fetal appearance.

The DiGeorge anomaly arises from a defect in thymus embryogenesis

The thymic epithelium is derived from the third and fourth pharyngeal pouches by the sixth week of human gestation. Subsequently the endodermal anlage is invaded by lymphoid stem cells, which undergo development into T cells.

A congenital defect in the organs derived from the third and fourth pharyngeal pouches results in the **DiGeorge anomaly**. The T cell deficiency is variable, depending on

Candida albicans in the mouth of a patient with SCID

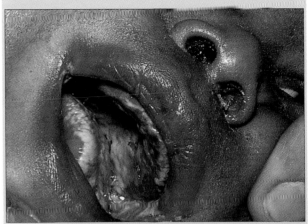

Fig. 16.9 *C. albicans* grows luxuriantly in the mouth and on the skin of patients with SCID.

DiGeorge anomaly

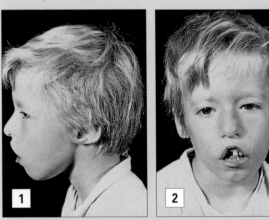

Fig. 16.10 Note the wide-set eyes, low-set ears, and shortened philtrum of upper lip.

how badly the thymus is affected; only in <1% of the patients, the T cell deficiency is so severe to cause SCID. Infants with DiGeorge anomaly have distinctive facial features (Fig. 16.10). They also have congenital malformations of the heart or aortic arch and neonatal tetany due to hypocalcemia resulting from the hypoplasia or aplasia of the parathyroid glands.

The majority of patients with DiGeorge anomaly have partial monosomy of 22q11.2 or 10p. Patients with DiGeorge anomaly who present with a SCID phenotype may be treated by thymus transplantation. Thymic tissues derived from unrelated infant donors at the time of heart surgery is treated to remove all lymphoid cells (to avoid graft-versus-host disease) and is implanted into muscular tissue of the affected patients. In spite of the complete HLA mismatch, lymphoid progenitors derived from hematopoietic stem cells of the patients, colonize the transplanted thymic tissue, mature there and are then exported to the periphery.

Disorders of immune regulation

Self-non self discrimination is an essential function of the adaptive immune system. Failure to recognize non-self antigens leads to increased susceptibility to infections, as observed in patients with congenital defects of T and/or B cell-mediated immunity. In contrast, defects in recognition and tolerance of self antigens are associated with auto-immunity. Finally, modulation of immune responses is important to maintain homeostasis. In some forms of primary immunodeficiency, the inability to clear pathogens results in persistent inflammatory reactions and may cause severe tissue damage.

Defective function of regulatory T (Treg) cells causes severe autoimmunity

Regulatory T cells (CD4$^+$ CD25$^+$) suppress immune responses to self-antigens in the periphery.

> **Q. What is the characteristic transcription factor of Treg cells?**
> A. FOXP3, which is expressed in the thymus.

Mutations of the *FOXP3* gene cause Immune dysregulation-polyendocrinopathy-enteropathy-X-linked (IPEX) syndrome, a severe, X-linked form of autoimmunity. Males with IPEX syndrome present in the first months of life with intractable diarrhoea, insulin-dependent diabetes and skin rash. Severe infections may follow because of breakage of the cutaneous and mucosal barriers. There is a lack of functional CD4$^+$ CD25$^+$ FOXP3$^+$ lymphocytes. Activated, self-reactive T lymphocytes infiltrate target organs (Fig. 16.11) and there are high levels of autoantibodies against insulin, other pancreatic antigens and enterocytes. In typical cases, the disease evolves rapidly. Treatment with immunosuppressive drugs is required to control autoimmune manifestations, however stem cell therapy is the only curative approach.

Gut mucosa of a patient with IPEX

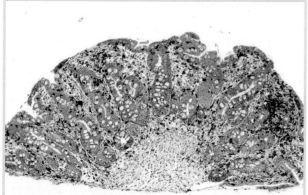

Fig. 16.11 The gut mucosa of patients with IPEX shows villous atrophy and severe infiltration by T cells, identified by staining for CD3.

Impaired apoptosis of self-reactive lymphocytes causes autoimmune lymphoproliferative syndrome (ALPS)

Apoptosis of autoreactive lymphocytes is important to preserve immune homeostasis. Interaction between FAS ligand (FasL), expressed by activated lymphocytes, and FAS (CD95), triggers intracellular signaling that ultimately results in activation of caspases and cell death. Mutations of FAS are the predominant cause of autoimmune lymphoproliferative syndrome (ALPS), with lymphadenopathy, hepatosplenomegaly and autoimmune cytopenia. There is an increased risk of malignancies (especially B-cell lymphomas), that occur in 10% of the patients with FAS mutations. Patients with ALPS have an increased number of 'double negative' T lymphocytes that express the αβ form of the TCR, but do not express CD4 or CD8 molecules. ALPS is most often inherited as an autosomal dominant trait, and is due to dominant-negative mutations that interfere with the signal transducing activity of FAS trimeric complexes. A rare variant of FAS is due to FasL mutations. In a few patients, mutations of caspase-8 and of caspase-10 have been also identified. Treatment is based on use of immunosuppressive drugs.

Congenital defects of lymphocyte cytotoxicity result in persistent inflammation and severe tissue damage

The cytotoxic activity of T cells and NK cells depends on the expression of cytolytic proteins that are assembled into granules and transported through microtubules to the lytic synapse that is formed upon contact with target cells. **Familial hemophagocytic lymphohistiocytosis (FHL)** includes a group of disorders characterized by impairment of the mechanisms of transport, docking or release of the lytic granules. Deficiency of perforin (see Fig. 10.12) is the most common form of FHL. In these diseases, persistence of the pathogen (most often, a virus) causes expansion of CD8$^+$ T cells that, while unable to mount a cytotoxic response, secrete increased amounts of TH1 cytokines, and IFNγ. Excessive amounts of IFNγ trigger macrophage activation, causing phagocytosis of blood elements and tissue damage. The disease is usually fatal, and treatment is based on immunosuppressive drugs (to reduce immune activation) and HSCT.

Similarly, **X-linked proliferative syndrome (XLP)** results from a failure to control the normal proliferation of Tc cells following an infection with Epstein–Barr virus (EBV), which causes infectious mononucleosis.

Affected males appear normal until they encounter EBV, when they develop either:

- fatal infectious mononucleosis;
- hypogammaglobulinemia (often with preserved levels of IgM);
- lymphoma; or
- aplastic anemia.

The defective gene on the X chromosome encodes an adapter protein of T and B cells called **SAP** or the **SLAM-associated protein**. SLAM is expressed on the surface of T and B cells. Its intracellular tail interacts with the adapter protein, SAP, which is required for cytolytic activity of T and NK cells. Furthermore, SAP is important also for the function of follicular helper T cells (T_{FH}), that govern trafficking of B lymphocytes to the germinal centers. Defective function of T_{FH} cells accounts for the hypogammaglobulinemia of XLP. Treatment is based on HSCT.

Immunodeficiency syndromes

Immunodeficiency syndromes include a heterogeneous group of disorders characterized by immune and extra-immune manifestations. The immunological abnormalities associated with these diseases may involve both adaptive and innate immunity.

Chromosomal breaks occur in TCR and immunoglobulin genes in hereditary ataxia telangiectasia

Hereditary ataxia telangiectasia (AT) is inherited as an autosomal recessive trait. Affected infants develop a wobbly gait (ataxia) at about 18 months and ultimately are wheel-chaired. Dilated capillaries (telangiectasia) appear in the eyes and on the skin by 6 years of age (Fig. 16.12). AT is accompanied by a variable T cell deficiency. About 70% of patients with AT are also IgA deficient and some also have IgG2 and IgG4 deficiency.

Q. In what other ways are IgA, IgG2, and IgG4 related (as opposed to IgM, IgG1, and IgG3)?
A. The IgA1, IgA2, IgG2, and IgG4 heavy chain genes all lie further downstream of the recombined VDJ gene than IgM, IgG1, and IgG3 (see Fig. 9.16). This may account for the selective deficiency in making the class switch to IgA, IgG2, and IgG4. Class switching involves the production and resolution of double-stranded DNA breaks.

The number and function of circulating T cells are greatly diminished, so cell-mediated immunity is depressed. Patients develop severe sinus and lung infections. Their cells exhibit chromosomal breaks, usually in chromosome 7 and chromosome 14, at the sites of the T cell receptor (TCR) genes and the genes encoding the heavy chains of immunoglobulins.

Ocular telangiectasias

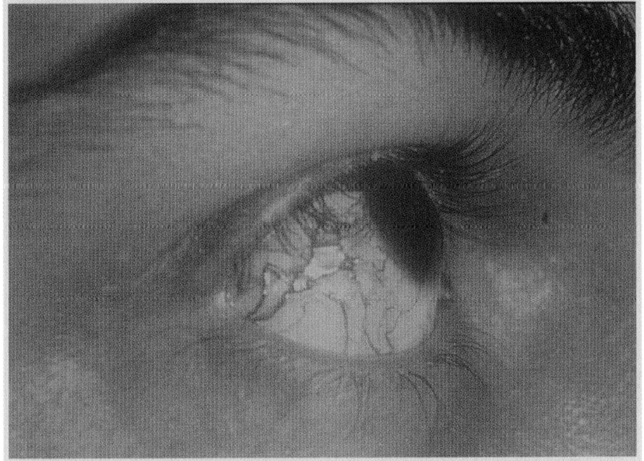

Fig. 16.12 Ocular telangiectasias in a patient with ataxia telangiectasia.

The cells of patients with AT are very susceptible to ionizing irradiation because the defective gene in AT encodes a protein involved in the repair of double-strand breaks in DNA. This defect leads to increased risk of malignancies, especially lymphoma and leukemia.

T cell defects and abnormal immunoglobulin levels occur in Wiskott–Aldrich syndrome

The **Wiskott–Aldrich syndrome (WAS)** is an X-linked immunodeficiency disease. Affected males with WAS:

- have a low number of platelets (thrombocytopenia), that are also unusually small in size;
- develop severe eczema as well as pyogenic and opportunistic infections;
- often have increased amounts of serum IgA and IgE, normal levels of IgG, and decreased amounts of IgM;
- have T cells with defective function.

The malfunction of cell-mediated immunity gets progressively worse. The T cells have a uniquely abnormal appearance, as shown by scanning electron microscopy, reflecting a cytoskeletal defect. They have fewer microvilli on the cell surface than normal T cells. Similar defects of cytoskeleton reorganization are observed in the patients' monocytes and dendritic cells, with severe impairment of filopodia formation and of migration in response to chemokines. Patients with WAS have also a severe defect of natural killer (NK) cytolytic activity which accounts for the higher rate of herpes virus infections.

The Wiskott–Aldrich Syndrome protein (WASp) plays a critical role in cytoskeleton reorganization. In T and NK cells, it participates at formation of the immunological synapse, favoring tight interaction of T lymphocytes with dendritic cells and B cells, and of NK cells with target cells.

Because of the severity of the disease, and because expression of the WAS gene is restricted to the hematopoietic system, definitive treatment is based on HSCT.

Deficiency of STAT3 causes impaired development and function of T_H17 cells in hyper-IgE syndrome

Hyper-IgE syndrome (HIES) can be inherited as an autosomal dominant or recessive trait; however, the clinical and immunological features of these forms are distinct. Autosomal dominant HIES is due to heterozygous mutations of the **signal transducer and activator of transcription 3 (*STAT3*)** gene. This is a transcription factor that is activated in response to activation of the JAK-STAT signaling pathway through cytokine and growth factor receptors that contain the gp130 protein. Biological responses to IL-6 and IL-10 are depressed, and development of T_H17 cells is impaired, resulting in poor secretion of IL-17 and IL-22. This causes impairment in immune defense against bacterial and fungal infections; in addition, production of antibacterial molecules (e.g. defensins) by epithelial cells is also affected. The clinical phenotype includes eczema, cutaneous, and pulmonary infections sustained by *S. aureus* (with formation of pneumatoceles), and *Candida* spp. Patients with STAT3 deficiency also show defective shedding of primary teeth, scoliosis, higher risk of bone fractures, joint hyperextensibility, and characteristic facial traits.

In contrast, the autosomal recessive HIES syndrome is due to mutations of the **dedicator of cytokinesis 8 (DOCK8)** gene, that encodes for a protein involved in cytoskeleton reorganization. Patients with DOCK8 deficiency suffer from severe infections from early life. Viral infections due to CMV, HPV, and HSV, and allergies are particularly common. There is also an increased risk of malignancies. *In vitro* proliferation of T cells to mitogens is markedly reduced. Immunoglobulin levels are variable, but IgG is often increased whereas IgM is low. The clinical and immunological phenotype of DOCK8 deficiency indicates that this is a combined immunodeficiency.

Genetic defects of phagocytes

Phagocytic cells (polymorphs and mononuclear phagocytes) are important in host defense against pyogenic bacteria and other intracellular microorganisms.

A severe deficiency of neutrophils (**neutropenia**) can result in overwhelming bacterial infection. **Severe congenital neutropenia** (SCN) is defined as a neutrophil count that is persistently less than 0.5×10^9 cells/L. A variety of genetic defects may cause SCN in humans. The majority of these patients have a severe block in myeloid development in the bone marrow. The most common form of SCN is due to mutation of the *ELA2* gene, encoding neutrophil elastase. In some cases, *ELA2* mutations cause cyclic neutropenia, with oscillations in the neutrophil count that reaches a nadir approximately every 21 days, resulting in periodicity of the infections.

Two groups of genetic defects affect phagocyte function without altering their development:

- chronic granulomatous disease (CGD); and
- leukocyte adhesion deficiency (LAD).

These disorders are clinically important in that they result in susceptibility to severe infections and are often fatal.

Chronic granulomatous disease results from a defect in the oxygen reduction pathway

Patients with CGD have defective **NADPH oxidase**, which catalyzes the reduction of O_2 to $\bullet O_2^-$ by the reaction: $NADPH + 2O_2 \rightarrow NADP^+ + 2 \bullet O_2^- + H^+$. They are therefore incapable of forming superoxide anions (O_2^-) and hydrogen peroxide in their phagocytes following the ingestion of microorganisms.

> **Q. What would be the consequence of a failure of superoxide generation?**
>
> A. Phagocytes cannot readily kill ingested bacteria or fungi, particularly catalase-producing organisms (see Fig. 7.18 and Chapter 14).

As a result, microorganisms remain alive in phagocytes of patients with CGD. This gives rise to a cell-mediated response to persistent intracellular microbial antigens, with formation of granulomas.

Children with CGD develop pneumonia, infections in the lymph nodes (lymphadenitis), and abscesses in the skin, liver, and other viscera. Infections due to *Staphylococcus aureus* are particularly common, however patients with CGD are uniquely prone to fungal (in particular *Aspergillus* and *Candida*) and mycobacterial infections. Treatment of CGD requires regular use of antibacterial and antifungal prophylaxis and aggressive management of infections. HSCT may provide a definitive cure.

LAD is due to defects of leukocytes trafficking

The receptor CR3 in the phagocyte membrane that binds to C3bi on opsonized microorganisms is critical for the ingestion of bacteria by phagocytes. This receptor is deficient in patients with **type 1 LAD** (LAD1), who consequently develop severe bacterial infections, particularly of the mouth and gastrointestinal tract. CR3 is composed of two polypeptide chains:

- an α chain of 165 kDa (CD11b); and
- a β chain of 95 kDa (CD18).

In LAD1, there is a genetic defect of the β chain, encoded by a gene on chromosome 21.

Two other integrin proteins share the same β chain as CR3 – namely lymphocyte functional antigen (LFA-1) and p150,95 (see Chapter 6); these proteins are also defective in LAD1.

LFA-1 is important in cell adhesion and interacts with intercellular adhesion molecule-1 (ICAM-1) on endothelial cell surfaces and other cell membranes. Because of the defect in LFA-1, phagocytes from patients with LAD1 cannot adhere to vascular endothelium and cannot therefore migrate out of blood vessels into areas of infection. As a result patients with LAD1 cannot form pus efficiently and this allows the rapid spread of bacterial invaders.

When leukocytes in the circulation enter an area of inflammation their speed of movement is greatly retarded by the interaction of **selectins** with their ligands (see Fig. 6.6). E-selectin interacts with Sialyl Lewis^x (SLeX), a fucosylated molecule that is expressed on the surface of neutrophils and monocytes. In **LAD2** a genetic defect of intracellular fucose transporter prevents fucosylation of membrane glycoproteins, including SLeX. Consequently, the leukocytes of patients with LAD2 cannot roll on the endothelium and fail to extravasate and reach inflamed tissues. Since fucose metabolism is important also in the central nervous system, patients with LAD2 also show mental retardation and dysmorphisms in addition to infections.

A third form of LAD (**LAD3**) is due to impaired integrin signaling that also involves platelets. These patients suffer from severe infections and increased bleeding. All forms of LAD are characterized by marked elevation of the leukocyte count in peripheral blood (leukocytosis); this reflects the response of the bone marrow to inflammatory stimuli (with increased production of myeloid cells) and inability of the leukocytes to leave circulation and reach peripheral tissues.

Immunodeficiencies with selective susceptibility to infections

Most forms of primary immunodeficiency disease (PID) are characterized by broad susceptibility to infections, such as bacterial infections in patients with antibody deficiency, defects of neutrophils or complement; and infections of viral, fungal or bacterial origin in patients with combined immunodeficiency. In contrast, some forms of PID are characterized by susceptibility to some specific pathogens. The study of these patients has shown the critical role played by some components of the immune system in the response to these pathogens.

Macrophage microbicidal activity is impaired by defects in IFNγ signaling

The destruction of intracellular microorganisms that flourish in macrophages depends on the activation of microbicidal activity in macrophages by IFNγ. When microorganisms are taken up by macrophages, the macrophages secrete IL-12, which then binds to the IL-12 receptor on T cells and induces secretion of IFNγ.

Children with genetic defects in the genes encoding IL-12, the IL-12 receptor (IL-12R), or the IFNγ receptor suffer from recurrent infection with non-pathogenic mycobacteria and, to a lesser extent, with salmonella. These various defects are inherited as autosomal recessive or autosomal dominant traits. Treatment with IFNγ is beneficial in patients with IL-12 and IL-12R mutations, whereas HSCT is the treatment of choice for patients with mutations in IFNγ receptor.

Defects of TLR-signaling cause susceptibility to pyogenic infections

Toll-like receptors (TLR) are a series of molecules that are expressed at the cell surface or at the membrane of endosomes, and mediate recognition of pathogen-associated molecular patterns, such as lipopolysaccharide, glycolipids, single- or double-stranded RNA (see Fig. 6.20). The classical pathway of TLR activation involves the adaptor molecules MyD88 and the intracellular kinases IRAK-4 and IRAK-1. Activation of this pathway upon binding of TLRs to their ligands, results in the induction of NFκB and production of inflammatory cytokines (IL-1, IL-6, TNFα, IL-12). Mutations of **IRAK4** and **MyD88** cause severe and invasive pyogenic infections early in life, often without significant inflammatory response. Infections tend to become less frequent later in life, when the adaptive immune system has matured.

TLR-3, -7, -8 and -9 can activate an alternative pathway that involves the adaptor molecule UNC-93B, resulting in the induction of type 1 interferons (IFNα -β). Mutations of **TLR3** and **UNC-93B** cause selective susceptibility to herpes simplex encephalitis due to infection by HSV-1. Severe viral infections are also observed in patients with complete deficiency of STAT1, a transcription factor that is activated following binding of type 1 interferon to the specific receptor, resulting in expression of IFN-dependent genes.

Genetic deficiencies of complement proteins

The proteins of the complement system and their interactions with the immune system are discussed in Chapter 4. Genetic deficiencies of almost all the complement proteins have been found in humans (Fig. 16.13) and these deficiencies reveal much about the normal function of the complement system.

Immune complex clearance, inflammation, phagocytosis, and bacteriolysis can be affected by complement deficiencies

Deficiencies of the classical pathway components, C1q, C1r, C1s, C4, or C2, result in a propensity to develop immune complex diseases such as systemic lupus erythematosus.

Q. Why should these deficiencies result in immune complex disease?

A. The classical complement pathway is required for the dissolution of immune complexes by covalent binding of

---

Genetic deficiencies of human complement

group	type	deficiency	hereditary		
			AR	AD	XL
I	immune complex disease	C1q	●		
		C1s, or C1r + C1s	●		
		C2	●		
		C4	●		
II	angioedema	C1 inhibitor		●	
III	recurrent pyogenic infections	C3	●		
		factor H	●		
		factor I	●		
IV	recurrent *Neisseria* infections	C5	●		
		C6	●		
		C7	●		
		C8	●		
		properdin			●
		factor D	●		
V	asymptomatic	C9	●		

Fig. 16.13 Genetic deficiencies of human complement. (AR, phenotypically autosomal recessive; AD, autosomal dominant; XL, X-linked recessive.)

C4b and C3b to components of the complex. It is also required for the transport of complexes on erythrocytes in humans (see Fig. 25.6).

Deficiencies of C3, factor H, or factor I result in increased susceptibility to pyogenic infections – this correlates with the important role of C3 in the opsonization of pyogenic bacteria.

Deficiencies of the terminal components C5, C6, C7, and C8, and of the alternative pathway components, factor D and properdin, result in remarkable susceptibility to infection with the two pathogenic species of the *Neisseria* genus: *N. gonorrhoeae* and *N. meningitidis*. This clearly demonstrates the importance of the alternative pathway and the macromolecular attack complex in the bacteriolysis of this genus of bacteria.

All of these genetically-determined deficiencies of complement components are inherited as autosomal recessive traits, except:

- properdin deficiency, which is inherited as an X-linked recessive; and
- C1 inhibitor deficiency, which is inherited as an autosomal dominant.

Hereditary angioneurotic edema (HAE) results from C1 inhibitor deficiency

The C1 inhibitor (C1INH) is responsible for dissociation of activated C1, by binding to C1r2C1s2. Deficiency of C1INH results in HAE (Fig. 16.14), that is inherited as an autosomal dominant trait. Patients have recurrent episodes of swelling of various parts of the body (angioedema):

- when the edema involves the intestine, excruciating abdominal pains and cramps result, with severe vomiting;
- when the edema involves the upper airway, the patients may choke to death from respiratory obstruction – angioedema of the upper airway therefore presents a medical emergency, which requires rapid action to restore normal breathing.

Hereditary angioneurotic edema

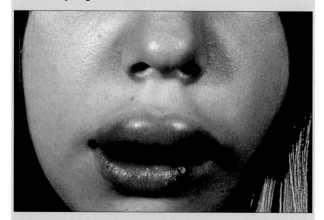

Fig. 16.14   This clinical photograph shows the transient localized swelling that occurs in this condition.

C1INH inhibits not only the classical pathway of complement, but also elements of the kinin, plasmin, and clotting systems.

The edema is mediated by two peptides generated by uninhibited activation of the complement and surface contact systems:

- a peptide derived from the activation of C2, called C2 kinin; and
- bradykinin derived from the activation of the contact system (Fig. 16.15).

The effect of these peptides is on the postcapillary venule, where they cause endothelial cells to retract, forming gaps that allow leakage of plasma (see Chapter 6).

There are two genetically determined forms of HAE:

- in type I, the C1INH gene is defective and no transcripts are formed; and
- in type II, there are point mutations in the C1INH gene resulting in the synthesis of defective molecules.

The distinction between type I and type II is important because the diagnosis of type II disease cannot be made by quantitative measurement of serum C1 inhibitor alone. Simultaneous measurements of C4 must also be done. C4 is always decreased in the serum of patients with HAE because of its destruction by uninhibited activated C1.

Pathogenesis of hereditary angioneurotic edema

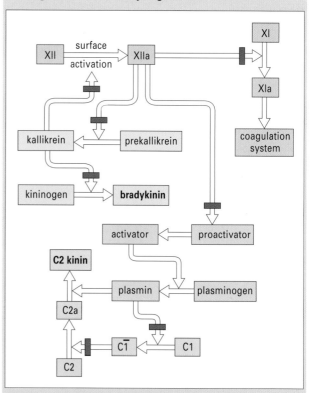

Fig. 16.15   C1 inhibitor is involved in inactivation of elements of the clotting, kinin, plasmin and complement systems, which may be activated following the surface-dependent activation of factor XII (Hageman factor). The points at which C1 inhibitor acts are shown in red. Uncontrolled activation of these pathways results in the formation of bradykinin and C2 kinin, which induce edema formation.

C1INH deficiency is not always genetically-determined, but may be acquired later in life. In particular, patients with autoimmune diseases or with B cell lymphoproliferative disorders (chronic lymphocytic leukemia, multiple myeloma, or B cell lymphoma) may produce autoantibodies to C1INH. C1INH brands are available for intravenous use to treat or prevent acute attacks of angioedema.

CRITICAL THINKING: HYPER-IgM IMMUNODEFICIENCY (SEE P. 438 FOR EXPLANATIONS)

A 3-year-old girl was brought to the emergency room because of fever and rapid respiration. She had had pneumonia once before at age 25 months. She had also had otitis media on ten different occasions, each time successfully treated with antibiotics. She had also suffered repeated episodes of tonsil and lymph node enlargement. A chest radiograph resulted in the diagnosis of left lower lobe pneumonia. Blood and sputum cultures contained *Streptococcus pneumoniae*. The white blood count was 13 500/mL of which 81% were neutrophils and 14% lymphocytes. Serum IgM was 470 mg/dL, IgG 40 mg/dL, and IgA and IgE were undetectable. Antibody to tetanus toxoid was undetectable. Blood typing was A positive, anti-B 1:320. The distribution of T, B and NK cells was normal, with 72%

CD3$^+$ T cells, 47% CD4$^+$, 23% CD8$^+$, 17% CD19$^+$, and 11% CD16$^+$ lymphocytes.

1 What clinical and laboratory tests lead to the suspicion that this child has hyper-IgM (HIgM) immunodeficiency and how do you conclude that it is not due to a mutation in CD40 ligand?

2 What is the most likely diagnosis in this case?

3 How do you explain that this child had no response to tetanus immunization and yet has a high titer for her age of antibody to blood group substance B?

4 What treatment would you recommend to the parents for this child and what would you say is her prognosis?

Further reading

Conley ME, Dobbs AK, Farmer DM, et al. Primary B cell immunodeficiencies: comparisons and contrasts. Annu Rev Immunol 2009;27:199–227.

Fischer A. Human primary immunodeficiency diseases. Immunity 2007;27:835–845.

Fischer A, Le Deist F, Hacein-Bey-Abina S, et al. Severe combined immunodeficiency. A model disease for molecular immunology and therapy. Immunol Rev 2005;203:98–109.

Frank MM. Complement disorders and hereditary angioedema. J Allergy Clin Immunol 2010;125:S262–S271.

Holland SM. Chronic granulomatous disease. Clin Rev Allergy Immunol 2010;38:3–10.

Klein C. Congenital neutropenia. Hematology Am Soc Hematol Educ Program 2009;344–350.

Notarangelo LD. Primary immunodeficiencies. J Allergy Clin Immunol 2010;125:S182–S194.

Pachlopnik Schmid J, Côte M, Ménager MM, et al. Inherited defects in lymphocyte cytotoxic activity. Immunol Rev 2010;235:10–23.

Sancho-Shimizu V, Zhang SY, Abel L, et al. Genetic susceptibility to herpes simplex virus 1 encephalitis in mice and humans. Curr Opin Allergy Clin Immunol 2007;7:495–505.

Thrasher AJ, Burns SO. WASP: a key immunological multitasker. Nat Rev Immunol 2010;10:182–192.

Zhang SY, Boisson-Dupuis S, Chapgier A, et al. Inborn errors of interferon (IFN)-mediated immunity in humans: insights into the respective roles of IFN-alpha/beta, IFN-gamma, and IFN-lambda in host defense. Immunol Rev 2008; 226:29–40.

CHAPTER 17

AIDS, Secondary Immunodeficiency and Immunosuppression

SUMMARY

- **Nutrient deficiencies often lead to impaired immune responses.** Malnutrition increases the risk of infant mortality from infection through reduction in cell-mediated immunity, including reduced numbers and function of $CD4^+$ helper cells and a reduction in levels of secretory IgA. Trace elements, iron, selenium, copper, and zinc are also important in immunity. Lack of these elements can lead to diminished neutrophil killing of bacteria and fungi, susceptibility to viral infections, and diminished antibody responses. Vitamins A, B6, C, E, and folic acid are likewise important in overall resistance to infection. Proper diet and nutrition, therefore, reduce morbidity and mortality caused by infection.

- **Some drugs selectively alter immune function.** Immunomodulatory drugs can severely depress immune functions. These drugs are often necessary to treat solid organ transplant patients and those with an autoimmune disease. Although necessary in such settings, these drugs are often broad acting, thereby increasing patients' susceptibility to a broad array of *opportunistic* infections caused by viruses, bacteria and fungi.

- **HIV is a primary cause of immunodeficiency.** Human immunodeficiency virus (HIV) is a retrovirus that predominantly targets $CD4^+$ T cells. Acute infection depletes CD4 T cell subsets and transiently suppresses circulating CD4 T cell numbers before the immune system establishes partial control of the virus and the chronic phase of infection begins. Though patients can remain in the chronic phase for an average of 10 years, without anti-retroviral drug treatment, CD4 T cell levels gradually fall, resulting in loss of cell-mediated immunity and susceptibility to life-threatening opportunistic infections. This final stage, AIDS (acquired immunodeficiency syndrome), is marked by low CD4 T cell counts, high HIV plasma levels, reactivation of other latent infections, and often, virus-associated malignancies such as Kaposi's sarcoma and non-Hodgkin's lymphoma.

- **Combination therapy for AIDS** with inhibitors of HIV reverse transcriptase, protease, and entry are reasonably successful, but associated with long-term toxicities in almost 50% of persons. An effective vaccine remains an elusive goal, in part due to the rapid mutation rate of the virus during reverse transcription.

Overview

Secondary immunodeficiencies are acquired and disrupt the development or function of an otherwise normal immune system. Unlike primary immunodeficiencies that are due to genetic abnormalities and often have a very defined presentation in the clinic, secondary defects are both more common and more heterogeneous. Therapeutic approaches for secondary immune deficiencies usually involve treating the primary extrinsic stressor, combined with increased vigilance for infection, as well as pharmacologic intervention or prophylaxis to address active or potential infections. Major causes of secondary immunodeficiency include:

- malnutrition;
- viral infection (e.g. HIV);
- iatrogenic immune suppression (e.g. post-organ transplant);
- cancer metastases or leukemias, especially those involving bone marrow;
- cancer treatments such as chemotherapy or irradiation;
- surgery or trauma;
- chronic disease, debility, or stress;
- advanced age.

Nutrient deficiencies

Globally, malnutrition is the most common cause of immunodeficiency. The connection between nutrition and immunity has a long historic record with periods of famine preceding periods of pestilence. As a primary diagnosis, malnutrition is a treatable problem that can range from severe protein-energy malnutrition (PEM) to marginal deficiencies in a single micronutrient. Immune responses are significantly impaired when calories, macronutrients or any key micronutrients are in limiting supply, leaving the undernourished at increased risk for infection.

Infection and malnutrition can exacerbate each other

Malnutrition and infection act synergistically to depress immunity and increase morbidity and mortality. Presence of infection often exacerbates the malnourished state by:

- increasing metabolic demands;
- decreasing appetite, thereby lowering intake of nutrients; and
- with gastrointestinal infection, decreasing nutrient absorption.

Once this cycle begins, it is self-propagating as infection compromises immunity, which then leads to more infection and debility (Fig. 17.1). At a population level, this may lead to decreased productivity, further decreasing economic and food resources and, again, driving the malnutrition and immune deficiency loop.

Risk factors for malnutrition include poverty, food scarcity, illiteracy, and chronic debilitation. The impacts of malnutrition are seen globally. The World Health Organization (WHO) estimates worldwide, 50% of childhood deaths are due to malnutrition, many in developing nations. However, malnutrition is not just a problem of the poorest countries. In the USA, it is estimated that less than 50% of the elderly are adequately nourished, and even within populations that consume adequate calories, poor dietary nutrient intake can cause marginal nutrient deficiencies with a significant detrimental impact on morbidity and mortality.

Addressing the individual impact of any single micronutrient on immune function is difficult as the malnourished often present with multiple deficiencies. In order to understand the role of nutrients in immune function, many studies have assessed the correlates of both PEM and individual micronutrients on infection rates and immune responses. For example, in one study of surgical and trauma patients, those who presented with lower levels of serum albumin were found to have an increased risk for infectious complications. In addition to such population studies, both *in vitro* studies on human immune cells and *in vivo* animal studies have helped elucidate the direct effects of malnutrition on immunity. In some cases, the mechanisms underlying the effects of single nutrient-deficient diets have been determined. We present an overview of these findings below.

Protein–energy malnutrition and lymphocyte dysfunction

Though not all of the underlying mechanisms are clear, multiple studies have correlated PEM with defects in all aspects of the immune system defense, but especially cell-mediated immunity. Lymphoid atrophy is a prominent morphological feature of malnutrition. The thymus, in particular, is a sensitive barometer in young children and the profound reduction in weight and size of the organ effectively results in **nutritional thymectomy**. Both increased apoptosis of immature CD4$^+$CD8$^+$ thymocytes and a decrease in proliferation contribute to thymic involution. Atrophy is evident in the thymus-dependent periarteriolar areas of the spleen and in the paracortical section of the lymph nodes. Decreases in the thymic hormones, thymulin and thymopoietin, accompany this loss in cellularity. Histologically:

- the lobular architecture is ill defined;
- there is a loss of corticomedullary demarcation;
- there are fewer lymphoid cells; and
- Hassall's corpuscles are enlarged and degenerate – some may be calcified.

Thus, with PEM there is a significant decrease in circulating T cell numbers, with CD4 T cells disproportionately affected giving a low CD4$^+$/CD8$^+$ ratio. Functional studies in mice fed protein-deficit diets have shown that both low T cell precursor number and decreased proliferative response of the remaining lymphocytes upon antigen encounter contribute to an inability to clear viral infection.

Mechanistically, PEM may contribute to lymphocyte functional deficits due to limits in the availability of the amino acid glutamine, required for both nucleotide synthesis and cytokine production, as well as by the increase in oxidative stress. PEM additionally causes imbalances in the neuroendocrine signals affecting lymphocyte survival. Glucocorticoids, released during stress, are increased with PEM, while leptin levels are decreased. Leptin, a hormone released from adipose tissues, has pleiotropic effects, but in mice it can protect thymocytes from glucocorticoid-induced apoptosis. It is not surprising then, that PEM significantly diminishes cell-mediated immunity.

B cell functional deficits are less pronounced in PEM. Although serum antibody levels are usually normal, clinical studies have found a reduction in the secretory IgA antibody

---

Malnutrition and infection exacerbate each other in a vicious circle

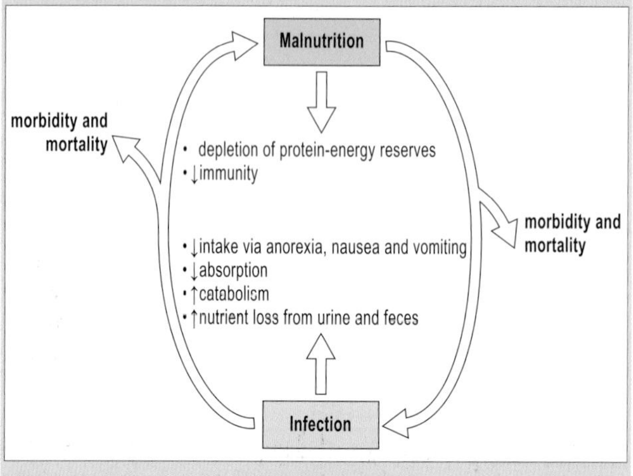

Fig. 17.1   Malnutrition and infection exacerbate each other in a vicious circle.

response to common vaccine antigens, which may contribute to a higher incidence of mucosal infections.

Nutrition also affects innate mechanisms of immunity

Poor nutrition also causes deficits in innate immune defenses, for example,

- a larger number of bacteria bind to epithelial cells of malnourished subjects;
- wound healing is impaired;
- the production of certain inflammatory cytokines, such as IL-2 and TNFα, is decreased;
- opsonization is decreased, largely because of a reduction in levels of various complement components – C3, C5, and factor B.

Q. How would a decrease in complement components affect innate immunity?
A. Decreased opsonization and killing of extracellular microorganisms increases susceptibility to bacterial infections (Chapter 4).

Deficiencies in trace elements impact immunity

Zinc is one of several trace elements essential for optimal immune system function. WHO estimates that about one third of the world's population is affected by some level of zinc deficiency. At particular risk are populations with plant-based diets, as fiber and phytate in plant foods inhibit zinc absorption. Similar to protein deficiencies, **zinc deprivation** can cause severe progressive involution of the thymus, with significant, rapid reduction in thymic weight, primarily due to cortical region loss. Zinc is a structural element both in the peptide hormone, thymulin, as well as in many transcription factors. Thus, reduction in the activity of thymulin contributes to thymic and lymphoid atrophy, and decreased activity of factors such as NFκB prevents adequate IL-2 and IFNγ production impairing cell-mediated immune responses. NK cell lytic activity is also diminished with zinc deficiency.

Iron deficiency results in a reduced ability of neutrophils to phagocytose or kill bacteria and fungi as well as decreased lymphocyte response to mitogens and antigens, and impaired NK cell activity. Iron is a double-edged sword as iron-dependent enzymes have crucial roles in lymphocyte and phagocyte function while iron bioavailability favors growth of many microorganisms.

Q. In what ways can neutrophils and macrophages restrict iron availability for microorganisms?
A. Soluble proteins such as lactoferrin produced by neutrophils reduce the availability of free iron in the phagolysosome. Macrophages have ion pumps (e.g. nRAMP) in their phagosomal membrane that remove iron from the phagosome (see Chapter 15).

Selenium, incorporated as the amino acid selenocysteine, is an important component of the antioxidants catalase and glutathione peroxidase. In vitro, selenium deficiency leads to decreased T cell responses, decreased NK cell function, and altered cytokine production. There is some correlation between low selenium levels and disease progression in HIV-infected patients, and with increased viral titers in patients receiving attenuated polio virus; however, the impact of selenium supplementation on anti-viral immunity remains unclear.

Vitamin deficiencies and immune function

Singular deficiencies in **vitamins B1, B6, and B12** are rare; however, as with all nutrients, severe deficits impact immune responses. In vivo studies examining the effects of B vitamin deficiencies, both in humans and animal models, typically show impairment of thymic and lymphoid cellularity, decreased proliferative responses, and decreased antibody production. **Vitamin C** and **vitamin E** have known antioxidant functions. Serum Vitamin C levels quickly diminish with stress or infection. Treatment of DCs in vitro with vitamin C can mediate p38 and NFκB activation augmenting IL-12 secretion. Vitamin E treatment of macrophages, via its antioxidant role, can decrease production of PGE_2.

Q. How might an increase on IL-12 secretion or a decrease in PGE_2 affect immune responses?
A. As PGE_2 normally suppresses IL-12 production, the overall increase in IL-12 would favor TH1 type responses.

Other work has likewise documented the immunoregulatory effects of **Vitamin A** on immune function. Vitamin A deficiency, which is endemic in developing nations, impairs epithelial and mucosal barriers, leading to hyperplasia, loss of mucus-producing cells, and susceptibility to gastrointestinal infection. Additionally, there is a reduction in the number and function of certain lymphocyte subsets, especially those of the gut-associated lymphoid tissue, contributing to overall defects in IgA levels.

Q. NFATc1, a member of the NFAT transcription factor family, is required for development of the B-1 B cell subset. Recent experiments using mice have shown that vitamin A deficiency severely reduces NFAT-c1 expression resulting in loss of the B-1 population. Why might this contribute to defects in mucosal immunity?
A. B1 cells are self-renewing cells that make significant contribution to the mucosal IgA response and are important in maintaining homeostasis with commensal gut bacteria.

Until the advent of antibiotics, cod liver oil and sunlight, both sources of **vitamin D**, were used as primary treatments for TB. Vitamin D deficiency can lead to increased infection rates and recent studies have begun to elucidate some of the molecular mechanisms behind the anti-infective role of vitamin D. Many cell types express the vitamin D receptor (VDR), and while vitamin D metabolites may modulate adaptive immune responses, they can also enhance innate immunity. Importantly, particularly for TB, signaling via the VDR may enhance both cathelicidin and defensin expression, thus boosting macrophage anti-microbial activity (Chapter 7).

Multiple studies in vitamin A-deficient animals have shown that supplementation of **vitamin A** or its metabolites enhances immune responses to vaccination and production of antibodies to both T-dependent and polysaccharide antigens. However, the health benefit of incorporating vitamin A supplements into vaccination programs for diseases such as measles, polio, diphtheria, pertussis and tetanus has been equivocal. There is some evidence that failure in some studies to actually correct the vitamin A deficiency may, in part, account for poor results. Finally, it is important to note that malnutrition due to insufficient intake or absorption is rarely one dimensional. Thus, interpretation of such studies where individual micronutrients are supplemented must take into account that other nutrient deficiencies may remain.

Obesity is associated with altered immune responses

Although the mechanisms remain unclear, obesity increases susceptibility to both nosocomial and post-surgical infections and increases risk of serious complications from common infections. Obese subjects and animals show alteration in various immune responses, including:

- cytotoxicity;
- NK activity; and
- the ability of phagocytes to kill ingested bacteria and fungi.

Altered levels of some micronutrients, lipids, and hormones may explain these immunological changes.

Immunodeficiency secondary to drug therapies

Several classes of drugs suppress immune function , either intentionally for therapeutic effect, or as an unwanted side effect.. For example, patients receiving organ transplants usually receive a variety of immunosuppressants to prevent rejection of the donor tissue and to treat graft-versus-host disease (GvHD, discussed in Chapter 21). Likewise, patients presenting with severe inflammatory, allergic, or autoimmune reactions often require therapeutic immunosuppression (Chapter 20 and Section 5). Pharmacological treatments that suppress immunity as a side effect include cancer treatments such as cytotoxic or anti-metabolite reagents that can also severely depress bone marrow hematopoiesis. Below, we will examine the different classes of immunosuppressive drugs commonly used and their impact on immune function.

Iatrogenic immune suppression post-organ transplantation

Due to genetic differences causing the immune system to perceive donor organs as foreign, recipients of organ transplants receive immunosuppressive regimens, often long-term. Essentially the goal of these treatments is to prevent an immune response against either the host or donor tissues while minimizing toxic side effects and susceptibility of the patient to infection. The primary effectors for both donor organ rejection and GvHD are T lymphocytes. Therefore, both prophylactic and therapeutic immunosuppressant drugs target the T cell branch of the immune system. We briefly summarize transplantation immunology and drugs that help prevent rejection below and Chapter 21 covers these subjects in more detail.

Approaches to suppress T cell-mediated damage include interfering with:

- T cell receptor signaling and activation;
- cytokine secretion;
- cytolytic function;
- T cell proliferation; and
- control of inflammatory mediators.

Drugs such as cyclosporin A and tacrolimus bind to cellular immunophilins and as a complex inhibit calcineurin (see Fig. 8.w1). This blockade dampens T cell signaling mediated by NFAT translocation and, in turn, decrease IL-2 and IFNγ production, impairing both T cell activation and proliferation. The drug sirolimus also binds an immunophilin; however, this interaction results in inhibition of the response to, rather than the production of IL-2, again blocking both proliferation and activation in some lymphocyte subsets.

Interference with cellular proliferation is another mechanism of immune suppression. Drugs such as azathioprine, or the more lymphocyte-specific inhibitor, mycophenolate mofetil prevent B and T cell proliferation by affecting DNA synthesis.

Glucocorticosteroids and their functional analogs are potent anti-inflammatory drugs with effects on all branches of the immune response. In light of their widespread use, we have included a more detailed discussion of this class of drugs below.

Glucocorticoids are powerful immune modulators

Among the pharmacological agents that dampen immune responses, the glucocorticoids have the broadest application. Glucocorticoids have pleiotropic effects that vary with both dose and duration of use; however, they are perhaps best known for their potent anti-inflammatory effect. They have been the front-line drugs for decades in the treatment of a variety of inflammatory and allergic conditions, and continue to be a major component of immunosuppressive regimens following organ transplantation.

Patients can receive glucocorticoids:

- systemically, for example, during the early period immediately post-organ transplant (Chapter 21);
- locally, for example as an inhalant for treatment of asthma (Chapter 23);
- topically, for example as for treatment of poison ivy-induced contact hypersensitivity (Chapter 23).

Glucocorticoids are naturally occurring steroids produced by the adrenal cortex. In response to chronic stress or to inflammatory cytokines, a cascade of hormone signals originating in the hypothalamus drives adrenal production of the immunomodulatory steroid, cortisol (Fig. 17.2 and see Fig. 11.17). Cortisol and its analogs are small steroid hormones that readily cross the cellular membrane and bind cytosolic glucocorticoid receptors. Activated glucocorticoid receptors enter the nucleus and can either directly bind DNA to affect gene transcription or regulate expression by disrupting other transcription factor complexes such as NFκB and AP-1 (Chapter 8).

The timeframe of the downstream effects of this transcriptional regulation ranges from several hours to several days, depending on the rate of protein turnover and de novo

The hypothalamus-pituitary-adrenal axis (HPA axis)

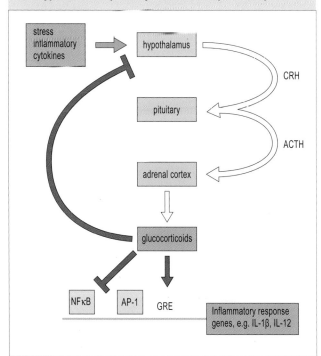

Fig. 17.2 The hypothalamus-pituitary-adrenal axis (HPA axis). Neuroendocrine signaling plays a key role in integrating feedback from the immune system to maintain homeostasis. Inflammatory cytokines trigger the hypothalamus to release corticotropin-releasing hormone (CRH). Increased CRH levels trigger pituitary production of adrenocorticotropic hormone (ACTH) that in turn signals the adrenal glands to increase glucocorticoid production. Glucocorticoids bound to their receptor can interfere with NFκB and AP-1 transcription factor complexes from binding to promoter regions. Additionally, they can interfere with transcription by directly binding to inhibitory glucocorticoid responsive elements (GRE). Under normal conditions, this signaling pathway serves as part of the negative feedback loop shutting down immune responses after infection is controlled.

protein expression that can vary among different pathways effecting changes in the cellular response. More rapid immunosuppressive effects of glucocorticoids can also occur. In T cells, for example, treatment with steroid analogues impedes activity of the tyrosine kinases, Fyn and Lck.

Q. How would suppression of Fyn and Lck affect T cell responses?

A. During TCR signaling, both Lck and Fyn are important in activation of both phospholipase C and the MAP kinase cascades (see Fig. 8.w1). Thus, prevention of tyrosine kinase activity would suppress T cell activation in response to antigens.

Functional effects of steroid treatment

Glucocorticoids have significant effects on both the innate and adaptive branches of the immune response. There is profound suppression of inflammatory cytokine secretion (IL-1β, IL-6, IL-8, TNFα, IL-12) and chemokine

expression. Both contribute to decreased recruitment of neutrophils and macrophages to sites of injury or infection. Glucocorticoids interfere with prostaglandin synthesis, COX2 production, and mast cell degranulation as well. Interestingly, while glucocorticoids enhance both phagocytosis of opsonized antigens and uptake via scavenger receptors, they reduce dendritic cell activation (upregulation of MHC class II and costimulatory B7 molecules).

Within the adaptive branch of immunity, profound downregulation of the inflammatory cytokines and the response of T cells to these cytokines preferentially shift the adaptive immune profile from TH1 toward a TH2-type (Chapter 11). In particular, glucocorticoids suppress both DC production of IL-12 and T cell expression of the IL-12 receptor. In contrast, the effect of corticosteroids on B cell responses is less profound. Thus, overall, humoral immune responses dominate cell-mediated responses during glucocorticosteroid treatment.

Q. After prolonged high steroid dosage there is a modest decrease in all immunoglobulin isotypes. Why should this be?

A. Lack of CD4+ T cell help for B cells will result in a general reduction in the numbers of mature B cells that develop.

While glucocorticoids are an invaluable tool, particularly for controlling inflammatory processes, they are often used for only short periods due to the risk of potent side effects. In administering any of the immunosuppressant drugs, physicians must weigh the therapeutic benefits against the risks of broad immunosuppression. Thus, the pharmacologic challenge that remains is to develop drugs that target only those immune responses involved in the disease process or organ rejection while leaving intact as much of the overall immune system functional as possible. This remains a somewhat elusive goal due to the highly integrated nature of the immune system wherein disturbance of one branch affects the function of the others.

Other causes of secondary immunodeficiencies

There are several other clinical conditions that lead to immune suppression and increased susceptibility to infection. Many chemotherapy regimens, as well as irradiation treatment for cancer, target rapidly dividing cells and cause loss of bone marrow precursor cells. Similarly, cancer metastases to the bone and leukemia involving bone marrow may decrease bone marrow output, or lead to generation of immature or atypical leukocyte populations. Major surgery and/or trauma, as well as chronic stressors or debility and advanced age all correlate with diminished immune function, in part due to the upregulation of endogenous glucocorticoids. Last, viral infections can cause loss of immune function.

Human immunodeficieny virus causes AIDS

Infection with human immunodeficiency virus (HIV) is second only to malnutrition in causing immune deficiency and is a significant cause of morbidity and mortality worldwide. HIV is a retrovirus whose primary cellular targets upon infection are CD4+ T cells, DCs, and macrophages.

Untreated, HIV leads to depletion of the immune system or acquired immunodeficiency syndrome (AIDS), leaving the host susceptible to fatal opportunistic infections. Disease caused by normally non-pathogenic infections, such as *Pneumocystis jirovecii* pneumonia, cytomegalovirus retinitis, and cryptococcal meningitis occur, as do cancers such as Kaposi's sarcoma and non-Hodgkin's lymphoma.

Present primarily in blood, semen, vaginal secretions, and breast milk of infected individuals, HIV is primarily transmitted via unprotected sex, contaminated needles/blood products, or vertically from mother-to-child during the perinatal period. Globally, more than 30 million people are living with the virus, with 2–3 million newly infected and an estimated 1.6–2.1 million deaths each year (WHO estimates, 2009). Over 25 million people have died from AIDS since the descriptions of the first cases in 1981.

There are two main variants, HIV-1 and HIV-2:

- HIV-2 is endemic in West Africa and appears to be less pathogenic;
- HIV-1 has several subtypes (or clades), which are designated by the letters A through K, and the

prevalence of the different clades varies by geographical region – over 90% of people infected with HIV-1 live in developing countries and spread is 80% by the sexual route.

HIV life cycle

HIV is a single-stranded RNA lentivirus. Each enveloped virion contains two copies of the 10-kilobase genome, each encoding nine genes flanked at each end by a long-terminal repeat sequence (LTR). The LTR are essential for integration of viral DNA into the host chromosome and also provide binding sites for initiating replication.

The HIV genome contains *gag* (core proteins), *pol* (reverse transcriptase, protease, and integrase enzymes), and *env* (envelope protein) genes (Fig. 17.3). In addition to these three main gene products, the virus encodes six regulatory and accessory proteins (Tat, Rev, Vpr, Vpu, Vif, and Nef). Alternatively spliced transcripts with overlapping open reading frames allow the coordinated expression of these proteins from the compact HIV genome.

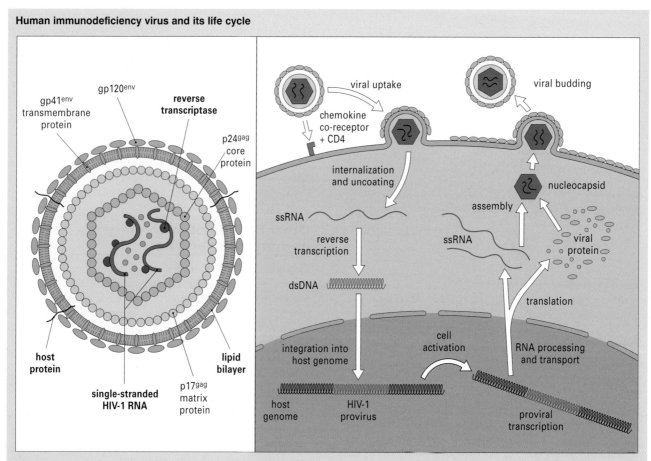

Fig. 17.3 After attachment to CD4 and a chemokine co-receptor (usually CCR5), the virus membrane fuses with the cellular membrane to allow entry into the cell. Following uncoating, reverse transcription of viral RNA results in the production of double-stranded DNA (dsDNA). This is inserted into the host genome as the HIV provirus, by a virally coded integrase enzyme, which is a target for new antiviral medications currently in development. Cell activation leads to transcription and the production of viral mRNAs. Structural proteins are produced and assembled. Free HIV viruses are produced by viral budding from the host cell, after which further internal assembly occurs with the cleavage of a large precursor core protein into the small core protein components by a virally coded protease enzyme, producing mature virus particles, which are released and can go on to infect additional cells bearing CD4 and the chemokine co-receptor.

HIV targets CD4 T cells and mononuclear phagocytes

HIV primarily targets CD4⁺ T cells, CD4⁺ macrophages, and some dendritic cells (DC). *Env* encodes a 160 kDa precursor of the envelope glycoproteins and proteolytic cleavage generates gp120 and gp41. Infection of the target cells requires initial attachment of gp120 to the major receptor, CD4. Viral entry also requires additional binding through co-receptors, most commonly the chemokine receptors CCR5 and CXCR4. Once bound to the cells, interaction via gp41 mediates cell-virus fusion. Upon entry of the HIV capsid, reverse transcription of the RNA genome generates cDNA that subsequently integrates into the host DNA. These latter two steps occur primarily within activated cells.

Differences in the envelope glycoprotein sequence determine whether the virus can utilize the chemokine receptors CCR5 or CXCR4, or both. HIV variants that utilize CCR5 or CXCR4 are referred to as R5 or X4 viruses, respectively. R5 viruses, therefore, can infect memory CD4 T cells and mononuclear phagocytes expressing CCR5. R5 tropism predominates early in HIV infection, while X4, R5, and R5/X4 dual tropic variants may be found in patients during later stages. Individuals homozygous for a 32 base pair deletion in the CCR5 allele (CCR5Δ32) are highly resistant to HIV infection by R5 viruses, but remain susceptible to infection with R4 virus. Other receptors for HIV include DC-SIGN on dendritic cells and galactosyl ceramide (GalC), a major binding site for infection within the brain, gut, and vagina.

Acute symptoms occur 2–4 weeks post infection

Disease is generally the result of infection by a single virion. With infection via a mucosal surface (~80% of infections), the initial target cell is likely a tissue DC or macrophage that can then transport virus to the draining lymphoid tissue. Migration of virus to lymphoid tissue allows productive infection of an activated CD4 T cell or macrophage, inducing cytokine release and further recruitment of activated cells. Recent studies have shown the gut-associated lymphoid tissues (GALT), a site rich with memory CCR5⁺CD4⁺ T cells, is an early locus of infection. HIV infection of GALT CD4 T cells quickly leads to their depletion. Approximately 2–4 weeks post infection, the patient experiences flu-like symptoms, with fever, swollen lymph nodes, malaise, occasionally rashes, headache, and nausea. During acute viremia plasma virus levels can reach up to 10 million copies/mL, with wide dissemination of the virus throughout tissues, often also accompanied by acute depletion of CD4 T cells in the blood and, importantly, establishment of HIV reservoirs. It is estimated that more than half of all memory CD4⁺ T cells are lost during this acute phase.

Viral latency is associated with chronic infection

Without anti-retroviral treatment, HIV levels peak 3–4 weeks post-infection, then gradually drop and plateau (Fig. 17.4). This reflects a combination of the decrease in readily available activated targets and, perhaps more importantly, control by the innate and adaptive immune responses. There is usually a moderate rebound in circulating CD4 T cell numbers at this point, though recent studies

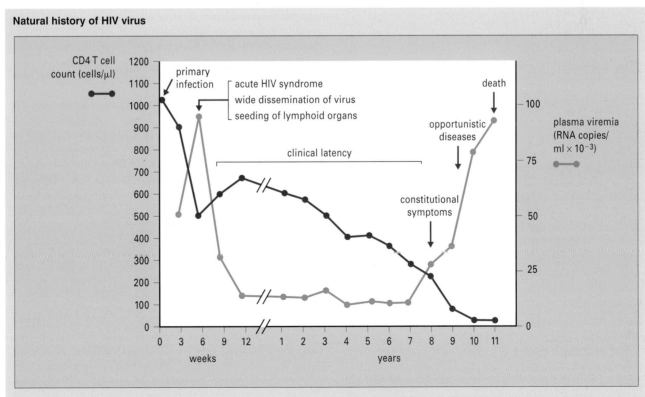

Natural history of HIV virus

Fig. 17.4 A typical course of HIV infection. *(Courtesy of Dr AS Fauci. Modified with permission from Pantaleo G, Graziosi C. N Engl J Med 1993;328:327–335. Copyright 1993 Massachusetts Medical Society. All rights reserved.)*

indicate GALT CD4 T cell populations do not recover. Simultaneously, the virus establishes stable viral reservoirs. This first consists of cells supporting low-level viral replication in lymphoid and other tissues, likely with efficient cell-to-cell propagation of the virus. The second reservoir is within CD4 T cells in which the HIV genome is integrated as a provirus, yet remains latent as a *silent* infection without viral protein transcription. Subsequent T cell activation can then stimulate virus production.

The plasma viral load after acute infection recedes (viral set point) can be an indicator for disease progression. The average period of stable infection is 10 years with mean plasma viral load of ~30 000 copies/mL. Rapid progressors can experience increases in viremia, CD4$^+$ cell depletion, and onset of opportunistic disease in as soon as 6 months. Plasma viral RNA levels of >100 000 copies/mL 6 months after infection are associated with a 10-fold greater risk of progression to AIDS with 5 years as compared to patients with HIV plasma load of <100 000 copies/mL. In contrast, long-term non-progressors (LTNP) generally have a lower viral set-point and may remain asymptomatic for more than 25 years with stable CD4 T cell numbers. During this chronic infection period active immune responses keep viral levels in check. Most infected individuals are asymptomatic during this period but can still transmit infectious virus to others.

HIV infection induces strong immune responses

Both humoral and cellular immune responses develop after infection. Detectable HIV-specific antibodies are evident in the first few weeks of infection. Production of neutralizing antibodies (which prevent virus-cell fusion and correlate with protection) does not occur until at least 12 weeks after infection. Therefore, although antibodies are sufficient to drive evolution of viral epitopes, they are insufficient to prevent disease progression.

The drop in HIV viremia to the set point level coincides with the expansion of HIV-specific CD8$^+$ T cells. In CD8 T cell-depleted animal models of infection, viral containment fails. Thus, as with many viruses, CD8 T cell responses are important components in the control of infection. These responses are usually against peptides derived from multiple viral proteins and comprise a considerable portion (up to 25%) of total CD8 T cells; however, neither the breadth nor the magnitude of CTL responses correlates with control of viremia. In contrast, the genetic background, specifically the HLA haplotype of the host, is important in determining viral control. Both the HLA-B*27 and HLA-B*57 class I alleles are associated with low viral set point and long-term asymptomatic control of infection. These patients are often LTNP and may have stable infection for >10 years.

HIV can evade the immune response

HIV is a rapidly mutating virus. Both error-prone reverse transcription and high recombination frequencies during reverse transcription combine with an extremely high virus production rate to generate genetic diversity. Particularly during acute infection, immune clearance via antibody and CTL recognition favor survival of virions with envelope or peptide sequence changes in regions targeted by host-protective epitopes. Additionally, the HIV protein Nef limits CTL detection of infected cells via selective downregulation of both HLA-A and HLA-B expression, reducing the surface display of viral epitopes. Viral escape, coupled with the existence of latent viral reservoirs undetectable by HIV-specific immune responses, prevents the immune system from eliminating HIV infected cells. Exacerbating this issue, the immune responses become progressively weaker over time.

> **Q. How does Nef mediated downregulation of only HLA-A and B, but not HLA-C and E promote viral immune evasion?**
> A. HLA-C and HLA-E are inhibitory signals for NK cells. Therefore Nef can decrease CTL recognition of infected cells without increasing susceptibility to NK cells (Chapter 10).

Immune dysfunction results from the direct effects of HIV and impairment of CD4 T cells

The chronic phase of HIV infection is marked by persistent generalized immune activation. Infected persons present with B cell polyclonal activation and hypergammaglobulinemia. Attachment of gp120 to mannose binding lectin and to subsets of Ig$^+$ B cells contributes to this activation. Inflammatory cytokines such as IFNα, IFNγ, IL-18, IL-15, and TNFα are elevated during acute infection. Finally, increased translocation of bacteria through the gut barrier, due to extensive HIV infection within the GALT and lamina propria, increases circulating LPS levels, activating many immune effectors via Toll-like receptors. In patients with high viral load, HIV-specific CTL typically contain low levels of intracellular perforin (see Figs 10.10 and 10.12) and have a poor proliferative capacity. During this chronic phase, CD8 T cells often express PD-1, a receptor associated with programmed cell death (Chapter 8). The points above are all consistent with persistent activation and eventual exhaustion of the supply of anti-HIV CD8 T cells that worsens over time.

Of equal if not greater impact on overall immune dysfunction from HIV infection, however, is the loss of the CD4 T cells. Though circulating CD4 T cell counts often rebound (at least quantitatively if not qualitatively) to pre-infection levels after the acute phase, they do not recover within the mucosal associated lymphoid tissues. Furthermore, in untreated patients, CD4 T cell levels eventually decline though they may remain above critical levels for a period of 6 months to 10 years.

CD4 T cell loss is due to direct killing by HIV and activation-induced apoptosis. Additionally, infected CD4 T cells present both gp120 and HIV peptide:HLA complexes on the cell surface leaving them subject to anti-HIV B and CTL clearance. Ongoing loss of CD4 T cell help ultimately contributes to the collapse of the CD8 T cell response as demonstrated experimentally by the ability to rescue anti-HIV CD8 T cell functionality by replacing the lost CD4 T cell population. However, progressive immunodeficiency is a hallmark of HIV and the eventual diminished CD4 T cell levels correlate tightly with the subsequent progression to advanced disease and death.

AIDS is the final stage of HIV infection and disease

Progression to this clinical stage includes a CD4 T cell count of <200/μL. As blood CD4 T cell counts gradually decline during the chronic phase, patients become susceptible to opportunistic infection and malignancies (see Fig. 17.4). Below 500 CD4 cells/μL, less severe conditions such as oral candidiasis, recurrent herpes virus outbreaks (e.g. shingles from varicella zoster virus and anogenital herpes from herpes simplex virus), and pneumococcal infections occur. CD4 T cell levels below 200/μL are associated with increased risk of life-threatening infections and malignancies including *Pneumocystis jirovecii* pneumonia and Kaposi's sarcoma, respectively. With CD4 levels below 50/μL, patients become vulnerable to additional systemic infection with organisms such as *Mycobacterium avium* complex. The three main organ systems affected are the respiratory system, gastrointestinal tract, and central nervous system.

Pneumonia *Pneumocystis jirovecii* (previously *P. carinii*) is the most common opportunistic respiratory infection (Fig. 17.5), but pulmonary bacterial infections, including *Mycobacterium tuberculosis*, also occur. Protozoa (cryptosporidia and microsporidia) are the most

Common features of late-stage HIV infection

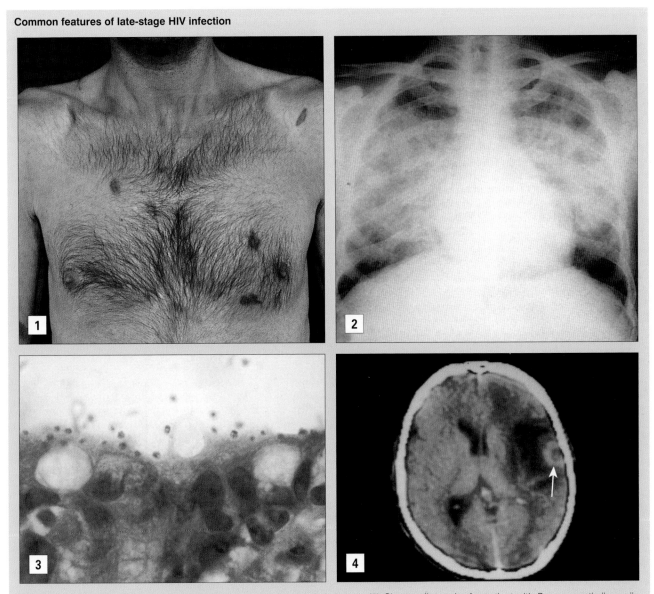

Fig. 17.5 (1) Multiple Kaposi's sarcoma lesions on the chest and abdomen. (2) Chest radiograph of a patient with *Pneumocystis jirovecii* pneumonia, showing bilateral interstitial shadowing. (3) Small bowel biopsy from a patient with diarrhea caused by cryptosporidia, showing intermediate forms of cryptosporidia (small pink dots) on the surface of the mucosa. (4) Computed tomography scan of the head of a patient with cerebral toxoplasmosis. The patient presented with a history of fits and weakness of the left arm and leg. Injection of contrast revealed a ring-enhancing lesion in the right hemisphere (arrow), with surrounding edema (dark area).

common pathogens isolated in patients with diarrhoea and weight loss (see Fig. 17.5). **Enteric bacteria** such as *Salmonella* and *Campylobacter* spp. may also afflict AIDS patients.

Neurological complications in AIDS are due to direct effects of HIV infection, opportunistic infections, or lymphoma. AIDS-related dementia once affected between 10–40% of patients with other manifestations of AIDS, but with more effective antiviral treatment has become less common. Neurological involvement can be due to a number of pathogens. ***Cryptococcus neoformans*** is a fungus and is the most common cause of AIDS-related meningitis. **Toxoplasmosis**, a protozoal infection, causes cysts in the brain and neurological deficit (see Fig. 17.5). **Cytomegalovirus** reactivation may cause inflammation of the retina, brain, and spinal cord and its nerve roots, and a **polyomavirus (JC virus)**, which infects oligodendrocytes in the brain, produces a rapidly fatal demyelinating disease – **progressive multifocal leukoencephalopathy**.

Kaposi's sarcoma (KS), caused by infection with **KS-associated herpes virus (KSHV)**, is the most common AIDS-associated malignancy (Fig. 17.5). KSHV infections, similar to CMV herpesvirus infections, are often asymptomatic in individuals with competent T cell immunity. With HIV co-infection, however, KSHV titers increase and KS emerges with multifocal lesions (see Fig. 17.5) of mixed cellularity often resulting in widespread involvement of skin, mucous membranes, viscera (gut and lungs) and lymph nodes. KSHV infection can also lead to development of B cell lymphomas, affecting the brain, gut, bone marrow, lymph nodes, spleen and body cavities such as the pericardial and pleural spaces. KSHV also causes two B cell lymphoproliferative diseases, multicentric Castleman's disease and primary effusion lymphoma.

Most of the opportunistic infections as well as malignancies, such as KS and Epstein–Barr virus-associated non-Hodgkin's lymphomas, are due to the inability of the immune response to suppress baseline levels of reactivation of latent organisms in the host and in some cases, to ubiquitous organisms to which we are continually exposed. They are difficult to diagnose and treatment often suppresses rather than eradicates them. Relapses are common and continuous suppressive or maintenance treatment is necessary.

An effective vaccine remains an elusive goal

Currently, treatment for HIV focuses on anti-viral drug cocktails that significantly reduce the patient's viral load. Due to the rapid rate of mutation in the viral genome during replication, single drug therapy nearly always leads to rapid drug resistance. However, by providing the patient with a cocktail of anti-viral drugs, each targeting a different aspect of the viral life cycle, it is possible to prolong the period of time before plasma viral load increases and T cell counts drop. Anti-retroviral therapies, unfortunately, are not a cure, nor can they prevent transmission of the virus.

Despite increasing characterization of adaptive immune responses, the correlates of protection remain to be fully defined, and this has left the field with mostly empiric approaches. Ideally, investigators will develop a vaccine that provides sufficient protection to prevent viral transmission. Encouraging early reports of persons repeatedly exposed to HIV who never became infected suggested that adaptive immune responses, particularly HIV-specific CD8 T cell responses, might be responsible for apparent protection, but this remains somewhat controversial. Such a vaccine will almost certainly also require the induction of broadly neutralizing antibody responses; something that candidate vaccines have yet to achieve. To date there have been clinical trials of numerous candidate HIV vaccines, but most would agree that an effective vaccine remains an elusive goal.

Q. Why is it difficult to identify suitable antigens that could be used in a neutralizing vaccine?
A. The very rapid rate of HIV mutation and the high rate of virus production mean that the virus can readily mutate to evade a specific immune response, and yet may develop variants that retain infectivity.

Many in the field believe that a vaccine that protects from disease progression, while not necessarily protecting from the initial infection, is a more realistic short-term goal. Toward this goal, investigators have focused on approaches that induce cellular immune responses, particularly CD8 T cells responses. However, there is increasing evidence suggesting that optimal efficacy will also need to elicit robust CD4 T cell responses to HIV.

As no cure or vaccine is currently available, our main weapon is prevention through health education and control of infection.

CRITICAL THINKING: SECONDARY IMMUNODEFICIENCY (SEE P. 438 FOR EXPLANATIONS)

A 52-year-old record producer developed a severe cough with increasing shortness of breath. He also had a fever, chest pain, and malaise. For the week before presentation he complained of pain on swallowing. His past medical history included gonorrhea and genital herpes within the previous 3 years. Over the previous 2 months he had suffered from persistent diarrhea and lost 9 kg in weight from a baseline of 68 kg. He lived with his girlfriend with whom he had been having unprotected intercourse for several years. There was no history of intravenous drug abuse.

On examination he was underweight and had enlarged lymph nodes in the neck, axillae, and groin. Plaques of *Candida albicans* were visible in his throat. There were abnormal breath sounds in his lungs. The results of his blood tests are shown in Table 1.

Table 1
Results of investigations on presentation

Investigation	Result (normal range)
hemoglobin (g/dL)	12.8 (13.5–18.0)
platelet count ($\times 10^9$/L)	128 (150–400)
white cell count ($\times 10^9$/L)	6.2 (4.0–11.0)
neutrophils ($\times 10^9$/L)	5.4 (2.0–7.5)
eosinophils ($\times 10^9$/L)	0.24 (0.4–0.44)
total lymphocytes ($\times 10^9$/L)	0.75 (1.6–3.5)
T lymphocytes CD4$^+$ ($\times 10^9$/L) CD8$^+$ ($\times 10^9$/L)	0.12 (0.7–1.1) 0.42 (0.5–0.9)
B lymphocytes ($\times 10^9$/L)	0.11 (0.2–0.5)
arterial blood gases PaO$_2$ (kPa) PaCO$_2$ (kPa) pH HCO$_3$ base excess	7.8 (>10.6) 5.52 (4.7–6.0) 7.39 (7.35–7.45) 25.6 –0.9
ECG	normal
chest radiography	bilateral diffuse interstitial shadowing
bronchoscopy with bronchoalveolar lavage	positive for *Pneumocystis jirovecii*

Because of his sexual history, the patient was counseled about having a human immunodeficiency virus (HIV) test, and consented. An enzyme-linked immunosorbent assay (ELISA, see Method box 3.2, Fig. 2) was positive for anti-HIV antibodies and a polymerase chain reaction (PCR) demonstrated HIV-1 RNA in the plasma.

Examination of an induced sputum specimen revealed *Pneumocystis jirovecii*, which together with the positive HIV ELISA is an AIDS-defining illness. Thus a clear diagnosis of acquired immune deficiency syndrome (AIDS) was made and the patient's *P. jirovecii* pneumonia was treated with oxygen by mask and parenteral co-trimoxazole. He was discharged from hospital taking oral co-trimoxazole.

Within 3 months he was seen again in accident and emergency with blurred vision and 'flashing lights' in his eyes. He was shown to have an infection of his retina with cytomegalovirus and was treated with injections of ganciclovir. The CD4 count at this time was 0.04×10^9/L. While receiving this treatment the patient became increasingly unwell and semiconscious. Investigations at this time are shown Table 2.

Continued

CRITICAL THINKING: SECONDARY IMMUNODEFICIENCY (SEE P. 438 FOR EXPLANATIONS) CONT.

Table 2
Results of investigations 3 months after presentation

Investigation	Result (normal range)
hemoglobin (g/dL)	10.4 (13.5–18.0)
platelet count ($\times 10^9$/L)	104 (150–400)
white cell count ($\times 10^9$/L)	4.1 (4.0–11.0)
neutrophils ($\times 10^9$/L)	4.2 (2.0–7.5)
eosinophils ($\times 10^9$/L)	0.24 (0.4–0.44)
total lymphocytes ($\times 10^9$/L)	0.62 (1.6–3.5)
T lymphocytes CD4$^+$ ($\times 10^9$/L) CD8$^+$ ($\times 10^9$/L)	0.03 (0.7–1.1) 0.40 (0.5–0.9)
B lymphocytes ($\times 10^9$/L)	0.09 (0.2–0.5)
chest radiography	minimal areas of diffuse shadowing
blood culture	negative
blood glucose (mmol/L)	7.6 (<10.0)
CSF from lumbar puncture Appearance	turbid
white cells (polymorphs/mm^3)	2500
protein (g/L)	4.2 (0.15–0.45)
glucose (mmol/L)	4.5 (> 60% blood glucose)
Indian ink stain	positive for cryptococcus

A diagnosis of cryptococcal meningitis was made and intravenous amphotericin was started. The patient did not respond to treatment and died shortly afterwards. At autopsy, *P. jirovecii* was isolated from his lungs and evidence of early cerebral lymphoma was noted.

1 What diagnostic tests are available for HIV infection?

2 Which of these tests should be used if HIV infection is suspected in a mother and her child infected vertically?

3 What serological and cellular indices can be used to monitor the course of HIV infection?

Further reading

Altfeld M, Allen TM, Yu XG, et al. HIV-1 superinfection despite broad CD8$^+$ T cell responses containing replication of the primary virus. Nature 2002;420:434–439.

Brenchley JM, Schacker TW, Ruff LE, et al. CD4$^+$ T cell depletion during all stages of HIV disease occurs predominantly in the gastrointestinal tract. J Exp Med 2004;200:749–759.

Cunningham-Rundles S, McNeeley DF, Moon A. Mechanisms of nutrient modulation of the immune response. J Allergy Clin Immunol 2005;115:1119–1128.

Day CL, Walker BD. Progress in defining CD4 helper cell responses in chronic viral infections. J Exp Med 2003;198:1773–1777.

International HIV Controllers Study. The major genetic determinants of HIV-a control affect HLA class I peptide presentation. Science 2010;330:1551–1557.

McElrath MJ, Haynes BF. Induction of immunity to human immunodeficiency virus type-1 by vaccination. Immunity 2010;33:542–554.

Migueles SA, Laborico AC, Shupert WL, et al. HIV-specific CD8$^+$ T cell proliferation is coupled to perforin expression and is maintained in nonprogressors. Nat Immunol 2002;3:1061–1068.

Paczesny S, Hanauer D, Sun Y, Reddy P. New perspectives on the biology of acute GVHD. Bone Marrow Transplant 2010;45:1–11.

Stahn C, Löwenberg M, Hommes DW, Buttgereit F. Molecular mechanisms of glucocorticoid action and selective glucocorticoid receptor agonists. Mol Cell Endocrinol 2007;275:71–78.

CHAPTER 18

Vaccination

SUMMARY

- **Vaccination applies immunological principles to human health.** Adaptive immunity and the ability of lymphocytes to develop memory for a pathogen's antigens underlie vaccination. Active immunization is known as vaccination.

- **A wide range of antigen preparations are in use as vaccines,** from whole organisms to simple peptides and polysaccharides. Living and non-living vaccines have important differences, living vaccines being generally more effective.

- **Adjuvants enhance antibody production,** and are usually required with non-living vaccines. They concentrate antigen at appropriate sites or induce cytokines.

- **Most vaccines are still given by injection,** but other routes are being investigated.

- **Vaccine efficacy needs to be reviewed from time-to-time**.

- **Vaccine safety is an overriding consideration.** When immunization frequencies fall, the population as a whole is not protected. Fears over the safety of the MMR vaccine resulted in measles epidemics and increases in incidence of rubella.

- **Vaccines in general use have variable success rates.** Some vaccines are reserved for special groups only and vaccines for parasites and some other infections are only experimental.

- **Passive immunization can be life-saving.** The direct administration of antibodies still has a role to play in certain circumstances, for example when tetanus toxin is already in the circulation.

- **Non-specific immunotherapy can boost immune activity.** Non-specific immunization, for example by cytokines, may be of use in selected conditions.

- **Immunization against a variety of non-infectious conditions is being investigated.**

- **Recombinant DNA technology will be the basis for the next generation of vaccines.** Most future vaccines will be recombinant subunit vaccines incorporated into viral or bacterial vectors. This should provide enhanced efficacy and safety.

Vaccination

Vaccines apply immunological principles to human health

Vaccination is the best known and most successful application of immunological principles to human health. It exploits the property of immunological memory to provide long lasting protection against infectious disease.

The first vaccine was named after Vaccinia, the cowpox virus. Jenner pioneered its use 200 years ago. It was the first deliberate scientific attempt to prevent an infectious disease and was based on the notion that infection with a mild disease (cowpox) might protect against infection with a similar but much more serious one (smallpox), although it was done in complete ignorance of viruses (or indeed any kind of microbe) and immunology.

It was not until the work of Pasteur 100 years later that the general principle governing vaccination emerged – altered preparations of microbes could be used to generate enhanced immunity against the fully virulent organism. Thus Pasteur's dried rabies-infected rabbit spinal cords and heated anthrax bacilli were the true forerunners of today's vaccines, whereas, until very recently, Jenner's animal-derived (i.e. 'heterologous') vaccinia virus had no real successors.

Even Pasteur did not have a proper understanding of immunological memory or the functions of the lymphocyte, which had to wait another half century.

Finally, with Burnet's clonal selection theory (1957) and the discovery of T and B lymphocytes (1965), the key mechanism became clear.

In any immune response, the antigen(s) induces clonal expansion in specific T and/or B cells, leaving behind a population of memory cells. These enable the next encounter with the same antigen(s) to induce a secondary response, which is more rapid and effective than the normal primary response.

While for many infections the primary response may be too slow to prevent serious disease, if the individual has been exposed to antigens from the organism in a vaccine before encountering the pathogenic organism, the expanded population of memory cells and raised levels of specific antibody are able to protect against disease. The principles of vaccination can be summarized as:

- priming of specific lymphocytes to expand the pool of memory cells;
- use of harmless forms of immunogen – attenuated organisms, subcellular fragments, toxoids or vectors;
- use of adjuvants to enhance immune responses; and
- production of safe, affordable vaccines to promote herd immunity.

Q. Rabies is one of the few diseases in which active immunization may be carried out after the individual becomes infected. What particular feature of rabies infection makes this a reasonable treatment?

A. The time between infection and the development of the disease is long, so an effective immune response has time to develop before virus reaches the CNS to produce symptoms.

Vaccines can protect populations as well as individuals

Vaccines protect individuals against disease, and if there are sufficient immune individuals in a population, transmission of the infection is prevented. This is known as **herd immunity**.

The proportion of the population that needs to be immune to prevent epidemics occurring depends on the nature of the infection:

- if the organism is highly infectious so that one individual can rapidly infect several non-immune individuals, as is

the case for measles, a high proportion of the population must be immune to maintain herd immunity;
- if the infection is less readily transmitted, immunity in a lower proportion of the population may be sufficient to prevent disease transmission.

Effective vaccines must be safe to administer, induce the correct type of immunity, and be affordable by the population at which they are aimed. Over the middle of the 20th century for many of the world's major infectious diseases, this was achieved with brilliant success, culminating in the official eradication of smallpox in 1980. Beyond this era progress was much slower and fears over vaccine safety made development more lengthy and costly. However, the advent of recombinant DNA technology has led to a number of significant advances in the first decade of the 21st century and a number of new, safe and effective vaccines have come onto the market during this period. Despite these successes for many diseases development of an effective vaccine has remained elusive, in particular, parasitic diseases and HIV.

Nevertheless, with the availability of new technologies and a greater understanding of the immunological principles that underlie effective vaccines, the future for new vaccine development looks brighter than it has for some years.

Antigen preparations used in vaccines

A wide variety of preparations are used as vaccines (Fig. 18.1). In general, the more antigens of the microbe retained in the vaccine, the better, and living organisms tend to be more effective than killed organisms. Exceptions to this rule are:

- diseases where a toxin is responsible for the pathology – in this case the vaccine can be based on the toxin alone;

The main antigenic preparations

type of antigen		vaccine examples
living organisms	natural	vaccinia (for smallpox) vole bacillus (for tuberculosis; historical)
	attenuated	polio (Sabin; oral polio vaccine)*, measles*, mumps*, rubella*, yellow fever 17D, varicella-zoster (human herpesvirus 3), BCG (for tuberculosis)*
intact but non-living organisms	viruses	polio (Salk)*, rabies, influenza, hepatitis A, typhus
	bacteria	*pertussis, typhoid, cholera, plague
subcellular fragments	capsular polysaccharides	pneumococcus, meningococcus, *Haemophilus influenzae*
	surface antigen	hepatitis B*
toxoids		tetanus*, diphtheria*
recombinant DNA-based	gene cloned and expressed	hepatitis B (yeast-derived)*
	genes expressed in vectors	experimental
	naked DNA	experimental
*standard in most countries		

Fig. 18.1 A wide range of antigenic preparations are used as vaccines.

- a vaccine in which microbial antigens are inserted into vector and expressed in a host cell.

Live vaccines can be natural or attenuated organisms

Natural live vaccines have rarely been used

Apart from vaccinia, no other completely natural organism has ever come into standard use. However:

- bovine and simian rotaviruses have been tried in children;
- the vole tubercle bacillus was once popular against tuberculosis, and
- in the Middle East and Russia *Leishmania* infection from mild cases is reputed to induce immunity.

Although it is possible that another good heterologous vaccine will be found, safety problems with this approach remain considerable. Nevertheless, the ability to genetically manipulate heterologous organisms can increase safety (for example, by removing genes responsible for virulence) and allow the creation of hybrid organisms capable of eliciting a strong immune response to the natural human pathogen. A recent example of the successful application of this approach is in the development of new rotavirus vaccines.

Attenuated live vaccines have been highly successful

Historically, the preferred strategy for vaccine development has been to attenuate a human pathogen, with the aim of diminishing its virulence while retaining the desired antigens.

This was first done successfully by Calmette and Guérin with a bovine strain (*Mycobacterium bovis*) of *Mycobacterium tuberculosis*, which during 13 years (1908–1921) of culture *in vitro* changed to the much less virulent form now known as BCG (bacille Calmette–Guérin), which has at least some protective effect against tuberculosis.

The real successes were with viruses, starting with the 17D strain of yellow fever virus obtained by passage in mice and chicken embryos (1937), and followed by a roughly similar approach with polio, measles, mumps, and rubella (Fig. 18.2)

Q. Why would passage of a virus in a non-human species be a rational way of developing a vaccine for use in humans?
A. The selective pressure on the virus to retain genes needed for virulence in humans and for human-to-human transfer is removed. Consequently some variants may lose these genes and are at no disadvantage in the animal, but will retain antigenicity for use as attenuated vaccine strains.

Just how successful the vaccines for polio, measles, mumps, and rubella are is shown by the decline in these four diseases between 1950 and 1980 (Fig. 18.3).

Attenuated microorganisms are less able to cause disease in their natural host

Attenuation 'changes' microorganisms to make them less able to grow and cause disease in their natural host. In early attenuated organisms, 'changed' meant a purely random set of mutations induced by adverse conditions of growth. Vaccine candidates were selected by constantly monitoring for

Live attenuated vaccines

	disease	remarks
viruses	polio	types 2 and 3 may revert; also killed vaccine
	measles	80% effective
	mumps	
	rubella	now given to both sexes
	yellow fever	stable since 1937
	varicella-zoster	mainly in leukemia
	hepatitis A	also killed vaccine
bacteria	tuberculosis	stable since 1921; also some protection against leprosy

Fig. 18.2 Attenuated vaccines are available for many, but not all, infections. In general it has proved easier to attenuate viruses than bacteria.

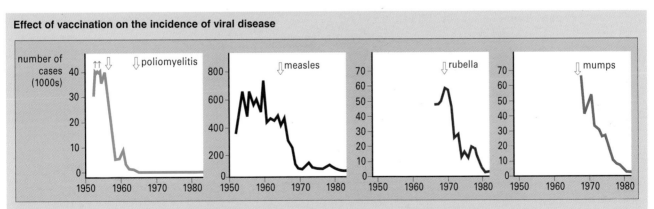

Effect of vaccination on the incidence of viral disease

Fig. 18.3 The effect of vaccination on the incidence of various viral diseases in the USA has been that most infections have shown a dramatic downward trend since the introduction of a vaccine (*arrows*).

retention of antigenicity and loss of virulence – a tedious process.

When viral gene sequencing became possible it emerged that the results of attenuation were widely divergent. An example is the divergence between the three types of live (Sabin) polio vaccine:

- type 1 polio has 57 mutations and has almost never reverted to wild type;
- types 2 and 3 vaccines depend for their safety and virulence on only two key mutations – frequent reversion to wild type has occurred, in some cases leading to outbreaks of paralytic poliomyelitis.

Those genes not essential for replication of the virus are mostly concerned with evasion of host responses and **virulence**, that is the ability to replicate efficiently and disseminate widely within the body, with pathological consequences. Many pathogenic viruses contain virulence genes that mimic or interfere with cytokine and chemokine function. Some of these have sequence homology to their mammalian counterparts and others do not.

> **Q. It is often found that attenuated viruses that are avirulent do not make good vaccines. Why should this be?**
> A. Inflammation induced by damage to the host has an adjuvant effect, leading to more effective presentation of the vaccine antigens.

Killed vaccines are intact but non-living organisms

Killed vaccines are the successors of Pasteur's killed vaccines mentioned above:

- some are very effective (rabies and the Salk polio vaccine);
- some are moderately effective (typhoid, cholera, and influenza);
- some are of debatable value (plague and typhus); and
- some are controversial on the grounds of toxicity (pertussis).

Figure 18.4 lists the main killed vaccines in use today. These are gradually being replaced by attenuated or subunit vaccines. However, in the case of polio, some countries are reverting to the use of killed vaccine which is safer than the attenuated vaccine, even though it is less effective. This choice only becomes relevant when the risk of contracting the disease is low in comparison with the risk of developing adverse reactions to the vaccine.

Inactivated toxins and toxoids are the most successful bacterial vaccines

The most successful of all bacterial vaccines – tetanus and diphtheria – are based on inactivated exotoxins (Fig. 18.5), and in principle the same approach can be used for several other infections. An inactive, mutant form of diphtheria toxin (CRM_{197}) has been used as the basis for a number of newly generated conjugate vaccines (see below).

Subunit vaccines and carriers

Aside from the toxin-based vaccines, which are subunits of their respective microorganisms, a number of other vaccines are in use which employ antigens either purified from microorganisms or produced by recombinant DNA technology (Fig. 18.6). For example, a recombinant Hepatitis B surface antigen synthesized in baker's yeast, has been in use since 1986.

Killed (whole organism) vaccines

disease		remarks
viruses	polio	preferred in Scandinavia; safe in immunocompromised
	rabies	can be given post-exposure, with passive antiserum
	influenza	strain-specific
	hepatitis A	also attenuated vaccine
bacteria	pertussis	brain damage in v. rare cases? replaced by safe acellular vaccine
	typhoid	about 70% protection
	cholera	combined with recombinant modified toxin
	plague	short-term protection only
	Q fever	good protection

Fig. 18.4 The principal vaccines using killed whole organisms.

Toxin-based vaccines

organism	vaccine	remarks
Clostridium tetani	inactivated toxin (formalin)	three doses, alum-precipitated; boost every 10 years
Corynebacterium diphtheriae		usually given with tetanus
Vibrio cholerae	recombinant modified toxin	combined with whole killed organism
Clostridium perfringens	inactivated toxin (formalin)	for newborn lambs

Fig. 18.5 The principal toxin-based vaccines. Note that there are no vaccines against the numerous staphylococcal and streptococcal exotoxins, or against bacterial endotoxins such as lipopolysaccharides.

Acellular pertussis vaccine consisting of a small number of proteins purified from the bacterium has been available for some years now, and has been shown to be effective, safer and less toxic than the whole killed-organism vaccine. It is usually administered as part of a DTaP (Diphtheria, Tetanus, Pertussis) combination vaccine routinely given to infants.

Conjugate vaccines are effective at inducing antibodies to carbohydrate antigens

Although protein antigens such as hepatitis B surface antigen are immunogenic when given with alum adjuvant (see below), for many types of bacteria, virulence is determined by the bacterial capsular polysaccharide, prime examples being *Neisseria meningitidis*, *Streptococcus pneumoniae*, and *Haemophilus influenzae B*. Such carbohydrate antigens, though they can be isolated and have been used for vaccination, are poorly immunogenic, particularly in infants under 2 years, and often do not induce IgG responses or long-lasting protection. Attempts to boost immunity by repeat administration of these vaccines can actually compromise immunity by depleting the pool of antibody-producing B cells.

Q. Why do polysaccharide antigens not induce IgG responses or lasting immunity?

A. Polysaccharide antigens are not processed for presentation to TH cells, so they do not induce class switching, affinity maturation, or generate memory T cells (see Chapters 8 and 9).

A major advance in the efficacy of subunit vaccines has been obtained by conjugating the purified polysaccharides to carrier proteins such as tetanus or diphtheria toxoid. These protein carriers, which can now be produced in highly purified form by recombinant DNA techniques, are presumed to recruit TH cells and the conjugates induce IgG antibody responses and more effective long lasting protection.

Starting with *Haemophilus influenzae* (Hib) in the early 1990s, conjugate vaccines for *Neisseria* meningitis strains A, C, Y and W-135 are also now in widespread usage. In the UK up until 1992 when the vaccine was introduced, Hib was the major cause of infantile meningitis leading to many hundreds of cases per year. The introduction of the vaccine led to a very rapid decline making Hib meningitis now a very rare occurrence (Fig. 18.7).

Antigens can be expressed from vectors

Many antigens can now be produced in recombinant form by cloning their genes into a suitable expression vector. This approach has been highly successful with the hepatitis B surface (HBsAg) antigen, cloned into yeast and this has now replaced the first-generation HBsAg vaccine, which was laboriously purified from the blood of hepatitis B carriers; it has also brought down the cost of the vaccine.

The most spectacular success with this approach, however, has been the development of the vaccines against human papilloma virus (HPV) infection. HPV has been established as the causative agent in cervical carcinoma and over 70% of cases are accounted for by the serotypes 16 and 18. Two new vaccines (trademarked Gardasil and Cervarix) have been developed using recombinant expression vectors that produce the viral surface protein L1. Aggregates of L1 spontaneously assemble into virus-like particles (VLP) that are highly immunogenic. Because these particles contain no nucleic acid the vaccine cannot lead to HPV infection and is very safe. Trials suggest that very high levels of protection against HPV infection and cervical carcinoma are afforded with these vaccines. A vaccine has been licensed in the UK for girls aged 9–15 and for women aged 16–26 since 2007, and in September 2008 HPV vaccination was adopted as part of the national immunization program for girls aged 12–13 across the UK.

Adjuvants enhance antibody production

The increasing use of purified or recombinant antigens has refocused attention on the requirement to boost immune responses through the use of adjuvants. These are often necessary as the antigens on their own are insufficiently immunogenic.

Work in the 1920s on the production of animal sera for human therapy discovered that certain substances, notably aluminum salts (alum), added to or emulsified with an antigen, greatly enhance antibody production – that is, they act as adjuvants. Aluminum hydroxide is still widely used with, for example, diphtheria and tetanus toxoids.

The difficulty with adjuvants is that they mediate their effect through stimulating the inflammatory response, generally necessary to produce a good immune response to

Subunit vaccines

	organism	remarks
virus	hepatitis B virus	surface antigen can be purified from blood of carriers or produced in yeast by recombinant DNA technology
bacteria	*Neisseria meningitidis*	capsular polysaccharides or conjugates of groups A, C, γ and W-135 are effective B is non-immunogenic
	Streptococcus pneumoniae	84 serotypes; capsular polysaccharide vaccines contain 23 serotypes; conjugates with five or seven bacterial serotypes now available
	Haemophilus influenzae B	good conjugate vaccines now in use

Fig. 18.6 Conjugate vaccines are replacing pure polysaccharides. *N. meningitidis* type B is non-immunogenic in humans because the capsular polysaccharide cross-reacts with self carbohydrates towards which the host is immunologically tolerant.

Introduction of the vaccine led to a rapid decline in Hib meningitis

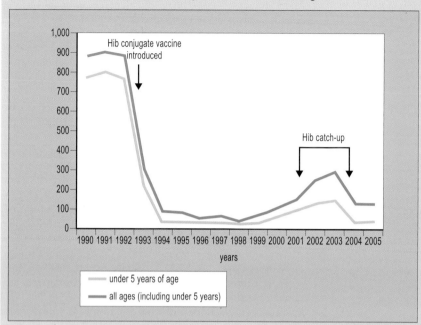

Fig. 18.7 Incidence of *H. influenzae* type B in children in England and Wales (1990–2004). Vaccination was initiated in 1992. There was an upsurge in cases after 1999, possibly because the vaccine was less effective when used in combination with other vaccines, but this was controlled with a further campaign, initiated in 2003. *(Based on data from the Health Protection Agency.)*

antigen. Unfortunately, the inflammatory response is often responsible for the side effects of immunization, such as pain and swelling at the injection site, and can lead to greater malaise, elevated temperature and/or 'flu-like symptoms'. These are often impediments to vaccine uptake, especially when the distress is caused in small infants who are the commonest vaccine recipients.

With modern understanding of the processes leading to lymphocyte triggering and the development of memory, it is hoped that better adjuvants can be developed. Considerable efforts have been made to produce better adjuvants, particularly for T cell-mediated responses. Figure 18.8 gives a list of these, most of which are still highly experimental or too toxic for use in humans. One recent exception however, is monophosphoryl lipid A (MPL). This compound is derived from chemical degradation of lipopolysaccharide (LPS), the major component of the cell wall of gram negative bacteria. MPL retains potent adjuvant activity but, unlike LPS itself, has low toxicity. It is combined with alum in an adjuvant product AS04, which is incorporated in the new HPV vaccine, Cervarix™. In another adjuvant formulation (AS02) MPL is combined with a saponin (QS21) in an oil-water emulsion. AS02 has proven to be of major importance in boosting the immunogenicity of the candidate malaria vaccine RS,S.

Adjuvants concentrate antigen at appropriate sites or induce cytokines

It appears that the effect of adjuvants is due mainly to two activities:

- the concentration of antigen in a site where lymphocytes are exposed to it (the 'depot' effect); and
- the induction of cytokines that regulate lymphocyte function.

Aluminum salts probably have a predominantly depot function, inducing small granulomas in which antigen is retained.

Newer formulations such as liposomes and immune-stimulating complexes (ISCOMs) achieve the same purpose by ensuring that antigens trapped in them are delivered to antigen-presenting cells (APCs).

Particulate antigens such as virus-like particles (polymers of viral capsid proteins containing no viral DNA or RNA) are highly immunogenic and have the useful property that they may also induce cross-priming (i.e. enter the MHC class 1 processing pathway though not synthesized within the APC, see Chapter 8).

Q. Many bacterial carbohydrates and glycolipids are good adjuvants, even though they are not good immunogens. Why should this be so?

A. The discovery of Toll-like receptors (TLRs, see Fig. 6.20) and other pattern recognition receptors, such as lectin-like receptors for carbohydrates (see Fig. 7.10), has provided an explanation for the long-known efficacy of many bacterial products as adjuvants. It is clear that they act mainly by binding to PRRs and stimulating the formation of appropriate cytokines by APCs.

Ligation of different PRRs may bias the response toward TH1 or TH2 cytokine production.

Not surprisingly cytokines themselves have been shown to be effective adjuvants, particularly when coupled directly to the antigen. Cytokines may be particularly useful in immunocompromised patients, who often fail to respond to normal vaccines. It is hoped that they might also be useful in directing the immune response in the desired direction, for example in diseases where only TH1 (or TH2) cell memory is wanted.

Adjuvants

adjuvant type	routinely used in humans	experimental* or too toxic for human use†
inorganic salts	aluminum hydroxide (alhydrogel) aluminum phosphate calcium phosphate	beryllium hydroxide
delivery systems		liposomes* ISCOMs* block polymers slow-release formulations*
bacterial products	*Bordetella pertussis* (with diphtheria, tetanus toxoids)	BCG *Mycobacterium bovis* and oil† (complete Freund's adjuvant) muramyl dipeptide (MDP)†
natural mediators (cytokines)		IL-1 IL-2 IL-12 IFNγ
ISCOMs, immune-stimulating complexes		

Fig. 18.8 A variety of foreign and endogenous substances can act as adjuvants, but only aluminum and calcium salts and pertussis are routinely used in clinical practice.

Vaccine administration

Most vaccines are delivered by injection

Administration by injection presents some risks, particularly in developing countries, where re-use of needles and syringes may transmit disease, particularly HIV. Alternatives to needle delivery do exist, however, and can be beneficial for use in mass vaccination programs and for improving compliance in those with 'needle phobia'. Mass vaccination, for many years, made use of multiuse jet injectors that fire a high-velocity liquid stream, which is very effective. Unfortunately, the possibility of cross-contamination from the reusable design has, in more recent years, limited their application. Efforts are now being made to develop disposable single use cartridges for such injectors, but inevitably at greater cost per vaccination.

Jet injectors can deliver vaccine intramuscularly, as with a needle, but they can also be used for cutaneous delivery, which should help to reduce the discomfort and potential for distress in infants. Cutaneous delivery is a highly effective method for vaccination; the skin harbors many Langerhans' cells, which are very active in antigen presentation to T cells in lymph nodes, to which they migrate when activated by exposure to antigen. They also help to initiate an inflammatory response through release of cytokines and chemical mediators, all of which can potentiate the vaccine.

The main difficulty with cutaneous delivery is penetrating below the outer, cornified layer of the skin. Techniques to improve this such as the uses of microneedle arrays (Fig. 18.9) are under development and may one day allow vaccination using skin patches, similar to those used currently for delivering (small molecule) drugs, such as contraceptives.

Mucosal immunization is a logical alternative approach

Because most organisms enter via mucosal surfaces, mucosal immunization makes logical sense. The success of the oral polio vaccine, the newly formulated rotavirus vaccine and an effective cholera vaccine indicates that it can be made to work. However, although live attenuated vaccines can be effective when delivered orally, most killed vaccines are not.

Q. What key problems would one expect to be associated with oral vaccines?
A. Antigens may be broken down by passage through the stomach and digestive system, but, more problematically, the intestinal immune system is designed to generate tolerance rather than an immune response against food antigens.

Immunization only occurs when pathogenic organisms invade the gut wall. This can be mimicked by providing an adjuvant. Toxins from pathogenic intestinal organisms (cholera and *Escherichia coli*) have been the most studied intestinal adjuvants. Because the native toxins are extremely potent, partially inactivating mutations have been introduced to prevent excessive intestinal stimulation. Although these adjuvants work in experimental models, it is difficult to achieve a reproducible balance between:

- adequate stimulation of an immune response; and
- excessive gut inflammation.

An alternative is to use recombinant bacteria engineered to express antigens of interest, but the same difficulty applies:

- if the bacteria are non-pathogenic they may not immunize;
- if the bacteria are too pathogenic they may cause unpleasant symptoms.

Microneedle array

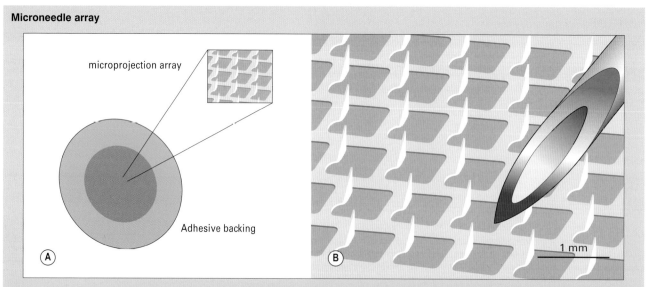

microprojection array

Adhesive backing

(A)

(B)

1 mm

Fig. 18.9 **A,** The size of an experimental microneedle array is shown. **B,** Scanning electron photomicrograph of a microprojection needle array which is coated with vaccine suspension and used to deliver antigen to the skin subcutaneously. A 25-gauge needle is shown (at right) for size comparison. *(Figure redrawn courtesy of J. Matriano (ALZA Corporation) with kind permission of Springer Science and Business Media).*

Several recombinant and partially attenuated salmonella strains have been used experimentally to explore this vaccine strategy.

Similar problems relate to nasal immunization, usually tried against upper respiratory infections such as influenza or respiratory syncytial viruses (RSV). With the exception below no nasal vaccine has entered *routine* use because of:

- difficulties in balancing attenuation against immunogenicity in the case of live RSV vaccine strains;
- the need for an adjuvant for an inactivated nasal influenza virus; and
- safety worries because of the proximity of the nasal mucosa to the brain through the cribriform plate.

A nasally delivered trivalent influenza vaccine using live attenuated virus though has been licensed since 2003 in the USA, and has been found to be safe and well tolerated, even in infants. Exceptionally perhaps, the success of this vaccine is partly due to the extra safety provided by the inability of the vaccine strain to replicate in cells other than those of the nasopharyngeal epithelium. Conversely, an inactivated nasal flu vaccine originally developed in Switzerland was withdrawn over safety concerns relating to its associated adjuvant.

Vaccine efficacy and safety

To be introduced and approved, a vaccine must obviously be effective, and the efficacy of all vaccines is reviewed from time to time. Many factors affect it.

An effective vaccine must induce the right sort of immunity:

- antibody for toxins and extracellular organisms such as *Streptococcus pneumoniae;*
- cell-mediated immunity for intracellular organisms such as the tubercle bacillus.

Where the ideal type of response is not clear (as in malaria, for instance), designing an effective vaccine becomes correspondingly more difficult. An effective vaccine must also:

- be **stable on storage** – this is particularly important for living vaccines, which normally require to be kept cold (i.e. a complete 'cold chain' from manufacturer to clinic, which is not always easy to maintain);
- have **sufficient immunogenicity** – with non-living vaccines it is often necessary to boost their immunogenicity with an adjuvant.

Live vaccines are generally more effective than killed vaccines.

Induction of appropriate immunity depends on the properties of the antigen

Living vaccines have the great advantage of providing an increasing antigenic challenge that lasts days or weeks, and inducing it in the right site – which in practice is most important where mucosal immunity is concerned (Fig. 18.10).

Live vaccines are likely to contain the greatest number of microbial antigens, but safety is an issue in a time of increasing concern about the side effects of vaccines.

Vaccines made from whole killed organisms have been used, but because a killed organism no longer has the advantage of producing a prolonged antigenic stimulus, killed vaccines have been frequently replaced by subunit vaccines. These can be associated with several problems:

- purified subunits may be relatively poorly immunogenic and require adjuvants;
- the smaller the antigen, the more histocompatibility complex (MHC) restriction may be a problem (see Chapters 5 and 8); and
- purified polysaccharides are typically thymus independent – they do not bind to MHC and therefore do not immunize T cells.

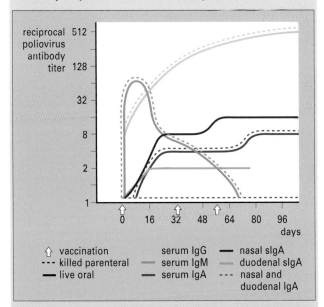

Antibody responses to live and killed polio vaccine

Fig. 18.10   The antibody response to orally administered live attenuated polio vaccine (solid lines) and intramuscularly administered killed polio vaccine (broken lines). The live vaccine induces the production of secretory IgA (sIgA) in addition to serum antibodies, whereas the killed vaccine induces no nasal or duodenal sIgA. As sIgA is the immunoglobulin of the mucosa-associated lymphoid tissue (MALT) system (see Chapter 2), the live vaccine confers protection at the portal of entry of the virus, the gastrointestinal mucosa. (*Courtesy of Professor JR Pattison, Ch. 26 in Brostoff J, et al., eds. Clinical immunology. London: Mosby; 1991.*)

These problems have been overcome in vaccines that are routinely used in humans by the use of adjuvants and by coupling polysaccharides either to:

- a standard protein carrier such as tetanus or diphtheria toxoid; or
- to a protein from the immunizing organism such as the outer membrane protein of pneumococci.

However, immunization even with the newer conjugate vaccines, especially when used in infants under 12 months, has shown that antibody levels wane after a number of years. For Hib this has indicated that a booster is required, generally given at around school-age, though ironically the tendency for meningococci to colonize healthy individuals can provide a boost to immunity in those who are immunized. This latter effect may become less common in the future with improved herd immunity, and therefore, a reduced frequency of carriage.

MHC restriction is probably more of a hypothetical than real difficulty because most candidate vaccines are large enough to contain several MHC-binding epitopes. Nevertheless, even the most effective vaccines often fail to immunize every individual – for example, about 5% of individuals fail to seroconvert after the full course of hepatitis B vaccine.

Most of the vaccines in routine use in humans depend on the induction of protective antibody. However, for many important infections, particularly of intracellular organisms

(e.g. tuberculosis, malaria, and HIV infection), cellular immune responses are important protective mechanisms.

In recent years there has therefore been much effort to develop vaccines to induce immunity of both CD4 and CD8 T cells. So far the use of DNA and viral vectors have been the routes most commonly explored because both of these strategies lead to the production of antigens within cells and therefore the display of processed peptide epitopes on MHC molecules.

Although these methods, particularly combined in prime-boost regimens, have been highly effective in experimental animal models, so far in humans it has proved difficult to induce high frequencies of long-lasting antigen-specific T memory cells.

Even in experimental animals the duration of protection may not be long-lasting, perhaps because protection by cellular mechanisms requires activated effector cells rather than resting memory cells. Such cells are not well maintained in the absence of antigen.

Vaccine safety is an overriding consideration

Vaccine safety is of course a relative term, with minor local pain or swelling at the injection site, and even mild fever, being generally acceptable. More serious complications may stem from the vaccine or from the patient (Fig. 18.11):

- vaccines may be contaminated with unwanted proteins or toxins, or even live viruses;
- supposedly killed vaccines may not have been properly killed;
- attenuated vaccines may revert to the wild type; and
- the patient may be hypersensitive to minute amounts of contaminating protein, or immunocompromised, in which case any living vaccine is usually contraindicated.

Although serious complications are very rare, vaccine safety has now become an overriding consideration, in part because of the very success of vaccines:

- because many childhood infectious diseases have become uncommon in developed countries, the populations of these countries are no longer aware of the potentially devastating effects of infectious diseases;
- unlike most drugs, vaccinations are given to people who have previously been perfectly well;
- the public is becoming increasingly aware of the possibilities of profitable litigation and companies correspondingly more defensive.

Q. Why is vaccine safety perceived as a less important issue when a vaccine is first introduced?
A. At the time of vaccine introduction the prevalence and danger associated with the infection is so great that any risks associated with the vaccine are relatively small.

MMR controversy resulted in measles epidemics

Anti-vaccine movements in the UK are essentially as old as vaccination itself, dating back to a few years after the introduction of smallpox vaccination by Jenner in 1796. In the modern era, difficulties concerning vaccine safety are well

Safety problems with vaccine

type of vaccine	potential safety problems	examples
attenuated vaccines	reversion to wild type	especially polio types 2 and 3
	severe disease in immunodeficient patients	vaccinia, BCG, measles
	persistent infection	varicella-zoster
	hypersensitivity to viral antigens	measles
	hypersensitivity to egg antigens	measles, mumps
killed vaccines	vaccine not killed	polio accidents in the past
	yeast contaminant	hepatitis B
	contamination with animal viruses	polio
	contamination with endotoxin	pertussis

Fig. 18.11 The potential safety problems encountered with vaccines emphasize the need for continuous monitoring of both production and administration.

The MMR controversy resulted in measles epidemics

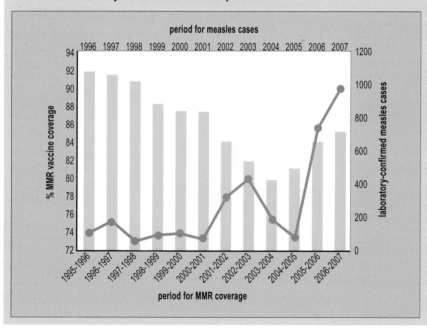

Fig. 18.12 The fall in uptake of the MMR vaccine in the UK to a low point in 2002, resulted in an upsurge in cases of measles. *(Data from BMJ 2008; 336:729.)*

illustrated by the controversy over MMR (measles, mumps, and rubella triple vaccine).

In 1998 a paper was published that received wide publicity in the UK media, purporting to support an association between MMR vaccination and the development of autism and chronic bowel disease. Although a large amount of subsequent work failed to substantiate these findings and the original paper has now been retracted, take-up of MMR in the UK and Ireland declined over several years and epidemics of measles occurred because of declining herd immunity (Fig. 18.12).

In 2004, the introduction of a new five-valent vaccine containing diphtheria and tetanus toxoids, acellular pertussis, *Haemophilus influenzae* type b, and inactivated polio virus threatened to result in decreased take-up in the UK, though the vaccine was shown to be safe and effective. It was argued that giving five immunogens simultaneously was 'too much' for the delicate immune system of infants. This argument is spurious, as most of the vaccines within it are subunits (except for inactivated polio). The whole vaccine therefore actually contains fewer antigens than the live bacteria and other organisms that infants encounter every day. Fortunately, the vaccine take up has remained high.

New vaccines can be very expensive

Although vaccination can safely be considered the most cost-effective treatment for infectious disease, new vaccines may be very expensive. The initial high cost is

Vaccines in general use

disease	vaccine	remarks
tetanus diphtheria pertussis polio (DTPP)	toxoid toxoid killed whole killed (Salk) or attenuated (Sabin)	given together in three doses between 2 and 6 months; tetanus and diphtheria boosted every 10 years
measles mumps rubella	attenuated	given together (MMR) at 12–18 months
Haemophilus influenzae type b	polysaccharide	new; may be given with DTPP

Fig. 18.13 Vaccines that are currently given, as far as is possible, to all individuals.

necessary to recoup the enormous development costs (US $200–400 million).

A good example is the recombinant hepatitis B vaccine, which was initially marketed in 1986 at US $150 for three doses. Although the cost has decreased greatly, even $1 is beyond the health budget of many of the world's poorer nations.

By contrast, the cost of the six vaccines included in the World Health Organization Expanded Program on Immunization (diphtheria, tetanus, whooping cough, polio, measles, and tuberculosis) is less than $1. The actual cost of immunizing a child is several times greater than this because it includes the cost of laboratories, transport, the cold chain, personnel, and research.

The Children's Vaccine Initiative, set up in 1990, is a global forum that aims to bring together vaccine researchers, development agencies, governments, donors, commercial and public sector vaccine manufacturers to seek means of delivering vaccines to the world's poorest populations who most need them.

Following major meningitis epidemics in Africa in 1996/7, the World Health Organization set up the Meningitis Vaccine Project in 2001, with a grant from the Bill and Melinda Gates Foundation. This project aimed to bring a new conjugate vaccine to Africa at a cost low enough that the affected countries could afford. This culminated in the production of MenAfriVac™ manufactured by the Serum Institute of India Ltd, and available at a cost of just $0.50 per dose. A major vaccination program for sub-Saharan Africa began at the end of 2010.

Vaccines in general use have variable success rates

The vaccines in standard use worldwide are listed in Figure 18.13. Four of them – polio, measles, mumps, and rubella – are so successful that these diseases are earmarked for eradication early in the 21st century. If this happens, it will be an extraordinary achievement, because mathematical modeling suggests that they are all more 'difficult' targets for eradication than smallpox was.

In the case of polio, where reversion to virulence of types 2 and 3 can occur, it has been suggested that it will be necessary to switch to the use of killed virus vaccine for some

years, so that virulent virus shed by live virus-vaccinated individuals is no longer produced.

For a number of reasons, other vaccines are less likely to lead to eradication of disease. These include:

- **the carrier state** – eradication of hepatitis B would be a major triumph, but it will require the breaking of the carrier state, especially in the Far East, where mother to child is the normal route of infection;
- **suboptimal effectiveness** – effectiveness of BCG varies markedly between countries, possibly due to variation in environmental mycobacterial species (tuberculosis is increasing, especially in patients with immune deficiency or AIDS), and the pertussis vaccine is only about 70–80% effective;
- **safety fears** – especially when the risk of infection is low, often lead to reduced levels of uptake. In the UK the spurious association of the MMR vaccine with autism has continued to affect the public's willingness to be vaccinated;
- **free-living forms and animal hosts** – the free-living form of tetanus will presumably survive indefinitely and it will not be possible to eradicate diseases that also have an animal host, such as yellow fever.

One of the future problems is going to be maintaining awareness of the need for vaccination against diseases that seem to be disappearing, while, as the reservoir of infection diminishes, cases tend to occur at a later age, which with measles and rubella could actually lead to worse clinical consequences.

Some vaccines are reserved for special groups only

In the developed world BCG and hepatitis B fall into this category, but some vaccines will probably always be confined to selected populations – travelers, nurses, the elderly, etc. (Fig. 18.14). In some cases this is because of:

- geographical restrictions (e.g. yellow fever);
- the rarity of exposure (e.g. rabies);
- problems in producing sufficient vaccine in time to meet the demand (e.g. each influenza epidemic is caused by a different strain, requiring a new vaccine).

Flu pandemics caused by emergence of totally novel influenza strains occur periodically, often caused by the

Vaccines restricted to certain groups

disease	vaccine	eligible groups
tuberculosis	BCG	tropics – at birth; UK – 10–14 years; USA – at-risk only
hepatitis B	surface antigen	at risk (medical, nursing staff, etc.); drug addicts; male homosexuals; known contacts of carriers
rabies	killed	at risk (animal workers); postexposure
meningitis yellow fever typhoid, cholera hepatitis A	polysaccharide attenuated killed or mutant killed or attenuated	travelers
influenza	killed	at risk; elderly
pneumococcal pneumonia	polysaccharide	elderly
varicella-zoster	attenuated	leukemic children

Fig. 18.14 Vaccines that are currently restricted to certain groups.

acquisition of genetic material from strains of flu that normally infect animals, such as equine or avian influenza.

In the recent past, major pandemic scares have surfaced in relation to avian and swine flu. Intensive efforts have been made to improve vaccine production methods such that sufficient vaccine is available to deal with such outbreaks. This has involved production of virus in cell culture rather than, conventionally, in chicken eggs, and the application of new immunogens based on VLPs consisting of recombinant antigen mixtures, not inactivated virus. Virosomes produced from purified, solubilized virus complexed with lipid vesicles have also been employed and possess enhanced immunogenicity compared to conventional vaccines. Virosomal vaccine has proven highly effective in elderly patients.

Both the hemagglutinin and neuraminidase antigens, which together make up the outer layer of the virus and are the antigens of importance in the vaccine, are however, subject to extensive variation. A vaccine effective against all strains of influenza would therefore be of tremendous value. A promising approach to this problem is to use chemical modification, such as glycosylation to reduce the immunodominance of the variable regions of these antigens, such that significant titers of antibody to invariant regions of these proteins may be induced.

Vaccines for parasitic and some other infections are only experimental

Some of the most intensively researched vaccines are those for the major tropical protozoal and worm infections (see Chapter 15). However, none has come into standard use, and some have argued that none will because none of these diseases induces effective immunity and 'you cannot improve on nature'.

Nevertheless, extensive work in laboratory animals has shown that vaccines against malaria, leishmaniasis, and schistosomiasis are perfectly feasible, and there is a moderately effective vaccine against babesia in dogs. In cattle an irradiated vaccine against lungworm has been in veterinary use for decades.

Q. Why, even with effective vaccines, will it be impossible to eradicate many parasitic diseases?
A. Many parasites have alternative species to humans as their host (see Chapter 15).

It remains possible, however, that the parasitic diseases of humans are significantly more difficult to treat, possibly because of the polymorphic and rapidly changing nature of many parasitic antigens. For example:

- none of the small animal models of malaria shows such extensive antigenic variation as *Plasmodium falciparum*, the protozoon causing malignant tertian malaria in humans;
- similarly, rats appear to be much easier to immunize against schistosomiasis than other animals, including possibly humans.

Part of the problem is that in the laboratory these parasites are usually not propagated in their natural host.

A vaccine against *Plasmodium falciparum*, has been one of the most sought after for over a generation, as the burden of disease and death in endemic malarial regions in Africa is huge. Malaria is unusual in that its life cycle offers a variety of possible targets for vaccination (Fig. 18.15). Over the years several trials of clinical malaria vaccine have been published, using antigens derived from either the liver or the blood stage, with only very moderate success.

During the last five years or so, however, a realistic candidate vaccine has emerged from a partnership begun in the early 1980s, between the pharmaceutical company GlaxoSmithKline (GSK) and the US Walter Reed Army Institute of Research (WRAIS). The vaccine known as RS,S is based on a genetically engineered version of the circumsporozoite (CS) protein that is expressed on sporozoites and liver stage schizonts (see Fig. 18.15). Recombinant CS protein is expressed in yeast cells as a fusion protein with the Hepatitis B surface antigen (HBsAg), the basis of the successful recombinant HepB vaccine. Co-expression of the fusion protein along with unmodified HBsAg, allows the formation of VLP-type aggregates of the antigens. To make this

Malaria vaccine strategies

stage	vaccine strategy
sporozoites	sporozoite vaccine to induce blocking antibody, already field-tested in humans
liver stage	sporozoite vaccine to induce cell-mediated immunity to liver stage
merozoites	merozoite (antigen) vaccine to induce blocking antibody
asexual erythrocyte stage	asexual stage (antigen) vaccine to induce other responses to red cell stage, and against toxic products ('anti-disease' vaccine)
gametocytes	vaccines to interrupt sexual stages – 'transmission-blocking' vaccine
gametes	

Fig. 18.15 A number of different approaches to malaria vaccines are being investigated, reflecting the complexity of both the life cycle of malaria and immunity to it.

preparation sufficiently immunogenic has required combination with the powerful new adjuvant AS02 (see above).

Phase II trials in Africa have shown a significant protective effect on both infection rate and clinical malaria development. A large phase III trial is now underway and, should the initial promise be realized, the first licensed antimalarial vaccine may become available by 2015.

Our understanding of how the RS,S vaccine elicits a protective immune response unfortunately remains poor, and the degree of protection provided is limited, but it is hoped that further research will result in an even more effective second generation vaccine in the future.

A problem with these chronic parasitic diseases is that of immunopathology. For example, the symptoms of *Trypanosoma cruzi* infection (Chagas' disease) are largely due to the immune system (i.e. autoimmunity). A bacterial parallel is leprosy, where the symptoms are due to the (apparent) overreactivity of TH1 or TH2 cells. A vaccine that boosted immunity without clearing the pathogen could make these conditions worse.

Another example of this unpleasant possibility is with dengue, where certain antibodies enhance the infection by allowing the virus to enter cells via Fc receptors.

Similarly, a HIV vaccine trial, which though promising in inducing a cell mediated-response, was aborted as the risk of

HIV infection in the vaccinated subjects was increased over the unvaccinated controls.

Other viral and bacterial vaccines that are also experimental are:

- attenuated shigella;
- Epstein–Barr virus surface glycoprotein;
- respiratory syncytial virus (RSV);
- group b *Streptococcus aureus*.

For many diseases there is no vaccine available

No vaccine is currently available for many serious infectious diseases, including staphylococci and streptococci, syphilis, chlamydia, leprosy, and fungal infections. The predominant problem is often the lack of understanding of how to induce effective immunity. HIV infection heads this list of diseases (see Chapter 17), which represent the major challenge for research and development in the coming decade (Fig. 18.w2)

Passive immunization can be life-saving

Driven from use by the advent of antibiotics, the idea of injecting preformed antibody to treat infection is still valid for certain situations (Fig. 18.16). It can be life-saving when:

- toxins are already circulating (e.g. in tetanus, diphtheria, and snake-bite);
- high-titer specific antibody is required, generally made in horses, but occasionally obtained from recovered patients.

At the opposite end of the scale, normal pooled human immunoglobulin contains enough antibody against common infections for a dose of 100–400 mg IgG to protect hypogammaglobulinemic patients for a month. Over 1000 donors are used for each pool, and the sera must be screened for HIV and hepatitis B and C.

In this light it is still somewhat surprising that the use of specific monoclonal antibodies, though theoretically highly attractive, has not yet proved to be an improvement on traditional methods, and their chief application to infectious disease at present remains in diagnosis.

One exception to this rule has been the monoclonal antibody Palivizumab™, launched in 1998, which has found application in prophylaxis against respiratory syncytial virus (RSV) infection, where the development of a vaccine has remained elusive. Palivizumab™ has proven effective in protecting high risk individuals, such as premature infants.

Antibody genes can now be engineered to form Fab, single chain Fv, or VH fragments (see Chapter 3). Libraries of these can be expressed in recombinant phages and screened against antigens of interest. Selected antibody fragments can be produced in bulk in bacteria, yeasts, or mammalian cells, for use *in vitro* or *in vivo*. This technology has helped in the production of human and humanized mouse monoclonal antibodies for therapeutic application.

Future vaccines

Without doubt the future generation of new, improved and safer vaccines lies in the exploitation of recombinant DNA technology and genetic engineering of pathogenic organisms

Passive immunization

disease	source of antibody	indication
diphtheria, tetanus	human, horse	prophylaxis, treatment
varicella-zoster	human	treatment in immunodeficiencies
gas gangrene, botulism, snake bite, scorpion sting	horse	post-exposure
rabies	human	post-exposure (plus vaccine)
hepatitis B	human	post-exposure
hepatitis A, measles	pooled human immunoglobulin	prophylaxis (travel), post-exposure

Fig. 18.16 Although not so commonly used as 50 years ago, injections of specific antibody can still be a life-saving treatment in specific clinical conditions.

and their antigens. A development of the ability to clone genes is the possibility of using a benign, non-pathogenic virus as a vector to display antigens to the immune system in a way that mimics their natural exposure but is without the risks associated with attenuated pathogens. The gene(s) encoding the desired antigen(s) is incorporated into the genetic material of the vector, which can then express the gene, and produce the antigen in situ. The vector can then be injected into the patient and in some cases also allowed to replicate.

Vaccinia is a convenient vector

A convenient vector that is large enough to carry several antigens is vaccinia. The modified Ankara strain (MVA) was used clinically for many years as a safe and immunogenic smallpox vaccine. Through prolonged growth in avian cells, MVA has deleted the genes required for it to replicate in human cells, which therefore makes it highly suitable for use as a vector.

The MVA strain of vaccinia is the basis of an experimental vaccine against TB (MVA-85A) in which the virus has been genetically engineered to express the 85A antigen of *Mycobacterium tuberculosis*.

Although the BCG vaccination has been available for many years and protects against severe infantile TB infection it is not effective at preventing the chronic lung disease found more typically in children and adults. This form of TB is responsible for a many as 2 million deaths a year worldwide, and has become an even greater problem since the spread of HIV and the concomitant immune suppression it induces.

The new vaccine began trials in 2002 in the UK and has been subsequently tested in clinical trials in the Gambia, South Africa, and Senegal. The results suggest that this vaccine may act as a very effective booster to BCG immunization. The full results of these trials should be available in 2012.

A number of other experimental vaccines using recombinant vaccinia have been tested, though none is yet in routine use. Many other viruses, such as adenovirus, alphavirus, polio and measles have also been proposed and tested experimentally as vaccine vectors. Adenovirus, for example, has been used to display antigens from HIV and used in clinical trials.

As an alternative to viral vectors, attenuated bacteria have the advantage that they have genomes large enough to incorporate many genes from other organisms, and so may be used as polyvalent immunogens. Recombinant forms of BCG, in particular, have been used for experimental bacterial vaccines.

'Naked' DNA can be transfected into host cells

One of the most intriguing possibilities for future development is the use of DNA for vaccination. Genes encoding antigens of interest cloned into a suitable expression plasmid vector are injected directly into muscle, injected sub-cutaneously, or coated onto gold micro-particles and 'shot' into the skin by pressurized gas – the **gene gun** (essentially a jet injector like those referred to above). Cells that take up the DNA express the encoded protein. The potential advantages of this approach are a long term exposure to the antigen, the possibility of stimulating both an antibody and cellular immune response and an adjuvant activity due to the presence of CpG dinucleotides in the recombinant DNA. This last is a potent activator of TLRs. Immunomodulatory genes (cytokines or co-stimuli) can also be incorporated into the DNA construct along with the genes coding for antigens, to generate and amplify the desired immune response. Uptake and expression of the DNA in APCs can induce long-lasting cellular and humoral immunity in experimental animals, but DNA vaccines have not yet fulfilled in humans the promise they have shown in animal model systems.

CRITICAL THINKING: VACCINATION (SEE P. 439 FOR EXPLANATIONS)

1 Why have attenuated vaccines not been developed for all viruses and bacteria?

2 'A vaccine cannot improve on nature'. Is this unduly pessimistic?

3 'The smallpox success story is unlikely to be repeated.' Is this true?

4 Will vaccines eventually replace antibiotics?

5 BCG: vaccine, adjuvant, or non-specific stimulant?

6 Why could an anti-worm vaccine do more harm than good?

7 By what means, other than their reaction with antibodies, might you identify antigens that could be used as vaccines?

Further reading

Almond JW. Vaccine Renaissance. Nat Rev Microbiol 2007;5:478–481.

Kaufmann SHE. The contribution of immunology to the rational design of novel antibacterial vaccines. Nat Rev Microbiol 2007;5:491–504.

Kusters I, Almond JW. Vaccine Strategies. In: Mahy DWJ, van Regenmortel MHV, eds. Desk Encyclopedia of General Virology. Oxford UK and San Diego USA: Academic Press; 2010:235–243.

Pollard AJ, Perret KP, Beverly PC. Maintaining protection against invasive bacteria with polysaccharide conjugate vaccines. Nat Rev Immunol 2009;9:213–220.

Immune Responses Against Tissues

CHAPTER 19

Immunological Tolerance

SUMMARY

- **Immunological tolerance is the state of unresponsiveness to a particular antigen** which is primarily established in T- and B-lymphocytes. The clonal receptors of lymphocytes are generated by random recombination of the many genes that code for the antigen binding regions. This creates the need to sort out dangerous receptors that could recognize and destroy self tissues. The breakdown of immunological tolerance to self-antigens is the cause of autoimmune diseases.

- **Immunological tolerance is achieved by many different mechanisms** operating on different cell types.

- **Central tolerance refers to the selection processes which T cell precursors undergo in the thymus** before they are released as mature naive T cells. Thymic epithelial cells and dendritic cells present self-antigens to the immature T cell precursors. Those T cell precursors that respond strongly to the self-antigens presented in the thymus undergo apoptosis. This is called negative selection. A specialized population of thymic epithelial cells is capable of expressing genes which are expressed in a strictly organ specific manner (e.g. insulin, which is expressed only in the pancreas and the thymus).

- **Peripheral tolerance refers to the diverse mechanism that enforce and maintain T-cell tolerance outside the thymus.** These include the prevention of contact between auto-reactive T-cells and their target antigens **(immunological ignorance)**, the **peripheral deletion** of auto-reactive T-cells by activation induced cell death or cytokine withdrawal, the incapacity of T cells to mount effector responses upon recognizing their target antigen **(anergy),** and the suppression of immune responses by **regulatory T cells.**

- **B cell tolerance** is established by several mechanisms including clonal deletion of autoreactive B cells, mostly in the bone marrow; the rearrangement of autoreactive B cell receptors **(receptor editing)** or by **B cell anergy.** In addition B-cell tolerance is maintained by tolerant T cells. The production of high-affinity class-switched antibodies depends on T-cell help. Therefore, if tolerance to a particular antigen is firmly established in the T-cell compartment, B-cells that recognize this antigen will usually remain tolerant.

- **To establish or re-establish tolerance** is a major goal for innovative treatments for autoimmunity, allergy and transplantation. In contrast, to overcome immunological tolerance is one major goal for innovative treatments against cancer.

Generation of autoreactive antigen receptors during lymphocyte development

The specificity of the antigen receptors of T cells and B cells is the result of random shuffling of the many genes that encode the antigen-binding site of these receptors. Theoretically, this process could generate more than 10^{15} different T-cell receptors, including some that can bind to autoantigens (Fig. 19.1). Similar considerations apply to B-cell receptors. Cells expressing such receptors are often called self-reactive lymphocytes. The immune system has to fulfill two contradictory requirements: on the one hand the repertoire of different antigen receptors needs to be as large as possible to avoid 'holes in the repertoire' that could be exploited by pathogens to evade immune detection. On the other hand, the receptor repertoire must be shaped to prevent the immune system from attacking the organism that harbors it. Any disturbance in this delicately balanced system can have pathogenic or even lethal consequences, either from infections or from the unwanted reaction with autoantigens or harmless external antigens as in allergy. This paradox was recognized at the beginning of the last century by Paul Ehrlich who coined the term 'horror autotoxicus' for the necessity to avoid immunological reactions against self-antigens. Tolerance is the process that eliminates or neutralizes such autoreactive cells, and a breakdown of this system can cause autoimmunity. To avoid autoreactivity the

The need for immunological tolerance

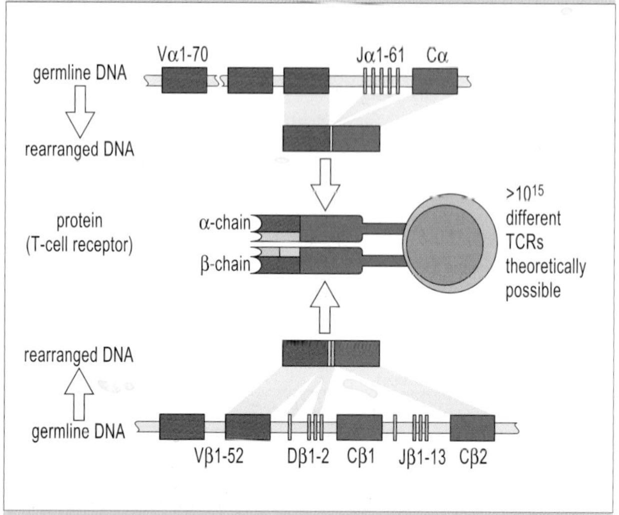

Fig. 19.1 Lymphocyte receptors are produced by random recombination of the many genes encoding for their heterodimeric receptors. Humans possess more than 70 different T cell receptor (TCR) $V\alpha$ gene elements, 61 $J\alpha$ gene elements, and one $C\alpha$ gene element in germline configuration. One $V\alpha$, $J\alpha$ and $C\alpha$ gene element is used to code for an individual TCRα chain. For the TCR β-chain there are 52 $V\beta$, 2 $D\beta$, 13 $J\beta$, and 2 $C\beta$ gene elements. Additional combinatorial possibilities are created by random insertion of N regions (V–J for the TCRα, and V–D, D–J for the TCRβ). The random combinations of these different elements allow for the generation of more than 10^{15} different TCRs. Similar numbers apply to B cell receptor heavy and light chains. Due to the random recombination of genetic elements useful, useless and harmful receptors will be produced. Selection processes are, therefore, required to establish a lymphocyte receptor repertoire that is able to recognize all microbial pathogens without inflicting damage to the organism that harbors it.

randomly generated repertoire of T- and B-cell receptors is censored by several different mechanisms. CD4$^+$ T$_H$ cells are pivotal for the multitude of immunological mechanisms that induce and maintain immunological tolerance. In this chapter we will discuss immunological tolerance in B cells and conventional $\alpha\beta$ TCR expressing T cells.

T cell tolerance

T cell tolerance is established at two levels. Immature thymocytes undergo harsh selection processes in the thymus. This is often called **central tolerance** and results in the deletion of most T cells with high affinity for self antigens. Mature T cells are also regulated to avoid self-reactivity. The mechanisms that reinforce T cell tolerance outside the thymus are collectively called **peripheral tolerance**.

Central T-cell tolerance develops in the thymus

The chief mechanism of T-cell tolerance is the deletion of self-reactive T cells in the thymus. Immature T cell precursors migrate from the bone marrow to the thymus. There, they proliferate, differentiate and undergo selection

processes before a selected few re-enter the blood stream as mature naive T cells. These differentiation and selection processes depend on interactions with thymic epithelial cells and dendritic cells in specialized microenvironments within the thymus (Fig. 19.2).

Generation of their clonal TCR is the first step in T cell development

In the thymus the T cell precursors – also called thymocytes – start to express the recombinase-activating gene (RAG) products and begin to rearrange their $\alpha\beta$ TCR genes. T cell precursors that enter the thymus express neither CD4 nor CD8 and are, therefore, called double negative (DN) thymocytes. The DN precursors actively proliferate, undergoing approximately 20 cell divisions and assemble the TCR β chain. Only those DN cells that have successfully rearranged a TCR β chain will progress to the next stage and express CD4 and CD8 simultaneously. These immature CD4$^+$CD8$^+$ double positive (DP) thymocytes start to reassemble TCR α chains and express T cell receptors (TCR). The randomly rearranged TCRs expressed by the DP thymocytes collectively constitute the organism's unselected TCR repertoire which is also called the germline repertoire. These thymocytes undergo processes of **positive and negative selection.** Less than 5% of them survive these selection events and are allowed to exit the thymus as naive mature T cells.

In addition to $\alpha\beta$ T cells, other lineages including natural killer T (NKT) cells and $\gamma\delta$ T cells also develop in the thymus. Although much less is known about thymic selection of $\gamma\delta$ T cells there are profound differences in the thymic development of $\gamma\delta$ T cells and $\alpha\beta$ T cells. Ligand mediated selection events do not seem to be required for the selection of the $\gamma\delta$ T cell repertoire. In contrast, instruction for particular effector functions occurs in the thymus for $\gamma\delta$ T cells. Given the many current uncertainties about $\gamma\delta$ T cell selection and NKT selection in the thymus, this section will deal exclusively with thymic selection of $\alpha\beta$ T cells.

Thymocytes are positively selected for their ability to interact with self MHC molecules

The DP T cells interact with thymic cortical epithelial cells that present peptides derived from endogenous proteins bound to major histocompatibility complex (MHC) molecules. Recognition of self-peptide/MHC complexes is vital for the DP T cells for two reasons:

- in the DP T cells RAG is active and TCR α chains are continuously rearranged to maximize the chance of producing a TCR capable of interacting with self MHC;
- only upon recognition of a peptide/MHC complex via the TCR is RAG expression halted and the cell is committed to express a particular $\alpha\beta$ TCR.

Moreover, recognition of a peptide/MHC complex via the TCR is necessary for the DP T cell to receive a survival signal. This is called **positive selection** (see Fig 19.2). Experiments have shown that T cells are positively selected by interaction with self-MHC to prepare them for subsequent activation by non-self-peptide/self-MHC complexes, indicating the biological benefit of positive selection.

T cell repertoire selection in the thymus

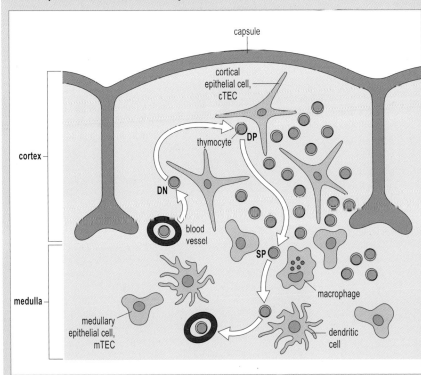

capsule

cortical epithelial cell, cTEC

thymocyte   DP

cortex

DN

blood vessel

SP

medulla

macrophage

medullary epithelial cell, mTEC

dendritic cell

Fig. 19.2 T cell precursors, the thymocytes, enter the thymic cortex through blood vessels. At this stage the thymocyte cells are called double negative (DN) because they express neither CD4 nor CD8. They proliferate and express *recombinase activating gene* products to assemble their TCRs. Thymocytes that have successfully rearranged a TCR β chain express both CD4 and CD8 (double positive, DP) and these reassemble α-chains to form the TCR. They interact with cortical thymic epithelial cells (cTECS). Recognition of a selecting ligand is necessary for thymocytes' survival, so-called positive selection. Positive selection also induces commitment to either the CD4⁺ or CD8⁺ lineage, the cells become single positive (SP) which move to the thymic medulla. Here they interact with antigen presenting cells, including medullary thymic epithelial cells (mTECs), capable of expressing tissue restricted antigens (TRAs). Thymocytes that react strongly with ligands presented by APCs in the thymic medulla undergo apoptosis. This is called negative selection. *(Adapted from Kyewsky B, Klein L, Ann Rev Immunol 2006;24:571–606.)*

Q. What determines whether a T cell will develop into a CD4⁺ T cell or a CD8⁺ cell?

A. It depends on whether the TCR interacts productively with a peptide/MHC I or a peptide/MHC II complex (see Chapter 2).

Accordingly mice that do not express MHC-class II molecules lack CD4⁺ T cells and mice that do not express MHC-class I molecules lack CD8⁺ T cells.

Positive selection occurs predominantly in the thymic cortex

Specialized APC, the cortical thymic epithelial cells (cTECs) are pivotal for positive selection. cTECs differ in their antigen processing machinery (cathepsins, proteasome subunits) from hematopoietic antigen presenting cells. Given that the number of different peptides that can be presented by any particular MHC molecule is much smaller than the number of different TCRs that undergo positive selection, each peptide must be involved in positively selecting many different T cells. Accordingly, experiments have demonstrated that the peptide on which a TCR is positively selected does not need to share sequence similarity with the peptides recognized by that same TCR in the periphery.

Note that positive selection depends on the recognition of self-peptides bound to self-MHC. The TCRs that are positively selected based on low-affinity interactions with self-peptide/MHC form the selected repertoire that ultimately recognizes microbial antigens, to protect the organism from infectious diseases. This is one illustration for the flexibility of antigen recognition by T cells. The peptides that mediate positive selection in the thymus are also presented outside the thymus where they support survival of mature T cells and may also act as co-agonists that enhance T cell activation by agonist peptides.

An immediate question is why T cells which were selected based upon self-recognition usually do not cause damage to the organism. One answer is that the threshold for TCR signaling is lower in immature DP T cells in the thymus than in mature T cells in the periphery. Thus, DP T cells can respond to low-affinity interaction with peptide/MHC complexes that would not trigger mature T cells. One important regulator of this TCR signaling threshold is the microRNA miR-181a that regulates the expression of several phosphatases involved in TCR signaling. DP T cells express much higher levels of miR181a than mature SP T cells.

Lack of survival signals leads to death by neglect

DP T cells whose receptors have a very low affinity for the peptide/MHC complexes they encounter during their approximately 3–4-day lifespan in the thymic cortex do not receive survival signals and undergo apoptosis in the thymus (see Fig. 19.w2). This is called **death by neglect**. Accordingly, T cells do not progress beyond the DP stage in mice that have been manipulated to lack expression of MHC molecules. Analyses of the germ line repertoire of TCRs have revealed that this unselected repertoire contains more self-MHC reactive TCRs than expected by chance. In other words: co-evolution of TCR and MHC molecules has shaped the germline αβ TCR repertoire to favor the generation of receptors that can interact with self-MHC.

Thymocytes are negatively selected if they bind strongly to self-peptides on MHC molecules

After positive selection and commitment to the CD4 or CD8 lineage in the thymic epithelium, thymocytes express the chemokine receptor CCR7 and migrate towards the central region of the thymus, the thymic medulla, where the CCR7 ligands CCL19 and CCL20 are produced. In the thymic medulla the thymocytes are probed for another 4–5 days. T cells whose receptors have a high affinity for the peptide/MHC complexes encountered in the medulla are autoreactive and therefore, potentially dangerous. They receive death signals and undergo apoptosis. This is called **negative selection** (see Fig 19.2). Experimental evidence suggests that the majority of the DP T cells which were positively selected are later eliminated by negative selection.

The relevance of negative thymic selection can be demonstrated by neonatal thymectomy. Mice that are thymectomized within the first three days after birth develop an autoimmune syndrome including sialadenitis, diabetes, autoimmune gastritis and hepatitis.

A library of self antigens is presented to developing T cells in the thymus

The induction of central tolerance requires the presence of autoantigens in the thymus. This poses an obvious problem for thymic selection: Some autoantigens, e.g. insulin are expressed in a tissue-specific manner, are frequently called tissue-restricted antigens (TRAs). The question, then, is (how) do TRAs get into the thymus for presentation to developing T cells? Some might be brought into the thymus by immigrating antigen presenting cells but it is highly unlikely that this would yield a reliable representation of the organism's TRAs. Moreover, developmentally regulated TRAs, e.g. antigens that are only expressed after puberty, would not gain access to the fetal thymus. The answer is that specialized cells in the thymus, the medullary thymic epithelial cells (mTECs) express proteins that are otherwise strictly tissue restricted. This has been called ectopic or **promiscuous gene expression** (Fig. 19.3).

MTECS express several hundreds or even thousands of functionally and structurally highly diverse antigens that represent almost all tissues in the body. Importantly, mTECs express not only tissue restricted antigens but also developmentally regulated antigens. Thus, gene expression in mTECs is uncoupled from spatial and developmental regulation. The exact mechanisms of this promiscuous gene expression are not yet fully understood. It has become clear that not all mTECs express all TRAs. Any particular TRA is expressed by less than 5% of mTECs.

Whereas mTECs are the only cells known to be capable of promiscuous gene expression, they are not the only cells important for negative selection. Thymic dendritic cells can take up TRAs expressed by mTECs and cross-present these TRAs to T cells. Recent intravital imaging studies have yielded the estimate that a thymocyte makes contact with approximately 500 dendritic cells during its sojourn in the thymic medulla. Although we do not have experimentally based quantitative estimates for thymocyte:mTEC contacts, the purging of self-reactive T cells in the thymic medulla is a remarkable achievement.

Medullary thymic epithelial cells express and present tissue restricted antigens

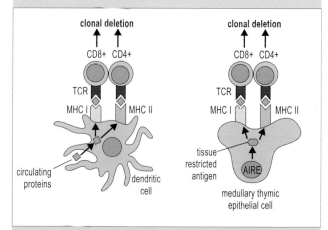

Fig 19.3 Different antigen presenting cell populations induce thymic tolerance. Dendritic cells and other conventional APCs present phagocytosed or endogenously synthesized proteins to T lymphocytes. T cells that express receptors with high affinity for these ubiquitous proteins will undergo apoptosis. Medullary thymic epithelial cells (mTECs) express the transcriptional autoimmune regulator, AIRE and, therefore, possess the unique capacity of expressing tissue restricted antigens (TRAs) ectopically in the thymus. This allows for intrathymic clonal deletion of T cells expressing TCRs with high affinities for antigens that are expressed in a tissue restricted manner outside the thymus. *(Adapted from Sprent J, Surh CD. Nature Immunol 2003;4:303–304.)*

Subtle quantitative alterations in the thymic expression of TRAs can be consequential. Murine intrathymic expression levels of autoantigens including insulin and myelin antigens correlate inversely with susceptibility to autoimmune diseases, type I diabetes and experimental autoimmune encephalitis (EAE) respectively. Similarly, in humans genetic variants resulting in low levels of intrathymic insulin-expression are strongly associated with susceptibility to type I diabetes.

Qualitative variations in TRAs expressed in mTECs have also been associated with autoimmune disease models. Differential splicing or the expression of embryonic, rather than mature variants of myelin autoantigens have been associated with strain-specific susceptibility to EAE and may well play a role in the pathogenesis of multiple sclerosis in humans.

AIRE controls promiscuous expression of genes in the thymus

What enables mTECs to express a broad array of TRAs independently of spatial or developmental regulation? mTECs express the transcriptional regulator **Aire (autoimmune regulator)**. Aire controls the expression of a large number of TRAs in mTECs (see Fig. 19.3).

Q. What effect do you think that disruption of the *Aire* gene would have?
A. Mice with targeted disruption of the *aire* gene have reduced promiscuous gene expression in mTECs and suffer from various autoimmune manifestations.

Immunological ignorance

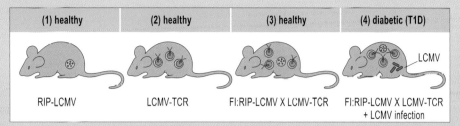

(1) healthy	(2) healthy	(3) healthy	(4) diabetic (T1D)
RIP-LCMV	LCMV-TCR	FI:RIP-LCMV X LCMV-TCR	FI:RIP-LCMV X LCMV-TCR + LCMV infection

Fig 19.4 Immunological ignorance was first demonstrated in transgenic mice. (**1**) One transgenic strain of mice expresses a viral (LCMV) antigen under the control of the rat insulin promotor (RIP) in pancreatic islets cells. These mice remain healthy. (**2**) Another strain expresses a transgenically encoded T cell receptor specific for the LCMV antigen (LCMV TCR). These mice also remain healthy. (**3**) F1 mice from a cross between the RIP-LCMV and LCMV TCR mice express the viral antigen in the pancreas and they have T cells that express the transgenic LCMV specific TCR. The transgenic T cells are not deleted in the thymus of these mice and they respond appropriately to LCMV antigen *in vitro* but, the mice remain healthy, indicating that the naïve LCMV-specific T cells do not get in contact with the LCMV antigen which is expressed in the pancreas. (**4**) When the F1 mice are infected with LCMV, the LCMV-specific T cells become activated in the secondary lymphatic organs by high concentrations of processed antigen and can then enter the pancreas and destroy the insulin synthesizing cells. Consequently, the mice succumb to immune mediated diabetes.

Similarly, in humans, point mutations in the gene coding for Aire are the cause of the rare monogenic autosomal recessive autoimmune polyendocrinopathy–candidiasis–ectodermal dystrophy (APECED) syndrome. APECED is characterized by high titres of several different autoantibodies that cause disease, mainly in endocrine organs. Together these findings strongly suggest that the autoimmune manifestations are caused by diminished expression of TRAs in thymic mTECs due to the Aire deficiency. Aire associates with a large number of partners to form distinct complexes that impinge on different steps of transcription. The different functions of Aire's partner proteins include chromatin structure and DNA-damage response, gene transcription, RNA processing, and nuclear transport. It is still unclear, however, how Aire controls promiscuous gene expression. Moreover, experimental evidence strongly suggests that additional yet unidentified transcriptional regulators must also be involved in promiscuous gene expression by mTECs.

Peripheral T-cell tolerance

Despite the intricate mechanisms of central tolerance induction in the thymus, approximately one third of the autoreactive clones are not deleted. Thus, a large number of low-avidity self-reactive T cells escapes into the periphery; thus, autoreactive T cells are part of the normal repertoire. For example, T cells that recognize insulin or myelin basic protein can be isolated from people without diabetes or multiple sclerosis. Despite their low avidity for self-antigen these cells are potentially dangerous and can cause autoimmune tissue destruction. Autoimmune diseases, however, are the exception rather than the norm. It follows that peripheral tolerance mechanisms must exist to prevent these autoreactive T cells from causing harm.

Immunological ignorance occurs if T cells do not encounter their cognate antigen

Immunological ignorance is maintained as long as autoreactive T-lymphocytes do not enter the tissue in which the autoantigen that they recognize is expressed. The autoreactive naive T cells are not tolerized and can be activated upon recognizing their cognate antigen.

The importance of immunological ignorance was demonstrated in mice that express a transgene-encoded TCR which recognizes a peptide derived from the lymphocytic choriomeningitis virus (LCMV). These mice were bred with another transgenic strain that expressed the viral peptide on the surface of their pancreatic islet cells. Surprisingly, diabetes did not develop in the offspring even though *in vitro* their T cells could kill cells that displayed the viral peptide (Fig. 19.4). The T cells in these double-transgenic mice were therefore, not tolerant *in vivo*, instead they were ignorant of their target cells.

When the mice were infected with LCMV, the transgenic T cells became activated, invaded the pancreas and destroyed the islet cells. Consequently the mice succumbed to diabetes. Importantly, LCMV-infection did not cause diabetes in those mice that expressed the transgenic TCR but not the LCMV-peptide in the pancreas. Once activated by LCMV infection, the hitherto ignorant autoreactive T cells (autoreactive because the LCMV-derived peptide was transgenically expressed in the pancreas) acquired the capacity to migrate into their target tissue where they recognized and destroyed the LCMV-peptide expressing islet cells (see Fig. 19.4).

Some self antigens are sequestered in immunologically privileged tissues

Self-reactive T cell lines that recognize autoantigens including myelin antigens and pancreatic antigens can easily be cloned from healthy humans. How, then, is autoimmune disease avoided in the presence of potentially pathogenic autoreactive T cells?

One explanation is the **sequestration** of potentially harmful T cells from the tissues in which their target self-antigens are expressed. Sequestration can be achieved when antigens are physically separated from

T cells (e.g. by the blood–brain barrier, see Chapter 12). The blood–brain barrier can be surmounted by activated lymphocytes, however, and many organs do not possess a physical barrier to prevent lymphocytes entering from the bloodstream. Instead, lymphocyte migration is controlled by chemokines, selectins and their receptors.

Lymphocyte activation enhances their migration into non-lymphoid tissues

Upon activation in secondary lymphatic organs naive T cells acquire effector functions and express a different set of chemokine receptors and adhesion molecules which then enables them to enter other organs, particularly in the context of inflammation. Naive T cells lacking those surface molecules, however, are excluded from non-lymphoid tissues so that under normal conditions, potentially autoreactive T cells will ignore their antigens, thereby maintaining self-tolerance. Should such cells be activated accidentally they would pose a permanent threat to the organism. DCs that are activated during infection are likely to present not only microbial but also self-antigens. The T cells activated in this process would gain the capacity to enter tissues and thus have lost their ignorance. Consequently, additional mechanisms must ensure the maintenance of immunological self tolerance.

Antigen presenting cells reinforce self tolerance

Dendritic cells can present antigen in a tolerogenic manner

Experiments designed to analyse CD4 and CD8 T-cell responses to antigens that were expressed in a tissue restricted manner (e.g. exclusively in the pancreas or the skin) revealed that self-Ag specific T cells accumulated in the draining lymph nodes as a result of reaction with self-antigen transported by DCs. Depending on the information received from the DC in addition to peptide presentation, the T_H cells may become

- activated;
- anergic;
- converted into a regulatory T cell; or
- undergo apoptosis.

The critical importance of DCs for the maintenance of tolerance has also been shown in experiments in which conditional DC depletion in mature mice resulted in spontaneous autoimmunity.

Q. What is the key requirement for T cell activation?
A. Co-stimulatory and instructive signals from mature DC are necessary for T cell activation (see Chapter 8).

Functional maturation of DCs, characterized by strong expression of MHC and co-stimulatory molecules is induced by microbial or self-derived stimuli, which are sometimes called danger signals (Fig. 19.5). In the absence of such stimuli immature DCs express MHC and costimulatory molecules at low levels and antigen presentation induces T cell anergy or deletion depending upon the expression of high or low levels of self-antigen respectively (see Fig. 19.w1). The signals that induce tolerogenic DC maturation as well

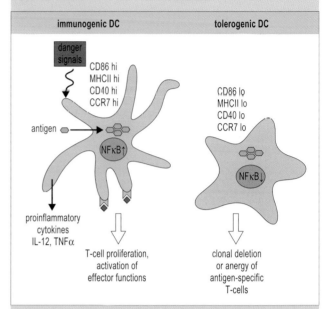

Critical role of APC for T-cell tolerance

Fig 19.5 Antigen presenting cells (APC) are critical for the decision between T-cell activation or tolerance. Upon antigen uptake the APC become activated if they sense exogenous or endogenous danger signals. Such classically activated APC present antigen in an immunogenic manner to T-lymphocytes and induce T-cell proliferation and effector functions. Such immunogenic DC, which have matured under inflammatory conditions (i.e. they have received signals via their TLRs or other pattern recognition receptors), upregulate co-stimulatory molecules (e.g. CD86, CD40), MHC class II molecules and CCR7. These changes increase their capacity to present antigen to T cells in an immunogenic manner. They also activate NFκB and express proinflammatory cytokines (e.g. IL-12) which instruct T-cell effector functions. If, in contrast, the APC do not receive danger signals they can still undergo homeostatic maturation. Such APC present antigen in a non-immunogenic manner to T cells and induce clonal deletion or anergy. Tolerogenic DC which are either immature or have matured under steady state conditions, express only low amounts of co-stimulatory and MHC-II molecules and do not secrete proinflammatory cytokines.

as the tolerogenic interactions between DC and T cells are only incompletely understood. Still there are some clear candidates. Several molecules have already been identified that are necessary for tolerogenic DC:T cell interactions. These include surface molecules such as E-cadherin, PD-1 L, CD103, CD152 (CTLA-4) and ICOS-L (CD275) and cytokines, including IL-10 and TGF-β.

Tolerogenic DCs mature under steady-state conditions

DC maturation under steady-state conditions can be triggered by disrupting DC-DC adhesion which is mediated by E-cadherin. Similar to DC maturation induced by microbial products, the disruption of DC-DC contacts induces upregulation of MHC class II, co-stimulatory molecules and chemokine receptors and this process requires the activation of β-catenin. In contrast to DCs that have matured upon sensing microbial products, the DCs that have matured under steady-state conditions do not produce pro-inflammatory cytokines. Consequently, when they present antigen to naive T$_H$ cells these DCs induce regulatory T cells rather than effector T cells. Activation of the Wnt-β-catenin signaling pathway in DCs is required for the expression of interleukin-10, transforming growth factor-β and retinoic acid-metabolizing enzymes that are important for the induction of Treg differentiation and the suppression of effector T cells. Mice that lack β-catenin expression selectively in DC develop more severe inflammation in a mouse model of inflammatory bowel disease. It is likely that other, currently unknown triggers and signaling pathways are also relevant for steady-state DC maturation.

Moreover, DCs receive instructive signals from tissue cells. Epithelial cells, for example, produce a host of molecules capable of instructing DC development towards immunogenic or tolerogenic effector functions. At steady state conditions, the production of thymic stromal lymphopoietin (TSLP), IL-25, and IL-33 dominates and these cytokines favor tolerogenic DC development. Responding to tissue trauma, the epithelial cells switch to producing IL-1, IL-6, TNF-α, and type I interferons which strongly favor immunogenic DC maturation. Several additional triggers are known that induce DCs to become tolerogenic. These include the uptake of apoptotic cells and certain immunosuppressive cytokines such as IL-10 and TGF-β1 or substances such as prostaglandin E2 or the vitamin D3 1α,25-dihydroxy-metabolite.

Regulatory T cells

Regulatory T cells (Treg) specialize in preventing and suppressing immune responses and are central for the prevention of autoimmune diseases. Usually, Tregs comprise approximately 10% of all CD4$^+$ T cells. An inborn lack of Treg cells is the cause of severe autoimmune inflammation in patients suffering from the IPEX (immunodysregulation, polyendocrinopathy, enteropathy, X-linked) syndrome. Treg cells do not only limit autoimmune responses, they also dampen responses against microbial and viral antigens, allergens, tumors, and allografts, and protect fetuses (semi-allografts) during pregnancy.

Regulatory T cells suppress immune responses

Neonatal thymectomy in mice results in an autoimmune syndrome that affects a number of different organs including the thyroid, stomach, ovaries, and testes. Adoptive transfer of CD4$^+$ T cells or CD4$^+$CD8$^+$ thymocytes from non-thymectomized syngeneic mice prevents autoimmune disease manifestations. These findings have three important implications:

- normal mice harbor self-reactive cells, which can cause autoimmune damage;
- normal mice produce CD4$^+$ T cells in the thymus, which can suppress the autoreactive cells;
- depletion of these suppressive cells can cause autoimmune disease.

It was, therefore, important to identify the CD4$^+$ subset capable of suppressing autoimmune disease. Subsequent experiments revealed that adoptive transfer of CD4$^+$ cells induced a range of autoimmune diseases in immunodeficient hosts provided that the transferred CD4$^+$ cells had been purged of cells that coexpress CD25 (the IL-2 receptor alpha chain). Co-transfer of CD4$^+$CD25$^+$ cells prevented autoimmunity. Accordingly, these CD4$^+$CD25$^+$ cells were named **regulatory T cells** (Treg). Further experiments demonstrated that the majority of these cells constitute a distinct, thymus-derived lineage of CD4$^+$ T cells. These thymus-derived Treg cells are usually called 'natural Treg cells'.

Since the seminal report of these findings numerous reports have confirmed that Tregs suppress immune responses against both self and non-self antigens *in vivo* and *in vitro*. When cultured *in vitro* Tregs do not proliferate and do not produce effector cytokines such as IL-2, TNF-α, IFNγ, or IL-4 upon stimulation via their TCR. This anergic state is not overcome by co-stimulatory signals.

When co-cultured with CD25$^-$ effector cells *in vitro*, Treg can suppress the proliferation of the effector cells. To be able to suppress, Tregs need to be stimulated via their TCR.

In addition to Treg cells, various other cell types can help to suppress immune responses by distinct effector mechanisms. Moreover, not all CD4$^+$CD25$^+$ T cells are Tregs.

Q. Which cells apart from Tregs express CD25?
A. CD25 is also expressed by activated T cells (see Fig. 8.18).

Therefore, Tregs cannot be discriminated from activated T$_H$ effector cells based on the expression of CD25 alone.

The transcription factor FoxP3 controls Treg development

Regulatory T cells express the transcription factor forkhead box P3 (FoxP3), a member of the forkhead/winged-helix family of transcription factors.

Q. The lethal X-linked recessive mouse mutant Scurfy is caused by a frameshift mutation in the FoxP3 gene. What effect do you think this would have on the immune system?
A. Male scurfy mice are characterized by hyperactivation of CD4$^+$ T cells, massive overproduction of numerous cytokines and extensive lymphocytic infiltration of multiple organs.

The same manifestations occur in FoxP3-null mice. Both scurfy mice and FoxP3-null mice are deficient in CD4$^+$CD25$^+$ regulatory T cells. In normal mice only CD4$^+$CD25$^+$ peripheral T cells and CD4$^+$CD25$^+$ thymocytes express FoxP3. Other T cells, resting or activated, do not express FoxP3. Forced expression of FoxP3 can convert CD4$^+$CD25$^-$ T cells into CD4$^+$CD25$^+$ T cells that can suppress the activation of other T cells. Thus, FoxP3 is essential for Treg differentiation and maintenance and is important for Treg effector functions. Consequently, the coexpression of CD4, CD25 and FoxP3 is widely used to identify murine Treg cells.

Defects in FoxP3 result in multi-system autoimmune diseases

Since the discovery of FoxP3 a multitude of studies in animal models of autoimmunity proved that a deficiency in CD4$^+$CD25$^+$FoxP3$^+$ Treg can accelerate the development or increase the severity of autoimmune disease. Conversely, in some models, disease could be prevented or even reversed through adoptive transfer of Treg.

Similarly, Treg isolated from human peripheral blood can suppress T cell proliferation and cytokine production *in vitro*. The human counterpart of the scurfy mutation is the IPEX (immune dysregulation, polyendocrinopathy, enteropathy, X-linked) syndrome mentioned above, which is caused by defects in FoxP3 expression resulting in a lack of Treg and has similar clinical manifestations to those observed in scurfy mice. IPEX patients suffer from autoimmune diseases, most prominently autoimmune diabetes (type I diabetes, T1D), thyroiditis, hemolytic anemia, and inflammatory bowel disease and allergic manifestations such as eczema. More than 90% of IPEX patients die from autoimmune diabetes at an early age. This demonstrates that (almost) all individuals harbor potentially diabetogenic autoreactive T cells in their peripheral repertoire. Usually, in healthy people, these autoreactive T cells are controlled by Tregs.

In contrast to murine T cells, *human* T cells express FoxP3 readily and transiently upon TCR signaling. Most of these cells do not possess immunosuppressive capacities. Thus, FoxP3 expression is not a reliable marker for human Treg cells. In fact, the stability of FoxP3-expression in natural Tregs is currently still a matter of debate.

Natural Treg cells differentiate in the thymus

During thymic development FoxP3 expression starts in CD4$^+$CD8$^+$ double positive thymocytes. Approximately 5% of the more mature CD4$^+$CD8$^-$ single positive thymocytes express FoxP3. These Treg cells which acquire their phenotype and functional capacities in the thymus and are released into the periphery as CD4$^+$CD25$^+$FoxP3$^+$ T cells, are called natural Treg cells or **nTregs** (Fig. 19.6).

The number of FoxP3$^+$ thymocytes is drastically reduced in mice that lack MHC class I or II expression. Thus, the nTregs must be subject to positive and negative selection based on the recognition of self-peptide/MHC complexes

Natural and induced Tregs

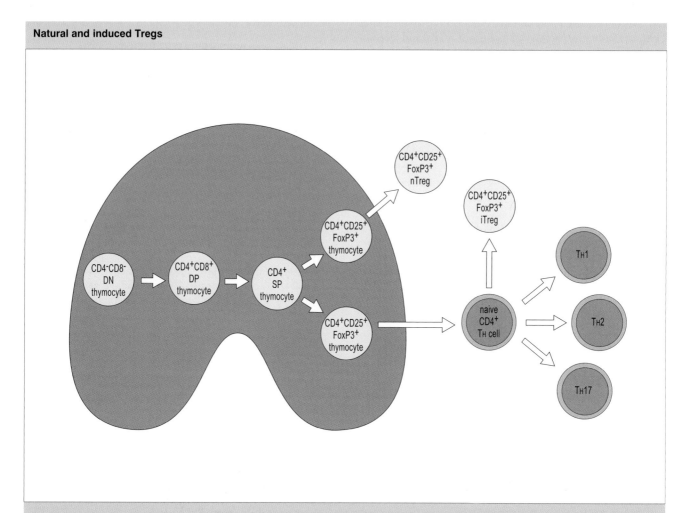

Fig 19.6 In mice CD4$^-$CD8$^-$ double negative (DN) T cell precursors enter the thymus and undergo several selection processes. At the CD4 single positive stage a population of thymocytes starts expressing FoxP3 and CD25. These cells leave the thymus as natural regulatory T cells (Treg) which comprise approximately 5–10% of all peripheral CD4$^+$ T cells. The CD4$^+$FoxP3$^-$CD25$^-$ thymocytes emigrate from the thymus as naive effector TH cells. Upon activation and instruction by APC they can assume different effector functions, broadly characterized as TH1, TH2, or TH17 cells. Some of the naive CD4$^+$FoxP3$^-$CD25$^-$ TH cells can also develop into CD4$^+$FoxP3$^+$CD25$^+$ induced Treg cells. These iTregs exert similar functions to the nTregs, however their FoxP3 expression is less stable.

presented by thymic APCs. Thus, the same cell types that mediate negative selection are also relevant for Treg generation. How, then, are nTregs selected during thymic development? TCR repertoire analyses do not support the notion that the Treg repertoire was skewed towards self-reactivity. Current evidence rather suggests that high affinity interactions of the TCR with self-peptide/MHC complexes in the thymus favors the recruitment of thymocytes into the Treg lineage.

iTreg cells differentiate in the periphery

In addition to the natural Tregs which differentiate in the thymus, mature T cells outside the thymus can also acquire Treg phenotype and function. These are called induced Treg cells (**iTregs**) (see Fig. 19.6). FoxP3 expression can be induced in naive CD4$^+$ cells *in vitro* by antigen recognition in the presence of TGF-β. There is a close developmental relationship between iTregs and TH17 cells. Antigen recognition in the presence of TGF-β induces FoxP3 expression if IL-6 is not present. In contrast, antigen recognition in the presence of TGF-β and IL-6 prevents FoxP3 expression, induces expression of the retinoic acid receptor (RAR) related orphan nuclear receptor RORγt expression and therefore, TH17 differentiation. The transcription factor IRF4 is necessary for the down-regulation of TGF-β-induced FoxP3 expression in response to IL-6 (Fig. 19.7).

Chronic antigen stimulation, particularly with suboptimal doses, *in vivo* also induces FoxP3 expression and iTreg differentiation.

> **Q. Which tissue of the body is normally subject to a high level of continuous antigen stimulation?**
> A. The intestine – large numbers of iTreg cells are present in the intestine where T cells are continuously stimulated by microbial antigens and resident cells produce TGF-β (see Fig. 12.12).

Methylation of the FoxP3 gene is less widespread in iTreg than in natural Treg cells. Consequently, iTreg differentiation is less stable and it is possible that iTregs lose their regulatory capacities and acquire alternative effector functions *in vivo*. In contrast to murine T cells, induction of FoxP3 by TGF-β does not induce regulatory capacities in human T cells.

Treg effector functions

Treg effector functions can be analyzed *in vivo* either by depletion or transfer of Treg cells or *in vitro*. When cultured *in vitro*, Tregs proliferate poorly upon stimulation via their TCR unless IL-2 is also added to the culture. Nevertheless, Treg proliferation can be demonstrated *in vivo*. Tregs need stimulation via their TCR to exert their immunosuppressive functions. Once activated, Treg cells suppress immune responses independent of their own antigen-specificity. This antigen-nonspecific immunosuppression has been called **bystander suppression**. Another characteristic of Treg action has long been known as **infectious tolerance**. The concept of infectious tolerance is based on *in vivo* transfer studies in which the adoptive transfer of Tregs induced the differentiation or selective outgrowth of Tregs in the host. These endogenous Tregs would maintain tolerance

even after the transferred Tregs were no longer detectable in the host.

Tregs can act on a number of different target cells including effector T cells and dendritic cells but also on numerous other cell types including B cells, macrophages, NK cells, NKT cells, mast cells, osteoblasts and osteoclasts. They produce or consume cytokines to modulate their target cells and Tregs are also capable of lysing target cells (Fig. 19.8).

Tregs secrete immunosuppressive cytokines

One possible mechanism of immunosuppression by Tregs would be the secretion of immunosuppressive cytokines (see Fig. 19.8). Indeed, three inhibitory cytokines, IL-10, TGF-β, and IL-35 are produced by Tregs and important for Treg development or effector function. Importantly, IL-10 and TGF-β are not exclusively produced by Tregs but can be produced by many different cell types. Moreover, most *in vitro* studies found IL-10 or TGF-β produced by Treg non-essential for Treg mediated suppression.

IL-10 is a potent suppressor of macrophage and T cell effector functions and critically important to dampen immune responses. Many cell types including TH2 and TH17 cells normally produce IL-10, and some TH1 cells start to

---

Close lineage relationship between TH17 and induced Tregs

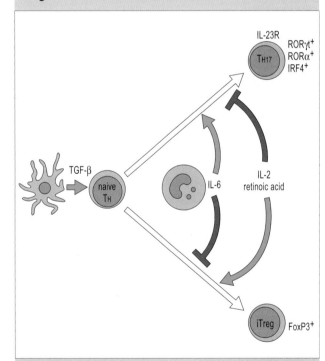

Fig 19.7 T cell differentiation depends largely on instructing cytokines provided by the APC upon T cell activation. TGF-β is an important instructive signal for the development of both TH17 and iTregs. If, in response to IL-6, the transcription factor IRF-4 suppresses FoxP3 expression while increasing RORγt expression, development of TH17 rather than iTreg cells ensues. In contrast, IL-2 or retinoic acid favor the development of iTreg and inhibit TH17 differentiation. The major transcription factors for the functional differentiation of TH17 and iTreg are shown.

Treg effector mechanisms

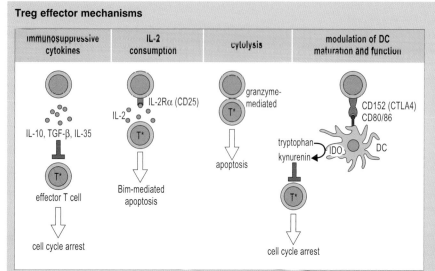

Fig 19.8 Treg cells employ different mechanisms to control effector T cells (T*). These include the secretion of immunosuppressive cytokines; the consumption of IL-2, leading to a lack of IL-2 to sustain proliferation and survival of effector T cells leading to Bim-mediated apoptosis, cytolysis of effector T cells and the modulation of DC maturation and function. IDO, indoleamine 2,3-dioxygenase. *(Adapted from Shevach EM, Immunity 2009;30:636 and Vignali DAA et al. Nature Reviews Immunology 2008;8:523.)*

produce it following chronic antigen stimulation. Therefore, the production of IL-10 by Treg is not critically required in many experimental settings. Mice that lack IL-10 expression specifically in Treg do not develop autoimmune disease manifestations spontaneously. Nevertheless, experimentally induced airway hypersensitivity is more severe in these mice than in their wild type littermates and Treg produced IL-10 seems to be most critical for the control of mucosal immune responses to environmental stimuli. The importance of Treg produced IL-10 seems to depend on the triggers and localization of the immune response.

TGF-β has immunosuppressive functions and is critically required for the differentiation of precursors into Treg cells *in vivo* and *in vitro*. TGF-β is also necessary to maintain FoxP3 expression of nTreg cells and thus for Treg cell homeostasis. In contrast, the relevance of Treg cell produced TGF-β as a mediator of Treg effector function *in vivo* remains unproven. In one particularly instructive experimental system Treg from TGF-β1-deficient mice were able to inhibit colonic inflammation that was induced by adoptive transfer of FoxP3-negative T cells. Importantly, administration of an anti-TGF-β mAb abrogated suppression of colitis mediated by TGF-β1-deficient Treg. These results show that TGF-β is absolutely required for suppression of colitis, but does not need to be produced by Tregs.

IL-35 is a heterodimeric member of the IL-12 family. It consists of an Ebi3 (Epstein–Barr virus-induced gene 3) subunit and p35, which is also known as IL-12. In mice IL-35 is selectively expressed by Treg and required for their optimal effector function.

The relevance of IL-35 for human Treg effector functions is less clear. Many different human cell types express p35. Resting human Tregs do not express Ebi3. Together, these findings make it unlikely that IL-35 is relevant for human Treg. However, IL-35 can induce naive human CD4+ T cells to produce IL-35 and acquire immunosuppressive capacities without expressing FoxP3.

Tregs also secrete other immunosuppressive soluble mediators, including galectin 10, that may be important for Treg effector functions.

Tregs can deplete IL-2

One important effect of Tregs on responder T cells is to inhibit the induction of mRNA for cytokines, including IL-2. Importantly, the addition of exogenous IL-2 does not rescue IL-2 mRNA production in the responder cells.

The consumption of IL-2 by Tregs can induce IL-2-deprivation mediated apoptosis of effector T cells. However, Tregs can block autoimmune disease even in IL-2 deficient mice and the importance of IL-2 consumption for Treg *effector function* is still a matter of debate.

Matters are complicated by the fact that IL-2 is important for the apoptosis of antigen-activated T cells. Hence, the lack of IL-2 or IL-2 signaling does not only result in Treg deficiency but also obliterates peripheral clonal deletion of receptor-activated T cells Therefore, the clinical manifestations of the IL-2 deficiency syndrome cannot be attributed completely to the loss of Tregs.

Cytolysis

Treg are cytotoxic to different cell types, including dendritic cells, CD8+ T, NK, and B cells. In different experimental systems Treg cytotoxicity depended on granzyme B-, perforin-, or Fas-FasL-dependent pathways. Treg-mediated DC death in lymph nodes has been demonstrated *in vivo* and limits the onset of CD8+ T cell responses.

Modulation of DC maturation and function

Some of the *in vitro* experiments to assess the suppressive function of Tregs are performed by stimulating the responder T cells with plate-bound antibodies in the absence of antigen presenting cells. Data from such experiments indicate that Tregs can act directly on responder T cells. *In vivo*, however, the modulation of DC/T interactions is also an important mechanism of Treg-mediated immunosuppression. Depletion of Treg cells *in vivo* results in increased DC maturation and elevated numbers of DC. Direct interactions between Treg cells and DCs have also been observed by intravital microscopy. During these interactions Treg cells can exert different effects on DC.

Loss of Treg effector functions

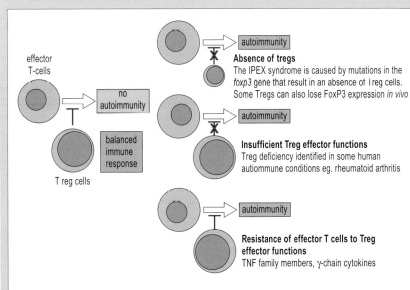

Fig 19.9 In the balanced steady state, Tregs prevent overshooting or unwanted immune responses. Mutations in the FoxP3 gene can result in a complete lack of Treg cells and lethal autoimmune disease manifestations. FoxP3 expression is unstable in iTregs and these cells can convert into effector T cells. Impaired Treg function could also contribute to the pathogenesis of autoimmune diseases. Effector T cells can become resistant to Treg mediated suppression. *(Adapted from Buckner JH, Nat Rev Immunol 2010;10:849).*

Direct cytolysis. *In vivo* studies have shown that Treg cells can induce the death of antigen-presenting DCs in lymph nodes in a perforin-dependent manner. This depletion of DCs limited the onset of CD8$^+$ T cell responses.

Treg cells can also modulate maturation and function of DCs and can probably also modulate the function of mononuclear phagocytes. *In vitro*, Treg cells can downregulate the expression of co-stimulatory molecules, including CD80 and CD86 by DC. By averting co-stimulatory interactions between DC and effector T cells the Treg cells can efficiently inhibit T-cell priming. CD152 (CTLA4) which is expressed constitutively by Treg cells plays an important role in reducing the DCs costimulatory capacity.

Q. What effect does CTLA4 expression have on T cell function, and how does it have its effects?
A. CTLA4 is a high affinity ligand for the costimulatory molecules CD80 and CD86, and ligation of CTLA4 inhibits T cell activation.

The effects of Treg cells on DC are severely reduced when blocking antibodies against CD152 are added or CD152-deficient Treg cells are used in these assays. Moreover, mice that lack CD152 expression selectively in Treg cells spontaneously develop systemic autoimmune disease. This latter finding clearly illustrates that CD152 is pivotal for Treg effector functions.

Treg cells can induce DCs to express indoleamine 2,3-dioxygenase (IDO), which depletes tryptophan resulting in the suppression of effector T cell responses. This interaction also depends on the interaction between CD152 and CD80/86 (see Fig. 19.8).

This list of Treg cell effector mechanisms is by no means complete. Many more molecules and cellular interactions have been identified that may be important for Treg effector function. Clearly there is not one dominant molecular or cellular interaction by which Tregs exert their effector functions. Instead, Treg cells use different effector functions to prevent or suppress different innate or adaptive immune

responses triggered by different stimuli at different anatomical locations. With few exceptions, the dramatic phenotype seen in scurfy mice or IPEX patients who lack FoxP3 does not develop when just one of the pathways mentioned in this section is absent. One such exception is the lack of CD152 which causes widespread lymphocytic infiltration of multiple organs. Moreover, IL-10 deficiency and the IL-2 deficiency syndrome, which cause a similar dramatic phenotype, are not solely attributable to disturbed Treg function.

Can loss of Treg function explain autoimmune disease?

Several pathological mechanisms have been proposed to explain why autoimmunity occurs despite the presence of Tregs. Could Tregs, despite being present in normal or even enhanced numbers have lost (some of) their effector functions? There is some evidence that Tregs can lose their function or that effector T cells become resistant to their action.

However, except for the IPEX syndrome (Fig. 19.9), in which FoxP3$^+$ Tregs are completely absent, there is currently no convincing evidence that reduced numbers of Tregs would cause autoimmune disease. In contrast, Tregs are frequently found in increased numbers at the site of autoimmune lesions.

T cell anergy

T cells that cannot be completely activated upon recognition of their cognate antigen are called anergic. The phenomenon of **T cell clonal anergy** was discovered in CD4$^+$ TH1 clones that failed to produce IL-2 and proliferate when stimulated *in vitro* with antigen in the absence of co-stimulatory signals. In such clones the anergic state may be maintained for several weeks. Characteristically, full effector functions can be rescued in anergic T cell clones by *in vitro* exposure to IL-2.

T cells with diminished proliferation and cytokine production can also be isolated *ex vivo*, e.g. after non-immunogenic peptide application, exposure to superantigens or prolonged exposure to antigen. This phenomenon is sometimes called **adaptive tolerance**. T cell clonal anergy induced *in vitro* differs from T cell anergy, or adaptive tolerance, *in vivo*. Nevertheless, some of the major molecular pathways leading to anergy seem to be similar *in vitro* and *in vivo*. Mice deficient for molecules known to be important for anergy induction *in vitro* are resistant towards the induction of T cell anergy *in vivo*.

One plausible explanation for the functional and molecular differences between clonal T cell anergy *in vitro* and *in vivo* is that several different pathways can induce and enforce T cell clonal anergy. To date, there are no surface marker(s) that would allow the reliable identification of anergic T cells.

The induction of anergy is an active process

T cells in which protein-synthesis is pharmacologically blocked cannot be rendered anergic. How, then, do T cells integrate signals received via the TCR, co-stimulatory receptors, and cytokine receptors to respond with activation, differentiation or anergy? Anergy induction can be described as a series of molecular switches all of which share three characteristics,

- they are present in naive T cells;
- they result in the suppression of *il2* gene expression;
- their actions are antagonized by signals emanating from CD28 or the IL-2R.

The transcription factor NFAT1 fulfils these criteria and is indeed central for anergy induction. Other molecules important for anergy induction have also been identified and include p27kip1, Tob.

In vitro, T-cell anergy can be overcome by the addition of exogenous IL-2 to the culture. The fate of *in vivo* anergized T cells is less clear. It has been shown that anergic T cells can survive for several weeks *in vivo*. Currently it is unknown if such cells will ultimately be removed or if they can be re-activated.

T cells can be deleted in the periphery

T cells that have survived thymic selection can still be deleted in the periphery. When TCR transgenic T cells are adoptively transferred into recipient mice that express the antigen recognized by the transgenic TCR, the transferred T cells will undergo apoptosis in the recipient mice. The transferred T cells survive if they lack the pro-apoptotic protein Bim (Bcl2 interacting mediator of cell death) or if they over-express the anti-apoptotic protein Bcl2 (Bim antagonizes Bcl2). Peripheral deletion not only enforces self-tolerance, it is also helps maintain lymphocyte homeostasis throughout life. At the height of the immune response against certain viruses, almost half of all CD8+ T cells in the blood of the infected patients can be specific for one dominant virus-derived peptide. The majority of these cells must be removed once the virus has been cleared.

Cytokine withdrawal can induce apoptosis

One mechanism of peripheral deletion results from the lack of growth factors, particularly IL-2, for which all activated T cells compete. Cytokine withdrawal triggers an intrinsic pathway of apoptosis involving activation of the Bim factor. Regulatory T cells can accelerate or induce cytokine-withdrawal induced apoptosis of effector T cells by consuming IL-2.

IL-2 is not only critically important for the proliferation and differentiation of naive T cells. When effector T cells are re-stimulated with large amounts of antigen, the addition of IL-2 induces apoptosis in the cycling T cells. This form of peripheral deletion has been called **activation induced cell death** (AICD) or **restimulation induced cell death** (RICD). Mice that are deficient in IL-2 or IL-2 signaling develop an autoimmune syndrome characterized by an abundance of activated T lymphocytes, multiple auto-antibodies and lymphocytic infiltration of several organs. Restimulation induced cell death is one explanation for the observation that the administration of high doses of antigen can induce tolerance. This phenomenon has been called **high dose tolerance**.

Thus, IL-2 has contradictory effects at different phases of the T-cell response. During priming IL-2 is critically required to support clonal expansion and differentiation and a lack of IL-2 at that stage will induce apoptosis. When already activated, an effector T cell simultaneously encountering high concentrations of antigen and IL-2, will undergo apoptosis. Therefore, IL-2 both initiates and terminates T-cell responses.

T cells can be killed by ligation of Fas

The death of T cells is also mediated by the pathway involving Fas (CD95) and its ligand (FasL or CD95L); engagement of the Fas receptor induces apoptosis. Since T cells express both Fas and its ligand on activation, the interaction between the two molecules can induce apoptosis. The importance of this mechanism for the maintenance of self-tolerance is illustrated by the fact that patients with defective Fas have a severe autoimmune lymphoproliferative disease. A similar phenotype including the accumulation of chronically activated T lymphocytes and the development of autoimmunity is caused by a Fas mutation in lpr mice and by a FasL mutation in gld mice.

Some tissues, such as the anterior chamber of the eye, the CNS and the testes normally express Fas ligand. Consequently, when CD95+ effector T cells enter these tissues, they undergo apoptosis and cannot damage the tissue.

B cell tolerance

B lymphocytes and plasma cells that produce antibodies that recognize self-antigens, so called auto-antibodies, pose a threat to the organism. Grave's disease, which is clinically characterized by overshooting production of thyroid hormones, is caused by autoantibodies that act as agonists for the receptor for thyroid stimulating hormone. Blistering skin diseases are caused by autoantibodies that recognize adhesion molecules in the epidermis. In addition to such organ-specific diseases autoantibodies can cause systemic autoimmunity as exemplified by the multi-organ autoimmune disease systemic lupus erythematosus (see Chapter 20).

Q. What process allows the generation of a vast number of diverse clonally distributed B cell receptors, during B cell development?

A. They are generated by random shuffling of the many genes that code for the antigen-binding site of the receptors (see Figs. 3.21 & 3.22).

Autoreactive receptors can be generated in this process and indeed a large percentage of immature B cells have been demonstrated to be autoreactive, creating a demand for immunological pathways that ensure tolerance induction and maintenance in B cells. How B cell tolerance is achieved and maintained differs in several important ways from the immunological pathways to T cell tolerance:

- first, B cells mature in the bone marrow and in mammals there is no B-cell equivalent of thymic repertoire selection in T cells;
- second, mature B cells change their receptors by random mutation in a process called affinity maturation. While affinity maturation serves to generate antibodies with increased affinity for harmful antigens these random mutations could also generate antibodies with high affinity for self antigens. The immune system must have developed mechanisms to prevent the generation of such high-affinity autoantibodies. Indeed, even after immunisation with foreign antigens that closely resemble self antigens, high affinity autoantibodies are usually not produced;
- third, the production of high affinity, class-switched antibodies depends on T cell help. Thus, B cell tolerance is taken care of in large part, if not completely, by T cell tolerance of self-antigens.

Altogether, less than 10% of the mature follicular B cells have been found to be autoreactive. B cell tolerance to autoantigens is established by clonal deletion, receptor editing, the induction of anergy, and the B cells' dependence on T cell help (Fig. 19.10).

B cells undergo negative selection in the bone marrow

Clonal deletion of B lymphocytes was first directly demonstrated in mice that expressed a transgenic BCR specific for a foreign antigen (hen egg lysosyme, HEL). These mice were bred with another strain of transgenic mice that expressed HEL. The F1 mice expressed both HEL and BCRs that recognized HEL. The HEL-specific B-cells were deleted (negatively selected) in the bone marrow of the F1 mice (see Fig. 19.10(1)). When HEL-specific mature B cells from mice that did not express the HEL-transgene were adoptively transferred into mice that expressed HEL, these B cells were also deleted in the recipient mice. Apoptosis of mature germinal centre B cells occurs rapidly, within 4–8 hours of encountering the self-antigen. When the BCR transgenic mice were also Bim-deficient, they survived in the recipient mice. Similar to T cells, the pro-apoptotic factor Bim is important for BCR-induced apoptosis. This is further illustrated by the fact that Bim-deficient mice spontaneously produce autoantibodies against DNA.

Receptor editing allows potentially self-reactive B cells to avoid negative selection

Death by apoptosis is not the only possible outcome for immature B cells in the bone marrow when the strength of signals received through the BCR exceeds a certain threshold. Internalization of the BCR is an important early step in the BCR-induced apoptosis program. This has a number of consequences relevant for BCR-induced apoptosis including a reduced expression of receptors for the cytokine B-cell-activating factor (BAFF) which is necessary to sustain B-cell survival. In contrast, expression of the genes that encode the key enzymes for V(D)J recombination, RAG1 and RAG2, continues. This offers B cells the chance to rearrange their VH or VL regions to replace the autoreactive one. This process is called **BCR editing** (see Fig. 19.10(2)). Approximately two days remain for the B cell to rearrange a less autoreactive receptor. If it fails to do so, it will undergo apoptosis, either in the bone marrow or upon arrival in the spleen. Single-cell PCR analyses reveal secondary rearrangements in roughly two thirds of the immature B cells in the bone marrow. As the frequency of cells with secondary rearrangements is only about 50% of all B cells in the spleen,

B cell tolerance mechanisms

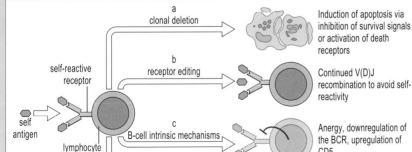

Fig 19.10 Autoreactive B cells can be controlled by clonal deletion (**1**), receptor editing (**2**), B-cell intrinsic mechanisms such as the induction of anergy (**3**) and the B cell-extrinsic mechanisms such as their dependence on T cell help and growth factors (**4**). *(Adapted from Goodnow CC et al. Nature 2005;435:590.)*

receptor editing does not always result in a useful, non-autoreactive BCR.

B cell anergy can be induced by self antigens

B cells can also become anergic upon recognizing a tolerizing self-antigen (see Fig. 19.10(3)). Anergic B cells lack the capacity to proliferate and produce antibodies in response to BCR signaling. In anergic B cells signaling via the BCR is uncoupled from NFκB, thus preventing B cell proliferation. At the same time BCR signaling still prevents apoptosis. Similar to other immature and naive B cells, anergic B cells have a very limited life span if they do not receive appropriate signals. The anergic state can be reversed if the B cell receives signaling via the BCR simultaneously with synergistic signals from another receptor. Such simultaneous signaling is likely to occur when the B cell encounters microbial rather than self antigens. One example is signaling both via the BCR and toll like receptors (TLRs). This would typically be the case when a B cell encounters a pathogen, e.g. gram-negative bacteria possessing LPS which triggers signaling via TLR4.

Another rescue pathway for anergic B cells is activation of phosphatidylinositol 3-kinase (PI3 kinase). Again, this would typically occur when the B cell encounters microbial antigens which are tagged with C3d, a cleavage product of the complement component C3.

Q. How can C3d enhance antigen presentation to a B cell?
A. Simultaneous binding of antigen to the BCR and binding of C3d to the complement receptor CD21 on the surface of the B cell gives a strong activation signal and reduces the requirement for antigen (see Fig. 9.5).

The dual signaling results in the activation of PI3 kinase and rescues the B cell from the anergic state.

B cell tolerance due to lack of T cell help

Perhaps the main mechanism to ensure B cell tolerance is the B cells' dependence on T cell help for high affinity isotype switched antibody production (see Fig. 19.10(4)). BCR signaling results in changes in gene expression that facilitate antigen presentation to T cells:

- enhanced CCR7 expression enables the B cells to migrate from the follicle towards the T cell zone in the secondary lymphatic organs;
- induction of CD86 increases the number of ligands for the co-stimulatory receptor CD28 on T cells;
- productive antigen-presentation to T cells results in the increased secretion of T-cell cytokines such as IL-4 and IL-21 that prevent B-cell apoptosis and support B-cell proliferation.

In vivo imaging studies have shown the formation of conjugates between T and B cells at the border between the follicle and the T-cell zone. Each of these contacts lasts for approximately 10–40 min and the B cells spend about 1.5 days in this perifollicular area. A T cell subset, the T follicular helper (TFH) cells express the chemokine receptors CXCR5 that enables them to migrate towards the B cell follicles. It also produces cytokines such as IL-4 and IL-21 that support B cell differentiation into antibody-secreting cells and it has the costimulatory receptor ICOS that enhances interactions with ICOSL+ B cells. Dysregulation of TFH development or function has been associated with autoimmunity. For example, mice with a mutation of the TFH regulatory protein Roquin have massively increased TFH numbers in their germinal centres and develop pathogenic autoantibodies.

The survival of germinal centre (GC) B cells also depends on repeated interactions between CD40 on B cells and its ligand CD154 on T cells. Injection of a blocking mAb against CD154 results in the dissolution of germinal centres within several days. To survive and differentiate into antibody producing cells, naive B cells need to receive two signals:

- signal one upon antigen binding to the BCR; and
- signal two from TH cells.

Only those B cells that present antigen which is recognized by a TH cell will receive anti-apoptotic signals from that T cell. Since the T cell repertoire has been largely purged of self-reactive receptors, a B cell recognizing and presenting a microbial antigen is much more likely to receive T cell help than a B cell that recognizes a self-antigen. Thus, both T- and B-cell tolerance must be overcome before high affinity autoantibodies can be produced.

CRITICAL THINKING: IMMUNOLOGICAL TOLERANCE (SEE P. 439 FOR EXPLANATIONS)

1. Figure 19.10 depicts four mechanisms to establish B cell tolerance. Compare these with the mechanisms used to establish T cell tolerance and explain similarities and differences.

2. The transcriptional regulator AIRE (autoimmune regulator) is considered to be critical for the establishment of self tolerance. Explain the experimental and clinical evidence on which this statement is based.

3. T-cell precursors undergo positive selection processes in the thymus. Explain 'positive selection'. There is no positive selection for B cells. Can you speculate why positive selection is required for T-cells but not for B-cells?

4. Explain how dendritic cells contribute to peripheral T cell tolerance.

5. Pathogens with exclusively peripheral-tissue tropism (such as papillomavirus) can evade immune responses. Can you explain which tolerance-mechanism is subverted by such pathogens?

6. Mice that express a transgene-encoded TCR which is specific for a self antigen usually do not develop autoimmune disease. How could you distinguish in an

Continued

CRITICAL THINKING: IMMUNOLOGICAL TOLERANCE (SEE P. 439 FOR EXPLANATIONS) CONT.

in vitro assay if the transgenic T cells were ignorant or anergic?

7 Patients with autoimmune diseases often have increased numbers of regulatory T cells (Tregs) in diseased

tissue – speculate about possible explanations for this seemingly paradoxical finding.

Further reading

Germain RN. Special regulatory T-cell review: A rose by any other name: from suppressor T cells to Tregs, approbation to unbridled enthusiasm. Immunology 2008;123:20–27.

Goldrath AW, Bevan MJ. Selecting and maintaining a diverse T-cell repertoire. Nature 1999;402:255–262.

Goodnow CC, Vinuesa CG, Randall KL, et al. Control systems and decision making for antibody production. Nat Immunol 2010;11:681–688.

Kamradt T, Mitchison NA. Tolerance and autoimmunity. N Engl J Med 2001;344:655–664.

Klein L, Hinterberger M, Wirnsberger G, Kyewski B. Antigen presentation in the thymus for positive selection and central tolerance induction. Nat Rev Immunol 2009;9:833–844.

Matzinger P, Kamala T. Tissue-based class control: the other side of tolerance. Nat Rev Immunol 2011;11:221–230.

Pulendran B, Tang H, Manicassamy S. Programming dendritic cells to induce T(H)2 and tolerogenic responses. Nat Immunol 2010;11:647–655.

Saibil SD, Deenick EK, Ohashi PS. The sound of silence: modulating anergy in T lymphocytes. Curr Opin Immunol 2007;19:658–664.

Sakaguchi S, Yamaguchi T, Nomura T, Ono M. Regulatory T cells and immune tolerance. Cell 2008;133:775–787.

Schwartz RH. T cell anergy. Annu Rev Immunol 2003;21:305–334.

Shevach EM. Mechanisms of FoxP3$^+$ T regulatory cell-mediated suppression. Immunity 2009;30:636–645.

von Boehmer H, Melchers F. Checkpoints in lymphocyte development and autoimmune disease. Nat Immunol 2010;11:14–20.

Autoimmunity and Autoimmune Disease

SUMMARY

- **Autoimmunity is associated with disease.** Autoimmune mechanisms underlie many diseases, some organ-specific, others systemic in distribution, and autoimmune disorders can overlap – an individual may have more than one organ-specific disorder, or more than one systemic disease.

- **Genetic factors play a role in the development of autoimmune diseases.** Twin studies show that there is a heritable component to autoimmunity. The vast majority of autoimmune diseases are polygenic but HLA genes are particularly important.

- **Self-reactive B and T cells persist even in normal subjects.** Autoreactive B and T cells persist in normal subjects, but in disease are selected by autoantigen in the production of autoimmune responses.

- **Controls on the development of autoimmunity can be bypassed.** Microbial cross-reacting antigens and cytokine dysregulation can lead to autoimmunity.

- **In most diseases associated with autoimmunity, the autoimmune process produces the lesions.** The pathogenic role of autoimmunity can be demonstrated in experimental models. Human autoantibodies can be directly pathogenic. Immune complexes are often associated with systemic autoimmune disease. Autoantibody tests are valuable for diagnosis and sometimes for prognosis.

- **Treatment of autoimmune disease has a variety of aims.** Treatment of organ-specific diseases usually involves metabolic control. Treatment of systemic diseases includes the use of anti-inflammatory and immunosuppressive drugs. Biological therapies using monoclonal antibodies against pro-inflammatory cytokines have revolutionized the treatment of the autoimmune rheumatic diseases. B cell-directed therapies have proved highly effective in many autoimmune diseases.

Like a highly trained army, the immune system has evolved to recognize and destroy foreign invading forces. Sometimes immune recognition fails resulting in 'friendly fire' against the body's own tissue. For example, 'friendly fire' directed against synovial tissue causes rheumatoid arthritis; whereas an attack on cells within the pancreas results in diabetes mellitus.

Non-specific inflammation (e.g. in response to infection) invariably leads to some degree of 'collateral' damage, but because of efficient clearance of the inciting pathogen and negative feedback loops, this is usually self-limited. In contrast, once initiated autoimmune reactions usually persist because the inciting self-antigen cannot be cleared without complete destruction of the target tissue. Furthermore, the tissue destruction resulting from the autoimmune attack may expose previously hidden antigens, leading to further autoantibody production. This phenomenon is known as epitope spread.

Autoimmunity and autoimmune disease

Because the repertoire of specificities expressed by the B cells and T cells is generated randomly, it includes many that are specific for self components. The body therefore requires self-tolerance mechanisms to distinguish between self and non-self determinants to avoid autoreactivity (see Chapter 19). However, such mechanisms may fail and a number of diseases have been identified in which there is autoimmunity, with copious production of autoantibodies and autoreactive T cells. The targets of the autoimmune 'attacks' vary widely as we shall see.

Not every 'autoimmune event' leads to clinically overt disease. For example, anti-nuclear antibodies may be observed in the healthy relatives of patients with systemic lupus eythematosus, as well as a small number of unrelated, healthy individuals.

Autoimmunity strictly refers to an inappropriate *adaptive* immune response, i.e. a loss of self-tolerance. Although the terms autoinflammatory and autoimmune are often used interchangeably, the two are not synonymous. Autoinflammatory diseases can occur without autoimmunity. For example, the periodic fever syndromes, which include familial Mediterranean fever and tumor necrosis factor receptor associated periodic syndrome (TRAPS), are caused by dysregulation of the *innate* immune system, without any adaptive immune response against 'self'. Conversely,

Pathological changes in Hashimoto's thyroiditis

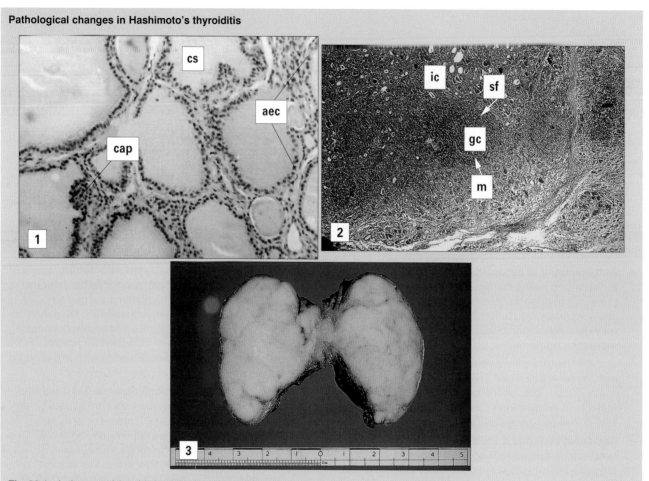

Fig. 20.1 In the normal thyroid gland (**1**), the acinar epithelial cells (aec) line the colloid space (cs) into which they secrete thyroglobulin, which is broken down on demand to provide thyroid hormones (cap, capillaries containing red blood cells). In the Hashimoto gland (**2**), the normal architecture is virtually destroyed and replaced by invading cells (ic), which consist essentially of lymphocytes, macrophages, and plasma cells. A secondary lymphoid follicle (sf), with a germinal center (gc) and a mantle of small lymphocytes (m), is present. H&E stain. × 80. (**3**) In contrast to the red color and soft texture of the normal thyroid, the pale and firm gross appearance of the Hashimoto gland reflects the loss of colloid and heavy infiltration with inflammatory cells. ((**2**) *Reproduced from Woolf N. Pathology: basic and systemic. London: WB Saunders; 1998.*)

autoimmune diseases need not be inflammatory; examples include immune thrombocytopenia, hemolytic anemia and myasthenia gravis.

Autoimmune conditions present a spectrum between organ-specific and systemic disease

Hashimoto's thyroiditis is highly organ-specific

One of the earliest examples in which the production of autoantibodies was associated with disease in a given organ is **Hashimoto's thyroiditis**. (Thyroiditis is a condition that is most common in middle-aged women and often leads to the formation of a goiter or hypothyroidism.) The gland is infiltrated, sometimes to an extraordinary extent, with inflammatory lymphoid cells. These are predominantly mononuclear phagocytes, lymphocytes and plasma cells, and secondary lymphoid follicles are common (Fig. 20.1). The gland often also has regenerating thyroid follicles.

The serum of patients with Hashimoto's disease usually contains antibodies to thyroglobulin. These antibodies are demonstrable by agglutination and by precipitin reactions when present in high titer. Most patients also have

antibodies directed against a cytoplasmic or microsomal antigen, also present on the apical surface of the follicular epithelial cells (Fig. 20.2), and now known to be thyroid peroxidase, the enzyme that iodinates thyroglobulin. The antibodies associated with Hashimoto's thyroiditis react only with the thyroid, so the resulting lesion is highly localized.

SLE is a systemic autoimmune disease

By contrast, the serum from patients with diseases such as systemic lupus erythematosus (SLE) reacts with many, if not all, of the tissues in the body. In SLE, one of the dominant antibodies is directed against the cell nucleus (see Fig. 20.2).

Hashimoto's thyroiditis and SLE represent the extremes of the autoimmune spectrum (Fig. 20.3):

- the common target organs in **organ-specific disease** include the thyroid, adrenal, stomach, and pancreas;
- the non-organ-specific diseases, often termed **systemic autoimmune diseases**, which include rheumatological disorders, characteristically involve the skin, kidney, joints, and muscle (Fig. 20.4).

Autoantibodies to thyroid

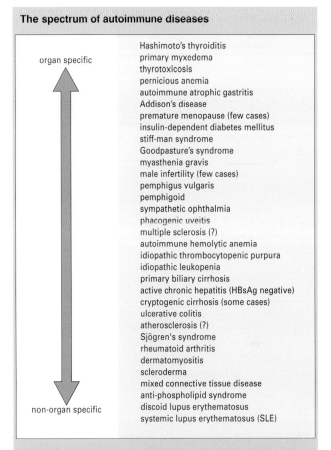

Fig. 20.2 Healthy, unfixed human thyroid sections were treated with patients' serum, and then with fluoresceinated rabbit anti-human immunoglobulin. (**1**) Some residual thyroglobulin in the colloid (RTg) and the acinar epithelial cells (AEC) of the follicles, particularly the apical surface, are stained by antibodies from a patient with Hashimoto's disease, which react with the cells' cytoplasm but not the nuclei (N). (**2**) In contrast, serum from a patient with systemic lupus erythematosus (SLE) contains antibodies that react only with the nuclei of acinar epithelial cells and leave the cytoplasm unstained. *(Courtesy of Mr G Swana.)*

The spectrum of autoimmune diseases

organ specific

Hashimoto's thyroiditis
primary myxedema
thyrotoxicosis
pernicious anemia
autoimmune atrophic gastritis
Addison's disease
premature menopause (few cases)
insulin-dependent diabetes mellitus
stiff-man syndrome
Goodpasture's syndrome
myasthenia gravis
male infertility (few cases)
pemphigus vulgaris
pemphigoid
sympathetic ophthalmia
phacogenic uveitis
multiple sclerosis (?)
autoimmune hemolytic anemia
idiopathic thrombocytopenic purpura
idiopathic leukopenia
primary biliary cirrhosis
active chronic hepatitis (HBsAg negative)
cryptogenic cirrhosis (some cases)
ulcerative colitis
atherosclerosis (?)
Sjögren's syndrome
rheumatoid arthritis
dermatomyositis
scleroderma
mixed connective tissue disease
anti-phospholipid syndrome
discoid lupus erythematosus
systemic lupus erythematosus (SLE)

non-organ specific

Fig. 20.3 Autoimmune diseases may be classified as organ-specific or non-organ-specific depending on whether the response is primarily against antigens localized to particular organs or against widespread antigens.

The location of the antigen determines where a disease lies in the spectrum

The autoantigen in organ-specific autoimmune disease is expressed only in that tissue. In contrast, autoantigens in systemic autoimmune disease are typically present in multiple tissues (if not ubiquitously) throughout the body. Examples include tRNA synthetases in myositis (which in spite of its name may also involve the skin, joints, lungs, and heart), small nuclear ribonucleoproteins (snRNPs) in SLE, and topoisomerases in systemic sclerosis. These small proteins play a vital role in the cellular 'machinery'. tRNA synthetases are involved in protein translation, snRNPs in mRNA splicing, and topoisomerases in DNA replication. Thus it is not difficult to appreciate the myriad clinical manifestations of an autoimmune 'attack' on these targets.

An individual may have more than one autoimmune disease

Autoimmune diseases 'hunt in packs'; in patients with an autoimmune disease, the chance of developing an additional autoimmune disease is significantly elevated. This holds true for both organ-specific and systemic autoimmune disease.

- Thyroid antibodies occur with a high frequency in patients with pernicious anemia who have gastric autoimmunity, and these patients have a higher incidence of thyroid autoimmune disease than the normal population. Similarly, patients with thyroid autoimmunity have a high incidence of stomach autoantibodies and to a lesser extent the clinical disease itself (pernicious anemia).
- Around 15% of patients with primary Sjögren's syndrome have concomitant autoimmune

hypothyroidism, and up to 40% have thyroid antibodies. Around 10% of SLE patients have thyroid antibodies in their serum.
- 30% of patients with SLE and Sjögren's syndrome have a second, third or even fourth autoimmune disease.

The systemic autoimmune rheumatic diseases show considerable overlap. This is typified by the so called 'overlap syndromes' in which patients exhibit mixed features of SLE, myositis, and scleroderma. Features of rheumatoid arthritis, notably an erosive arthritis, are present in 5% of patients with SLE. In these diseases immune complexes are deposited systemically, particularly in the kidney, joints, and skin, giving rise to widespread lesions.

The mechanisms of immunopathological damage vary depending on where the disease lies in the spectrum:

- where the antigen is localized in a particular organ, type II hypersensitivity (e.g. autoimmune hemolytic anemia) and type IV cell-mediated reactions, as in type 1 insulin-dependent diabetes, are most important (see Chapters 24–26);
- in systemic disorders such as SLE, type III immune complex deposition leads to inflammation through a variety of mechanisms, including complement activation and phagocyte recruitment. In rheumatoid arthritis immune complexes directly stimulate production of cytokines such as TNFα.

Two types of autoimmune disease

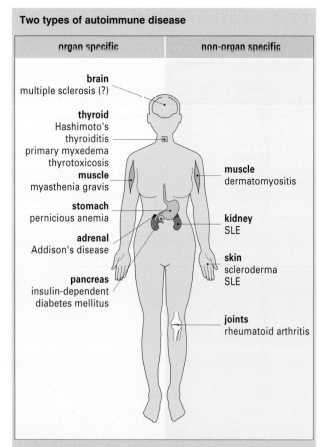

Fig. 20.4 Although the non-organ-specific diseases characteristically produce symptoms in the skin, joints, kidney, and muscle, individual organs are more markedly affected by particular diseases, for example the kidney in SLE and the joints in rheumatoid arthritis.

Overlap between thyroid and gastric autoimmunity

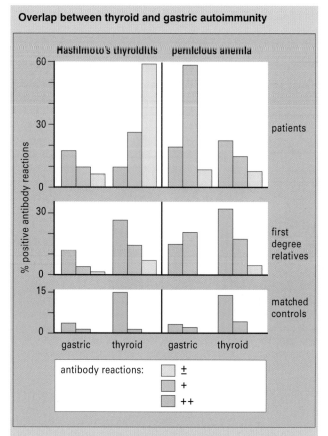

Fig. 20.5 Genetic factors affect the predisposition to autoimmunity and selection of the target organ in the relatives of patients with Hashimoto's thyroiditis and pernicious anemia. (*Data adapted from Doniach D, Roitt IM, Taylor KB. Ann NY Acad Sci 1965;124:605.*)

Genetic factors in autoimmunity

There is an undoubted familial incidence of autoimmunity. This is largely genetic rather than environmental, as may be seen from studies of identical and non-identical twins. Thus if one of a pair of identical twins gets SLE, there is a 25% chance the other will develop it. If the twin is not identical the concordance rate is only 2–3%.

Within families, clustering of distinct autoimmune diseases has been reported. A large population-based survey found that families with a proband with rheumatoid arthritis were more likely to manifest other autoimmune disorders. This finding holds true for relatives of patients with other autoimmune diseases, such as multiple sclerosis, which suggests the presence of shared pathogenic factors across the autoimmune diseases. However, the majority of individuals with autoimmune disease will not have an affected first degree relative. Thus whilst genetic factors are important in the pathogenesis of autoimmunity, they are usually not sufficient to cause disease without additional environmental influences.

Within the families of patients with organ-specific autoimmunity, not only is there a general predisposition to develop organ specific antibodies, other genetically controlled factors tend to select the organ that is mainly affected. Thus, although relatives of patients with Hashimoto's thyroiditis and families of patients with pernicious anemia both have a higher than normal incidence and titer of thyroid autoantibodies, the relatives of patients with pernicious anemia have a far higher frequency of gastric autoantibodies (Fig. 20.5), indicating that there are genetic factors that differentially select the stomach as the target within these families.

Usually, several genes underlie susceptibility to autoimmunity

Clearly, the vast majority of autoimmune diseases are not single gene disorders. Rather, they occur as a result of the complex interplay of multiple genetic and environmental factors. Evidence from genome-wide association studies has demonstrated that many genes contribute to disease susceptibility, i.e. autoimmunity is usually polygenic. Thus the effect of variation in any one gene is by itself typically small.

There is emerging interest in how epigenetic modifications of DNA and associated histones may provide explanations of the molecular basis of complex polygenic disease traits such as autoimmunity. Epigenetic changes may occur as a result of environmental stimuli, but may also be partly heritable.

HLA associations in autoimmune disease

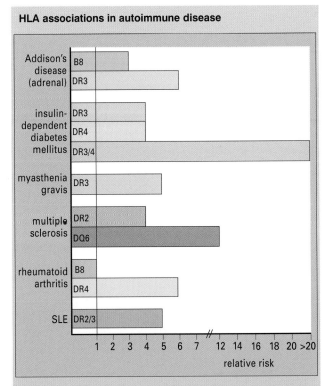

Fig. 20.6 The relative risk is a measure of the increased chance of contracting the disease for individuals bearing the HLA antigen, relative to those lacking it. Virtually all autoimmune diseases studied have shown an association with some HLA specificity. The greater relative risk for Addison's disease associated with HLA-DR3 as compared with HLA-B8 suggests that DR3 is closely linked to or even identical with the 'disease susceptibility gene'. In this case it is not surprising that B8 has a relative risk greater than 1, because it is known to occur with DR3 more often than expected by chance in the general population, a phenomenon termed linkage disequilibrium. Both DQ2 and DQ8 are also associated with type 1 diabetes mellitus, and are usually found in conjunction with the extended haplotype containing the DR3/4 disease-associated alleles. Rheumatoid arthritis is linked to a pentamer sequence in DR1 and certain subtypes of DR4, but not to any HLA-A or HLA-B alleles.

Certain HLA haplotypes predispose to autoimmunity

Further evidence for the operation of genetic factors in autoimmune disease comes from their tendency to be associated with particular HLA specificities (Fig. 20.6). For most autoimmune diseases, the MHC region which is located on the short arm of chromosome 6, provides the strongest genetic component to disease susceptibility. Recent high-density genome mapping in multiple autoimmune diseases has demonstrated complex, multilocus effects that span the entire region, with both shared and unique loci across diseases.

In some autoimmune disorders single HLA genes appear to determine disease susceptibility (e.g. HLA-B27 and ankylosing spondylitis). In others, such as rheumatoid arthritis, complex interactions between alleles at multiple genes within the HLA are involved. Rheumatoid arthritis shows no associations with the HLA-A and -B loci haplotypes, but is associated with a nucleotide sequence known as the

'shared epitope' (encoding amino acids 70–74 in the DRβ chain) that is common to DR1 and major subtypes of DR4; the MHC association with rheumatoid arthritis is restricted to patients who are positive for antibodies to citrullinated peptides. The nucleotide sequence of the shared epitope is also present in the dnaJ **heat-shock proteins** of various bacilli and EBV gp110 proteins, suggesting an interesting possibility for the induction of autoimmunity by a microbial cross-reacting epitope (see below). The plot gets deeper, though, with the realization that HLA-DR molecules bearing this sequence can bind to another bacterial heat-shock protein, dnaK, and to the human analog, namely hsp73, which targets selected proteins to lysosomes for antigen processing.

The haplotype B8, DR3 is common in both the organ-specific diseases and systemic autoimmune diseases like SLE and myositis, though Hashimoto's thyroiditis tends to be associated more with DR5. Interestingly, for type 1 diabetes mellitus, DQ2/8 heterozygotes have a greatly increased risk of developing the disease (see Fig. 20.6).

Genes of the MHC including HLA-A1, B8, and DR3 have been linked to SLE, although over a dozen other genes (including those regulating interferon α) have shown a stronger linkage.

Genes outside the HLA region also confer susceptibility to autoimmunity

Although HLA risk factors tend to dominate, autoimmune disorders are genetically complex and genome-wide searches for mapping the genetic intervals containing genes for predisposition to disease also reveal a plethora of non-HLA genes (Fig. 20.7) affecting:

- loss of tolerance;
- lymphocyte activation (receptor signaling pathways and co-stimulation);
- microbial recognition;
- cytokines and cytokine receptors;
- end-organ targeting.

One of the commonest genes outside of the HLA region to be associated with autoimmune disease is the protein tyrosine phosphatase gene (PTPN22), which is expressed in lymphocytes. The minor allele of PTPN22 (Trp620) is associated with type 1 diabetes, rheumatoid arthritis, autoimmune thyroiditis and SLE. Crohn's disease, in contrast, is linked to the more common allele (Arg620). The minor allele results in gain of function and results in inhibition of B and T cell activation and homozygous individuals have a profound defect in lymphocyte receptor signaling. The mechanisms by which this leads to autoimmunity are not clear, but possibilities include failure to delete autoreactive T cells in the thymus, impaired regulatory T cell function, and ineffective clearance of pathogens. It is interesting to note that two alleles with contrasting effects on lymphocyte receptor signaling are associated with distinct autoimmune diseases.

Autoimmunity and autoimmune disease

Despite the complex selection mechanisms operating to establish self tolerance during lymphocyte development, the body contains large numbers of lymphocytes, which are potentially autoreactive.

Some genetic loci associated with autoimmune disease

Chromosomal location	Candidate genes	Function of protein encoded by gene	Diseases
1p13	PTPN22	T & B cell receptor signalling	RA, T1D, SLE, IBD, AT
	CD2/CD58	T cell activation	RA, MS
1p31	IL23R	Component of IL-23 receptor	IBD, Psoriasis, AS
1q23	CRP	Innate immunity	SLE
	FCGR2A	Phagocytosis and immune complex clearance	SLE
	FCGR2B	B cell regulation. Phagocytosis of immune complexes	SLE
	FCGR3A	Expressed on natural killer cells. Mediates antibody-dependent cellular cytotoxicity	SLE
	FCGR3B	Clearance of immune complexes	SLE, AAV
1q32	IL10	Downregulates immune responses	IBD, T1D, SLE
1q41-42	PARP	Apoptosis	SLE
	TLR5	Innate immunity	SLE
2q33	CTLA4	Transmits inhibitory signals to T cells	RA, T1D
2q35-37	PDCD1	Transmembrane protein; activation leads to cytokine inhibition and control of cellular activation & antibody production	SLE
5q33	IL12B	p40 subunit common to both IL-12 and IL-23	IBD, Psoriasis
6p21	MHC region : multiple genes e.g. TNF-α, C2, C4	multiple	majority of autoimmune diseases
6q23	TNFAIP3	Induced by TNF and pattern recognition activation. Inhibits NF-κB signalling	RA, SLE, Psoriasis
10p15	IL2RA	IL-2 receptor α chain	MS, T1D, SLE, Grave's disease, AAV

Fig. 20.7 CRP, C reactive protein; CTLA4, cytotoxic T lymphocyte-associated protein 4; FCGR, Fc gamma receptor; IL, interleukin; MHC, major histocompatibility complex; PARP, poly-ADP-ribose polymerase; PDCD1, programmed cell death 1; PTPN22, protein tyrosine phosphatase, non-receptor type 22; TLR5,: toll-like receptor 5; TNF-α, tumor necrosis factor α; AAV, ANCA-associated vasculitis; AS, ankylosing spondylitis; AT, autoimmune thyroiditis; IBD, inflammatory bowel disease; MS, multiple sclerosis; RA, rheumatoid arthritis; SLE, systemic lupus erythematosus; T1D, type 1 diabetes mellitus.

Thus, many autoantigens, when injected with adjuvants, make autoantibodies in normal animals, demonstrating the presence of autoreactive B cells, and it is possible to identify a small number of autoreactive B cells (e.g. anti-thyroglobulin) in the normal population.

Autoreactive T cells are also present in normal individuals, as shown by the fact that it is possible to produce autoimmune lines of T cells by stimulation of normal circulating T cells with the appropriate autoantigen (e.g. myelin basic protein [MBP]) and IL-2.

Autoantibody production alone does not equal autoimmune disease

Healthy individuals may have autoantibodies without clinical disease. For example, 13% of healthy individuals have significant levels of anti-nuclear antibodies (ANA) and their prevalence in the general population aged over 60 rises to 20–30%. Transiently positive ANA may occur following infection. In patients who eventually develop autoimmune disease, autoantibody production may predate clinical disease by years – in one study autoantibodies preceded the onset of clinical manifestations by up to 9 years.

The autoantibodies typically appear in a stereotyped order, providing insight into the sequential pathogenic changes that occur as SLE develops. Antinuclear antibodies, antibodies to Ro, and antibodies to beta2 glycoprotein 1 appear first; anti-dsDNA antibodies typically appear 1–2 years before symptom onset; antibodies to Sm and RNP appear in the months immediately preceding symptoms. Similarly rheumatoid factors and anti-CCP antibodies have been identified in the serum of individuals years before they develop clinically overt rheumatoid arthritis.

Progression to autoimmune disease occurs in stages

These findings allow us to conceptualize autoimmune disease as a multistep process. The first stage is predisposition of an individual to autoimmunity by his or her genes, and other factors such as female hormones. The second phase is initiated by an event, probably stochastic or perhaps caused by an environmental trigger such as infection or ultraviolet radiation, leading to loss of self-tolerance and autoantibody production. This however is not alone sufficient to cause disease. A further step is required before progression to a third phase involving tissue damage by the autoimmune attack. This autoimmune attack leads to further release of self-antigens, which are not removed in the normal efficient manner (see below), and propagation of the autoimmune response, resulting in the clinical manifestations of disease. The earliest clinical features of systemic autoimmune diseases such as SLE or RA are usually non-specific such as fatigue or constitutional symptoms. This prodrome typically precedes the development of the classic disease phenotype by weeks to months.

During the propagation phase, not only is there an autoimmune response to an increasing number of autoantigens (demonstrated by the sequential development of multiple autoantibodies in patients with SLE), but also to more epitopes within each antigen – a phenomenon termed **epitope spread**. Epitope spread can be involve multiple epitopes on the same molecule (intramolecular spread), or epitopes on different molecules associated as part of a macromolecular complex (intermolecular spread). The latter provides a mechanism for how antibodies to non-protein self antigens such as DNA and phospholipid can occur.

Autoimmunity results from antigen-driven self-reactive lymphocytes

Given that autoreactive B cells exist, the question remains whether they are stimulated to proliferate and produce autoantibodies by interaction with autoantigens or by some other means, such as non-specific polyclonal activators or idiotypic interactions (see below and Fig. 20.8).

Evidence that B cells are selected by antigen comes from the existence of high-affinity autoantibodies, which arise through somatic mutation, a process that requires both T cells and autoantigen. In addition, patients' serum usually contains autoantibodies directed to epitope clusters occurring on the same autoantigenic molecule. Apart from the presence of autoantigen itself, it is very difficult to envisage a mechanism that could account for the co-existence of antibody responses to different epitopes on the same molecule. A similar argument applies to the induction, in a single individual, of autoantibodies to organelles (e.g. nucleosomes and spliceosomes, which appear as blebs on the surface of apoptotic cells) or antigens linked within the same organ (e.g. thyroglobulin and thyroid peroxidase).

The most direct evidence for autoimmunity being antigen driven comes from studies of the Obese strain chicken, which spontaneously develops thyroid autoimmunity. If the thyroid gland (the source of antigen) is removed at birth, the chickens mature without developing thyroid autoantibodies (Fig. 20.9). Furthermore, once thyroid autoimmunity has developed, later removal of the thyroid leads to a gross decline of thyroid autoantibodies, usually to undetectable levels.

Comparable experiments have been carried out in the non-obese diabetic (NOD) mouse, which models human autoimmune diabetes – chemical destruction of the β cells leads to decline in pancreatic autoantibodies.

Possible model of T cell help via processing of intermolecular complexes in the induction of autoimmunity

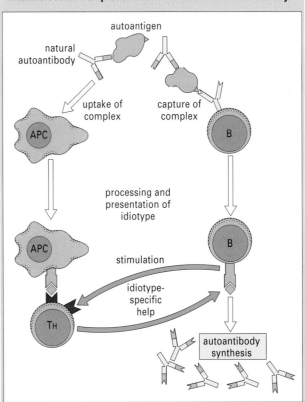

Fig. 20.8   An immune complex consisting of autoantigen (e.g. DNA) and a naturally occurring (germline) autoantibody is taken up by an antigen-presenting cell (APC), and peptides derived by processing of the idiotypic segment of the antibody (Id) are presented to Tн cells. B cells that express the 'pathogenic' autoantibody can capture the complex and so can receive T cell help via presentation of the processed Id to the Tн cell. Similarly, an anti-DNA-specific B cell that had endocytosed a histone–DNA complex could be stimulated to autoantibody production by histone-specific Tн cells.

Effect of neonatal thyroidectomy on Obese chickens

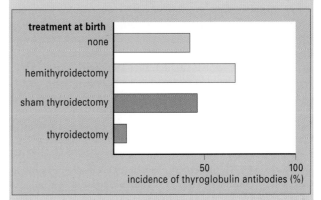

Fig. 20.9   Because removal of the thyroid at birth prevents the development of thyroid autoantibodies, it would appear that the autoimmune process is driven by the autoantigen in the thyroid gland. (Based on data from de Carvalho et al. J Exp Med 1982;155:1255.)

In organ-specific disorders, there is ample evidence for T cells responding to antigens present in the organs under attack. But in non-organ-specific autoimmunity, identification of the antigens recognized by T cells is often inadequate. However, histone-specific T cells are generated in patients with SLE and histone could play a 'piggyback' role in the formation of anti-DNA antibodies by substituting for natural antibody in the mechanism outlined in Figure 20.8.

Another possibility is that the T cells do not 'see' conventional peptide antigen (possibly true of anti-DNA responses), but instead recognize an antibody's idiotype (an antigenic determinant on the V region of antibody).

In this view SLE, for example, might sometimes be initiated as an 'idiotypic disease', following the model shown in Figure 20.8. In this scheme, autoantibodies are produced normally at low levels by B cells using germline genes. If these then form complexes with the autoantigen, the complexes can be taken up by APCs (including B cells) and components of the complex, including the antibody idiotype, presented to T cells. Idiotype-specific T cells would then provide help to the autoantibody-producing B cells.

Evidence for the induction of anti-DNA and glomerulonephritis by immunization of mice with the idiotype of germline 'natural' anti-DNA autoantibody lends credence to this hypothesis.

The 'waste disposal' hypothesis of SLE

Antibodies to nuclear components are the serological hallmark of SLE. The question arising from this observation is how nuclear components normally hidden are detected by the immune system as antigen. The answer appears to lie with apoptosis. There is strong evidence that SLE (and possibly other autoimmune diseases) are diseases of failure of clearance of apoptotic cells, i.e. due to decreased macrophage 'scavenger' function. When a cell undergoes apoptosis (programmed cell death), blebs of cellular material are formed on the cell surface. Antigens normally buried deep within the cell (and so not detected by the immune system) are exposed on the cell surface. In healthy individuals these apoptotic cells are efficiently cleared. However, in SLE apoptosis is defective; it has been demonstrated that scavenging of apoptotic debris *in vitro* by macrophages from lupus patients is less efficient than by macrophages from healthy controls. Thus the antigens contained within the apoptotic blebs may trigger an autoimmune response. Apoptotic blebs vary in size; larger blebs contain antigens including Sm, Mi-2, Ro-60, and La, whilst smaller blebs contain fodrin, Jo-1, Ro-52, and ribosomal P. Antibodies against all of these targets can be found in systemic autoimmune diseases such as SLE, Sjögren's syndrome, and myositis (Fig. 20.10).

A defective complement pathway may also contribute to ineffective clearance of apoptotic cells as C1q binds to cell debris, allowing macrophages with C1q receptors to engulf the apoptotic cells. Complement deficiency in SLE is usually attributed to consumption as a secondary consequence of immune complex formation. However, it is clear that in a very small number of patients complement deficiency is the cause rather than the effect of SLE. In patients with these rare genetic disorders of deficiency of complement components (including C1q, C2 and C4, as discussed previously), there is a hugely increased risk of developing a lupus-like disease. Reduced

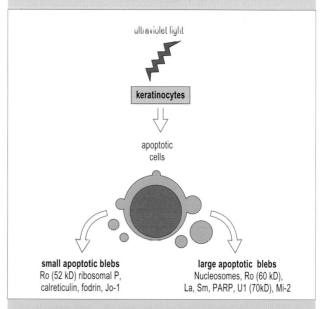

Induction of surface blebs during apoptosis

Fig. 20.10 Apoptosis of keratinocytes exposed to ultraviolet light is illustrated. The different constituents of developing small and large surface blebs during apoptosis are shown. PARP denotes poly-ADP-ribose polymerase. *(Based on Rahman A, Isenberg DA: Systemic lupus erythematosus. N Engl J Med, 2008; 358:929–939.)*

clearance of immune complexes by the spleen has been demonstrated in a patient with C2 deficiency and SLE. This problem was correctable with transfusions of fresh-frozen plasma containing C2. The C1q knock-out mouse also provides evidence for the role of complement in clearance of apoptotic cells. This mouse develops a lupus-like glomerulonephritis, and renal biopsy reveals multiple apoptotic fragments.

The clustering of the lupus autoantigens in apoptotic blebs provides an elegant explanation for how epitope spread occurs in SLE. Intermolecular epitope spread occurs when molecules in close physical proximity are taken up by an APC. Uptake of an apoptotic cell by an APC will result in presentation of the antigens from the surface of the apoptotic cell. Thus the apoptotic cell acts as a cellular platform or 'scaffold' physically linking the multiple autoantigens targeted by the immune response in SLE.

Induction of autoimmunity

Normally, naive autoreactive T cells recognizing cryptic self epitopes are not switched on because the antigen is presented on 'non-professional' APCs such as pancreatic β-islet cells or thyroid epithelial cells which lack co-stimulator molecules, or because it is presented only at low concentrations on 'professional' APCs. However the normal mechanisms that maintain self-tolerance may be bypassed.

Molecular mimicry by cross-reactive microbial antigens can stimulate autoreactive lymphocytes

Infection with a microbe bearing antigens that cross-react with the cryptic self epitopes (i.e. have shared epitopes) will load the professional APCs with levels of processed

Cross-reactive antigens induce autoimmune TH cells

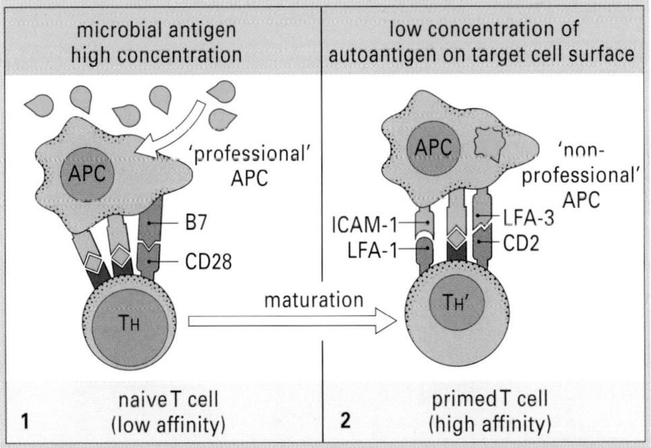

Fig. 20.11 The inability of naive TH cells to recognize autoantigen on a tissue cell, whether because of low concentration or low affinity, can be circumvented by a cross-reacting microbial antigen at higher concentration or with higher innate affinity, together with a co-stimulator such as B7 on a 'professional' APC; this primes the TH cells (**1**). Due to increased expression of accessory molecules (e.g. LFA-1 and CD2) the primed TH cells now have high affinity and, because they do not require a co-stimulatory signal, they can interact with autoantigen on 'non-professional' APCs such as organ-specific epithelial cells to produce autoimmune disease (**2**).

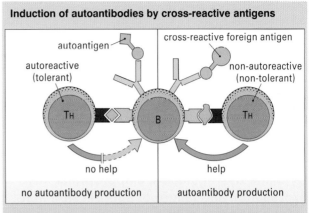

Fig. 20.12 The B cell recognizes an epitope present on autoantigen, but coincidentally present also on a foreign antigen. Normally the B cell presents the autoantigen, but receives no help from autoreactive TH cells, which are functionally deleted. If a cross-reacting foreign antigen is encountered, the B cell can present peptides of this molecule to non-autoreactive T cells and thus be driven to proliferate, differentiate, and secrete autoantibodies.

peptides that are sufficient to activate the naive autoreactive T cells. Once primed, these T cells are able to recognize and react with the self epitope on the non-professional APCs because they:

- no longer require a co-stimulatory signal; and
- have a higher avidity for the target, due to upregulation of accessory adhesion molecules (Fig. 20.11).

Cross-reactive antigens that share B cell epitopes with self molecules can also break tolerance, but by a different mechanism. Many autoreactive B cells cannot be activated because the CD4+ TH cells they need are unresponsive, either because:

- these TH cells are tolerized at lower concentrations of autoantigens than the B cells; or
- because they recognize only cryptic epitopes. However, these 'helpless' B cells can be stimulated if the cross-reacting antigen bears a 'foreign' carrier epitope to which the T cells have not been tolerized (Fig. 20.12). The autoimmune process may persist after clearance of the foreign antigen if the activated B cells now focus the autoantigen on their surface receptors and present it to normally resting autoreactive T cells, which will then proliferate and act as helpers for fresh B cell stimulation.

Molecular mimicry operates in rheumatic fever

An example of a disease in which such molecular mimicry may operate is rheumatic fever, in which autoantibodies to heart valve antigens can be detected. These develop in a small proportion of individuals several weeks after a streptococcal infection of the throat. Carbohydrate antigens on the streptococci cross-react with an antigen on heart valves, so the infection may bypass T cell self tolerance to heart valve antigens. Historically many concepts about autoimmunity arose

because the early immunologists often had a background in infectious diseases, and brought with them ideas about cross-reactivity and molecular mimicry extrapolated from rheumatic fever. However, the evidence for molecular mimicry in most chronic autoimmune diseases is lacking or absent. A notable exception is post-infective polyneuropathy.

There is circumstantial evidence for molecular mimicry in anti-neutrophil cytoplasmic antibody (ANCA) associated vasculitis (AAV). Antibodies to lysosomal membrane protein-2 (LAMP-2) are a subtype of ANCA found in most patients with pauci-immune focal necrotizing glomerulonephritis (FNGN). The autoantibodies to LAMP-2 commonly recognize an epitope with 100% homology to the bacterial adhesion FimH. Rats injected with FimH develop antibodies to LAMP-2 and pauci-immune FNGN. Furthermore, many humans with pauci-immune FNGN have evidence of recent infection with fimbriated organisms.

Shared B cell epitopes between *Yersinia enterolytica* and the extracellular domain of the thyroid stimulating hormone (TSH) receptor have been described.

In some cases foreign antigen can directly stimulate autoreactive cells

Another mechanism to bypass the tolerant autoreactive TH cell is where antigen or another stimulator directly triggers the autoreactive effector cells.

For example, lipopolysaccharide or Epstein–Barr virus causes direct B cell stimulation and some of the clones of activated cells will produce autoantibodies, though in the absence of T cell help these are normally of low titer and affinity. However, it is conceivable that an activated B cell might pick up and process its cognate autoantigen and present it to a naive autoreactive T cell.

Infection may trigger relapse in autoimmune disease

Many autoimmune diseases have a relapsing-remitting phenotype, characterized by periods of disease activity punctuated by periods of quiescence. This relapsing-remitting phenotype suggests there may be some varying influence on the autoimmune process. Clinical observation suggests that infections appear to trigger increased autoimmune disease activity, although proving a causal link is difficult. In Wegener's granulomatosis relapses are closely correlated with recent infection, and chronic *Staphylococcus aureus* nasal carriage is linked with more frequent relapses of upper respiratory tract disease. Whether infection increases the supply of auto-antigen or causes a general stimulation of the immune response through cytokine stimulation is unclear.

Cytokine dysregulation, inappropriate MHC expression, and failure of suppression may induce autoimmunity

It appears that dysregulation of the cytokine network can also lead to activation of autoreactive T cells, and as noted earlier genes affecting cytokines and their receptors (e.g. IL2RA) are implicated in autoimmune disease by genome-wide association studies.

One experimental demonstration of this is the introduction of a transgene for interferon-γ (IFNγ) into pancreatic β-islet cells. If the transgene for IFNγ is fully expressed in the cells, MHC class II genes are upregulated and autoimmune destruction of the islet cells results. This is not simply a result of a non-specific chaotic IFNγ-induced local inflammatory milieu because normal islets grafted at a separate site are rejected, implying clearly that T cell autoreactivity to the pancreas has been established.

The surface expression of MHC class II in itself is not sufficient to activate the naive autoreactive T cells, but it may be necessary to allow a cell to act as a target for the primed autoreactive TH cells. It was therefore most exciting when cells taken from the glands of patients with Graves' disease were found to be actively synthesizing class II MHC molecules (Fig. 20.13) and so were able to be recognized by CD4$^+$ T cells.

In this context it is interesting that isolated cells from several animal strains that are susceptible to autoimmunity are also more readily induced by IFNγ to express MHC class II molecules than cells from non-susceptible strains.

The argument that imbalanced cytokine production may also contribute to autoimmunity receives further support from the unexpected finding that tumor necrosis factor (TNF; introduced by means of a TNF transgene) ameliorates the spontaneous SLE-like disease of F1 (NZB × NZW) mice. Furthermore, serological (and less commonly clinical) features of SLE have developed in humans treated with TNF blockade.

Aside from the normal 'ignorance' of cryptic self epitopes, other factors that normally restrain potentially autoreactive cells may include:

- regulatory T cells;
- hormones (e.g. steroids);
- cytokines (e.g. transforming growth factor-β [TGFβ]); and
- products of macrophages.

Deficiencies in any of these factors may increase susceptibility to autoimmunity.

The feedback loop on TH cells and macrophages through the pituitary–adrenal axis is particularly interesting because defects at different stages in the loop turn up in a variety of autoimmune disorders (Fig. 20.14).

For example, patients with rheumatoid arthritis have low circulating corticosteroid levels compared with controls. After surgery, although they produce copious amounts of IL-1 and IL-6, a defect in the hypothalamic paraventricular nucleus prevents the expected increase in adrenocorticotropin (ACTH) and adrenal steroid output.

Human thyroid sections stained for MHC class II

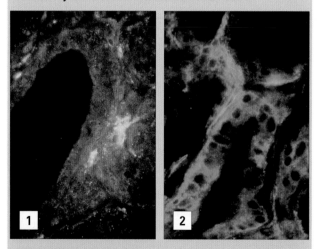

Fig. 20.13 (1) Normal thyroid with unstained follicular cells, and an isolated dendritic cell that is strongly positive for MHC class II. (2) Thyrotoxic (Graves' disease) thyroid with abundant MHC class II molecules in the cytoplasm, indicating that rapid synthesis of MHC class II molecules is occurring.

Defects in the cytokine/hypothalamic-pituitary-adrenal feedback loop in autoimmunity

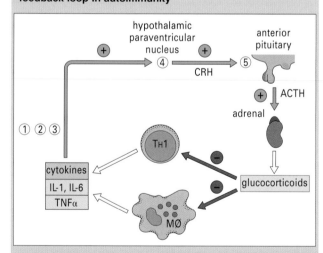

Fig. 20.14 Production of IL-1 is defective in the NOD mouse (**1**) and diabetes-prone BB rat (**2**); the disease can be corrected by injection of the cytokine. The same is true for the production of TNFα by the NZB × W lupus mouse (**3**). Patients with rheumatoid arthritis have a poor hypothalamic response to IL-1 and IL-6 (**4**). The hypothalamic–pituitary axis is defective in the Obese strain chicken and in the Lewis rat, which is prone to the development of Freund's adjuvant-mediated experimental autoimmune disease (**5**). (CRH, corticotropin releasing hormone, MØ, macrophage.)

There is currently intense interest focused on the role of Tregs. Patients with rheumatoid arthritis, for example, reveal a deficiency of Treg function (see below and Fig. 20.w5).

A subset of CD4 regulatory cells present in young healthy mice of the NOD strain, which spontaneously develop IDDM, can prevent the transfer of disease provoked by injection of spleen cells from diabetic animals into NOD mice congenic for the severe combined immunodeficiency trait; this regulatory subset is lost in older mice.

Pre-existing defects in the target organ may increase susceptibility to autoimmunity

We have already noted the sensitivity of target cells to upregulation of MHC class II molecules by IFNγ in animals susceptible to certain autoimmune diseases. Other evidence also favors the view that there may be a pre-existing defect in the target organ.

In the Obese strain chicken model of spontaneous thyroid autoimmunity, not only is there a low threshold of IFNγ induction of MHC class II expression by thymocytes, but when endogenous TSH is suppressed by thyroxine treatment, the uptake of iodine into the thyroid glands is far higher in the Obese strain than in a variety of normal strains. Furthermore, this is not due to any stimulating effect of the autoimmunity because immunosuppressed animals show even higher uptakes of iodine (Fig. 20.15).

Interestingly, the Cornell strain (from which the Obese strain was derived by breeding) shows even higher uptakes of iodine, yet these animals do not develop spontaneous thyroiditis. This could be indicative of a type of abnormal thyroid behavior, which in itself is insufficient to induce

autoimmune disease, but does contribute to susceptibility in the Obese strain.

Other situations in which the production of autoantigen is affected are:

- diabetes mellitus, in which one of the genetic risk factors is linked to a transcription factor controlling the rate of insulin production; and
- rheumatoid arthritis, in which the agalacto IgG glycoform is abnormally abundant.

The post-translational modification of arginine to citrulline, producing a new autoantigen in rheumatoid arthritis, represents yet another mechanism by which autoimmunity can be evoked.

> **Q. What evidence from rheumatoid arthritis supports the view that autoimmune diseases have a multifactorial etiology?**
> A. Defects in hypothalamic feedback, Tregs and post-translational modification of antigens (glycosylation and citrulline formation) as well as a strong MHC association have all been identified.

Autoimmune processes and pathology

Autoimmune processes are often pathogenic. When autoantibodies are found in association with a particular disease there are three possible inferences:

- the autoimmunity is responsible for producing the lesions of the disease;
- there is a disease process that, through the production of tissue damage, leads to the development of autoantibodies;
- there is a factor that produces both the lesions and the autoimmunity.

Autoantibodies secondary to a lesion (the second possibility) are sometimes found. For example, cardiac autoantibodies may develop after myocardial infarction.

However, sustained production of autoantibodies rarely follows the release of autoantigens by simple trauma. In most diseases associated with autoimmunity, the evidence supports the first possibility, that the autoimmune process produces the lesions.

Human autoantibodies can be directly pathogenic

When investigating human autoimmunity directly rather than using animal models, it is of course more difficult to carry out experiments. Nevertheless, there is much evidence to suggest that autoantibodies may be important in pathogenesis, as discussed below.

Autoantibodies can give rise to a wide spectrum of clinical thyroid dysfunction

A number of diseases have been recognized in which autoantibodies to hormone receptors may actually mimic the function of the normal hormone and produce disease. Graves' disease (thyrotoxicosis) was the first disorder in which **anti-receptor antibodies** were clearly recognized.

The phenomenon of neonatal thyrotoxicosis provides us with a natural 'passive transfer' study, because the IgG

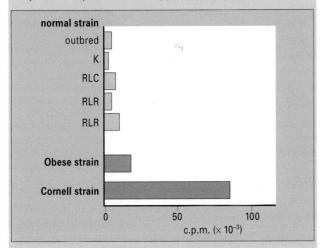

Thyroid ^{131}I uptake in TSH-suppressed chickens

normal strain
outbred
K
RLC
RLR
RLR
Obese strain
Cornell strain

0   50   100
c.p.m. (× 10⁻³)

Fig. 20.15 Thyroid ^{131}I uptake in Obese strain chickens and in the related Cornell strain is abnormally high compared with that in normal strains. Endogenous TSH production was suppressed by administration of thyroxine; therefore the experiment measured TSH-independent ^{131}I uptake. Values were far higher than normal in Obese strain chickens, which spontaneously develop thyroid autoimmunity, and even higher in the non-autoimmune Cornell strain from which the Obese strain was bred. This abnormality was not due to immune mechanisms because immunosuppression actually increased ^{131}I uptake into the thyroid gland.

The spectrum of autoimmune thyroid disease

thyroid disease	thyroid destruction	cell division		thyroid hormone synthesis	
		stimulation	inhibition	stimulation	inhibition
Hashimoto's thyroiditis					
Hashimoto's persistent goiter					
autoimmune colloid goiter					
Graves' disease					
non-goitrous hyperthyroidism					
'hashitoxicosis'					
primary myxedema					

Fig. 20.16 Responses involving thyroglobulin and the thyroid peroxidase (microsomal) surface microvillous antigen lead to tissue destruction, whereas autoantibodies to TSH (and other?) receptors can stimulate or block metabolic activity or thyroid cell division. 'Hashitoxicosis' is an unconventional term that describes a gland showing Hashimoto's thyroiditis and Graves' disease simultaneously.

antibodies from the thyrotoxic mother cross the placenta and react directly with the TSH receptor on the neonatal thyroid. Many babies born to thyrotoxic mothers and showing thyroid hyperactivity have been reported, but the problem spontaneously resolves as the antibodies derived from the mother are catabolized in the baby over several weeks.

Whereas autoantibodies to the TSH receptor may stimulate cell division and/or increase the production of thyroid hormones, others can bring about the opposite effect by inhibiting these functions, a phenomenon frequently observed in receptor responses to ligands that act as agonists or antagonists.

Different combinations of the various manifestations of thyroid autoimmune disease – chronic inflammatory cell destruction, and stimulation or inhibition of growth and thyroid hormone synthesis – can give rise to a wide spectrum of clinical thyroid dysfunction (Fig. 20.16).

A variety of other diseases are associated with autoantibodies

Myasthenia gravis provides an example of a disease where some of the autoantibodies can act as a receptor antagonist, blocking the acetyl choline receptor on the post-synaptic membrane of the neuromuscular junction, thus causing muscle weakness and fatigability. A parallel with neonatal hyperthyroidism has been observed – **antibodies to acetylcholine receptors** from mothers who have myasthenia gravis cross the placenta into the fetus and may cause transient muscle weakness in the newborn baby.

A similar phenomenon is seen in 5% of women who have anti-Ro antibodies (which are found in both SLE and Sjögren's syndrome). These antibodies can cross the placenta into the fetal circulation causing heart-block and/or transient lupus-like rash in the neonate, providing direct evidence of their pathogenity. This is known as the neonatal lupus syndrome.

ANCA are thought to be directly pathogenic in ANCA-associated vasculitides by causing neutrophil degranulation leading to endothelial damage. ANCA directed against myeloperoxidase (MPO) are commonly found in microscopic polyangiitis. Knockout mice lacking murine MPO (muMPO)

can be immunized with muMPO to produce antibodies to muMPO and passive transfer of these antibodies into suitable recipients produces necrotizing arteritis, focal necrotizing crescenteric glomerulonephritis and alveolar capillaritis and hemorrhage reminiscent of human disease.

Somewhat rarely, **autoantibodies to insulin receptors and to α-adrenergic receptors** can be found, the latter associated with bronchial asthma.

Neuromuscular defects can be elicited in mice injected with serum **containing antibodies to presynaptic calcium channels** from patients with the Lambert–Eaton syndrome, while **sodium channel autoantibodies** have been identified in the Guillain–Barré syndrome.

Yet another example of autoimmune disease is seen in rare cases of male infertility where **antibodies to spermatozoa** lead to clumping of spermatozoa, either by their heads or by their tails, in the semen.

In pernicious anemia an autoantibody interferes with the normal uptake of vitamin B₁₂

Vitamin B_{12} is not absorbed directly, but must first associate with a protein called intrinsic factor; the vitamin–protein complex is then transported across the intestinal mucosa.

Early passive transfer studies demonstrated that serum from a patient with pernicious anemia (PA), if fed to a healthy individual together with intrinsic factor–B_{12} complex, inhibited uptake of the vitamin.

Subsequently, the factor in the serum that blocked vitamin uptake was identified as **antibody against intrinsic factor**. It is now known that plasma cells in the gastric mucosa of patients with PA secrete this antibody into the lumen of the stomach (Fig. 20.17).

Antibodies to the glomerular capillary basement membrane cause Goodpasture's disease

Goodpasture's disease is characterized clinically by rapidly progressive glomerulonephritis and pulmonary haemorrhage. Patients with Goodpasture's disease have circulating

Failure of vitamin B₁₂ absorption in pernicious anemia

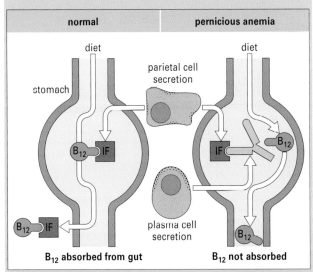

normal	pernicious anemia

Fig. 20.17 Normally, dietary vitamin B_{12} is absorbed by the small intestine complexed with intrinsic factor (IF), which is synthesized by parietal cells in gastric mucosa. In pernicious anemia, locally synthesized autoantibodies, specific for intrinsic factor, combine with intrinsic factor to inhibit its role as a carrier for vitamin B_{12}.

Upregulation of heat-shock protein 60 in endothelial cells at a site of hemodynamic stress

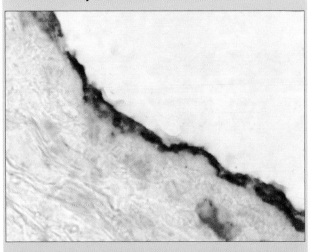

Fig. 20.18 Hsp60 expression (red) co-localized with intercellular adhesion molecule-1 (ICAM-1) expression (black) by endothelial cells and cells in the intima (macrophages) at the bifurcation of the carotid artery of a 5-month-old child. × 240. *(Photograph kindly provided by Professor G Wick.)*

antibodies to the **glomerular capillary basement membrane** which bind to the kidney and lung (see Fig. 25.3). Evidence for the direct pathogenity of these antibodies was demonstrated by the passive transfer of antibodies eluted from renal biopsy specimens into primates (whose renal antigens were similar to humans). The injected monkeys subsequently died from glomerulonephritis. Subsequent work has shown that these antibodies bind to the several non-collagenous-1 (NC-1) domains of type IV collagen in the GBM. Moreover, immunization of animals with NC-1 domains induces glomerulonephritis, providing a causal link between autoantigen and antibody.

Blood and vascular disorders caused by autoantibodies include AHA and ITP

Autoimmune hemolytic anemia (AHA) and idiopathic thrombocytopenic purpura (ITP) result from the synthesis of **autoantibodies to red cells and platelets**, respectively.

The primary antiphospholipid syndrome characterized by recurrent thromboembolic phenomena and fetal loss is triggered by the reaction of **autoantibodies with a complex of β_2-glycoprotein 1 and cardiolipin**.

The β_2-glycoprotein is an abundant component of atherosclerotic plaques, and there is increasing attention to the idea that autoimmunity may initiate or exacerbate the process of lipid deposition and plaque formation in this disease, the two lead candidate antigens being **heat-shock protein 60** (Fig. 20.18) and the low density lipoprotein, **apoprotein B**.

Immune complexes appear to be pathogenic in systemic autoimmunity

In the case of SLE, it can be shown that complement-fixing complexes of antibody with DNA and other nucleosome components such as histones are deposited in the kidney

(see Fig. 25.3), skin, joints, and choroid plexus of patients, and must be presumed to produce type III hypersensitivity reactions as outlined in Chapter 25. A variety of different antibodies have been eluted from the kidney biopsies of patients with SLE. These include anti-dsDNA (nucleosomes), anti-Ro and anti-Sm/RNP. Whilst placing these antibodies at the scene of the crime, their mere presence does not prove they 'pulled the trigger'. However, experiments using murine monoclonal anti-dsDNA antibodies in a rat kidney perfusion system, and other evidence from the use of human hybridoma derived anti-dsDNA antibodies in SCID mice, provides compelling evidence that some anti-dsDNA antibodies are genuinely pathogenic.

It has been proposed that anti-dsDNA/nucleosome antibodies bind to the negatively charged surface of the renal glomerulus via a histone (positively charged) 'bridge'. The histone is part of the nucleosome complex. The formation of immune complexes at the glomerular surface membrane is thought to induce an inflammatory response leading to the kidney damage so frequently seen in patients with SLE, though the precise mechanisms have yet to be elucidated.

Autoantibodies to IgG provoke pathological damage in rheumatoid arthritis

The erosions of cartilage and bone in rheumatoid arthritis are mediated by macrophages and fibroblasts, which become stimulated by cytokines from activated T cells and immune complexes generated by a vigorous immunological reaction within the synovial tissue (Fig. 20.19).

The complexes can arise through the self-association of IgG rheumatoid factors specific for the Fcγ domains – a

Pathology of rheumatoid arthritis

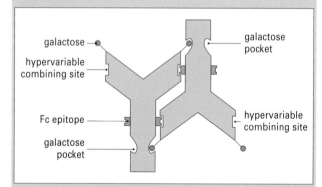

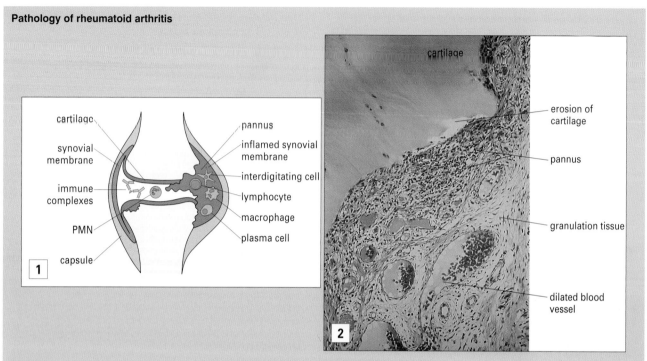

Fig. 20.19 In the rheumatoid arthritis joint an inflammatory infiltrate is found in the synovial membrane, which hypertrophies forming a 'pannus' (**1** and **2**). This covers and eventually erodes the synovial cartilage and bone. Immune complexes and neutrophils (PMNs) are detectable in the joint space and in the extra-articular tissues where they may give rise to vasculitic lesions and subcutaneous nodules. *(Histological section reproduced from Woolf N. Pathology: basic and systemic. London: W.B. Saunders; 1998.)*

Self-associated IgG rheumatoid factors forming immune complexes

Fig. 20.20 The binding between the Fab on one IgG rheumatoid factor and the Fc of another involves the hypervariable region of the combining site. As it has been established that the Fab oligosaccharides, which occur on approximately one in three different immunoglobulin molecules, are not defective with respect to glycosylation in rheumatoid arthritis, a Fab galactose residue could become inserted in the Fc pocket left vacant by a galactose-deficient Cγ2 oligosaccharide, so increasing the strength of intermolecular binding. The stability and inflammatory potency of these complexes is increased by binding IgM rheumatoid factor and Clq.

process facilitated by the striking deficiency of terminal galactose on the biantennary N-linked Fc oligosaccharides (Fig. 20.20). This agalacto glycoform of IgG in complexes can exacerbate inflammation through reaction with mannose-binding lectin and production of TNFα.

Evidence for directly pathogenic T cells in human autoimmune disease is hard to obtain

Adoptive transfer studies have shown that T$_H$1 cells are responsible for directly initiating the lesions in experimental models of organ-specific autoimmunity.

In humans, evidence for a pivotal role of T cells in the development of autoimmune disease includes:

- the production of high-affinity, somatically mutated IgG autoantibodies characteristic of T-dependent responses;
- the isolation of thyroid-specific T cell clones from the glands of patients with Graves' disease;
- the beneficial effect of ciclosporin in prediabetic individuals; and
- the close associations with certain HLA haplotypes.

However, it is difficult to identify a role for the T cell as a pathogenic agent as distinct from a T$_H$ function in the organ-specific disorders.

Indirect evidence from circumstances showing that antibodies themselves do not cause disease, such as in babies born to mothers with type 1 diabetes mellitus, may be indicative.

The central role of T$_H$1 cells in some autoimmune diseases has been challenged

Many autoimmune diseases such as rheumatoid arthritis were thought to be primarily driven by T$_H$1 cells. For this reason, the proposal to use rituximab (a monoclonal antibody against the CD20 molecule which is expressed on

B cells but not plasma cells) in rheumatoid arthritis was initially met with great skepticism. However, Rituximab's success in the treatment of RA has emphasized that B cells play a key role its pathogenesis, and has led some to doubt that RA is 'TH1 driven'. However, the precise mechanisms by which B cell depletion has a therapeutic effect are unclear. B cells are more than simply precursors to antibody producing plasma cells – they also act as antigen presenting cells, interacting with T cells in several ways. Thus rituximab's efficacy in RA cannot be used as proof that T cells are not important in its pathogenesis.

TH17 cells – a new player in autoimmunity?

Recent interest has focused on the role of TH17 cells in autoimmunity. Their initial discovery came about when it was noted that deletion of key TH1 molecules such as IL12 and IFN-γR did not abrogate EAE and collagen induced arthritis (CIA) in mice. In fact, these animals showed enhanced susceptibility, casting doubt on the role of TH1 cells as the fundamental players in autoimmunity. This led to the identification of a new cytokine IL23 – knockout of IL23 is protective against experimentally induced autoimmunity and IL23 was subsequently shown to induce IL-17 from activated T cells. Such IL-23 driven TH cells show a unique pattern of gene expression (which differs from that of IL-12 driven TH1 cells), and are now known to be TH17 cells. Whilst TGFβ, IL1β, and IL6, and not IL23, are the key cytokines for the induction of TH17 cells, IL23 is important for their maintenance; IL-23 deficient mice show normal numbers of TH1 cells but a reduction in TH17 cells.

In humans, high levels of IL-17 and its receptor are found in the synovial fluid and tissue of patients with RA. However, the number of TH17 cells is not elevated in the synovial fluid or PBMCs with RA compared to healthy controls. Multiple SNPs in the IL23 receptor gene region, as well as other genes involved in the IL23/TH17 pathway, are associated with inflammatory bowel disease. The results of trials of anti-IL-17 monoclonal antibodies in patients with RA and MS will help clarify the role of TH17 cells in these diseases.

Autoantibodies for diagnosis, prognosis, and monitoring

Whatever the relationship of autoantibodies to the disease process, they frequently provide valuable markers for diagnostic purposes. A particularly good example is the test for mitochondrial antibodies, used in diagnosing primary biliary cirrhosis (Fig. 20.21). Historically, exploratory laparotomy was needed to obtain this diagnosis, and was often hazardous because of the age and condition of the patients concerned. Some other diagnostically useful antibodies are listed below:

- antibodies to cyclic citrullinatated peptides (CCP) have a higher specificity than rheumatoid factor in the diagnosis of RA;
- the presence of anti-nuclear antibodies is one of the revised ACR criteria for SLE, but is non-specific. In contrast anti-dsDNA antibodies (also one of the ACR criteria) are highly specific for SLE, being present in 70% of SLE patients but in less than 0.5% of controls. Anti-Sm antibodies are found in 10% of Caucasian

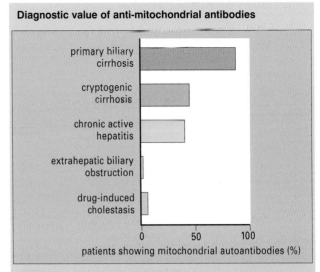

Diagnostic value of anti-mitochondrial antibodies

patients showing mitochondrial autoantibodies (%)

Fig. 20.21 Mitochondrial antibody tests using indirect immunofluorescence, together with percutaneous liver biopsy, can be used to assist in the differential diagnosis of these diseases. Many patients with primary biliary cirrhosis, but less than half of patients with cryptogenic cirrhosis or chronic active hepatitis, have anti-mitochondrial antibodies. The antibodies are rare in the other diseases.

and 30% of Afro-Caribbean SLE patients; like dsDNA antibodies they have a high specificity for SLE;
- autoantibodies often have predictive value. For instance, individuals testing positively for antibodies to both insulin and glutamic acid decarboxylase have a high risk of developing type 1 diabetes mellitus.

Prognosis and disease subtype:

- in rheumatoid arthritis, CCP antibodies are associated with a poor prognosis and predict erosive disease;
- within the context of a patient with SLE the presence of specific autoantibodies are associated with specific disease manifestations. For example, anti-La antibodies are associated with features of Sjögren's syndrome; anticardiolipin antibodies and anti-beta2 glycoprotein1 antibodies with thrombosis and miscarriage; anti-dsDNA antibodies with glomerulonephritis; anti-RNP with pulmonary hypertension, and anti-Ro with photosensitivity and the neonatal lupus syndrome.

Disease monitoring:

- anti-dsDNA antibodies can be used as a measure of disease activity in SLE. A rising titer of anti-dsDNA antibodies often heralds a disease flare, especially if accompanied by a falling C3 level, and should prompt the clinician to monitor the patient more frequently;
- similarly, a rising ANCA titer may indicate impending relapse in AAV. However, the association between ANCA titer and disease activity in AAV is much less robust than that between anti-dsDNA antibody titer and lupus activity.

Treatment of autoimmune diseases

Many autoimmune diseases can be treated successfully. Often, in organ specific autoimmune disorders, the symptoms can be corrected by metabolic control. For example:

- hypothyroidism can be controlled by administration of thyroxin;
- type 1 diabetes mellitus can be controlled by administration of insulin;
- in pernicious anemia, metabolic correction is achieved by injection of vitamin B_{12};
- in myasthenia gravis metabolic correction is achieved by administration of cholinesterase inhibitors.

If the target organ is not completely destroyed, it may be possible to protect the surviving cells by transfection with *FasL* or *TGFβ* genes.

Where function is completely lost and cannot be substituted by hormones, as may occur in lupus nephritis or chronic rheumatoid arthritis, tissue grafts or mechanical substitutes may be appropriate. In the case of tissue grafts, protection from the immunological processes that necessitated the transplant may be required.

Conventional immunosuppressive therapy with antimitotic drugs at high doses can be used to damp down the immune response, but, because of the dangers involved, tends to be used only in organ or life-threatening disorders such as SLE, myositis and ANCA-associated vasculitis (AAV).

Advances in treatment have transformed the 5 year survival rate in severe systemic autoimmune diseases such as SLE and AAV from around 50% and less than 10% respectively in the mid 20th century to over 90% today. However, the costs of this success in controlling autoimmune disease activity are the adverse effects of immunosuppressants, especially glucocorticoids. Most of the early mortality in SLE or AAV is now due to infection secondary to immunosuppressive therapy rather than from uncontrolled autoimmune disease. Long term use of drugs such as cyclophosphamide and azathioprine also increases the risk of infertility and possibly malignancy. The challenge now is to minimize treatment toxicity. This is likely to be achieved through several means. Firstly, the rational design of targeted therapies (in contrast to the 'shot-gun' approach of non-specific cytotoxics such as cyclophosphamide) should reduce the toxicity of treatment regimes. Secondly, it should become possible to identify patients through means of biomarkers in whom immunosuppression can be safely reduced. Some such biomarkers have already been identified but require further validation before translation into clinical practice. For example, CD8+ T cell transcription signatures from blood samples taken at time of diagnosis in patients with AAV and SLE identify subgroups of patients with high and low risk of subsequent relapse.

The most recent treatments for autoimmune disease are antibodies that target individual elements of the immune system, including:

- TNFα and IL-6 in rheumatoid arthritis;
- B cells in several autoimmune diseases (RA, SLE, AAV);
- co-stimulatory interactions in rheumatoid arthritis;
- trans-endothelial migration in multiple sclerosis.

Less well-established approaches to treatment may become practicable

As we understand more about the molecular mechanisms underlying autoimmunity, targeted therapy is becoming increasingly possible (Fig. 20.22):

- several centers are trying out autologous stem cell transplantation following hematoimmunoablation with cytotoxic drugs for patients with severe SLE and vasculitis;
- repeated injection of Cop 1 (a random copolymer of alanine, glutamic acid, lysine, and tyrosine) reduces relapse rate in relapsing–remitting multiple sclerosis. Cop 1 was originally designed to simulate the postulated 'guilty' autoantigen, MBP, and induce experimental autoimmune encephalitis; paradoxically it had the opposite effect. This suggests it is possible to achieve antigen-specific immune suppression.
- eculizumab, a monoclonal antibody against complement component C5, has been used successfully in paroxysmal nocturnal hemoglobinuria. It may prove effective in SLE;

Targeted therapeutic approaches in systemic lupus erythematosus

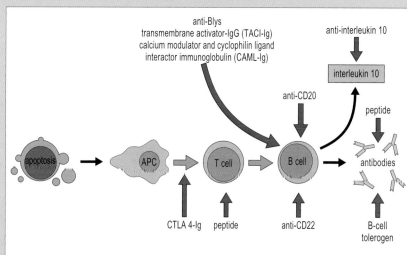

Fig. 20.22 This simplified diagram, which is based on our increased understanding of the immunologic events thought to occur in lupus, indicates the targets of current therapeutic interventions. (APC, antigen-presenting cell; BlyS, B-lymphocyte stimulator; CAML, calcium modulator and cyclophilin ligand; CTLA-4-Ig, cytotoxic T-lymphocyte-associated protein 4 IgG1; TACI-Ig, transmembrane activator and CAML interactor immunoglobulin.) *(Based on Rahman A, Isenberg DA: Systemic lupus erythematosus. N Engl J Med 2008; 358:929–930.)*

- TH cell subsets show considerable plasticity *in vivo*. Manipulation of the balance between pro-inflammatory TH17 cells and anti-inflammatory regulatory T cells may prove fruitful. Therapeutic interventions to increase the numbers of Tregs might increase self-tolerance and 'put the brakes' on inflammatory cascades. Adoptive transfer of polyclonal Tregs can prevent the onset of diabetes in NOD mice. However, it has become clear that successful treatment of *established* autoimmune disease by adoptive transfer of Tregs is antigen-specific; only Tregs specific for pancreatic antigens (and not polyclonal T regs) can reverse diabetes in NOD mice. This presents difficulties for treatment in human disease, where the inciting antigen is rarely known;
- inhibition of the activation or differentiation of TH17 cells, and/or blockade of linked cytokines such as IL17A and IL-23 may prove valuable. Trials of anti-IL17 monoclonal antibodies are already underway;
- small molecule therapies have the advantage of being cheaper to manufacture than monoclonal antibodies, of particular relevance in an era of spiraling healthcare costs. Kinases are intracellular enzymes that play a crucial role in signal transduction pathways controlling a number of cellular functions. Kinase inhibitors have been successfully used in oncology, but may also prove effective in autoimmune diseases. For example, a splenic tyrosine kinase inhibitor, reduces severity of antibody-mediated glomerulonephritis in rats, and is being trialled in RA.

The prospects for these new treatments either individually or in combination with therapeutic antibodies is very positive.

CRITICAL THINKING: AUTOIMMUNITY AND AUTOIMMUNE DISEASE (SEE P. 440 FOR EXPLANATIONS)

Miss Jacob, a 30-year-old Caribbean woman, was seen in a rheumatology clinic with stiff painful joints in her hands, which were worse first thing in the morning. Other symptoms included fatigue, a low-grade fever, a weight loss of 2 kg, and some mild chest pain. Miss Jacob had recently returned to the UK from a holiday in Jamaica and was also noted to be taking the combined oral contraceptive pill. Past medical history of note was a mild autoimmune hemolytic anemia 2 years previously.

On examination Miss Jacob had a non-specific maculopapular rash on her face and chest, and patchy alopecia (hair loss) over her scalp. Her mouth was tender and examination revealed an ulcer on the soft palate. She had moderately swollen and tender proximal interphalangeal joints. Her other joints were unaffected, but she had generalized muscle aches. The results of investigations are shown in the table.

Investigation	Result
radiograph of hands	soft tissue swelling, but no bone erosions
chest radiograph	a small pleural effusion at the right lung base
full blood count	a mild normocytic, normochromic anemia and mild lymphocytopenia
C-reactive protein levels	normal
erythrocyte sedimentation rate	raised
rheumatoid factor	negative
serum IgG levels	raised
anti-nuclear antibodies (ANA)	positive by immunofluorescence
anti-double-stranded DNA, anti-RNA, and anti-histone	positive by ELISA antibodies
complement (C3 and C4) levels	low
skin biopsy from an area unaffected by the rash	deposition of IgG and complement components at the junction between dermis and epidermis (lupus 'band' test)

A diagnosis of systemic lupus erythematosus (SLE) was made. Miss Jacob was treated with hydroxychloroquine, an anti-malarial, for the rash and the arthritis.

At a follow-up appointment urinalysis showed protein and red cells. Serum creatinine was mildly elevated as was her blood pressure. A renal biopsy showed membranous lupus nephritis. She was prescribed oral corticosteroids, mycophenolate mofetil and an angiotensin converting enzyme (ACE) inhibitor, which improved her renal function and blood pressure. Her physician also gave advice regarding birth control and pregnancy, and regular check-ups were arranged.

1 What is the immunological mechanism leading to the glomerulonephritis?

2 Are immune complexes the main mediator of systemic damage?

3 What is the mechanism for the vasculitis seen in SLE?

4 Are anti-double-stranded DNA (anti-dsDNA) antibodies pathognomonic of SLE?

Further reading

Arbuckle MR, McClain MT, Rubertone MV, et al. Development of autoantibodies before the clinical onset of systemic lupus erythematosus. N Engl J Med 2003;349:1526–1533.

Betterle C, Greggio NA, Volpato M. Clinical Review 93: Autoimmune polyglandular syndrome type 1. J Clin Endocrinol Metab 1998;83:1049–1055.

Edwards JC, Szczepanski L, Szechinski J, et al. Efficacy of the novel B cell targeted therapy, rituximab, in patients with active rheumatoid arthritis. N Engl J Med 2004;350:2572–2581.

Damsker JM, Hansen AM, Caspi RR. Th1 and Th17 cells: adversaries and collaborators. Ann N Y Acad Sci 2010;1183:211–221.

Rioux JD, Goyette P, Vyse TJ, et al. International MHC and Autoimmunity Genetics Network: Mapping of multiple susceptibility variants within the MHC region for 7 immune-mediated diseases. Proc Natl Acad Sci USA 2009;106:18680–18685.

Keymeulen B, Vandemeulebroucke E, Ziegler AG, et al. Insulin needs after CD3-antibody therapy in new-onset type 1 diabetes. N Engl J Med 2005;352:2598–2608.

Levine JS, Subang R, Nasr SH, et al. Immunization with an apoptotic cell-binding protein recapitulates the nephritis and sequential autoantibody emergence of systemic lupus erythematosus. J Immunol 2006;177:6504–6516.

McGaha TL, Sorrentino B, Ravetch JV. Restoration of tolerance in lupus targeted inhibiting receptor expression. Science 2005;307:590–593.

Notley CA, Ehrenstein MR. The yin and yang of regulatory T cells and inflammation in RA. Nat Rev Rheumatol 2010;6:572.

Park H, Li Z, Yang XO, et al. A distinct lineage of CD4 T cells regulates tissue inflammation by producing interleukin 17. Nat Immunol 2005;6:1133–1141.

Rahman A, Isenberg DA. Systemic lupus erythematosus. N Engl J Med 2008;358:929–939.

Roitt IM, Doniach D, Campbell PN, Vaughan-Hudson R. Auto-antibodies in Hashimoto's disease (lymphadenoid goitre). Lancet 1956;(ii):820–821.

Suber T, Rosen A. Apoptotic cell blebs: repositories of autoantigens and contributors to immune context. Arthritis Rheum 2009;60:2216–2219.

Wakeland EK, Liu K, Graham RR, Behrens TW. Delineating the genetic basis of systemic lupus erythematosus. Immunity 2001;15:397–408.

Zenewicz LA, Abraham C, Flavell RA, Cho JH. Unraveling the genetics of autoimmunity. Cell 2010;140:791–797.

Further references

Botto M, Dell'Agnola C, Bygrave AE, et al. Homozygous C1q deficiency causes glomerulonephritis associated with multiple apoptotic bodies. Nat Genet 1998;19:56–59.

Carr EJ, Clatworthy MR, Lowe CE, et al. Contrasting genetic association of IL2RA with SLE and ANCA-associated vasculitis. BMC Med Genet 2009;10:22.

Davies KA, Erlendsson K, Beynon HL, et al. Splenic uptake of immune complexes in man is complement dependent. J Immunol 1993;151:3866–3873.

Ding B, Padyukov L, Lundström E, et al. Different patterns of associations with anti-citrullinated protein antibody-positive and anti-citrullinated protein antibody-negative rheumatoid arthritis in the extended major histocompatibility complex region. Arthritis Rheum 2009;60:30–38.

Herrmann M, Voll RE, Zoller OM, et al. Impaired phagocytosis of apoptotic cell material by monocyte-derived macrophages from patients with systemic lupus erythematosus. Arthritis Rheum 1998;41:1241–1250.

Isenberg DA, Manson JJ, Ehrenstein MR, et al. Anti-dsDNA antibodies- at journey's end? Rheumatology 2007;46:1052–1056.

Kain R, Exner M, Brandes R, et al. Molecular mimicry in pauci-immune focal necrotizing glomerulonephritis. Nat Med 2008;14:1088–1096.

Lerner RA, Glassock RJ, Dixon FJ. The role of anti-glomerular basement membrane antibody in the pathogenesis of human glomerulonephritis. J Exp Med 1967;126:989–1004.

Lin JP, Cash JM, Doyle SZ, et al. Familial clustering of rheumatoid arthritis with other autoimmune diseases. Hum Genet 1998;103:475–482.

Mattey DL, Dawes PT, Clarke S, et al. Relationship among the HLA-DRB1 shared epitope, smoking, and rheumatoid factor production in rheumatoid arthritis. Arthritis Rheum 2002;47:403–407.

McKinney E, Lyons PA, Carr EJ, et al. A CD8+ T cell transcription signature predicts prognosis in autoimmune disease. Nat Med 2010;16:586–591.

Niewold TB, Hua J, Lehman TJ, et al. High serum IFN-alpha activity is a heritable risk factor for systemic lupus erythematosus. Genes Immun 2007;8:492–502.

Pinching AJ, Rees AJ, Pussell BA, et al. Relapses in Wegener's granulomatosis: the role of infection. Br Med J 1980;281:836–838.

Rioux JD, Goyette P, Vyse TJ, et al. Mapping of multiple susceptibility variants within the MHC region for 7 immune-mediated diseases. Proc Natl Acad Sci USA 2009;106:18680–18685.

Silman AJ, Newman J, MacGregor AJ. Cigarette smoking increases the risk of rheumatoid arthritis: Results from a nationwide study of disease-discordant twins. Arthritis Rheum 1996;39:732–735.

Stone JH, Merkel PA, Spiera R, Seo P, et al. Rituximab versus cyclophosphamide for ANCA-associated vasculitis. N Engl J Med 2010;363:221–232.

Tan EM, Feltkamp TE, Smolen JS, et al. Range of antinuclear antibodies in "healthy" individuals. Arthritis Rheum 1997;40:1601–1611.

Wakeland EK, Liu K, Graham RR, Behrens TW. Delineating the genetic basis of systemic lupus erythematosus. Immunity 2001;15:397–408.

Weinblatt M, Kavanaugh A, Genovese M, et al. An oral spleen tyrosine kinase (Syk) inhibitor for rheumatoid arthritis. N Engl J Med 2010;363:1303–1312.

Yamada H, Nakashima Y, Okazaki K, et al. Th1 but not Th17 cells predominate in the joints of patients with rheumatoid arthritis. Ann Rheum Dis 2008;67:1299–1304.

CHAPTER 21

Transplantation and Rejection

SUMMARY

- **Transplantation is the only form of treatment** for most end-stage organ failure.

- **The barrier to transplantation** is the genetic disparity between donor and recipient.

- **The immune response in transplantation depends on a variety of factors.** Host versus graft responses cause transplant rejection. Histocompatibility antigens are the targets for rejection. Minor antigens can be targets of rejection even when donor and recipient MHC are identical. Graft versus host reactions result when donor lymphocytes attack the graft recipient.

- **Rejection results from a variety of different immune effector mechanisms.** Hyperacute rejection is immediate and caused by antibody. Acute rejection occurs days to weeks after transplantation. Chronic rejection is seen months or years after transplantation.

- **HLA matching is one of two major methods for preventing rejection of allografts.** The better the HLA matching of donor and recipient, the less the strength of rejection.

- **Successful organ transplantation depends on the use of immunosuppressive drugs.** 6-MP, azathioprine, and MPA are antiproliferative drugs. Ciclosporin, tacrolimus, and sirolimus are inhibitors of T cell activation. Corticosteroids are anti-inflammatory drugs used for transplant immunosuppression. Antibodies to the IL2 receptor, or to leukocytes, are widely used.

- **The ultimate goal in transplantation is to induce donor-specific tolerance.** There is evidence for the induction of tolerance in humans and novel methods for inducing tolerance are being developed. Alloreactive cells can be made anergic. Immune privilege can be a property of the tissue or site of transplant.

- **Shortage of donor organs and chronic rejection limit the success of transplantation.** Living donation is one way to overcome the shortage of donor organs. Alternative approaches are being investigated. The favored animal for xenotransplantation is the pig.

Transplantation is the only form of treatment for most end-stage organ failure, and it is a central topic for immunologists for two reasons:

- the first is that transplantation is an important clinical procedure;
- the second is that transplantation has proved an important tool for understanding immunological mechanisms – for example, the major histocompatibility complex (MHC; see Chapter 5) was first described in the context of transplantation, and transplantation models continue to be widely used as tools in basic as well as applied immunology.

As a clinical procedure, transplantation is used to replace tissues or organs that have failed. The first successful transplants were those of the cornea, first described in 1906.

Q. Why in retrospect was corneal transplantation more likely to be successful than transplantation of other tissues?

A. The cornea is an immunologically privileged site (see Figs 12.w1–12.w3).

World War II provided an important impetus, with the problems of skin grafting airmen who had extensive burns motivating a number of scientists, most notably Peter Medawar, to investigate the immunological basis of graft rejection.

The subsequent demonstration by the Medawar group that it was possible to manipulate a recipient animal so that it accepted grafts from an unrelated donor animal encouraged the subsequent clinical development of transplantation. The discovery (by Calne and others) of immunosuppressive drugs and agents then allowed the widespread practice of transplantation in the last three to four decades of the 20th century.

In modern practice many transplants are performed routinely (Fig. 21.1). In addition to routine transplantation of the cornea, kidney, heart, lungs, and liver there is increasing interest in transplanting other organs, such as whole pancreas or islet cells for diabetes mellitus and also small bowel.

In general most transplants use organs from dead donors (**cadaveric transplants**), though there is an increasing number of living donors (usually related to the recipients) for kidney transplantation (see below).

Hematopoietic stem cell transplantation

Hematopoietic stem cell transplants are performed for two main reasons. One is to treat children who have inherited immune deficiencies. These children are very prone to infection, and will normally die young as a consequence. However, if they are given stem cells from a healthy donor, the infused stem cells can replace the defective bone marrow stem cells. The stem cells can then mature and into fully effective immune cells, thus giving the child a functioning immune system.

The second major application is for patients with leukemia. It is possible to eradicate the patient's leukemic cells with chemotherapy and radiotherapy. However, this also results in destruction of the patient's stem cells in the bone marrow and circulation. The patient therefore becomes immunodeficient and will die of infection. Stem cell transplantation can 'rescue' the patient by providing a fresh source of stem cells. In some cases the stem cells are autologous (in which they are harvested before chemotherapy, stored, and then infused back into patients after the therapy is over). In these settings there is no risk of graft versus host disease (see below). However, there is a risk that leukemic cells will be present in the stored stem cells, and will then grow in the patient. In other cases the stem cells come from a well matched donor. This removes the chance of carry over of leukemic cells, but does run the risk of graft verus host disease. In some forms of leukemia it has been shown that there is a graft versus leukemic effect, in which the allogeneic T cells mount a response against any leukemic cells remaining in the patient and prevent them from growing.

Genetic barriers to transplantation

The main immunological problem with transplantation is that the grafted organ or tissue is seen by the immune system as 'foreign' and is recognized and attacked – leading to rejection of the organ.

Transplantation is normally performed between individuals of the same species who are not genetically identical, and the antigenic differences are known as **allogeneic differences**, and result in an **allospecific immune response** (Fig. 21.2).

However, it is also possible in experimental circumstances (and possibly in the future in the clinical setting) to perform grafting between different species. This is

Clinical transplantation	
organ transplanted	**examples of disease**
cornea	keratoconus, dystrophies, keratitis
kidney	end-stage renal disease
heart	heart failure
lung/heart–lung	pulmonary hypertension, cystic fibrosis
liver	cancer, cirrhosis, biliary atresia
stem cells (bone marrow/ peripheral blood)	leukemia, immunodeficiency
skin (autografts)	burns
pancreas	diabetes mellitus
pancreatic islets	diabetes mellitus
small bowel	cancer, intestinal failure
neuronal cells	Parkinson's disease
haemotopoietic stem cells	potentially many diseases

Fig. 21.1 Organs and tissues shown in blue are routinely transplanted to treat various conditions. Transplantation of other organs (shown in yellow) is being developed, but has yet to be routinely applied in most centers.

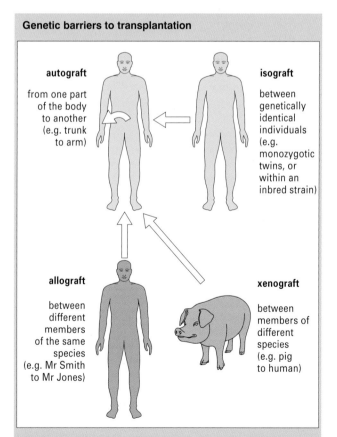

Genetic barriers to transplantation

autograft
from one part of the body to another (e.g. trunk to arm)

isograft
between genetically identical individuals (e.g. monozygotic twins, or within an inbred strain)

allograft
between different members of the same species (e.g. Mr Smith to Mr Jones)

xenograft
between members of different species (e.g. pig to human)

Fig. 21.2 The genetic relationship between the donor and recipient determines whether or not rejection will occur. Autografts or isografts are usually accepted, whereas allografts and xenografts are not.

termed **xenotransplantation**, and the antigenic differences between donor and recipient form the **xenogeneic barrier**.

Transplantation can also be performed within an individual (e.g. skin grafting), when it is known as an **autograft**.

Syngeneic or **isografts** can be performed between genetically identical individuals. This can occur clinically for identical twins, but is more commonly seen in experimental settings with inbred strains of animals.

In the case of autografts and isografts there should be no antigenic differences between donor and recipient, and so no immune response. This can be readily illustrated using transplantation of skin or organs between inbred strains of animals (Fig. 21.3).

Graft rejection

Host versus graft responses cause transplant rejection

Immune recognition of the antigenic differences between the donor organ and the recipient will, unless treated, lead to an immune response in which the host immune system responds to, and attacks, the donor tissue.

> **Q. What are the main genetic differences that are recognized by the host, and why should this be so?**
> A. Differences in MHC molecule allotypes are most important. The reason is that all nucleated cells express MHC molecules, and the T cell receptor on host T cells has a basic structure that interacts with and recognizes MHC molecules. Also the MHC class I and class II molecules have an extremely high level of genetic variability (see Chapter 5).

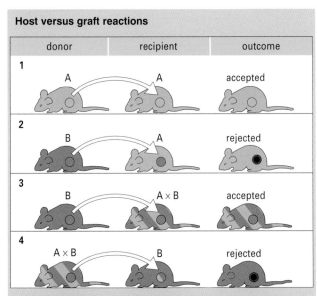

Host versus graft reactions

	donor	recipient	outcome
1	A	A	accepted
2	B	A	rejected
3	B	A × B	accepted
4	A × B	B	rejected

Fig. 21.3 Grafts between genetically identical animals are accepted. Grafts between genetically non-identical animals are rejected with a speed that is dependent on where the genetic differences lie. For example, syngeneic animals that are identical at the MHC locus accept grafts from each other (**1**). Animals that differ at the MHC locus reject grafts from each other (**2**). The ability to accept a graft is dependent on the recipient sharing all the donor's histocompatibility genes; this is illustrated by the difference between grafting from parental to (A × B) F$_1$ animals (**3**) and vice versa (**4**). Animals that differ at loci other than the MHC reject graft from each other, but much more slowly.

The nature of the host versus graft response is discussed in more detail below.

Similar to any other adaptive immune response, the immune response against a graft shows memory of previous encounters with an antigen. Therefore, once an animal has rejected an organ graft for the first time, if a second graft is performed from the same species or donor then it is rejected more rapidly (**second set rejection**).

There is a high frequency of T cells recognizing the graft

One of the main features of the immune response against a transplanted organ is that it is much more vigorous and strong than the response against a pathogen, such as a virus. This is largely reflected by the frequency of T cells that recognize the graft as foreign and react against it.

Thus, in a naive or unimmunized individual fewer than 1/100 000 T cells respond upon exposure to a virus or a protein immunization; however, 1/100–1/1000 T cells respond to allogeneic antigen-presenting cells (APCs). This is reflected in the strong T cell response (proliferation) seen when naive T cells are stimulated with allogeneic dendritic cells (Fig. 21.4)

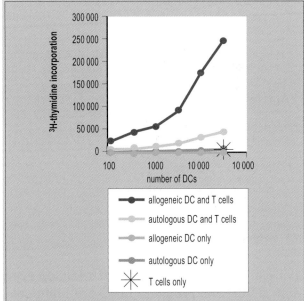

Measuring the strength of the alloresponse

legend:
- allogeneic DC and T cells
- autologous DC and T cells
- allogeneic DC only
- autologous DC only
- T cells only

Fig. 21.4 The strength of the alloresponse can be measured in a mixed lymphocyte reaction. In this assay T cells from an individual were mixed with varying numbers of dendritic cells (DCs) from either the same (autologous DC) or a different (allogeneic DC) donor. The dendritic cells were irradiated to prevent their proliferation. As a control cultures were included that contained just the dendritic cells or just the T cells. Five days later, T cell proliferation was measured by incorporation of ^{3}H-thymidine, which is incorporated into the DNA of dividing cells. There is strong proliferation of T cells exposed to allogeneic dendritic cells, even though these T cells have not been exposed to the allogeneic cells, i.e. it represents a primary immune response.

Histocompatibility antigens are the targets for rejection

Early experiments showed that the bulk of the allospecific response is against molecules of the MHC. We now know that these molecules are the MHC class I or class II molecules (see Chapter 5), which are responsible for presenting antigen (in the form of peptides) to either:

- CD8 T cells (MHC class I); or
- CD4 cells (MHC class II).

As discussed in Chapter 8, MHC molecules are highly polymorphic, and it is these polymorphic differences that are seen by alloreactive T cells.

Indirect recognition is important in chronic rejection

In a primary alloresponse (see Fig. 21.4), most of the alloreactive CD4 or CD8 T cells directly recognize the donor MHC molecules.

However, there are other forms of alloresponse, including:

- those against **minor MHC antigens** (see below); or
- the **indirect response** in which the recipient CD4 T cells recognize donor MHC molecules that have been processed by recipient APCs and are presented as peptides in the context of recipient MHC class II molecules (Fig. 21.5).

The indirect response is very similar to conventional T cell recognition of normal antigens, such as those from a pathogen, which are processed by host APCs and presented in the context of host MHC molecules.

> **Q. How frequent do you expect the T cells that recognize graft allogeneic molecules encoded outside the MHC to be?**
>
> A. The frequency of allospecific T cells in an unimmunized individual capable of recognizing donor tissue by the indirect pathway is low, equivalent to the frequency of reactivity to any normal antigen.

Nevertheless, the indirect pathway of recognition is important during chronic rejection, when the number of donor-derived professional APCs is no longer high enough to stimulate a direct immune response. It is also important in the rejection of corneal grafts because the cornea lacks large numbers of APCs.

Minor antigens can be targets of rejection even when donor and recipient MHC are identical

Although the MHC is the major target of the alloimmune response, there are also minor histocompatibility antigens. These can serve as targets of rejection even when the MHC is identical between donor and recipient.

The nature of most minor histocompatibility antigens is unknown, though they are assumed to be normal polymorphic molecules, peptides from which bind to host MHC and induce an immune response. In some cases they are expressed in a tissue-specific manner.

Perhaps the best studied minor histocompatibility antigen system is the H-Y system. These are antigens encoded by the Y chromosome, and so are expressed only on male cells. Thus,

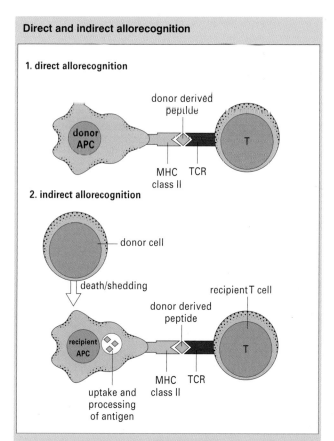

Direct and indirect allorecognition

Fig. 21.5 **(1)** In direct allorecognition the CD4 or CD8 T cell directly recognizes the donor APC, with the T cell receptor (TCR) binding donor MHC molecules bearing donor peptide. **(2)** Indirect allorecognition is more similar to conventional T cell recognition, in that the recipient CD4 T cells recognize foreign (donor derived) antigen that has been taken up and processed by recipient APCs. The TCR therefore recognizes recipient MHC bearing donor peptide. CD8 cells only see alloantigen by the direct pathway.

following immunization, it is possible to demonstrate immune responses and rejection of male organs or skin following transplantation mediated by female animals (2X chromosomes) against male cells (X and Y chromosome). It is not possible to show responses against female antigens by male animals because the male animals have one X chromosome, and so are tolerant to all antigens encoded on it (Fig. 21.6).

Graft versus host reactions result when donor lymphocytes attack the graft recipient

Although it is usual to think of the immune response recognizing and destroying the transplanted organ, the situation is different when competent immune cells are transplanted into a recipient. This can happen during bone marrow transplantation, when normal donor T cells may be infused into the recipient. In such circumstances the T cells can recognize the MHC molecules and/or minor histocompatibility antigens of the recipient as foreign, and produce an immune response against the recipient. This is known as **graft versus host disease (GvHD)**.

GvHD can be lethal, causing damage in particular to the skin and gut. It can be demonstrated in animal models by

H-Y minor histocompatibility antigens

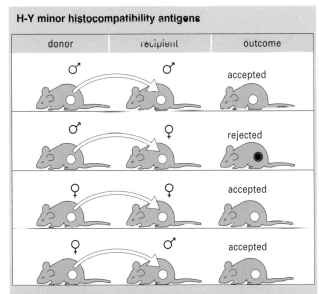

Fig. 21.6 The H-Y antigens are minor histocompatibility antigens expressed on male animals only. Their existence can be demonstrated by skin grafting between animals of the same strain. As would be expected grafts from female mice are always accepted, while those from male mice are accepted on male recipients, but not female recipients.

Graft versus host disease

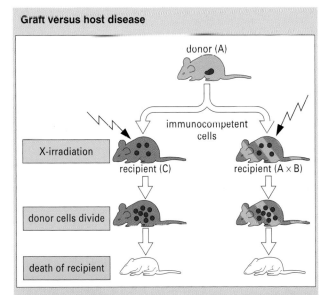

Fig. 21.7 Graft versus host disease is caused by immunocompetent cells reacting against their host animal. Immunocompetent cells from a donor of type A are injected into an immunosuppressed (X-irradiated) host of type C, or a normal (A × B) F_1 recipient. The immunosuppressed individual is unable to reject the cells and the F_1 animal is fully tolerant to parental type A cells. In both cases the donor cells recognize the foreign tissue types B or C of the recipient. They divide and react against the recipient tissue cells and recruit large numbers of host cells to inflammatory sites. Very often the process leads to the death of the recipient.

transfer of bone marrow to irradiated recipient animals (Fig. 21.7). It can be avoided by:

- careful matching of the donor and recipient;
- removal of all T cells from the graft; and
- immunosuppression.

Immune effector mechanisms in graft rejection

Rejection of organs or tissues can occur at various times, each of which is associated with different immune effector mechanisms (Fig. 21.8). These are:

- hyperacute rejection, which occurs within minutes to hours and is principally mediated by antibody;
- acute rejection, which usually occurs in days to weeks in animal models and is initiated by alloreactive T cells; and
- chronic rejection, which is seen months to years following transplantation.

Hyperacute rejection is immediate and mediated by antibody

Hyperacute rejection is seen when the recipient animal has pre-existing antibodies that are reactive with the donor tissue. This may be because:

- the individual has been sensitized to the donor MHC, for example by previous transplants, multiple blood transfusions or pregnancy;
- the animal may have natural pre-existing antibodies (e.g. as a result of ABO blood group incompatibility).

A special case is seen in xenotransplantation, where humans and Old World monkeys and apes all have pre-existing antibodies to a carbohydrate antigen α-galactosyl. This

carbohydrate is expressed on cell surface proteins of all other donors. Therefore, a xenotransplant of a cellular organ from a pig (or most other species) into a primate is at risk of hyperacute rejection.

Hyperacute rejection is seen within minutes of connecting the circulation into the transplanted organ. It is caused by the pre-existing antibodies binding to the endothelial cells lining the blood vessels and by initiating immune effector functions.

Q. Which immune effector functions would be activated following binding of antibody to the endothelium?
A. Complement will be activated, by the classical pathway (see Chapter 4).

Complement activation can lead to death of the endothelium, or, when the damage is sub-lethal, activation of the endothelial cells. This not only causes an inflammatory response, increasing vascular leakage, but can also cause blood coagulation The result is rapid destruction of the graft (Fig. 21.9).

Prevention of hyperacute rejection is performed by carefully avoiding transplanting an organ into an individual with pre-existing antibodies to that tissue. This is done by:

- ABO matching individuals; and
- cross-matching the donor and recipient.

This involves incubating donor leukocytes with recipient serum in the presence of complement; cell death indicates the presence of anti-donor antibody and is a contraindication to proceeding with transplantation. Such cross-matching is normally performed immediately before surgery. There is

Tempo of rejection response

type of rejection	time taken	mechanisms of rejection
hyperacute rejection	minutes to hours	preformed anti-donor antibodies
acute rejection	days to weeks	activation of alloreactive T cells
chronic rejection	months to years	slow cellular response, response of organ to injury, unknown causes

Fig. 21.8 Rejection of organs or tissues can occur at various times, each of which is associated with different immune effector mechanisms, ranging from antibody mediated to acute and chronic cellular responses.

Renal histology showing hyperacute graft rejection

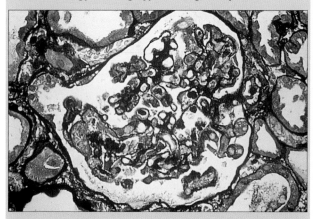

Fig. 21.9 Hyperacute rejection is caused by pre-existing antibody at the time of transplantation. There is extensive necrosis of the glomerular capillary associated with massive interstitial hemorrhage. This extensive necrosis is preceded by an intense polymorphonuclear infiltration, which occurs within the first hour of the graft's revascularization. The changes shown here occurred 24–48 hours after this. H&E stain. × 200.

increasing success in transplanting across ABO incompatible barriers, though this requires very careful preparation of the recipient.

Acute rejection occurs days to weeks after transplantation

Acute rejection is normally seen days to weeks after transplantation, and is caused by activation of allospecific T cells capable of damaging the graft.

Donor dendritic cells (sometimes called passenger leukocytes) play an important role in triggering acute rejection. Dendritic cells that are present in the organ, following transplantation into the recipient, migrate to the lymph nodes draining the organ and stimulate a primary alloimmune response.

The importance of these dendritic cells can be shown by 'parking experiments' in which:

- a kidney is transplanted from one strain of rat to another under cover of immunosuppression (to prevent rejection) (Fig. 21.10);
- the kidney is kept in that animal long enough to ensure that all the resident dendritic cells have migrated out of the organ;

Importance of passenger leukocytes in graft sensitization

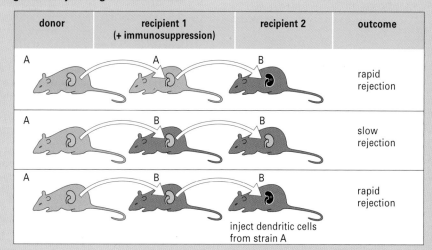

Fig. 21.10 The role of passenger leukocytes (dendritic cells) can be shown by 'parking' experiments in which kidneys are grafted from a rat of strain A into a recipient of strain B. Immunosuppression is used to prevent the animal from rejecting the graft. After a period the grafts are then retransplanted into a fresh strain B rat. There is very slow rejection of the graft (when compared to the rapid rejection seen when the kidney is transferred first into a strain A rat), which is thought to be due to the inability of the kidney from the strain A rat to immunize the strain B recipient due to the loss of dendritic cells during the period when the graft was 'parked' in the first strain A animal. The slow rejection probably occurs via the indirect pathway. The rejection occurs at the normal rapid tempo if strain A dendritic cells are injected into the recipient animal at the same time as the graft, suggesting that dendritic cells are capable of sensitizing the animal to the graft.

- the kidney is then transplanted into a third animal, of the same strain as the original recipient, where it shows prolonged graft survival.

However, if the third animal is injected with donor-derived dendritic cells there is rapid graft rejection. These data highlight the contribution of donor dendritic cells in initiating the alloresponse.

Although the direct pathway is thought to predominate in acute rejection, the indirect alloresponse, though significantly weaker, can also cause acute rejection in some animal models.

Once activated the T cells migrate to the organ and lead to tissue damage by standard immunological effector mechanisms (Fig. 21.11). These include:

- the generation of Tc cells; and
- the induction of delayed-type hypersensitivity reactions. The role of the T cells in graft rejection can be demonstrated by depletion studies in which antibodies

against T cell subsets are administered *in vivo*. Both of the major T cell subsets, CD4+ and CD8+, can cause graft rejection.

If the animal or patient has already been exposed to the alloantigens expressed by the graft, and as a consequence has been immunized, there will be alloreactive memory cells. This will lead to a much more rapid (accelerated) rejection of the graft (Fig. 21.12).

Chronic rejection is seen months or years after transplantation

In vascularized organs chronic rejection presents as occlusion of blood vessels, which on histological analysis show a thickening of the intima, similar in some respects to the thickening seen as a result of atherosclerosis (Fig. 21.13). Smooth muscle cell proliferation is often seen, together with a macrophage infiltrate (together with some lymphocytes).

Renal histology showing acute graft rejection

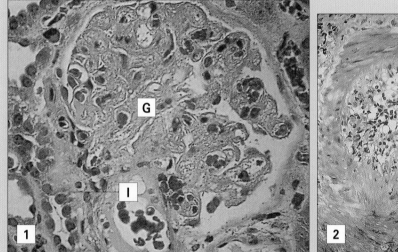 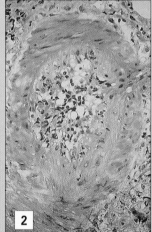 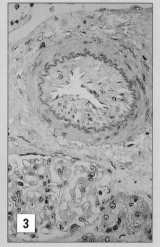

Fig. 21.11 (**1**) Small lymphocytes and other cells are accumulating in the interstitium of the graft. Such infiltration (I) is characteristic of acute rejection and occurs before the appearance of any clinical signs. H&E stain. (**2**) H&E stain of acutely rejecting kidney showing vascular obstruction. (**3**) van Gieson's stain of acutely rejecting kidney showing the end stage of this process. (G, glomerulus.)

Graft rejection displays immunological memory

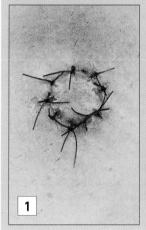 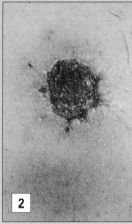 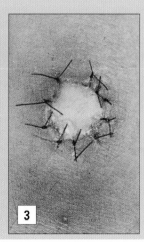

Fig. 21.12 A human skin allograft at day 5 (**1**) is fully vascularized and the cells are dividing, but by day 12 (**2**) is totally destroyed. A second graft ('second-set' graft) from the same donor shown here on day 7 (**3**) does not become vascularized and is destroyed rapidly. This indicates that sensitization to the first graft produces immunological memory.

Chronic rejection

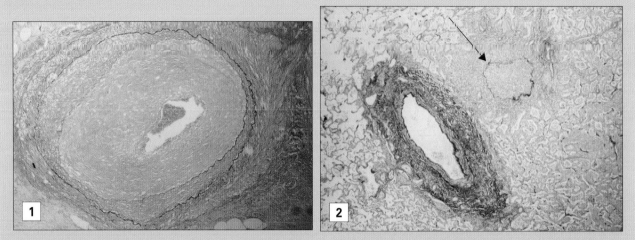

Fig. 21.13 Grafts that survive acute rejection are still capable of undergoing chronic rejection. (**1**) Section taken from a patient with chronic rejection of their heart graft. The lumen of the blood vessel in the heart has been narrowed as a result of thickening of the wall of the vessel, limiting the blood supply to the heart. (**2**) Section taken from a patient with chronic rejection of the lung, showing obliterative bronchiolitis (*arrow*) blocking the airways. *(Kindly supplied by Professor Marlene Rose, Imperial College London, Harefield Hospital, and Dr Margaret Burke, Pathology Department, Royal Brompton Hospital and Harefield Hospital.)*

This eventually leads to blockage of the blood vessels and subsequent ischemia of the organ.

A number of mechanisms can lead to chronic rejection. They include:

- a low-grade T cell response (mainly of the indirect allospecific pathway as a result of the loss of passenger leukocytes that activate T cells with direct pathway specificity);
- antibody can also be involved in chronic rejection, as indicated by the deposition of complement components (C4d) in tissues.

Non-immunological processes are also important, such as:

- the response of the graft to injury caused at the time of transplantation or by acute rejection episodes;
- recurrence of the original underlying disease; and
- drug-related toxicities (e.g. the immunosuppressive drug ciclosporin A is nephrotoxic and can damage the kidneys).

In some cases, initiation of chronic rejection may be immunological in nature, but its progression is due to non-immunological mechanisms.

Chronic rejection responds poorly to current immunosuppressive therapy. Therefore, although there has been considerable improvement in overall graft survival over the past decades, this improvement is mostly seen in the first year following transplantation – the subsequent survival of grafts has hardly altered over the past 20–30 years (Fig. 21.14). This indicates the need to improve the treatment of chronic rejection.

HLA matching is important to prevent rejection

The two major methods for preventing rejection of allografts are:

- to match the donor and recipient to minimize the antigenic differences; and
- to use immunosuppressive regimens that block the immune response against the organ.

However, in animal models (and hopefully in the clinic) there are techniques that can induce tolerance to an organ such that the immune system of the recipient 'learns' to treat the donor organ as 'self' and not destroy it. As discussed below, the ability to induce donor-specific tolerance is the 'Holy Grail' of transplantation immunology.

The better the HLA matching of donor and recipient, the less the strength of rejection

The major antigenic differences recognized by the alloimmune response are found on the MHC molecules (HLA in humans). These highly polymorphic molecules have a vital role in presenting antigens to T cells.

There are many different alleles of the MHC molecules, and one way to reduce the strength of a rejection response is to match the donor and recipient so that they share as many alleles as possible. In general matching is now performed using molecular techniques, with polymerase chain reactions (PCR) that are specific for the different alleles.

In humans HLA matching is rarely perfect between unrelated donors because of the difficulty in matching all MHC class I and class II gene loci and the high level of polymorphism at each locus.

Q. How many MHC loci would need to be matched to obtain a perfect match in a human population?
A. There are three HLA class I loci (HLA-A, HLA-B, and HLA-C), and one individual can express up to six different HLA class I molecules (for each antigen there will be a maternally derived and a paternally derived version). Similarly, there are three class II loci (HLA-DR, HLA-DP, and HLA-DQ), and again the maternal and paternal chromosomes would normally be different. In other words there are 12 potentially different loci.

Long-term survival of kidney grafts

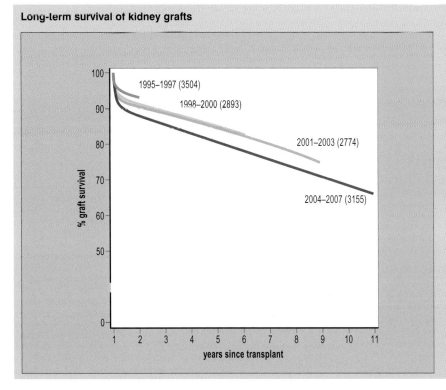

Fig. 21.14 The graph shows the survival of kidney grafts in patients transplanted from heart-beating donors in the UK 1995–2007. For comparison survival in the UK transplant program 1975–1979 is also included. There has been a considerable improvement in graft survival since 1975, but most of the improvement is seen in the first year. After that time the half-life of graft survival is similar for all patient groups. *(Data from Statistics and Audit Directorate, NHS Blood and Transplant, 2009.)*

The extensive polymorphism means that there can hundreds of variants of each antigen. For example the number of (protein) variants of the HLA molecules identified up to April 2011 was: HLA-A 1176; HLA-B 1641; HLA-C 808; HLA-DRA 2, -DRB 774; HLA-DQA 27, -DQB 106; HLA-DPA 16, -DPB 129.

Therefore, even before one considers other polymorphic molecules associated with the HLA locus, there is considerable complexity, which makes it highly unlikely for there to be a complete match.

In cases where the transplant is between living related donors (such as brothers and sisters) there is a greater opportunity for a match because in general the HLA locus is inherited en bloc as a single set (or haplotype) from each parent.

Loci outside the MHC can also lead to rejection (the minor histocompatibility antigens). However, there is no attempt to match for these antigens because there is little possibility of getting a good match and the effect of matching any single minor antigen is too small to be significant.

It should be noted that even when siblings are perfectly matched at the MHC locus they will not be matched (unless they are identical twins) for the minor histocompatibility antigens.

The importance of HLA matching is not always crucial

HLA matching is very important in bone marrow transplantation (where a large potential donor pool can reduce the risk of GvHD) and has a significant influence on the outcome in kidney transplantation. For other organs the importance is less clear, for example:

- in corneal transplantation there is no benefit of HLA matching;
- for those organs where transplantation is essential to maintain life (such as heart and liver) there is no possibility of waiting for a well-matched organ to become available.

Immunosuppressive drugs

The success of organ transplantation is entirely dependent on the use of immunosuppressive drugs that control the alloimmune response. Although rejection episodes still occur, they are usually kept in check by the drugs so that lasting damage is minimized.

Over recent decades there has been a marked improvement in short-term success rates, such that over 90% of kidney transplants are functioning 1 year after transplantation. The major reason for these improved success rates is the advent of more powerful immunosuppressive agents.

Q. What problems would you expect to result from long-term immunosuppression?

A. These drugs cause blanket suppression of the immune system so transplant recipients are more prone to opportunistic infections and have a raised incidence of malignancy. This is the reason for continuing interest in strategies to promote specific immunological tolerance (see below).

Despite the continuing interest in strategies to promote specific immunological tolerance, clinical transplantation is likely to require non-specific immunosuppression for some years to come. The present challenge is to use the currently available agents intelligently to minimize side effects while preserving graft function.

The commonest cocktail of drugs used for kidney transplant patients involves three agents, each of which has a distinct mode of action:

- a drug that inhibits T cell activation;
- an antiproliferative; and
- an anti-inflammatory agent.

Usually three agents are used in the early post-transplant period while the anti-donor immune response is at its peak. Increasingly monoclonal antibodies are also being used for preventing rejection.

Numerous clinical trials are addressing the safety of withdrawing one of these three agents within weeks or months of transplantation. It appears that maintenance immunosuppression with two drugs is safe and has an improved side effect profile.

Induction of donor-specific tolerance

Although generalized immunosuppression has been highly successful in preventing graft rejection, it comes at a price. This includes:

- the non-specific toxicity of the drugs;
- the need to stay indefinitely on medication; and
- the consequences of generalized immunosuppression such as the increased incidence of cancer and infection.

It would therefore be desirable to induce tolerance to the graft whereby the immune system specifically becomes non-responsive to the donor antigens, yet is still capable of responding normally to other antigens.

Tolerance to grafts was first demonstrated by Peter Medawar's group. They showed that, if allogeneic cells were injected into a neonatal animal, when the animal became adult it would be tolerant to tissue from the donor and would accept grafts without the need for immunosuppression.

There have been numerous examples of inducing tolerance to grafts in animal models since, but it has been difficult to translate this into the clinical setting.

One of the difficulties in the clinical setting is to demonstrate that tolerance really exists. In an animal model it is relatively easy to demonstrate tolerance by:

- performing a second graft (so showing that the immune system will no longer respond to the antigen); or
- demonstrating that an irrelevant third party graft is still rejected (demonstrating that graft survival is not due to a generalized immunosuppression).

However, this is more difficult in humans.

There is evidence for the induction of tolerance in humans

There are two sources of evidence for the induction of tolerance in humans.

First there are patients who have received grafts, but are no longer on immunosuppressive regimens because they cannot tolerate the drugs. They can show long-term graft survival. This is not formal evidence of tolerance, but it is highly suggestive that some people can have an operational tolerance whereby they fail to destroy their organ graft.

Second, it is possible to look at the frequency of alloreactive T cells in patients with grafts. In some groups there is a reduced frequency of these cells, but the response to other antigens remains normal (Fig. 21.15). Again, this is not a formal proof of tolerance because it is not yet known how the in-vitro assays relate to the response in patients. However, it does indicate that it might be possible to develop tests that will allow us to monitor the development of tolerance in patients, and so know how to tailor treatment to the individual (e.g. removing them from immunosuppression when indicated).

Third, there are now studies that do demonstrate long term graft survival (and so apparent tolerance) in patients

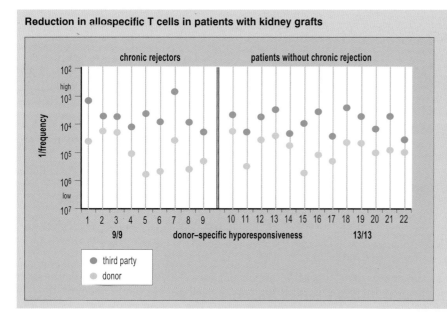

Reduction in allospecific T cells in patients with kidney grafts

Fig. 21.15 The graph shows the frequency of T cells capable of producing IL-2 from patients with long-term kidney grafts that react with cells bearing the donor alloantigen or control (third party) alloantigens. The data show two groups of patients – those with evidence of chronic rejection and those without. Both groups of patient show a reduced frequency of T cells capable of recognizing alloantigen from the donor of the organ when compared to the frequency against third party alloantigen. This indicates that the patients show a degree of reduced reactivity to alloantigens.

that have received joint renal and hematopoetic stem cell transplants. These patients had a short course of immuno-supression, and have since seen long term graft survival with no rejection. While the number of patients treated is limited, these data are very encouraging.

Novel methods for inducing tolerance are being developed

There are various ways in which tolerance (or the appearance of tolerance) can occur. Most of these are discussed in more detail in Chapter 19. An understanding of the mechanisms by which tolerance is induced and maintained allows the development of novel methods for inducing tolerance.

Central tolerance results from deletion of T cells in the thymus and is the most important form of tolerance induction for preventing autoimmunity. It has been harnessed for the induction of tolerance in experimental systems by transplanting the thymus from the donor into the recipient. This approach may be particularly useful in the context of xenotransplantation, where there is an opportunity to manipulate the donor and/or recipient before grafting of the organ.

Alloreactive cells can be made anergic

In the peripheral organs tolerance induction can result from deletion. However, it is also possible for alloreactive cells to be anergized. Anergy describes a state in which the cell is not deleted, but has been rendered unresponsive to further stimulation by the same antigen.

Q. What mechanism causes T cells to become anergic in the presence of an antigen presented on an appropriate MHC molecule?
A. Presentation of the antigen by a non-professional APC that lacks the ability to provide co-stimulatory signals (see Fig. 8.18).

Blockade of co-stimulatory molecules such as CD80 and CD86 with agents like CTLA-4–Ig (a fusion protein between CTLA-4, a ligand for CD80 and CD86, and the Fc part of an antibody molecule) can be used to induce anergy in alloreactive cells (Fig. 21.16). However, it should be noted that the situation can be more complex than this. In many APCs cross-linking of CD80 and CD86 with CTLA-4–Ig results in upregulation of an immunomodulatory enzyme indoleamine 2,3-dioxygenase (IDO). This enzyme catabolizes tryptophan, and as a result prevents T cell activation both as a result of:

- depriving T cells of this essential amino acid; and
- the products of tryptophan breakdown acting directly on the T cells.

The role of IDO in immune regulation was first recognized in the placenta, where it protects the fetus from immunological rejection – inhibition of IDO causes rejection of histoincompatible fetuses.

Another alternative is to induce a regulatory response to the alloantigen. The phenomenon of T cell regulation has long been recognized (Fig. 21.17), and can be shown in experimental models by transferring T cells from a tolerant animal to a naive recipient, and showing that this results in a transfer of the tolerance. Several types of T cell are capable of regulating the immune response, and strategies that seek to expand these cells may be one method to induce tolerance *in vivo*.

Limitations on transplantation

Two major issues limit success of transplantation:

- the first is the shortage of donor organs – this means that not everyone who would benefit from a transplant receives one, and, given the high success rate of

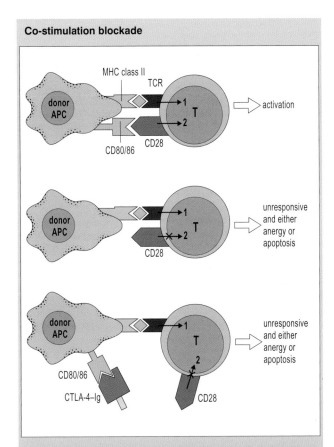

Co-stimulation blockade

Fig. 21.16 For full T cell activation to occur the T cell needs to receive two signals – signal 1 through the T cell receptor binding the appropriate peptide–MHC complex (which provides antigenic specificity) and signal 2 through co-stimulatory molecules (the most important of which for naive T cells is CD28 on the T cell binding CD80, or CD86 on the APC). Interaction of a T cell with an APC that lacks CD80 or CD86, so that signal 1 only is received, fails to activate the T cell and can result in apoptosis or anergy of the lymphocyte. In experimental or clinical settings it is possible to block the CD28 interaction with CD80/86 by addition of a soluble molecule, CTLA-4–Ig, which consists of the extracellular part of CTLA-4 (an alternative ligand for CD80/86) fused to the Fc of immunoglobulin. This molecule prevents the interaction of CD28 with CD80/86. It can also result in upregulation of immunoregulatory enzyme, indoleamine 2,3-dioxygenase (IDO), as described in the text.

Tolerance to grafts can be transferred by regulatory cells

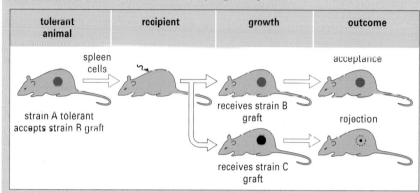

Fig. 21.17 An animal of strain A that has been made tolerant to a graft B can contain regulatory cells. If these cells are removed from the animal and transferred to a lightly irradiated strain A recipient, and this animal is then given a skin graft from strain B, then that graft may be accepted. In most cases this tolerance is specific, so if the second mouse received a graft of strain C it would be rejected.

transplantation, an increasing number of patients would benefit;

- the second problem is chronic rejection, which results in a continual loss of transplanted organs and necessitates patients remaining on immunosuppression, with the consequences of drug toxicity, systemic immunosuppression, increased incidence of malignancy, and infection.

The second of these problems, chronic rejection, would be solved if we were able to induce tolerance to grafts in patients. To do this it is necessary that:

- we develop assays that will allow us to determine when tolerance has been induced; and
- translate the therapies developed in animal models to the clinic.

These assays are still under development but may involve measuring the frequency of alloreactive and/or regulatory T cells in patients, as well as other immunological biomarkers. At present it is not clear which tolerance induction procedure is most likely to work in clinical transplantation, and further work in primate models is needed to address this issue.

Alternative approaches to overcoming the shortage of donor organs are being investigated

Although it is very important to increase the donor pool, the approaches discussed above will never provide all the organs needed. Alternatives include:

- the development of artificial mechanical organs;
- in the longer term, use of cloning and/or tissue engineering strategies to make artificial biological organs; and
- xenotransplantation (the use of animal organs).

CRITICAL THINKING: KIDNEY TRANSPLANTATION (SEE P. 440 FOR EXPLANATIONS)

Mrs X has diabetes mellitus, and this caused severe damage to her kidneys. This complication is called diabetic nephropathy, and is one of the major indications for kidney transplantation. Mrs X was on dialysis treatment, but this was not working well for her and she was advised that she would benefit from renal transplantation. However, it proved very difficult to find a suitable cadaveric donor for Mrs X and it was suggested that a family member might donate an organ. All her immediate family – her husband, five children, and two brothers – agreed to be considered as donors.

The HLA types and blood groups of the family members are shown in the table. On the basis of these tests a donor was selected and the transplant was performed.

Despite successful surgery, the kidney soon turned dark and swelled. This started to happen within a few minutes of the restoration of blood flow through the transplant, and necessitated the immediate removal of the graft.

Four years later Mrs X was still very ill on dialysis, no cadaveric donor was available, and it was decided to try again with a living related transplant. Another member of the family was selected to donate a kidney and it functioned well from the onset. Mrs X was given triple immunosuppression. She had only one rejection episode at about 3 weeks after grafting, and this was treated successfully with anti-rejection therapy. There were no other problems.

Continued

CRITICAL THINKING: KIDNEY TRANSPLANTATION (SEE P. 440 FOR EXPLANATIONS) CONT.

Person	Age	Relationship to patient	HLA genotypes			Blood group genes phenotype
			A	B	DR	
Mrs X	46	the patient	1 2	8 44	3 4	BODd BRh$^+$
Mr X	52	husband	2 3	14 7	8 2	AOdd ARhr
Anne	25	daughter	2 3	44 7	4 2	AOdd ARhr
Bert	24	son	1 2	8 14	3 8	ABDd ABRh$^+$
Chas	21	son	1 3	8 7	3 2	BOdd BRhr
Dave	15	son	2 1	44 60	4 9	BODd BRh$^+$
Edna	13	daughter	1 2	8 14	3 8	AODd ARh$^+$
Fred	48	brother	1 2	8 44	3 4	ABDd ABRh$^+$
Gary	56	brother	2 2	44 14	4 15	BODD BRH$^+$

The kidney continued to work for 8 years, but its function gradually declined from the fourth year onwards. It seemed there was little the doctors could do to prevent this worsening situation, and Mrs X eventually had to return to dialysis.

1 What are the difficulties in finding a donor organ?

2 Comment on the HLA relationships between Mrs X and her brothers.

3 Comment on the relationships between the children of Mrs X.

4 Classify each member of the family in terms of their HLA relationship to Mrs X (HLA identical, HLA haplotype match, complete HLA mismatch).

5 In terms of HLA matching alone, who was the best donor for Mrs X?

6 Consider what effect the blood group antigens had on the choice of donor. From whom could kidneys have been transplanted, and who would not have been suitable?

7 Of those who had a compatible blood group, who would you have chosen as the best donor? Explain your reasoning.

8 The outcome of the transplantation was a disaster! By what mechanism was the graft attacked?

9 Why was Mrs X at a greater risk of this untoward reaction?

10 What laboratory tests are used to avoid this rejection reaction, and what seems to have gone wrong on this occasion?

11 Four years after the first transplant it was decided to try again with a living related donor. Of all the family members, who would you have chosen as the donor and whose kidney was most likely to survive in Mrs X?

12 What is triple therapy immunosuppression?

13 What type of rejection occurred at 3 weeks after transplantation, and what immunological mechanisms were involved?

14 What is anti-rejection therapy?

15 There were no other problems with Mrs X. Can you think of some of the problems that might arise in a transplant recipient?

16 Why did the function of the transplant gradually decline, and why could the doctors not stop this process?

Discussion points

1 What are the ethical issues involved in this form of transplantation?

2 What novel forms of immunotherapy might be available in the future to prevent rejection of grafts?

CHAPTER 22

Immunity to Cancers

SUMMARY

- **The immune system can potentially survey the body for some types of developing tumor.**

- **Tumors can induce immunity.** Mice, rats, hamsters, and frogs can be immunized against tumors. In most tumors of animals, tumor immunity elicited by immunization is specific (or strongest) to the individual tumor that was used to immunize.

- **Tumor antigens have been characterized by three means – immunization-challenge experiments, T cell reactivity, and antibody reactivity.** Immunization-challenge experiments have uncovered the immunogenicity of heat-shock

protein-chaperoned antigenic peptides. Antigens identified by reactivity to T cells and antibodies include individual tumor-specific mutated antigens, cancer testes antigens, differentiation antigens, and viral tumor antigens.

- **Vigorous anti-tumor immune responses are compromised by regulatory mechanisms.** Tumors elicit immunity in their primary host, and such immunity is downregulated. Regulatory cells such as $CD25^+ CD4^+$ T cells and inhibition of activated anti-tumor T cells through T cell molecules such as CTLA-4 are involved in downregulation of tumor immunity.

Immune surveillance and protection from cancer

Cancer appears to have engaged the minds of immunologists almost since the beginning of immunology itself. Ehrlich, who opined on all things immunological, believed that the immune system could protect the host from cancer.

Burnet and Thomas refined that idea into the immune surveillance hypothesis of cancer. The hypothesis lived in limbo for several decades, failing to thrive and failing to die, until very recently when the work of Old, Schreiber, and their colleagues demonstrated that mice with a compromised immune status were more prone than immunocompetent mice to develop an array of cancers.

The immune surveillance hypothesis is often regarded as the intellectual underpinning of cancer immunology. Although the hypothesis itself has contributed little to our attempts to treat cancer through immunological means, it has profound implications for understanding the functions of the immune system.

Does infection have an anti-cancer effect?

German physicians in the 19th century noted dramatic regressions of cancer in occasional patients who developed streptococcal infections. These anecdotes led to a systematic exploration of infections/fever as an immunotherapeutic modality by William Coley, a New York City surgeon.

The work of Coley and his predecessors, suggesting that non-specific stimulation of the immune system, such as by an infection, can have an anti-cancer effect, remains a key idea in cancer immunology. It is only a small exaggeration to say that every idea in cancer immunity has been interpreted at some time or another, in terms of Coley's observations.

Tumor immunity in the primary host

Entirely unrelated to these two lines of enquiry, the study of cancer immunity saw a revival at the hands of those who were transplanting chemically induced tumors into the many inbred mice that began to be available in the 1950s. These investigators 'showed "highly successful" immunization against the "transplantable tumors" and expressed great hopes about cancer vaccination'.

In hindsight, these successful immunizations were simply a result of allogeneic differences between tumors and the host strain of mouse, a theme that played a seminal role in definition of the MHC, but had no relevance for cancer immunity.

Q. What will happen when a tumor from a mouse of one MHC haplotype is transplanted into a recipient with a different haplotype on the first occasion or the second?
A. A transplantation rejection reaction will ensue, and these reactions display specificity and memory (see Chapter 21).

355

Immunogenicity of chemically induced tumors

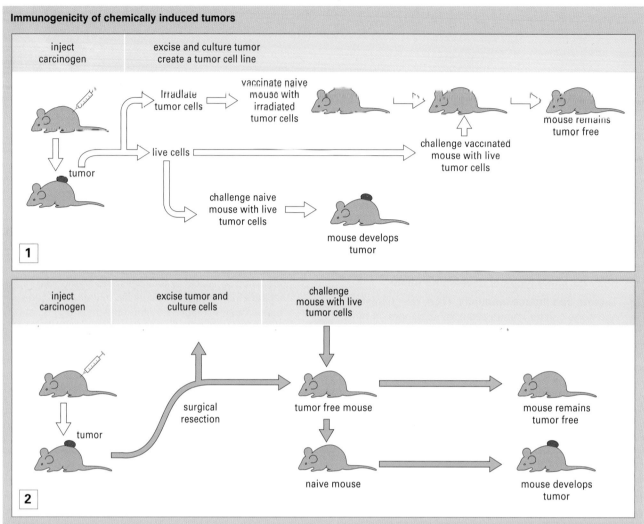

Fig. 22.1 (1) Mice immunized with tumor cells are protected against subsequent tumor growth. (2) The primary animal that develops the tumor is also immune to subsequent challenges with the same tumor.

Nonetheless, amidst the barrage of experiments where MHC-mismatched tumors were transplanted into mice, were the experiments of Ludwik Gross, and later those of Prehn and Main, and of George and Eva Klein, who showed that, even when MHC-matched tumors were used to immunize mice, protection against subsequent tumor growth could be achieved (Fig. 22.1). These studies led to two principles, which have informed much of cancer immunology since and are discussed below.

Cancers elicit protective immunity in the primary and syngeneic host

Mice and rats of a given haplotype can be immunized with irradiated cancer cells that arose in animals of the same haplotype. When they are challenged with live cancer cells, they are able to resist the tumor challenge. The following further observations and deductions have been derived from these results.

- The immunogenicity of tumors has provided the foundation stone for the idea of **tumor-specific antigens**. If one could immunize, then antigens must exist.

- Tumor immunity depends on many factors. The degree of tumor immunity depends upon the type of cancer and the method of its induction, or lack of induction. UV-induced cancers are highly immunogenic, methyl-cholanthrene-induced tumors less so, and spontaneous tumors even less so. Nonetheless, immunogenicity of tumors has been demonstrated in all model systems tested.

- The primary animal develops immunity to subsequent tumor challenge. Furthermore it is also immune to subsequent challenges with the same tumor (see Fig. 22.1).

- Protective immunity is only seen in prophylactic immunization and not therapeutic immunization – once a mouse has been implanted with a tumor, immunization with irradiated cancer cells (derived from the growing tumor) does nothing to mitigate tumor growth (Fig. 22.2). Exploration of differences between prophylaxis and therapy has led to fundamental insights into tumor immunity.

It is obviously not possible to test immunogenicity of tumors in humans by the transplantation-challenge experimental

Difference between prophylaxis against future tumors and therapy of pre-existing tumors

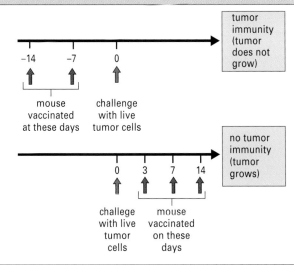

Fig. 22.2 Protective immunity is only seen in prophylactic immunization and not therapeutic immunization – once a mouse has been implanted with a tumor, immunization with irradiated cancer cells (derived from the growing tumor) does nothing to mitigate tumor growth.

Relative risk of tumors in immunosuppressed kidney transplant

tumor type	approximate relative risk
Kaposi's sarcoma	50–100
non-Hodgkin's lymphoma	25–45
carcinoma of the liver	20–35
carcinoma of the skin	20–50
carcinoma of the cervix	2.5–10
melanoma	2.5–10
lung	1–2

Fig. 22.3 In all forms of immunodeficiency the relative risk of developing tumors in which viruses are known to play a role is greatly increased. This is the case for all those listed except cancer of the lung. The relative risks vary in different studies according to the duration of follow-up and the presence of co-factors such as sunlight for skin cancer.

paradigm. There is no other reliable method of determining immunogenicity of tumors. It is therefore impossible to comment on the immunogenicity of human tumors. Much of the work in human cancer immunity has been done with melanomas leading to suggestions that, among human tumors, melanomas are particularly immunogenic. This is an erroneous belief – melanomas are simply the easiest human tumors to culture *in vitro* and hence the easiest to study.

Specific immunity may develop to induced and spontaneous tumors

When mice are immunized against a given fibrosarcoma, they are rendered immune to that fibrosarcoma, but only to that individual fibrosarcoma or lines derived from it. If the mice are challenged with another fibrosarcoma, even one induced by the same carcinogen, tumor growth is unaffected by the prior immunization.

The most extensive interrogation of the individually distinct antigenicity of chemically induced tumors was carried out by Basombrio and Prehn. They induced fibrosarcomas in 25 syngeneic BALB/c mice using methyl-cholanthrene and tested the immunogenicity of each one against all other tumors in an immunization-challenge model. They concluded that, even though all tumors were induced at the same time, in the same strain of mice of the same age by the same carcinogen and were histologically all fibrosarcomas, they were antigenically individually distinct. Independent tumors induced by the same carcinogen in the same mouse are also antigenically distinct.

Q. What can you infer about the nature of the immune response to tumors from this observation?
A. It must involve the adaptive immune system.

Spontaneous tumors are also antigenically distinct

Cross-reactivity among tumors does occur occasionally. Typically, such cross-reactive immunity has been observed to be significantly weaker than the individually specific antigenicity. Efforts at characterization of such cross-reactive tumor-protective antigens have not made much headway, except in the case of virally induced tumors. In contrast, there has been considerable success in identification of individually distinct antigens.

In addition to these experimental studies, several clinical observations point to the existence of tumor-protective immunity in humans. These include the increased relative risk of cancers in patients who are immunosuppressed because they are kidney transplant recipients (Fig. 22.3) or for a variety of other reasons (Fig. 22.4).

Q. The observation that immunosuppressed individuals are more susceptible to tumors can be explained in at least two different ways. Suggest what these explanations might be.
A. The individual may be unable to control virus infections that lead to cancer (oncogenic viruses), or they may be unable to survey and control primary tumors that arise by mutation. The explanations are not mutually exclusive.

Characterization of tumor antigens

The two broad approaches to the identification of tumor antigens are shown in Figure 22.5 and discussed individually below. Not surprisingly, the approaches have yielded results that are not fully concordant. These differences have helped highlight a fascinating interplay between immunity and tolerance to tumors, discussed below.

Tumor viruses and immunodeficiency

cause of immunodeficiency	common tumor types	viruses involved
inherited immunodeficiency	lymphoma	EBV
immunosuppression for organ transplants or due to AIDS	lymphoma cervical cancer skin cancer liver cancer Kaposi's sarcoma	EBV papilloma viruses probably papilloma viruses hepatitis B and C viruses human herpes virus 8
malaria	Burkitt's lymphoma	EBV
autoimmunity	lymphoma	EBV

Fig. 22.4 Skin cancer is the most common form of tumor in absolute numbers in organ transplant recipients. In other forms of immunodeficiency, tumors of the immune system dominate. Most normal adults carry both Epstein–Barr virus (EBV) and many papilloma viruses throughout life with no ill effects because they have antiviral immunity.

Comprehensive list of major types of tumor antigen

	category of antigen	individual antigens	tumors in which identified	activity in mouse models	human vaccine trials
tumor transplantation (mouse models)	heat-shock protein–peptide complexes	Gp96	fibrosarcoma, lung carcinoma, lymphoma, prostate carcinoma, etc.	+	phase III trials in renal carcinoma, melanoma underway
		Hsp70	fibrosarcoma, colon carcinoma	+	phase II trials in CML underway
		Hsp90, CRT Hsp110, 170	fibrosarcoma colon carcinoma	+	none yet
T cell/antibody (SEREX) reactivity (mostly human studies, some mouse models)	cancer/testes antigens	NY-ESO-1 MAGE, etc.	melanomas other tumors	N/A**	a number of phase I, II trials completed and underway
	differentiation antigens (lineage-specific)	melan A tyrosinase Gp100 PSA, etc.	melanomas (except PSA) (prostate carcinoma)		
	antigens with broader expression	human – CEA, MUC, HER2, G250	many tumors, except G250 (renal carcinoma only)		
		murine – P1A, gp70	many tumors	–	N/A
	common tumor-specific antigens	mutated p53, mutated ras, BCR-ABL, etc. papilloma virus?	many tumors	N/T*** exc. a single positive study with p53	no significant ongoing clinical effort
	unique tumor-specific antigens (mutations)	human – MUM-1, 2, β-catenin, HLA-A2-R170I, ELF2m, myosin-m, caspase-8, KIAA0205, HSP70-2m CDK4*, TRP2*, NA17A*	melanoma	N/A	N/A
		murine – Erk2, RNA helicase ribosomal proteins L9, L11	fibrosarcomas squamous cell carcinomas	+	none
	viral antigens	(see Fig. 22.5)			

CML, chronic myeloid leukemia; SEREX, serological analysis of recombinant cDNA expression libraries; *expressed on >1 melanoma, but not on any normal tissues; N/A**, not applicable; N/T***, not tested

Fig. 22.5 A comprehensive list of the major types of tumor antigen.

Tumor-specific antigens defined by immunization all belong to the family of HSPs

When tumors were biochemically fractionated and individual protein fractions tested for their ability to elicit protective tumor immunity, a number of tumor-protective antigens were identified in diverse tumor models, such as mouse sarcomas, melanomas, colon and lung carcinomas, and rat hepatomas.

Interestingly, regardless of the tumor models used, all antigens were found to belong to the family of proteins known as the **heat-shock proteins** (HSPs), which:

- could elicit protective immunity;
- were of the HSP90 (gp96 and HSP90), HSP70 (HSP110 and HSP/c70), calreticulin, and HSP170 (also known as grp170) families.

HSPs must be isolated directly from tumors to be immunologically active

Two aspects of HSP-elicited tumor immunity are notable.

- First, HSPs are present in normal tissues as well as tumors, and normal tissue-derived HSPs do not elicit rejection. They must be isolated from tumors to be immunologically active.
- Second, HSPs elicit immunity specifically against the individual tumors from which they are isolated.

These two observations suggested that HSPs in tumors differ from those in normal tissues and that HSPs in each tumor differ from the same molecules in other tumors.

This conundrum was resolved by the demonstration that the HSP molecules chaperone peptides in a peptide-binding pocket, much as the MHC molecules do, although the structural details of the pockets in HSP and MHC differ (Fig. 22.6). The specificity of immunogenicity derives from the peptides rather than the HSP itself – dissociation of HSP-associated peptides from HSPs abrogate the tumor rejection activity.

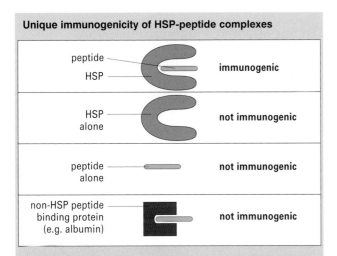

Unique immunogenicity of HSP-peptide complexes

peptide / HSP	immunogenic
HSP alone	not immunogenic
peptide alone	not immunogenic
non-HSP peptide binding protein (e.g. albumin)	not immunogenic

Fig. 22.6 HSP molecules chaperone peptides in a peptide-binding pocket. The specificity of immunogenicity derives from the peptides rather than the HSP itself – dissociation of HSP-associated peptides from HSPs abrogated the tumor rejection activity.

HSPs can chaperone many different peptides hence the HSP-chaperoned peptides contain among them any tumor-specific antigenic epitopes present in the tumor cell or the antigenic fingerprint of the tumor from which the HSPs are isolated.

HSP molecules bind to APCs and target peptides with high efficiency

The HSP molecule itself plays at least two crucial roles other than chaperoning peptides:

- HSPs bind antigen-presenting cells (APCs) such as macrophages and dendritic cells (DCs) through HSP receptors such as CD91 and thus target the peptides chaperoned by them into the APCs with high efficiency;
- further, the HSP-chaperoned peptides, once introduced into the APC, follow the endogenous as well as the exogenous pathway of antigen presentation and are processed and re-presented by the MHC I and MHC II molecules of the APCs (Fig. 22.7).

Q. How can an APC present internalized antigen via MHC class I molecules?
A. It can do this via the mechanism of cross-presentation.

It is by this mechanism that immunization with tumor-derived HSPs elicits a CD8 as well as CD4 response against the tumors. In addition, the HSP molecules stimulate the APCs to mediate maturation of DCs and secretion of an array of cytokines that provide the innate milieu for the adaptive response.

'Tumor-specific antigens' recognized by T cells show a wide spectrum of specificity

Many studies have identified tumor-reactive T cells in blood or within a tumor, and these findings have thus supported the idea of tumor antigens.

The work of Thierry Boon and his colleagues first made it technically possible to identify the CTL epitopes of cancer cells being recognized by the tumor-reactive T cells.

Although the idea of tumor-specific antigens in mouse models of cancer was based on tumor rejection *in vivo* and thus had connotations of tumor specificity, the tumor antigens defined by tumor-reactive T cells show a wider spectrum of specificity, and their connection with tumor immunity *in vivo* is tenuous.

The T cell-defined tumor antigens of murine tumors have been defined in a mastocytoma, two fibrosarcomas, a squamous cell carcinoma, and a colon carcinoma because these tumor lines are in popular use. Similarly, much of the corresponding work in human tumors has been carried out in melanomas because melanoma cell lines are easier to establish in culture, rather than because of any unique immunogenicity of human melanomas.

The tumor antigens identified as T cell epitopes fall into the following categories (see Fig. 22.5).

Cancer/testes antigens are expressed only in testes

Cancer/testes (CT) antigens, as the name suggests, are expressed on cancer cells and in testes, but not in other normal adult tissues. MAGE, BAGE, GAGE, and NY-ESO1 are examples of this class of antigen. Individual epitopes

Mechanism of specific immunogenicity of HSP-peptide complexes

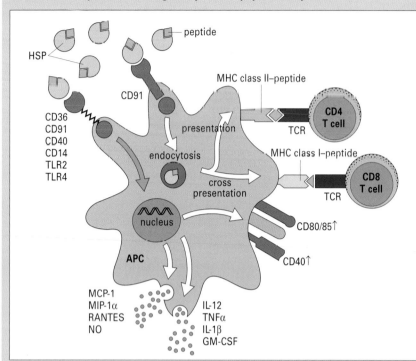

Fig. 22.7 Once introduced into the APC, the HSP-chaperoned peptides follow the endogenous class I as well as the exogenous class II pathway of antigen presentation and are processed and represented by the MHC class I and MHC II molecules of the APCs. HSP ligation induces production of chemokines and cytokines, and upregulation of CD40 and CD80/85. (MCP-1, monocyte chemotactic protein-1; MIP-1α, macrophage inflammatory protein-1α.) *(Redrawn from Srivastava P. Nat Rev Immunol 2002;2:185–194. Copyright 2002, Nature Reviews Immunology.)*

within CT antigens have been defined for CD8 as well as CD4 lymphocytes. Clinical trials with the MAGE antigen are currently underway.

Differentiation antigens are lineage specific and not tumor specific

Differentiation antigens, which are lineage specific, but not tumor specific, are expressed on normal tissues (melanocytes) as well as tumors (melanomas). Examples of such antigens include MART-1/Melan-A, tyrosinase, gp100, Trp1, and Trp2. Individual epitopes within differentiation antigens have been defined for CD8 as well as CD4 lymphocytes. Most differentiation antigens have been identified in human melanomas but in randomized clinical trials, there is little evidence that immunization with them confers clinical benefit to cancer patients.

Unique tumor-specific antigens have been characterized in melanomas

Individually tumor-specific or unique antigens presented by MHC class I or class II molecules have been characterized in human melanomas (see Fig. 22.5).

In terms of their specificity, these antigens are most similar to the individually tumor-specific antigens of murine tumors defined by tumor transplantation studies. Immunization with these antigens renders the mice resistant to tumor challenge. They are the only tumor antigens that have been shown to possess this essential property. The defined unique antigens of human tumors have not been tested for clinical activity.

T cell epitopes of viral antigens have been identified

T cell epitopes of viral antigens of virus-induced tumors have been identified such as:

- the T antigen of SV40 and the polyoma viruses;
- the E6 and E7 antigens of the human papilloma viruses that cause cervical cancer; and
- a number of antigens of EBV (Fig. 22.8).

Some of these, such as the HPV antigens, are used for prophylactic vaccination (see Chapter 18) and are being tested for clinical activity in human tumors.

'Tumor-specific antigens' defined by antibodies are rarely tumor specific

The search for antibodies that discriminate between cancer cells and normal cells has a long pedigree and has been carried out with the whole range of tools starting from antisera to panning antibody libraries. This search has been largely unsuccessful and rarely have tumor-specific antibodies been generated. Most anti-tumor antibodies, like anti-tumor T cells, happen to recognize CT antigens, differentiation antigens, and even more broadly distributed common antigens (see Fig. 22.5).

Antibodies to a B cell surface antigen, CD20, epidermal growth factor receptor, and HER2/Neu have now been approved for treatments, respectively, of B lymphoma, colorectal cancers, and breast cancers. Although these antibodies have shown some efficacy in the treatment of certain cancers at certain stages, they:

- do not recognize tumor-specific antigens;
- are actually used as pharmacological rather than immunological reagents.

Microorganisms and human tumors

tumor	organism
adult T cell leukemia	human T leukemia virus-I (HTLV-I)
Burkitt's lymphoma and lymphoma in immunosuppression	EBV
cervical cancer	human papilloma viruses (HPV 16 and 18, and others)
liver cancer	hepatitis B and C
nasopharyngeal cancer	EBV
skin cancer	probably human papilloma viruses
stomach cancer	*Helicobacter pylori*

Fig. 22.8 EBV causes Burkitt's lymphoma in endemic malaria areas of Africa and nasopharyngeal carcinoma in China, suggesting that co-factors, either genetic or environmental, are required for tumor development. *Helicobacter pylori* is the only bacterium so far known to be involved in the etiology of human cancer.

Antibodies used in the diagnosis of cancer may not be tumor specific

As serum antibodies are technically easy to measure, they have always attracted the attention of diagnosticians (Fig. 22.w2). Thus, antibody to carcinoembryonic antigen (CEA) is often used as a marker for progression or status of certain carcinomas; however, CEA or other such antigens are not tumor-specific antigens and diagnostic markers need not necessarily have the specificity required of a 'tumor-specific antigen'.

Anti-tumor immune responses

Successful tumor immunity is rare in patients who have cancer

Mechanisms of tumor immunity have been examined mostly in mouse models, partly because successful tumor immunity is rare in patients who have cancer. Moreover, as successful tumor immunity is rare in the tumor-bearing setting in mouse models, much of the work has been done in a prophylactic setting, which is not applicable to the human situation.

Not surprisingly, the pathways to elicitation of immune response to tumors are straightforward (Fig. 22.9). The tumor inoculum (with its antigenic load) is taken up by the APCs at the site of immunization and is cross-presented by them to the naive CD8 cells in the draining lymph nodes. Both responses are generally necessary in the mouse models tested and both responses have been shown to be present in the cancer patients studied.

Antibodies have not generally been shown to be protective in the natural setting.

NK cell activity has been demonstrated most commonly, but its necessity has rarely been examined critically. In the few studies where it has been examined, it appears that NK cells play a crucial role in the immune response to cancers. Clearly, the cytokines necessary for the effector functions of CD4, CD8, and NK cells, such as IL-2, IFNγ, IL-12, and others, are necessary as well.

Despite an immune response, tumors continue to grow

Despite clear evidence for the existence of tumor-specific antigens and the immune response elicited by them, tumors generally continue to grow. In this regard, Ehrlich made a curious observation that remains at the center of cancer immunity. He noted that animals with already growing tumors were strangely resistant to a second tumor challenge even as the first tumor kept growing (Fig. 22.10). This phenomenon, termed **concomitant immunity** as early as 1908, remained relatively unexamined until recently.

Concomitant immunity shows two aspects of tumor immunity

Concomitant immunity shows two aspects of tumor immunity:

- first, a growing tumor elicits in the primary host a tumor-protective immune response;
- second, although this response is sufficient to eliminate a nascent tumor, it fails to eliminate the tumor that elicited the response.

It was shown that concomitant immunity was tumor specific and operational only within a narrow window of 7–10 days after tumor implantation; if the second tumor was implanted beyond this time, it was not rejected. The lack of immunity beyond the narrow window was attributable to a new population of suppressor T cells that appeared at that time (Fig. 22.11). Similar to the phenomenon of concomitant immunity, it was also noted that mice in the process of rejecting an allograft were unable to concomitantly reject a growing tumor bearing the same alloantigens as the allograft.

Q. How do you interpret the observation above?
A. One would expect an allograft to be rejected in these circumstances, therefore there is something about the tumor that allows it to evade a normal allospecific rejection reaction.

A working diagram of the possible mechanism of tumor immunity

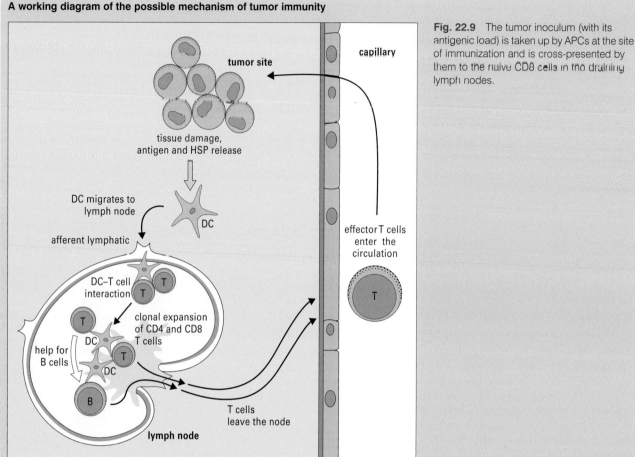

Fig. 22.9 The tumor inoculum (with its antigenic load) is taken up by APCs at the site of immunization and is cross-presented by them to the naive CD8 cells in the draining lymph nodes.

Immunization is effective prophylactically but rarely as therapy

The findings discussed above fit in well with the observations that, although naive mice can be immunized successfully using irradiated tumor cell vaccines in almost any tumor model, the same irradiated cell vaccine is ineffective at treating established tumors.

Prophylaxis is relatively effective, even if begun as late as 3 days before tumor implantation, but therapy is ineffective even if begun as early as 2 days after tumor implantation (see Fig. 22.2).

It is easy, and incorrect, to infer from these observations that the tumor-bearing mice or cancer patients are generally immunosuppressed. Tumor-bearing mice generally mount a vigorous immune response to model antigens and even unrelated tumors, almost until the very end of their lives. Similarly, patients with cancer do not generally succumb to the opportunistic infections that are the hallmark of general immunosuppression.

The naive state and tumor-bearing state are essentially different

Collectively, the observations above have shaped the thinking that, immunologically the tumor-bearing host is in a radically different state compared with the naive host.

What are the mechanisms behind this change of status? They are exactly the same as envisaged for the mechanisms

for the initiation and maintenance of peripheral tolerance. None of the explanations is fully satisfactory by itself, but each perhaps contributes to the final state of tolerance in some measure. Immune unresponsiveness per se is addressed in detail in Chapter 19. Aspects that are of specific relevance to tumor immunity include:

- inhibitory cytokines including TGFβ and IL-10;
- inhibition of T cell activity through CTLA-4 and PD1;
- down-regulation of the immune response through regulatory T cells;
- resistance to recognition by down-regulation of MHC class I molecules; and
- generation of antigen-loss variants.

Downregulation of MHC I molecule expression may result in resistance to recognition and lysis

A number of studies have shown:

- downregulation of expression of one or more MHC class I alleles;
- loss of β2-microglobulin; or
- loss or downregulation of any of the several components of the antigen processing machinery.

Although these alterations are clearly likely to inhibit recognition of tumor cells by T cells, they are also more likely to make tumors more susceptible to NK cells.

Conoomitant immunity

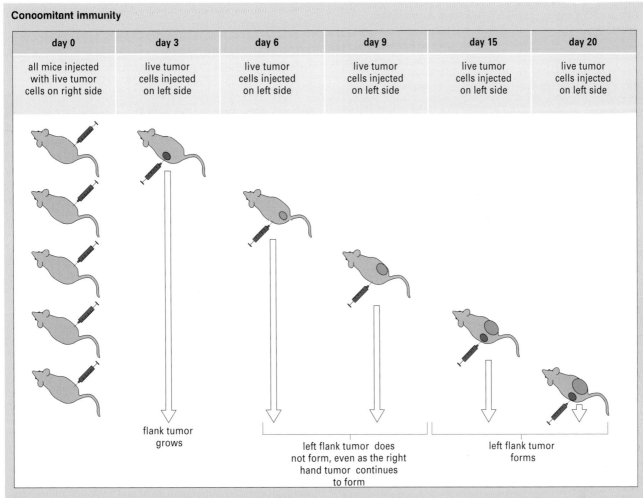

day 0	day 3	day 6	day 9	day 15	day 20
all mice injected with live tumor cells on right side	live tumor cells injected on left side	live tumor cells injected on left side	live tumor cells injected on left side	live tumor cells injected on left side	live tumor cells injected on left side

flank tumor grows

left flank tumor does not form, even as the right hand tumor continues to form

left flank tumor forms

Fig. 22.10   Animals with already growing tumors are resistant to a second tumor challenge even as the first tumor continues to grow.

On the whole, it is not clear what effect, if any, these alterations have on the net ability of a tumor to escape the immune response *in vivo*.

Generation of antigen-loss variants is another mechanism that no doubt plays a role to some degree in the immunological escape of tumor cells. However, because we do not yet have a significant knowledge of the identity of truly tumor-protective antigens, the role of antigen-loss variants cannot be critically examined.

T cell activity is inhibited through CTLA-4

An exciting explanation for unresponsiveness is the role of inhibition of T cell activity through CTLA-4.

Q. What are the functions of CD28 and CTLA-4 (CD152) on T cells?
A. CD28 transduces co-stimulatory signals to the T cell, while CTLA-4 also ligates B7, but is inhibitory (see Fig. 22.12).

CTLA-4 inhibits the T cell by raising the stimulatory threshold or by inhibiting the proliferative drive of T cells (Fig. 22.12). The biological role of CTLA-4 appears to lie in limiting the T cell response to foreign antigens as well as to autoantigens.

Administering antibodies to CTLA-4 (that inhibit CTLA-4:B7 interactions) to mice bearing a broad array of tumors inhibited tumor growth, even when the antibody was administered after the tumors were visible and palpable (Fig. 22.w3). Such activity was generally seen only against the more immunogenic tumors and not against a poorly immunogenic melanoma (e.g. B16). In that instance, combination of anti-CTLA-4 antibody with a vaccine consisting of irradiated melanoma cells that were also transfected with the cytokine granulocyte–macrophage colony stimulating factor (GM-CSF), resulted in a stronger anti-tumor response than by anti-CTLA-4 antibody or the vaccine alone. Clinical development of this idea is discussed below.

Similar results have been observed in other tumor models. These results support the notion derived from studies on concomitant immunity that progressive tumor growth results in the generation of inhibitory influences on the anti-tumor immune response.

Abrogation of CD25⁺ cells leads to protective tumor immunity

The notion that progressive tumor growth results in the generation of inhibitory influences on the anti-tumor immune response is further supported by the recent work on the CD25⁺ CD4⁺ Treg cells (see Chapter 11). These cells have been shown to suppress CD8⁺ T cell responses in general, including autoimmune responses.

Effector CD8 and suppressor CD4 cells in concomitant immunity

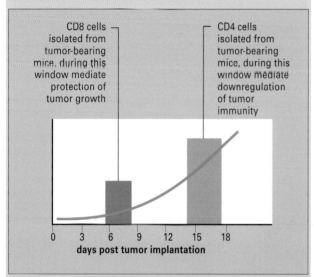

CD8 cells isolated from tumor-bearing mice, during this window mediate protection of tumor growth

CD4 cells isolated from tumor-bearing mice, during this window mediate downregulation of tumor immunity

days post tumor implantation

Fig. 22.11 Concomitant immunity is tumor specific and operational only within a narrow window of 7–10 days after tumor implantation. If the second tumor is implanted beyond this time, it is not rejected. The lack of immunity beyond the narrow window is attributable to a new population of suppressor T cells that appear at that time.

Mechanism of action of anti-CTLA-4 antibody

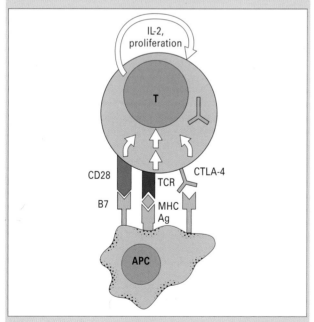

IL-2, proliferation

T

CD28

TCR

CTLA-4

B7

MHC
Ag

APC

Fig. 22.12 CTLA-4 inhibits the T cell by raising the stimulatory threshold or by inhibiting the proliferative drive of T cells.

Recent studies have shown that abrogation of the $CD25^+$ subpopulation (through anti-CD25 antibodies or through genetic manipulation) in tumor-bearing mice leads to a robust T cell response and protective tumor immunity even in an aggressive tumor model such as the B16 melanoma.

Conversely, re-addition of these cells can suppress the anti-tumor immune response.

Results consistent with these have been observed in patients with melanoma whose regulatory $CD4^+$ T cells specifically inhibit the $CD8^+$ activity against autologous melanoma cells, but not against other targets.

More recent studies have examined this paradigm through the prism of the $CD25^+$ T cells. In a study of patients with ovarian cancer, such cells were shown to be associated with a higher risk of death and reduced survival. Interestingly, the $CD25^+$ T cells were shown to migrate preferentially to the solid tumors and the ascites, but rarely to the draining lymph nodes.

Such results indicate that, despite the poor clinical outcomes in advanced cancer, the host does mount a vigorous anti-tumor immune response, which is compromised by regulatory mechanisms. Manipulation of such regulatory mechanisms for enhancing cancer immunity is bound to influence the fine balance between tolerance and autoimmunity. In certain contexts, that may be a reasonable price to pay.

Immunotherapy for human cancer

Animal models are limited in the translation of therapy

There exists a 'common wisdom' but incorrect belief, that treatment of cancers of mice is easy and has no bearing on treatment of human cancers. Mouse tumors are hard to cure – not a single publication reports curing a mouse with stage IV disseminated disease.

Most approaches study prophylactic vaccination in mice, a smaller number begin treatment on the day of tumor challenge, and only a handful of studies begin treatment more than 10 days after tumor challenge. In most mouse tumor models, mice die within 4–6 weeks of tumor challenge, and thus the window of treatment is extremely narrow.

Most approaches to immunotherapy of human cancer have either never been tested in appropriate mouse models or have failed to show anti-tumor activity when tested. It is important to bear this in mind while examining the three major categories of approaches to immunotherapy of human cancer, discussed below.

Antibodies have been used successfully

As antibodies are the oldest known immunological reagents, it is only to be expected that the first, and thus far among the most successful, approaches to human cancer immunotherapy has been made using these reagents.

Nearly 20 years ago, Ronald Levy and colleagues treated patients with B cell lymphomas using individual patient's tumor-specific anti-idiotypic antibodies on the premise that the antibodies will recognize and help eliminate their targets – the surface immunoglobulin on the monoclonal lymphomas. The treatment was successful clinically, leading to significant objective tumor regressions, but was limited by the re-emergence of escape variants that did not express the idiotype. This approach has not been pursued further, but remains a powerful reminder of what true tumor-specific antibodies can do to real-life tumors.

Vaccination approaches to immunotherapy of human cancer currently being tested

vaccine	cancer
unique antigen (individually patient-specific) approaches	
idiotypes + KLH + GM-CSF	B lymphoma
intact autologous irradiated tumor cells + BCG	colon cancer
intact autologous haptenated irradiated tumor cells	melanoma
intact autologous GM-CSF transfected tumor cells	melanoma, renal cancer, lung cancer
autologous tumor lysates	renal cancer
HSP–peptide complexes	melanoma, renal cancer, colon cancer, chronic myeloid leukemia
shared tumor antigen approaches	melanoma
allogeneic irradiated cell lines	melanoma
differentiation antigens	melanoma
cancer/testes antigens	

Fig. 22.13 Several vaccination approaches are currently being pursued.

Selected antibodies are now approved for clinical use, but these represent pharmacological rather than immunological use of antibodies and include antibodies to:

- CD20 – rituximab – against B cell lymphoma;
- HER2/Neu – trastuzumab (Herceptin®) – against breast cancer;
- epidermal growth factor receptor – cetuximab (Erbitux®) – against colon cancer.

It is ironic that the anti-tumor antibodies that may recognize truly or relatively tumor-specific molecules, and that were the earliest hopes of much of the efforts in this area, have yet to enter the phase of randomized clinical testing. Such antibodies are difficult to characterize and therefore have been slow in development.

Vaccination can be used to treat cancer

Although the term vaccination is typically used to indicate prophylactic vaccination, cancer researchers use it to indicate the treatment of someone who already has cancer, with agents that stimulate anti-cancer immune response. Several vaccination approaches are currently being pursued (Fig. 22.13).

The idiotypes of B lymphomas have been used as vaccines

Following the use of anti-idiotypic antibodies and the attendant limitations discussed above, the idiotypes of B lymphomas have been used as vaccines. In this approach, a patient's idiotype is determined by polymerase chain reactions from the tumor tissues, and a synthetic idiotype, conjugated to a carrier such as keyhole limpet hemocyanin, is administered along with GM-CSF. A phase III trial in patients with follicular B lymphoma has been completed recently. Of the 117 patients who were in complete remission after chemotherapy, median time to relapse for the 76 vaccinated patients was 44.2 months, compared with 30.6 months for the 41 who received placebo. This was the first, and thus far, the only vaccine that has shown significant clinical activity in B cell lymphoma. For obvious reasons, this approach is limited to B lymphoma and related hematological malignancies.

Q. Which other group of cells is (theoretically) susceptible to anti-idiotypic targeting of tumor therapy?
A. The recombined T cell receptor is also expressed on specific clones of cells. The limitations that apply to the therapy of B cell lymphomas (mutation escape) also apply here, and it is in any case more difficult to generate antibodies to the T cell receptor.

Immunotherapy with DCs presenting a prostate antigen shows clinical benefit

In such studies, DCs are isolated from a cancer patient, pulsed with antigenic peptides, whole proteins, or tumor lysates and infused back into the patient. The most advanced clinical trials with this approach have been carried out in patients with prostate cancer, using the protein prostatic acid phosphatase because of the prostate-specific distribution of this protein, and because of its low homology with non-prostate proteins. Patients' antigen presenting cells are pulsed with a fusion protein consisting of prostatic acid phosphatase and GM-CSF, and are re-infused into the patient. In a randomized Phase 3 trial in 512 subjects, prostate cancer patients who received the acid phosphatase pulsed autologous APCs (Sipuleucel-T) showed a median survival of 25.8 months as compared to 21.7 months for patients who received placebo. This trial formed the basis of the FDA approval of this treatment for patients with asymptomatic or minimally symptomatic prostate cancer.

Immunization with HSP–peptide complexes demonstrates clinical benefit

The role of HSP–peptide complexes in eliciting tumor immunity has been discussed earlier.

The successful murine studies have been translated into a series of phase I and II trials involving patients with pancreatic, gastric, stomach, and renal cancers, and with melanoma, B lymphoma, and chronic myelogenous leukemia.

In these trials, surgically obtained tumor specimens (or leukemia cells obtained by leukopheresis) from a given patient are used as the starting material for preparation of gp96–peptide or hsp70–peptide complexes specifically for that patient (Fig. 22.14).

In a randomized phase 3 study in subjects with non-metastatic renal cell carcinoma, no difference was seen in recurrence-free survival between patients who received the autologous tumor-derived gp96–peptide vaccine (vitespen) and those who received no treatment. However, in

Treatment of cancer patients with HSP–peptide complexes

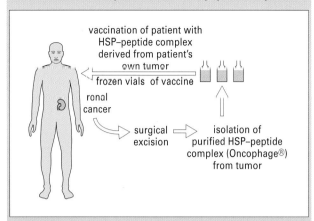

Fig. 22.14 Surgically obtained tumor specimens from a given patient are used as the starting material for preparation of gp96–peptide or HSP70–peptide complexes specifically for that patient.

Adoptive immunotherapy with T cells

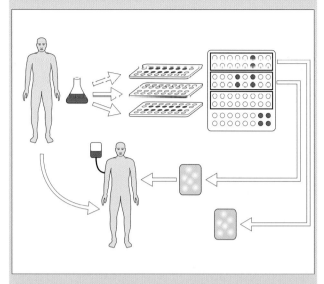

Fig. 22.15 Lymphocytes removed from a patient with a tumor are expanded *in vitro*. Cells that recognize the tumor are selected and reinfused into the original patient. Adoptive therapy with allogeneic lymphocytes may also be carried out. *(Redrawn from Dudley ME, Rosenberg SA. Adoptive-cell-transfer therapy for the treatment of patients with cancer. Nat Rev Cancer 2003;3:666–675. Copyright 2002, Nature Reviews Cancer, Macmillan Magazines Ltd.)*

the sub-set of patients with stage I and II disease the risk of recurrence among the 125 patients who received vitespen was approximately half the corresponding risk in 115 untreated patients ($p=0.056$). Moreover, in a sub-set of subjects with intermediate-risk disease the risk of recurrence among the patients who received vitespen was significantly reduced. Based on these data, the gp96–peptide vaccine vitespen was approved for use for intermediate-risk non-metastatic renal cell carcinoma patients in Russia.

Adoptive immunotherapy using T cells: the clinical benefits

Adoptive immunotherapy using T cells has a successful pedigree in murine models of cancer (Fig. 22.15). Clinical experience with bone marrow transplant recipients also provides a strong rationale for the approach.

Patients undergoing high-dose chemotherapy lose their bone marrow and are re-constituted with allogeneic stem cells, which engraft in the recipient. However, the T cells from the donor may see the normal tissues of the host as foreign, thus causing graft versus host disease (GVHD).

Interestingly, patients who develop GVHD also have a lower cancer relapse or graft versus tumor (GVT) incidence. The clinical experience with GVHD and GVT has long remained a compelling piece of evidence for the premise that T cells can eliminate human cancers *in vivo* (Fig. 22.16).

A number of studies have isolated tumor-infiltrating T cells from cancer patients, expanded them *in vitro* and infused the expanded cells back into the patients. Such studies have shown remarkable shrinkage of tumors in significant proportions of patients in non-randomized clinical studies.

In a variation of this approach, cloned T cells with defined specificity have been expanded to very large numbers and infused into patients with melanoma, showing dramatic tumor shrinkage.

However, hurdles to expansion of T cells as well as their effector functions *in vivo* remain, and there is considerable ongoing experimental effort to engineer T cells that will retain specificity and autonomy of growth and will be relatively refractory to downregulatory influences of the host.

Inhibition of downregulation of immune modulation is clinically valuable

The role of downregulation of tumor immunity in progressive tumor growth in mouse models has been discussed above. Inhibition of such downregulation is an attractive target of translation and antibodies to CTLA-4 are under clinical testing in this regard. A number of phase I and II clinical trials using antibodies to CTLA-4 have been completed in patients with melanoma and ovarian and renal cancer.

The most dramatic results have been obtained in patients who had previously been vaccinated with autologous GM-CSF transfected tumor cells as part of another study and had not shown significant response to that vaccination. When these patients were treated with anti-CTLA-4 antibody, they showed dramatic tumor shrinkage and infiltration of the tumors with lymphocytes and granulocytes.

Interestingly, patients previously immunized with differentiation antigen vaccines and who received the same anti-CTLA-4 antibody did not show clinical responses.

The synergy between vaccination with GM-CSF transfected tumor cells and administration of anti-CTLA-4 antibody was also previously seen in a mouse model of melanoma. Further clinical exploration of this attractive strategy is now in progress.

Graft versus host disease and graft versus tumor

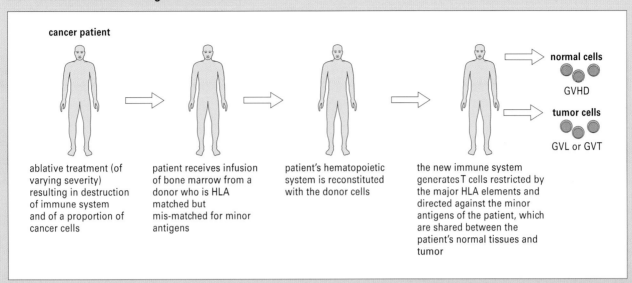

cancer patient

ablative treatment (of varying severity) resulting in destruction of immune system and of a proportion of cancer cells

patient receives infusion of bone marrow from a donor who is HLA matched but mis-matched for minor antigens

patient's hematopoietic system is reconstituted with the donor cells

the new immune system generates T cells restricted by the major HLA elements and directed against the minor antigens of the patient, which are shared between the patient's normal tissues and tumor

normal cells
GVHD

tumor cells
GVL or GVT

Fig. 22.16 Graft versus host disease (GVHD) and graft versus leukemia (GVL) effects. Both responses are restricted by the MHC alleles and directed against the minor antigens. The minor antigens are the same between the patient's normal tissues and tumor, hence the GVHD (immune response against normal tissues) and GVL (immune response against leukemia or other tumor) are generally inextricably linked. (GVT, graft versus tumor.)

CRITICAL THINKING: IMMUNITY TO CANCERS (SEE P. 441 FOR EXPLANATIONS)

1 Animals can be easily immunized against cancers. Why then do the same cancers grow progressively and kill their hosts?

2 Heat-shock proteins do not differ between tumors and normal tissues. Yet, HSP preparations isolated from tumors elicit tumor immunity, whereas similar preparations from normal tissues do not. Explain the mechanistic basis of this phenomenon.

3 How have tumor antigens been defined? How many classes of tumor antigen have been defined thus far?

4 Explain the phenomenon of concomitant immunity.

5 Discuss the evidence that the immune response to tumors is downregulated in tumor-bearing mice and in patients with cancer.

Further reading

Belli F, Testori A, Rivoltini L, et al. Vaccination of metastatic melanoma patients with autologous tumor-derived heat shock protein gp96–peptide complexes: clinical and immunologic findings. J Clin Oncol 2002;20:4169–4180.

Coulie PG, Karanikas V, Lurquin C, et al. Cytolytic T-cell responses of cancer patients vaccinated with a MAGE antigen. Immunol Rev 2002;188:33–42.

Egen JG, Kuhns MS, Allison JP. CTLA-4: new insights into its biological function and use in tumor immunotherapy. Nat Immunol 2002;3:611–618.

Fehervari Z, Sakaguchi S. CD4$^+$ Tregs and immune control. J Clin Invest 2004;114:1209–1217.

Ho WY, Blattman JN, Dossett ML, et al. Adoptive immunotherapy: engineering T cell responses as biologic weapons for tumor mass destruction. Cancer Cell 2003;3:431–437.

Klein G. The strange road to the tumor-specific transplantation antigens (TSTAs). Cancer Immun 2001;1:6.

North RJ. Down-regulation of the antitumor immune response. Adv Cancer Res 1985;45:1–43.

Scanlan MJ, Gure AO, Jungbluth AA, et al. Cancer/testis antigens: an expanding family of targets for cancer immunotherapy. Immunol Rev 2002;188:22–32.

Srivastava PK. Do human cancers express shared protective antigens? or the necessity of remembrance of things past. Semin Immunol 1996;8:295–302.

Srivastava PK. Interaction of heat shock proteins with peptides and antigen presenting cells: chaperoning of the innate and adaptive immune responses. Annu Rev Immunol 2002;20:395–425.

Van Der Bruggen P, Zhang Y, Chaux P, et al. Tumor-specific shared antigenic peptides recognized by human T cells. Immunol Rev 2002;188:51–64.

Wick M, Dubey P, Koeppen H, et al. Antigenic cancer cells grow progressively in immune hosts without evidence for T cell exhaustion or systemic anergy. J Exp Med 1997;186:229–238.

Hypersensitivity

CHAPTER 23

Immediate Hypersensitivity (Type I)

SUMMARY

- **The classification of hypersensitivity reactions is based on the system proposed by Coombs and Gell.**

- **Historical observations have shaped our understanding of immediate hypersensitivity.** The severity of symptoms depends on IgE antibodies, the quantity of allergen, and also a variety of factors that can enhance the response including viral infections and environmental pollutants.

- **Most allergens are proteins.**

- **Production of IgE depends on genotype.** In genetically predisposed individuals, IgE production occurs in response to repeated low-dose exposure to inhaled allergens such as dust mite, cat dander, or grass pollen.

- **Allergens are the antigens that give rise to immediate hypersensitivity and contribute to asthma rhinitis or food allergy.**

- **Mast cells and basophils contain histamine.** IgE antibodies bind to a specific receptor, FcεRI, on mast

cells and basophils. This Fc receptor has a very high affinity, and when bound IgE is cross-linked by specific allergen, mediators including histamine, leukotrienes, and cytokines are released.

- **Multiple genes have been associated with asthma in different populations.** Multiple genetic loci influence the production of IgE, the inflammatory response to allergen exposure, and the response to treatment. Polymorphisms have been identified in the genes, in promoter regions, and in the receptors for IgE, cytokines, leukotrienes, and the β_2-receptors.

- **Skin tests are used for diagnosis and as a guide to treatment.**

- **Several different pathways contribute to the chronic symptoms of allergy.**

- **Immunotherapy can be used for hayfever and anaphylactic sensitivity.**

- **New approaches are being investigated for treating allergic disease.**

Classification of hypersensitivity reactions

The adaptive immune response provides specific protection against infection with bacteria, viruses, parasites, and fungi. Some immune responses, however, give rise to an excessive or inappropriate reaction – this is usually referred to as **hypersensitivity**.

The term hypersensitivity evolved from the observations of Richet and Portier one hundred years ago, who described the catastrophic result of exposing a pre-sensitized animal to systemic antigen. The resulting outcome, termed **anaphylaxis**, became the prototype of immediate hypersensitivity responses.

Coombs and Gell in 1963 proposed a classification scheme in which allergic hypersensitivity of the type described by Portier and Richet was termed type I, and broadened the definition of hypersensitivity to include:

- **Immediate (Type I) hypersensitivity responses** are characterized by the production of IgE antibodies against

foreign proteins that are commonly present in the environment (e.g. pollens, animal danders, or house dust mites) and can be identified by wheal and flare responses to skin tests which develop within 15 minutes.

- **Antibody-mediated (Type II) hypersensitivity reactions** occur when IgG or IgM antibodies are produced against surface antigens on cells of the body. These antibodies can trigger reactions either by activating complement (e.g. autoimmune hemolytic anemia) or by facilitating the binding of natural killer cells (see Chapter 24);.

- **Immune complex diseases (Type III hypersensitivity)** involve the formation of immune complexes in the circulation that are not adequately cleared by macrophages or other cells of the reticuloendothelial system. The formation of immune complexes requires significant quantities of antibody and antigen (typically microgram quantities of each). The classical diseases of this group are systemic lupus erythematosus (SLE),

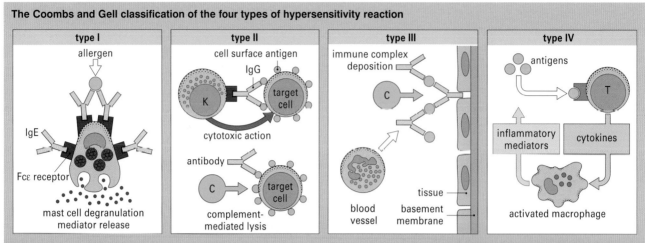

The Coombs and Gell classification of the four types of hypersensitivity reaction

Fig. 23.1 In type I hypersensitivity, mast cells bind IgE via their Fc receptors. On encountering allergen the IgE becomes cross-linked, inducing degranulation and release of mediators that produce allergic reactions. In type II, antibody is directed against antigen on an individual's own cells (target cell) or foreign antigen, such as transfused red blood cells. This may lead to cytotoxic action by K cells, or complement-mediated lysis. In type III, immune complexes are deposited in the tissue. Complement is activated and polymorphs are attracted to the site of deposition, causing local tissue damage and inflammation. In type IV, antigen-sensitized T cells release lymphokines following a secondary contact with the same antigen. Cytokines induce inflammatory reactions and activate and attract macrophages, which release inflammatory mediators.

chronic glomerulonephritis, and serum sickness (see Chapter 25).

- **Cell-mediated reactions (Type IV hypersensitivity)** are those in which specific T cells are the primary effector cells (see Chapter 26). Examples of T cells causing unwanted responses are:

  - contact sensitivity (e.g. to nickel or plants such as poison ivy);
  - the delayed hypersensitivity responses of leprosy or tuberculosis;
  - the exaggerated response to viral infections such as measles; and
  - the persistent symptoms of allergic disease.

The original Coombs and Gell classification is shown in Figure 23.1.

In the past several years it has become apparent that the Coombs and Gell classification artificially divided mechanistically related antibody reactions (such as types I, II, and III), which contribute to the pathophysiology of many common immune-mediated diseases, while including the T cell-mediated reactions of delayed-type hypersensitivity (DTH) in a common classification (termed type IV).

Based on our current understanding of the underlying pathways of inflammation triggered by antigen exposure and the disease conditions observed, common mechanisms appear to operate in types I, II, and III hypersensitivity. These common mechanisms involve the engagement by antibody–antigen complexes with cellular receptors for the Fc region of antibodies (termed **Fc receptors**).

Historical perspective on immediate hypersensitivity

The first allergic disease to be defined was seasonal hayfever caused by pollen grains (which have a defined season of weeks or months) entering the nose (rhinitis) and eyes (conjunctivitis). In severe cases patients may also get seasonal asthma and seasonal dermatitis. Charles Blackley, in 1873, demonstrated that pollen grains placed into the nose could induce symptoms of rhinitis. He also demonstrated that pollen extract could produce a wheal and flare skin response in patients with hayfever.

The **wheal and flare skin response** is an extremely sensitive method of detecting specific IgE antibodies. The timing and form of the skin response is indistinguishable from the local reaction to injected histamine. Furthermore, the immediate skin response can be effectively blocked with antihistamines.

In 1903, Portier and Richet discovered that immunization of guinea pigs with a toxin from the jellyfish *Physalia* could sensitize them so that a subsequent injection of the same protein would cause rapid onset of breathing difficulty, influx of fluid into the lungs, and death. They coined the term **anaphylaxis** (from the Greek *ana*, non, and *phylaxos*, protection) and speculated about the relationship to other hypersensitivity diseases. They noted that:

- human anaphylaxis had no familial characteristics (unlike most of the other allergic diseases); and
- natural exposure to inhaled allergens did not cause anaphylaxis or urticaria.

Subsequently, it became clear that injection of any protein into an individual with immediate hypersensitivity to that protein can induce anaphylaxis. Thus, anaphylaxis occurs when a patient with immediate hypersensitivity is exposed to a relevant allergen in such a way that the antigen enters the circulation rapidly.

Q. In what circumstances can large amounts of allergen enter the circulation rapidly?

A. Following direct injection of the antigen into the tissue, such as a bee sting, a therapeutic injection for hyposensitization, or injection of a drug, e.g. penicillin.

Anaphylaxis may also occur as a result of eating an allergen such as peanut or shellfish, or following the rupture of hydatid cysts with the rapid release of parasite antigens (Fig. 23.2).

Anaphylaxis and urticaria

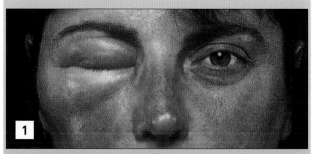

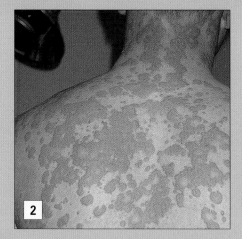

Fig. 23.2 (1) The anaphylactic response to bee venom in a patient who has IgE antibodies to the venom protein, phospholipase A. The immediate reaction occurs within 20 minutes and is mediated by the release of histamine and other mediators from mast cells. The patient shown had been stung on the face, but the reaction can become generalized, leading to a fall in blood pressure, generalized urticaria, and/or bronchospasm (i.e. anaphylaxis). (2) Diffuse urticaria on a patient with severe chronic urticaria. The lesions have a raised edge and come up within minutes or hours. The lesions almost always resolve within 12 hours leaving no trace on the skin.

The term **allergen** was first used by von Pirquet in 1906 to cover all foreign substances that could produce an immune response. Subsequently, the word 'allergen' came to be used selectively for the proteins that cause 'supersensitivity'. Thus, **an allergen is an antigen that gives rise to immediate hypersensitivity.**

Characteristics of type I reactions

Most allergens are proteins

Substances that can give rise to wheal and flare responses in the skin and to the symptoms of allergic disease are derived from many different sources (see http://www.allergen.org/). When purified they are almost all found to be proteins and their sizes range from 10–40 kDa. These proteins are all freely soluble in aqueous solution, but have many different biological functions including digestive enzymes, carrier proteins, calycins, and pollen recognition proteins.

Any allergen can be described or classified by its source, route of exposure, and nature of the specific protein (Fig. 23.3).

Extracts used for skin testing or *in-vitro* measurement of IgE antibodies are made from the whole material, which contains multiple different proteins, any of which can be an allergen. Indeed, it is clear that individual patients can react selectively to one or more of the different proteins that are present in an extract.

> **Q. Name one genetic factor that determines whether an individual can make an immune response to a specific allergen.**
> A. The individual's MHC haplotypes determine which antigens and antigen fragments are presented to T cells.

Estimates of exposure can be made either by visual identification of particles (e.g. pollen grains or fungal spores) or by immunoassay of the major allergens (e.g. Fel d1 or Der p1).

IgE is distinct from the other dimeric immunoglobulins

In 1921, Küstner, who was allergic to fish, injected his own serum into the skin of Prausnitz, who was allergic to grass pollen but not fish, and demonstrated that it was possible to passively transfer immediate hypersensitivity (the Prausnitz–Küstner or P–K test). Prausnitz also noticed that an immediate wheal and flare occurred at the site of passive sensitization when he ate fish. This showed that some protein or part of fish proteins sufficient to trigger mast cells can be absorbed into the circulation.

Over the next 30 years it was established that P–K activity was a general property of the serum of patients with immediate hypersensitivity and that it was allergen specific (i.e. it behaved like an antibody).

In 1967 Ishizaka and his colleagues purified the P–K activity from a patient with ragweed hayfever and proved that this was a novel isotype of immunoglobulin – IgE. However, it was obvious that the concentration of this immunoglobulin isotype in serum was very low i.e. ≤ 1 µg/mL.

IgE is distinct from the other dimeric immunoglobulins because it has:

* an extra constant region domain;
* a different structure to the hinge region; and
* binding sites for both **high-** and **low-affinity IgE receptors, FcεRI** and **FcεRII**, respectively (see Fig. 3.19).

The primary cells that bear FcεRI are **mast cells** and **basophils**, which are the only cells in the human that contain significant amounts of histamine.

Low-affinity receptors for IgE – FcεRII or CD23 – are also present on B cells and may play a role in antigen presentation.

In addition in atopic dermatitis dendritic cells in skin can express a high-affinity receptor for IgE, but this receptor lacks the β chain of FcεRI.

The properties of IgE can be separated into three areas:

* the characteristics of the molecule including its half-life and binding to IgE receptors;
* the control of IgE and IgG antibody production by T cells; and
* the consequences of allergen cross-linking IgE on the surface of mast cells or basophils.

Properties of allergens

source	airborne particles	dimension of airborne particle (μm)	allergen		
			name	MW (kDa)	function/homologies
dust mite – *Dermatophagoides pteronyssinus*	feces	10–40	Der p1 Der p2	25 13	cysteine protease (epididymal protein)
cats – *Felis domesticus*	dander particles	2–15	Fel d1	36	uteroglobin
German cockroach – *Blattella germanica*	frass, saliva and other debris	≥ 5	Bla g2 Bla g4 Bla g5	36 21 23	aspartic protease calycin glutathione-*S*-transferase
rat – *Rattus norvegicus*	urine on bedding ?	2–20	Rat n1	19	pheromone binding protein
grass	pollen	30	Lol p1	29	not known
fungi – *Alternaria alternata,* *Aspergillus fumigatus*	spores spores	14 × 10 2	Alt a1 Asp f1	28 18	not known mitogillin

Fig. 23.3 Patients who become 'allergic' to one of the well-recognized sources of allergens have actually produced an IgE antibody response to one or more of the proteins produced by mites, trees, grass, cats, or fungi. The proteins are predominantly water soluble with a molecular weight (MW) ranging from 10–40 kDa. In many cases the function of the proteins is known, but it is not clear whether function such as enzymic activity alters the ability of these proteins to induce an allergic response. The properties of the particles carrying these allergens are very important because they influence both how much becomes airborne, and also where the allergen is deposited in the respiratory tract. The dimensions of the particles airborne vary from ≤2 μm for *Aspergillus* or *Penicillium* spores to ≥20 μm for mite fecal pellets and some pollen grains. (Sizes are given as diameter in μm. For a full list of allergens see http://www.allergen.org/.)

The half-life of IgE is short compared with that of other immunoglobulins

The concentration of IgE in the serum of normal individuals is very low compared to all the other immunoglobulin isotypes. Values range from <10–10 000 IU/mL, and the international unit (IU) is equivalent to 2.4 ng. Most sera contain <400 IU/mL (i.e. <1 μg/mL). The reasons why serum IgE is so low include:

- serum IgE has a much shorter half-life than other isotypes (~2 days compared with 21–23 days for IgG);
- IgE is produced in small quantities and is only produced in response to a select group of antigens (allergens and parasites); and
- IgE antibodies are sequestered on the high-affinity receptor on mast cells and basophils.

Q. What fundamental reason explains the low production of IgE?

A. The class switch from IgM to IgE happens infrequently and is controlled by T cells. The position of the IgE constant region gene is towards the distal end of the Ig gene stack (see Fig. 9.17), but the position alone cannot explain the infrequency of the switch to IgE.

The half-life of IgE in the serum has been measured both by injecting radiolabeled IgE and by infusing plasma from allergic patients into normal and immune-deficient patients.

The half-life of IgE in serum is less than 2 days; by contrast, IgE bound to mast cells in the skin has a half-life of approximately 10 days.

The low quantities of IgE in the serum must reflect a more rapid breakdown of IgE, as well as removal from the circulation by binding onto mast cells.

The most important site of breakdown of IgE is thought to be within **endosomes** where the low pH facilitates breakdown of free immunoglobulin by cathepsin.

Serum is constantly being taken up by endocytosis. Many macromolecules including IgE degrade in the endosome. One major exception is IgG, which is protected by binding to the neonatal Fc gamma receptor, FcγRn (Fig. 23.4).

IgG4 is transferred across the placenta, but IgE is not

In cord blood the concentration of IgE is very low, generally <1 IU/mL (i.e. <2 ng/mL). Thus, there appears to be almost no transfer across the placenta.

By contrast, IgG, including IgG4 antibodies to allergens such as those from dust mite or cat, are very efficiently transferred across the placenta. This process also involves endocytosis and receptor-mediated transport.

Passive transfer of IgE to the fetus may be blocked because IgE is broken down in the endosomes, or because an Fc receptor that is essential for transport is absent on the cells that comprise the placental tissues. In prenatal transfer, IgG is protected in endosomes by binding to FcγRn.

Endocytosis of plasma

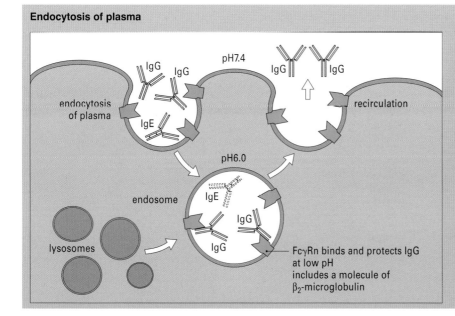

Fig. 23.4 Endocytosis of plasma contributes to the short half-life of IgE as plasma proteins are taken up and the pH falls because of lysosomes combining with the endosome. At low pH IgG including IgG4 molecules bind to the neonatal Fc γ receptor (FcγRn). By contrast, IgE molecules do not bind to FcγRn so are not protected and are digested by cathepsin. As the endosomes recirculate, the pH rises to 7.4 and the undamaged IgG molecules are released into the circulation. The FcγRn includes a molecule of β_2-microglobulin. In keeping with this model the half-life of IgG is shorter than normal in mice that have had the gene for β_2-microglobulin removed (or knocked out).

T cells control the response to inhalant allergens

IgE production is dependent on Th2 cells

Experiments in animals have established that the production of IgE is dependent on T cells. It is also clear that T cells can suppress IgE production.

T cells that suppress Th2 responses including IgE production:

- act predominantly by producing interferon-γ (IFNγ); and
- are produced when the animal (e.g. mouse, rat, or rabbit) is primed in the presence of Freund's complete adjuvant.

This adjuvant, which includes bacterial cell walls and probably bacterial DNA, is a very potent activator of macrophages.

With the discovery of Th1 and Th2 cells, it became clear that IgE production is dependent on Th2 cells and that any priming that generates a Th1 response will inhibit IgE production.

The main cytokines that are specifically relevant to a Th1 response include:

- interleukin-12 (IL-12) produced by macrophages; and
- IFNγ produced by T cells.

By contrast, the primary cytokines relevant to a Th2 response are:

- IL-4 and IL13;
- IL-5; and
- IL-10 (Fig. 23.5).

It is clear from experiments in mice and humans that the expression of the gene for IgE is dependent on IL-4. Thus, if immature human B cells are cultured with anti-CD40 and IL-4, they will produce IgE antibodies.

Cytokines regulate the production of IgE

In humans IgE antibodies are the dominant feature of the response to a select group of antigens and most other immune responses do not include IgE.

The classical allergens are inhaled in very small quantities (5–20 ng/day) either perennially indoors or over a period of weeks or months outdoors. Immunization of mice with repeated low-dose antigen is a very effective method of inducing IgE responses.

By contrast, the routine immunization of children with diphtheria and tetanus toxoid does not induce persistent production of IgE antibodies. This is clear because we do not routinely take precautions against anaphylaxis when administering a booster injection of tetanus.

> **Q. In which tissues do Th2-type immune responses predominate, and in which tissues are Th1 responses promoted?**
> A. Th2 responses predominate in mucosal tissues, whereas Th1 responses predominate in the skin and CNS (see Chapter 12).

As T cells differentiate, Th1 cells express the functional IL-12 receptor with the IL-12 β2 chain. By contrast, Th2 cells express only part of the IL-12 receptor and this part is non-functional.

IL-4 is important in the differentiation of Th2 cells and is also a growth factor for these cells. Because it is produced by Th2 cells, it is at least in part acting on the cell that produced it (i.e. in an autocrine fashion). The interaction of IL-4 with T cells can be blocked either with:

- an antibody to IL-4; or
- a soluble form of the IL-4 receptor (IL-4R).

The release of soluble IL-4R from T cells may be a natural mechanism for controlling T cell differentiation. However, recent evidence suggests that in-vivo responses are controlled by T cells producing either IL-10 or transforming growth factor-β (TGFβ).

Both IgE and IgG4 are dependent on IL-4

The genes for immunoglobulin heavy chains are in sequence on chromosome 14. The gene for ε occurs directly following the gene for γ4. Both of these isotypes are

T cell differentiation during human immune responses

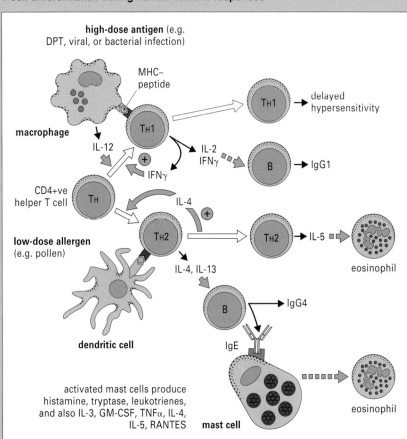

Fig. 23.5 The differentiation of TH cells depends on the antigen source, the quantity of allergen, and the cytokines produced. Bacterial antigens or a high dose of antigen will induce IL-12 from macrophages. In addition, the developing TH1 cells produce IFNγ, which further enhances the production of TH1 cells. Low-dose antigen without adjuvant will induce TH2 cells, which produce both IL-4 and IL-5. IL-4 plays a role in (i) enhancing the growth of TH2 cells; (ii) the expression of the gene for IgE. In turn IgE binds to the high-affinity receptor for IgE (FcεRI) on mast cells. IL-5 plays a critical role in the production of eosinophils.

Immunoglobulin genes on chromosome 14: two models of rearrangement to allow expression of the IgE gene

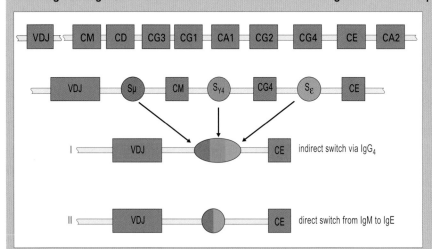

Fig. 23.6 Switch regions and heavy chain genes for immunoglobulin are arranged sequentially on chromosome 14. Both Cγ4 and Cε expression are dependent on IL-4 produced by T cells. The switch region of IgE often includes elements from Sγ4 indicating that the switching occurs sequentially. However, IgG4 responses can occur without IgE antibody responses.

dependent on IL-4 and they may be expressed sequentially (Fig. 23.6).

The mechanisms by which IgG4 is controlled separately from IgE are not well understood, but this may include a role for IL-10. Thus, immunotherapy for patients with anaphylactic sensitivity to honey bee venom will induce IL-10 production by T cells, decreased IgE, and increased IgG4 antibodies to venom antigens.

Recently, it has been shown that children raised in a house with a cat can produce an IgG response, including IgG4 antibody, without becoming allergic. A modified TH2 response (increased IgG4 and decreased IgE) therefore

Modified TH2 response

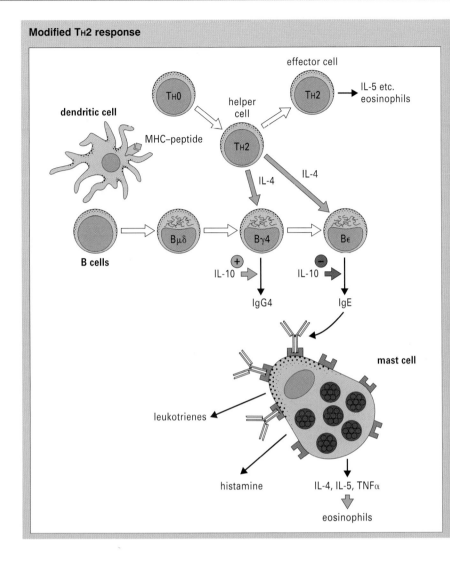

Fig. 23.7 The TH2 response includes T effector cells as well as help for IgE and IgG4 antibody production. In turn IgE plays a major role in triggering mast cells. However, increasing evidence shows that higher doses of allergen (e.g. bee venom, cat dander, or rat urine) can induce a modified or tolerant TH2 response. This response includes IgG4 antibodies, but not IgE. The cytokine IL-10 may well play a role in enhancing IgG4 antibody while suppressing production of IgE.

represents an important mechanism of tolerance to allergens (Fig. 23.7). IgG4 antibody responses without IgE antibody are a feature of immunity/tolerance to insect venom, rat urinary allergens, and food antigens as well as cat allergens.

Characteristics of allergens

Allergens have similar physical properties

In mice a wide range of proteins can be used to induce an IgE antibody response. The primary factors that influence the response are:

- the strain of mouse;
- the dose; and
- adjuvants used.

Thus, repeated low-dose immunization with alum or pertussis (but not complete Freund's adjuvant) will produce IgE responses. However, the dose necessary to induce an optimal response varies greatly from one strain to another.

The allergens that have been defined have similar physical properties (i.e. freely soluble in aqueous solution with a molecular weight of 10–40 kDa), but are diverse biologically. Cloning has revealed sequence homology between allergens and proteins including calycins, pheromone binding proteins,

enzymes, and pollen recognition proteins. Although many of the allergens have homology with known enzymes, this is not surprising because enzymic activity is an important property of proteins in general. Some important allergens, for example Der p2 from mites, Fel d1 from cats, and Amb a5 from ragweed pollen, have neither enzymic activity nor homology with known enzymes. Thus, enzymic activity is not essential for immunogenicity.

Nevertheless, the group I allergens of dust mites are cysteine proteases and in several model situations it has been shown that this enzymic activity influences the immunogenicity of the protein. Thus cleavage of CD23 or CD25 on lymphocytes by Der p1 can enhance immune responses. Alternatively, it has been shown that Der p1 can disrupt epithelial junctions and alter the entry of proteins through the epithelial layer. The interest in this property is increased because many different mite allergens are inhaled together in the fecal particles so the enzymic activity of one protein (i.e. Der p1) could facilitate either the physical entry or the immune response to other mite proteins.

The primary characterization of allergens relates to their route of exposure. The routes includes:

- inhaled allergens;
- foods;

- drugs;
- antigens from fungi growing on the body (e.g. *Aspergillus* spp.); and
- venoms.

The routes are important because they define the ways in which the antigens are presented to the immune system. Antigen presentation may well be the site at which genetic influences play the biggest role, the properties of the different groups of allergen need to be considered separately.

The inhalant allergens cause hayfever, chronic rhinitis, and asthma

The inhalant allergens are the primary causal agents in hayfever, chronic rhinitis, and asthma among school-aged children and young adults and they play an important role in atopic dermatitis.

Allergens can only become airborne in sufficient quantity to cause an immune response or symptoms when they are carried on particles. Pollen grains, mite fecal particles, particles of fungal hyphae or spores, and animal skin flakes (or dander) are the best defined forms in which allergens are inhaled (Fig. 23.8).

In each case it is possible to define the approximate particle size and the quantity of protein on the particle as well as the speed with which the proteins in the particle dissolve in aqueous solution (see Fig. 23.3).

Thus, for grass pollen, mite fecal pellets, and cat dander:

- the relevant allergens are present in high concentrations within the particles (up to 10 mg/cm^3);
- the particles are 'large' (i.e. 3–30 μm diameter); and
- the allergens elute rapidly in aqueous solution.

The allergens within these particles will be delivered to the nasal epithelium and the local lymph nodes because a large proportion of particles of this size will impact on the mucous membrane during passage of inhaled air through the nose.

Small quantities of inhalant allergen cause immediate hypersensitivity

Estimates of the quantity of mite or pollen-derived proteins inhaled vary from 5–50 ng/day. Thus exposure to some allergens may be as little as 1 μg/year. This is important because it probably explains:

- why the immune response is consistently of this one kind (i.e. immediate hypersensitivity); and
- why no respiratory diseases, other than asthma, have been associated with these allergens.

The quantities inhaled also seriously restrict the models about how allergens contribute to asthma. Inhaling a small number (i.e. 10–100) of 'large' particles (10–30 μm in diameter) per day could produce local areas of inflammation but would not be expected give rise to alveolitis, acute bronchospasm, or progressive lung fibrosis.

Only a small number of food proteins are common causes of allergic responses

Although many food proteins can occasionally give rise to IgE responses, only a small number are common causes of food allergy. These include egg, milk, wheat, soy, tree nuts, peanut, fish, and shellfish. In contrast to inhaled allergens,

these proteins are often eaten in very large quantities (i.e. ≈10–100 g/day). In general only a small fraction of these food proteins is absorbed. However, small peptides can be freely absorbed and may be recognized by T cells and even by IgE antibodies in a minority of individuals. Nevertheless, the bulk of the allergic and anaphylactic responses to foods are thought to be related to food proteins that have not been digested, either triggering mast cells in the intestine or entering the circulation.

Q. Recent evidence from Dr Sampson and his colleagues has shown that some children produce IgE antibodies against linear epitopes on food allergens. What implication does this have for induction of allergy in cooked food?

A. Denaturation of a protein by heat will not destroy linear epitopes, consequently cooking will not alter the allergenicity.

Particles carrying airborne allergens – mite fecal pellets and pollen grains

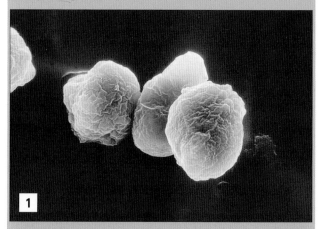

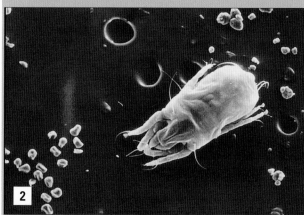

Fig. 23.8 The dust mite is the most important source of allergen in house dust, largely as fecal particles (**1**). A mite is shown in (**2**) with pollen grains lower left and fecal particles upper right. The mite is approximately 300 μm in length (i.e. just visible but not small enough to become airborne). Mite fecal particles are approximately 10–40 μm in diameter and become airborne during domestic disturbance. Pollen grains are similar in size to mite fecal particles (i.e. approximately 30 μm in diameter). The important allergic sources of pollen (i.e. grass, ragweed, and trees) are wind pollinated and the grains are designed to travel in the air for long distances.

Desensitization can be used to control type I hypersensitivity

Given the importance of T cells to the control of IgE antibody production and their potential role in the recruitment of inflammatory cells, it is logical to try treatments which directly 'desensitize' T cells. The approaches used include treatments with modified allergens, including:

- allergen molecules modified *in vitro* by formaldehyde or glutaraldehyde (allergoids);
- site-directed mutagenesis;
- allergens combined with two to four molecules of CpG;
- peptides of 12–35 amino acids.

Therapeutic trials have been carried out with peptides from ragweed pollen antigens and the cat allergen Fel d1. The results show that peptide recognition is restricted by the HLA-DR type of the patient, which means that a wide range of peptides are necessary for treatment. In addition, there is clear evidence that peptides can produce a significant response in the lungs (Fig. 23.9) indicating that T cells in the lung can contribute to an asthmatic response.

Late asthmatic response to peptides from cat allergen

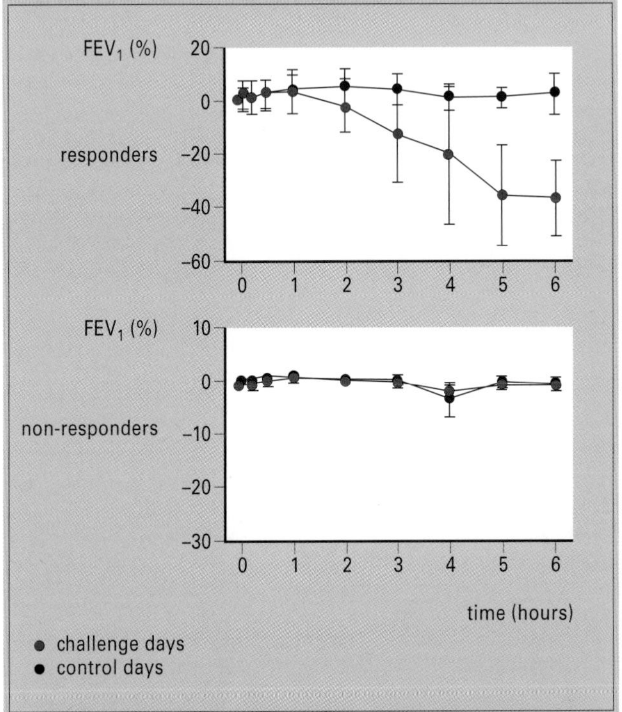

● challenge days
● control days

Fig. 23.9 Late asthmatic reactions induced in cat allergic patients by the intradermal injection of peptides derived from the cat allergen, Fel d1. The nine responders show a mean fall in forced expiratory volume in 1 second (FEV_1) of approximately 30%. The response to the peptides is MHC-restricted and correlated with the ability of the patients' T cells to respond to these peptides *in vitro*. On challenge days (red filled circle) injection of peptides was associated with a fall in FEV_1 which did not occur on the control days (black filled circle). Data are shown for nine responders (upper graph) and 31 non-responders (lower graph). *(Courtesy of Dr Mark Larché from J Exp Med 1999;189:1885.)*

Mediators released by mast cells and basophils

The only human cell types that contain histamine are mast cells and basophils. In addition, these are the only cells that express the high-affinity receptor for IgE (FcεRI) under resting conditions.

The primary and most rapid consequence of allergen exposure in an allergic individual is cross-linking of IgE receptors on mast cells and basophils:

- basophils are circulating polymorphonuclear leucocytes that are not present in normal tissue, but can be recruited to a local site by cytokines released from either T cells or mast cells;
- mast cells cannot be identified in the circulation, but are present in connective tissue and at mucosal surfaces throughout the body.

Mast cells in different tissues are morphologically and cytogenetically distinct.

Both the cells that contain histamine and the biology of these cells may be very different in other species. For example:

- in the rabbit the histamine content of the peripheral blood is almost all in platelets;
- in the mouse there are few if any circulating basophils; and
- in rats the degranulation of mast cells appears to be one granule at a time.

By contrast, in human mast cells and basophils the granules fuse with the exterior membrane and release their contents as a solution. The membrane of the granule then becomes part of the plasma membrane (Fig. 23.10).

Mast cells in different tissues have distinct granule proteases

Mast cells were originally identified by Ehrlich who named them based on the distinctive, tightly packed granules. (*Mast* means well fed, or fattening, in German.) Mast cells in different tissues can be distinguished by staining for proteases, and the content of these enzymes may be relevant to their role in allergic diseases. The granule proteases of mast cells have been cloned and sequenced and are distinct for two types of mast cell (Fig. 23.11):

- mucosal mast cells are characterized by the presence of tryptase without chymase (MCT);
- by contrast, connective tissue mast cells contain both chymase and tryptase (MCTC).

These enzymes may play a direct role in the lung inflammation of asthma, either by breaking down mediators or, in the case of tryptase, by acting as a fibroblast growth factor. Basophils contain very little of either of these proteases.

Staining of basophils in tissue sections requires special fixation and staining. Without this staining the granules in basophils cannot be identified and the cells appear as neutrophils (i.e. polymorphonuclear cells without eosinophilic or basophilic granules).

Human basophils

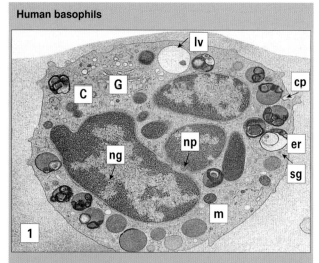

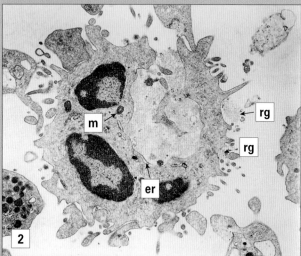

Fig. 23.10 Basophils are circulating mononuclear cells that have multilobed nuclei and distinctive granules that stain with metachromatic stains (**1**). Basophils can be recruited into local tissues such as the skin, nose, lungs, or gut by allergic and other immune responses. (**2**) A basophil degranulating 4 minutes after adding allergen. The degranulation that releases histamine occurs by fusion of the granule membrane with the external membrane of the cell. (C, centriole; cp, coated pit; er, endoplasmic reticulum; np, nuclear pore; G, Golgi apparatus; lv, lucent vesicle; m, mitochondria; ng, nuclear granule; rg, residual material from granules; sg, small granules.) *(Courtesy of Robin Hastie.)*

Differences between mast cell populations

	MMC	CTMC
location in vivo	gut and lung	ubiquitous
life span	< 40 days (?)	> 40 days (?)
T cell dependent	+	–
number of Fcε R$_1$ receptors	25 × 10^5	3 × 10^4
histamine content	+	++
cytoplasmic IgE	+	–
major AA metabolite LTC$_4$: PGD$_2$ ratio	25:1	1:40
DSGG/theophylline inhibits histamine release	–	+
major proteoglycan	chondroitin sulfate	heparin

Fig. 23.11 (**1**) There are at least two subpopulations of mast cell, the mucosal mast cells (MMCs) and the connective tissue mast cells (CTMCs). The differences in their morphology and pharmacology suggest different functional roles *in vivo*. MMCs are associated with parasitic worm infections and, possibly, allergic reactions. In contrast to the CTMC, the MMC is smaller, shorter lived, T cell dependent, has more Fcε receptors, and contains intracytoplasmic IgE. Both cells contain histamine and serotonin in their granules; the higher histamine content of the CTMC may be accounted for by the greater number of granules. Major arachidonic acid (AA) metabolites (prostaglandins [PGs] and leukotrienes [LTs]) are produced by both mast cell types, but in different amounts. For example, the ratios of production of the leukotriene LTC$_4$ to the prostaglandin PGD$_2$ are 25:1 in the MMC and 1:40 in the CTMC. The effect of drugs on degranulation is different between the two cell types. Sodium cromoglycate (DSCG) and theophylline both inhibit histamine release from the CTMC, but not from the MMC. (This may have important implications in the treatment of asthma.) Note that some of these data come from rodent studies and may not apply to humans. (**2**) Tryptase is a tetramer of 134 kDa that may comprise as much as 25% of the mast cell protein. Chymase is a monomer of 30 kDa. The relative proportions of these proteases in mast cells define MC$_T$ and MC$_{TC}$ populations, which have different distributions in human tissues. Basophils have very low amounts of both proteases. (The suffixes T and TC represent tryptase and chymase present in the respective cells.)

Cross-linking of FcεRI receptors results in degranulation

The process of degranulation in human mast cells and basophils involves fusing of the membrane of the granules containing histamine with the plasma membrane (see Fig. 23.10). The granule contents rapidly dissolve and are secreted, leaving behind a viable degranulated or partially degranulated cell. This process is initiated in most cases by cross-linking of two specific IgE molecules by their relevant allergen.

When two IgE receptors (FcεRI) are cross-linked, signal transduction through the γ chains of the receptor (see Fig. 23.12) leads to influx of calcium, which initiates both degranulation and the synthesis of newly formed mediators (Fig. 23.12).

Other mechanisms can be involved. Experimentally, degranulation can be triggered through FcεRI by using:

- anti-IgE;
- lectins such as phytohemagglutinin (PHA) or concanavalin A (Con A); or
- formyl-met-leu-phe (FMLP).

Mast cell mediator release

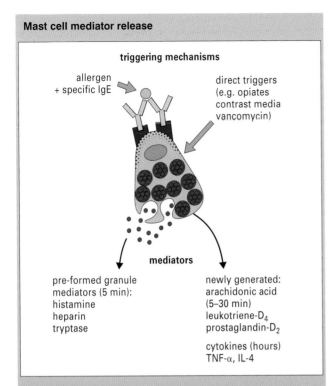

Fig. 23.12 Mast cells release mediators after cross-linking of the IgE receptors on their surface. Preformed mediators are released rapidly while arachidonic acid metabolites such as leukotriene D₄ and prostaglandin D₂ are released more slowly. Mast cells can also be triggered by opiates, contrast media, vancomycin, and the complement components C3a and C5a. The mediators, which are also released by basophils, include histamine, TNFα, and IL-4. Histamine released by mast cells can be measured in serum following anaphylaxis or extensive urticaria, but it has a half-life in minutes. By contrast, tryptase can be measured in serum for many hours after an anaphylactic reaction.

Q. Give an example of a mediator that can cause mast cell degranulation without cross-linking FcεRI.

A. Typical examples include the complement components C5a and C3a (see Fig. 6.18).

Drugs such as codeine or morphine, the antibiotic vancomycin, and contrast media used for imaging the kidneys also degranulate mast cells. Acute reactions to these agents, which are not thought to involve IgE antibodies, are referred to as **anaphylactoid**.

Genetic associations with asthma

Hayfever, asthma, and atopic dermatitis are common in allergic families. So that children with one allergic parent have a 30% chance of developing allergic disease; those who have two allergic parents have as high as a 50% chance.

Systematic studies of allergic diseases are complicated because the phenotypes for diseases, such as hayfever and asthma, are not well defined and depend on the approach used to make the diagnosis. Although on average, total IgE values increase progressively from normal, in hay fever, asthma, and atopic dermatitis, the individual values vary widely (Fig. 23.13).

Asthma defined by a patient questionnaire is therefore less specific than asthma defined by testing of specific or non-specific bronchial hyperreactivity. Furthermore, studies on asthma are complicated because several aspects are under genetic control, including

- IgE antibody responses;
- the inflammatory response to allergens;
- repair mechanisms; and
- bronchial reactivity.

Indeed, it is important not to confuse simple genetic diseases like cystic fibrosis or hemophilia with complex traits such as asthma or type II diabetes mellitus.

IgE levels and atopic disease

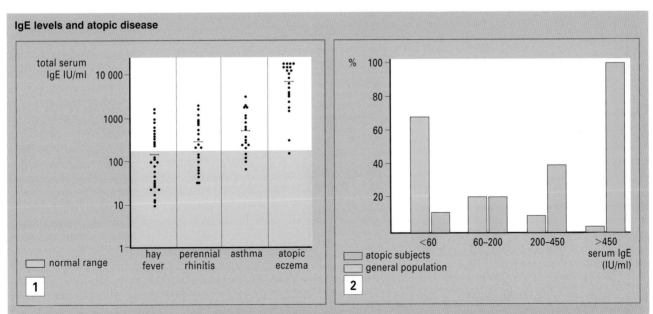

Fig. 23.13 **(1)** The serum concentration of IgE (which is around 100 IU/mL) is only approximately 0.001% that of IgG (around 10 mg/mL) and comprises less than 0.001% of the total immunoglobulin. Levels in atopic patients tend to be raised, and this is especially so in atopic eczema (the International Unit [IU] for IgE equals 2.4 ng). **(2)** The higher the level of IgE, the smaller the percentage of the population is affected, but the greater the likelihood of atopy. Where the level is greater than 450 IU/mL the majority of subjects are atopic.

Genetic influences over asthma and allergic diseases	
allergen specific	HLA related
IgE	total production
	FcεRI
	FcεRII
cytokines	IL-4 promoter and receptor
	IL-5
	IL-10
	IFNγ
	TGFβ promoter
	IL-11
	IL-13 and receptor
leukotriene pathway	five lipoxygenase activating protein (FLAP)
	lipoxygenase
	LTC$_4$ synthase
β$_2$-adrenergic receptor	leukotriene receptors – LTRI, LTRII
chemokines	polymorphisms
	CCR3 receptor

Fig. 23.14 Allergic diseases run in families, but the inheritance is not simple. Population-based studies have established that the inheritance of allergic diseases is influenced by multiple genes. Some of these, such as HLA-linked control of the response to pollen antigens or genes controlling total IgE, are related to the immune response. However, many others are related to the mechanisms of inflammation (e.g. IL-4 and IL-5 gene polymorphisms) or to the response to treatment (e.g. leukotriene receptor genes or polymorphisms of the β$_2$-adrenergic receptor).

It is therefore not surprising that multiple genes (currently at least 50), have been associated with asthma in different populations.

A further major problem in interpreting genetic analyses of allergic disease comes from the progressive increase in the incidence of asthma between 1960 and 2000. Clearly this increase cannot be attributed to genetic change and implies that some of the genes identified would influence asthma only in the presence of other changes either in the environment or in lifestyle. This is referred to as a gene–environment interaction.

The genetics of asthma has been studied both by genomic screening and by using candidate genes. Genomic screening identifies regions of the genome that link to asthma so that this region can be examined to identify specific genes.

If a candidate gene is identified, it is possible to examine the gene for polymorphisms that link to asthma. However, a brief consideration of the possible targets (Fig. 23.14)

makes it clear how complex the analysis of asthma is likely to be, and indeed is proving to be. Typical examples include polymorphisms of the promoter region for IL-4 and polymorphisms of the gene for IL-5.

Q. What effect might polymorphism in these genes have?
A. The level of production of IL-4, and the activity of IL-5, will vary between individuals, each of which will affect the type of immune response that develops – TH1 versus TH2 – either of which could directly influence the inflammatory response that occurs as a result of exposure to allergens.

A further series of polymorphisms have been identified that influence the response of asthma to treatment. These include:

- variants of the β$_2$-adrenergic receptor α chain; and
- genetic differences that influence the therapeutic response to leukotriene antagonists.

At present, it appears that the overall effects are too complex to be of any practical significance. Certainly it is most unlikely that gene transfer will ever be of significance therapeutically. However, as genetic screening becomes easier, pharmacogenetics may become an important method for identifying the best drugs for individual patients.

Skin tests for diagnosis and to guide treatment

The primary method for diagnosing immediate hypersensitivity is skin testing. The characteristic response is a **wheal and flare** (Figs 23.15 and 23.16):

- the wheal is caused by extravasation of serum from capillaries in the skin, which occurs as a direct effect of histamine and is accompanied by pruritus (also a direct effect of histamine);
- the larger erythematous flare is mediated by an axon reflex.

This skin response takes 5–15 minutes to develop and may persist for 30 minutes or more. Techniques for skin testing include:

- a prick test, in which a 25-gauge needle or a lancet is used to introduce ~0.2 μL of extract into the dermis;
- an intradermal injection of 0.02–0.03 mL.

All allergen injections have the potential to cause anaphylaxis and for safety reasons the intradermal test, which introduces approximately 100 times more extract, should always be preceded by a prick test.

Skin tests are evaluated by the size of the wheal compared to a positive (histamine) and negative (saline) control. In general, a 3 × 3 mm wheal in children and a 4 × 4 mm wheal in adults can be considered a positive response to a prick test.

A positive skin test indicates that the patient has specific IgE antibodies on the mast cells in their skin. In turn this implies that bronchial or nasal challenge would also be positive if sufficient antigen were administered.

In most cases (i.e. ≈80%) where the skin prick test is positive, IgE antibody will be detectable in the serum. However, blood tests for IgE antibody are generally less sensitive than intradermal skin tests.

Skin tests

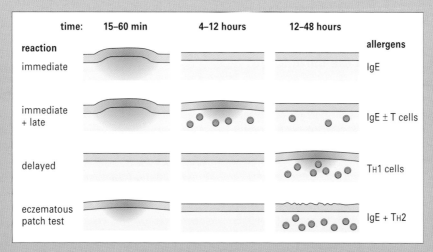

Fig. 23.15   Skin tests are carried out by introducing 0.02 mL of extract intradermally. With allergens such as pollen, cat, or dust mite, the positive reaction is an immediate (i.e. within 20 min) wheal, which in some cases is followed by an indurated response occurring late (i.e. at 4–12 hours). Non-allergic individuals make no discernible reaction to testing with these allergens. A delayed skin response is the commonest form of positive response to tuberculin, tetanus, and mumps, or to fungi such as *Trichophyton* and *Candida* spp. The skin typically shows no reaction up to 12 hours and then gradually develops an erythematous, indurated, delayed hypersensitivity response, which is maximal at 24–48 hours. Patch tests are performed by applying a gauze pad with allergen to a patch of skin that has been mildly abraded. This procedure may give an immediate wheal response, but this is followed at 24–48 hours by an indurated, erythematous response, which has many of the features of eczema. The patch test is not a diagnostic test, but has provided extensive information about the role of allergens in atopic dermatitis.

Skin test reactions

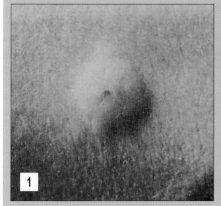

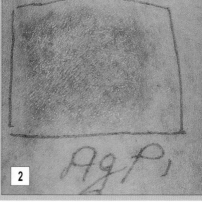

Fig. 23.16   (**1**) A type-I hypersensitivity reaction produces a raised wheal 5–7 mm in diameter and with a well-defined edge after about 15 minutes. (**2**) An erythematous and eczematous skin response 48 hours after the application of 5 μg of the mite allergen Der p1 to the skin of a patient with atopic dermatitis who had 56 IU/mL of IgE antibody to the dust mite *Dermatophagoides pteronyssinus*. Biopsy of the patch site revealed an infiltrate of eosinophils, basophils, and lymphocytes.

Q. Suggest explanations for the higher sensitivity of the skin test.
A. Most IgE is located on the high-affinity receptor on mast cells. Its half-life is 10 days on the mast cell as opposed to 2 days in blood. Sensitized mast cells can react to concentrations of allergen as low as 10^{-5} micrograms.

Positive skin tests are common

Epidemiologically, sensitization to a relevant inhalant allergen is a 'risk factor' for allergic disease. An individual with a positive skin test to grass pollen is therefore up to ten times more likely to have hayfever during the grass pollen season (odds ratio ≥ 10) than a skin test-negative individual. Equally an individual with a positive skin test to dust mite

or cat allergen is more likely to have asthma (odds ratios 2.0 to >6.0). It is assumed that allergen exposure contributes to the risk, but that the relationship is not simple.

Positive skin tests are common, and in individual cases may not be relevant, because the patient is not exposed to the allergen, for example:

- grass pollen is not relevant to understanding symptoms occurring during autumn;
- equally skin tests to cat dander or cockroach allergens may not be relevant if the patient has moved to an area or house where those allergens are not present.

In addition, up to one-third of skin test-positive individuals do not experience symptoms when they are exposed to the relevant allergen.

Following a strongly positive skin test, the skin response may return at 6–12 hours as an indurated late response which involves both the prolonged effects of mediators and a cellular influx.

Pathways that contribute to the chronicity of allergic diseases

The release of histamine that occurs within 15 minutes after allergen exposure can only explain a proportion of allergic disease. The chronic inflammation in the lungs of patients with asthma and in the skin of patients with atopic dermatitis cannot be explained by histamine because:

- the time course is too long;
- there is a cellular infiltrate in these tissues; and
- there are major differences in disease between patients who have apparently similar titer and specificity of IgE in their serum.

Several different pathways contribute to chronic symptoms and can alter the severity or chronicity of allergic disease.

- Local recruitment of mast cells and basophils, combined with increased 'releasability' of these cells, allows an increased response to the same allergen challenge – this mechanism plays a major role in the increased symptoms in the nose during the pollen seaseon.
- Release of leukotrienes, chemokines and cytokines from mast cells, or basophils; these mediators can have direct effects on blood vessels and smooth muscles. In addition IL-5, tumor necrosis factor (TNFα), and chemokines are each thought to contribute to the recruitment of inflammatory cells.
- T cells can be recruited to local tissues and can release a wide range of cytokines which have direct inflammatory effects.

Atopic dermatitis and the atopy patch test

Patients with atopic dermatitis (AD) have the highest levels of both specific IgE and total IgE. Thus IgE antibodies of ≥100 IU/mL (class 6), specific for dust mite, cockroach, pollens, or fungi, are common. Equally total IgE levels in patients with severe AD are usually ≥2000 IU/mL. However, there are still major disagreements about the importance of allergen exposure to the symptoms of this disease. This is because:

- the time course of the disease is chronic;
- injection of allergen into the skin causes a wheal and flare response, and doesn't consistently cause eczema;
- the disease is multi-factorial, including a role for food allergy, skin infection, genetic variations in skin barrier function (based on filaggrin), and also inhalant allergens.

The atopy patch test provides an important model of the ways in which allergen applied to the skin can induce eczema.

Epidermal spongiosis and a dermal infiltrate are features of a positive patch test

The infiltration of cells into the skin that occurs in the 24 hours after an allergen is applied can be studied in several ways:

- by local intradermal injections;
- by applying a patch of allergen on gauze that stays on the skin for 2 days; or

- by fixing a chamber containing allergen over a denuded area of skin.

The skin chamber allows repeated sampling whereas the other two techniques require biopsy of the skin.

In the **patch test** 10 µg allergen is applied on a gauze pad 2.5 cm², and the biopsy is carried out at 24 or 48 hours. A positive patch response induces:

- macroscopic eczema;
- spongiosis of the epidermis (a hallmark of eczema); and
- an infiltrate of cells into the dermis (see Fig. 23.16).

The cellular infiltrate includes eosinophils, basophils, and lymphocytes.

With persistent allergen at a site (i.e. 6 days), the eosinophils degranulate locally. This is in keeping with the evidence that the skin of patients with eczema contains large quantities of the eosinophil granule major basic protein (MBP), even though very few whole eosinophilic cells are visible (Fig. 23.17).

Biopsy of patch tests also yields T cells that are specific for the allergen used, which in most cases has been dust mite, thus establishing that antigen-specific T cells are present in the skin after antigen challenge.

Answering whether allergen-specific T cells are present at local sites is important because T cells could play a role both as effector cells and in the recruitment of other cells.

Establishing whether T cells play an effector role is also relevant to the nose in rhinitis, the lungs in asthma, the conjunctiva in hayfever, as well as the skin in atopic dermatitis.

Biopsy of patch test sites has also established that the Langerhans' cells in the skin of patients with eczema express FcεRI. It is assumed that these cells use IgE antibodies to help capture allergens and to increase the efficiency of antigen presentation.

Therefore, in any analysis of the factors influencing the severity of allergic disease (e.g. response to pharmacological treatment or response to immunotherapy), it is necessary to consider the relevance of both mast cells and effector T cells.

Allergens contribute to asthma

The causal role of bee venom in anaphylaxis or grass pollen in seasonal hayfever is obvious because:

- these diseases occur in individuals who have positive skin tests; and
- the symptoms are directly related to increased exposure.

By contrast, the role of inhaled allergens in chronic asthma is less obvious because exposure is perennial, the patients are often not aware of the relationship, and only a proportion of skin test-positive individuals develop asthma.

The evidence that allergens derived from dust mites, cats, dogs, the German cockroach, or the fungus *Alternaria* spp. contribute to asthma comes from several different lines of evidence:

- the epidemiological evidence that positive skin tests or serum IgE antibodies are a major risk factor for asthma;

Eosinophil major basic protein in the skin of atopic dermatitis

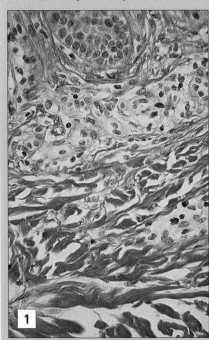
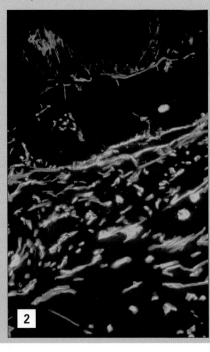

Fig. 23.17 Skin biopsy from a patient with severe atopic dermatitis. The hematoxylin and eosin (H&E) stain (**1**) shows an inflammatory infiltrate, but very few intact eosinophils are present. The same section stained with antibodies to eosinophil major basic protein (MBP) (**2**) shows extensive deposition of MBP in the dermis, demonstrating that eosinophils had degranulated in the skin. *(Courtesy of Dr K Lieferman.)*

- bronchial challenge with nebulized extracts can produce both rapid bronchospasm, within 20 minutes, and a late reaction in 4–8 hours, which is characterized by renewed mediator production and a cellular infiltrate;
- reduced exposure to allergens can lead to decreased symptoms and decreased non-specific bronchial reactivity – this avoidance can be achieved either by moving patients to an allergen-free unit or by controlling exposure in the home.

Bronchi in the lungs of patients with asthma are characterized by increased mast cells, lymphocytes of the TH2 type, eosinophils, and products of eosinophils. In addition, there is increased mucus production secondary to goblet cell hyperplasia, epithelial desquamation, and collagen deposition below the basement membrane. These changes are a reflection of chronic inflammation, and it is generally considered that eosinophils play a major role in these events (Fig. 23.18).

Q. Some recent evidence has shown that anti-IL-5 treatment has limited effects on asthma, though it decreases circulating eosinophils. How do you interpret this result?
A. In part this can be explained because other cells contribute in the inflammation in asthma, however, in addition eosinophils in the nases can be recruited and maintained by cytokines other than IL-5.

BAL analysis after allergen challenge demonstrates mast cell and eosinophil products

Analysis of bronchoalveolar lavage (BAL) after an allergen challenge demonstrates the presence of products derived from mast cells and eosinophils.

Q. What products would you expect to detect in BAL following challenge?
A. Histamine, prostaglandins, and leukotrienes from mast cells; major basic protein (MBP) and eosinophil cationic protein (ECP) from eosinophils (see Chapter 2).

Furthermore, MBP is present in biopsies of the lungs and can produce epithelial change typical of asthma *in vitro* (Fig. 23.19).

The subepithelial collagen deposition present in many patients with asthma is probably a reflection of fibroblast responses to local inflammation.

Although it has been suggested that these changes, which are referred to as 'remodeling', can lead to progressive decreases in lung function, the evidence for this view is not clear. In particular, progressive loss of lung function is unusual in asthma and there are no studies showing a correlation between the extent of collagen deposition and changes in lung function. Nonetheless, inhaled corticosteroids, which can block many different aspects of inflammation, are an effective long-term treatment that can control asthma. The effects of corticosteroids include:

- blocking the delayed response in the lungs;
- inhibiting influx of eosinophils, basophils, and lymphocytes;
- reducing eosinphil production in the bone marrow;
- inhibiting transcription of genes for IL-5, TNFα, and some chemokines;
- reducing T cell activity.

Locally active corticosteroids are widely used in seasonal rhinitis, perennial rhinitis, asthma, and atopic dermatitis. In addition, courses of systemic corticosteroids are used for the treatment of exacerbations of asthma.

Inflammatory response in asthmatic bronchi

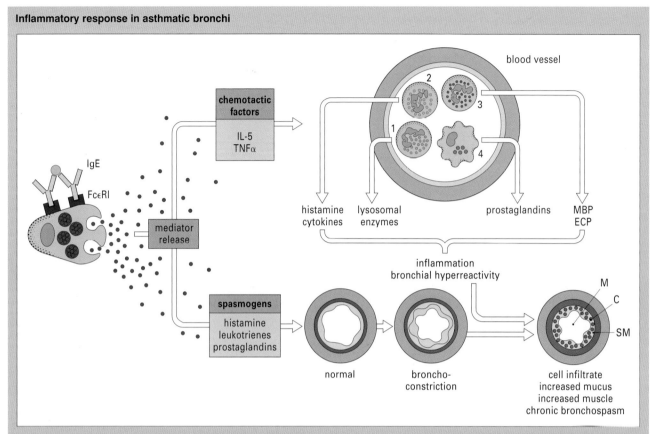

Fig. 23.18 Mast cells release factors that can induce immediate bronchospasm (e.g. histamine and LTD$_4$), but also release chemotactic factors such as LTB$_4$, IL-5, and TNFα. The spasmogens can induce edema, increased mucus, and smooth muscle constriction, resulting in an immediate decrease in airway conductance and a fall in FEV$_1$. By contrast, chemotactic factors recruit cells out of the circulation including eosinophils, neutrophils, lymphocytes, and macrophages. These cells can chronically modify the lung with goblet cell hyperplasia, collagen deposition below the basement membrane, and possibly smooth muscle hyperplasia. In addition, these cells and their products produce non-specific bronchial hyperreactivity. Thus, chronic bronchospasm includes elements of hypersecretion, inflammatory infiltrate, thickening of the walls of the small bronchi, and bronchial smooth muscle spasm. Evidence for this inflammatory response can be obtained from increased exhaled nitric oxide; increased eosinophils or eosinophil cationic protein (ECP) in induced sputum; and experimentally from biopsies of the lung. (1, neutrophils; 2, basophils; 3, eosinophils; 4, monocytes; C, cells; M, mucus; SM, smooth muscle.)

Bronchial hyperreactivity is a major feature of asthma

Non-specific bronchial hyperreactivity (BHR) is present in patients with asthma and is a major feature of the disease. Thus, airway obstruction, induced by cold air or exercise, and nocturnal asthma all correlate with non-specific bronchial reactivity. BHR can be demonstrated by challenging the lungs with histamine, methacholine, or cold air.

The mechanism by which exercise or cold air induces a bronchial response is thought to be evaporation of water with associated cooling of the epithelium. However, it is unclear whether this process triggers nerve endings directly or by causing local mediator release.

Evidence for inflammation of the lungs of patients with asthma is indirect

Bronchoscopy is not possible in patients with asthma except as a research procedure. Therefore the only evidence for inflammation of the lungs that can be obtained routinely is indirect:

- peripheral blood or nasal smear eosinophils are increased in most patients presenting with an acute episode of asthma (Fig. 23.20);
- nasal secretions may contain increased ECP and IL-8 (CXCL8).

Additional evidence about inflammation in the lungs can be obtained either from exhaled air or from condensates of exhaled air. Nitric oxide (NO$^\bullet$) gas is increased in patients with asthma, and this decreases following systemic or local corticosteroid treatment.

Q. Why should NO$^\bullet$ be increased in the lungs of asthmatic patients?
A. Macrophage activation causes synthesis of inducible nitric oxide synthase (iNOS) and consequent NO$^\bullet$ production in the lungs (see Fig. 7.19).

In addition, the pH of the condensate decreases during acute episodes. The increased exhaled NO$^\bullet$ may reflect upregulation of the enzyme iNOS. In many studies exhaled NO appears to be closely related to allergic inflation. In adults further information about the inflammation in the 'respiratory tract' can be obtained from computed

Localization of MBP in the lung of a severe asthmatic

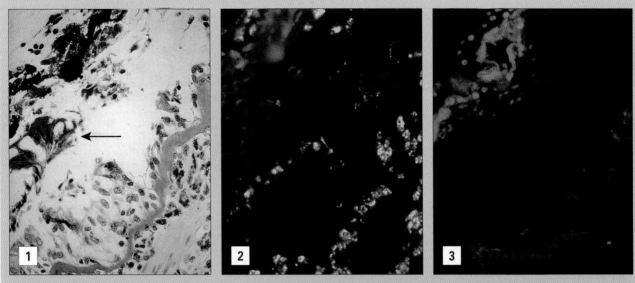

Fig. 23.19 (**1**) Respiratory epithelium showing striking submucosal eosinophil infiltration and a cluster of desquamated epithelial cells in the bronchial lumen (arrowed) next to a 'stringy' deposit of soot. H&E stain. (**2**) The same section stained for major basic protein (MBP) showing immunofluorescent localization in infiltrating eosinophils. MBP deposits are also seen on desquamated epithelial cells on the luminal surface. (**3**) A control section stained with normal rabbit serum does not stain eosinophils or bronchial tissue, but does show some non-specific staining of the sooty deposit. *(Courtesy of Dr G Gleich, reprinted from J. Allergy Clin. Immunol. 1982;70:160–169, with permission from American Academy of Allergy Asthma and Immunology.)*

Nasal eosinophils

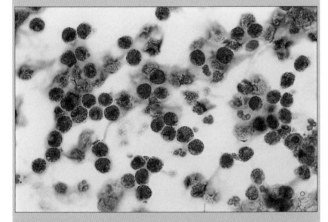

Fig. 23.20 Nasal smear from an 8-year-old boy presenting with acute asthma. Most of the cells are eosinophils – polymorphonuclear cells with a cytoplasm that stains red using H&E stain. He was known to be allergic to dust mites and had recently had a rhinovirus infection as judged by polymerase chain reaction on nasal secretions.

tomography (CT) of the nasal sinuses. Extensive opacification of the sinuses is present in approximately one-third of patients presenting with acute asthma. This reflects both:

- chronic sinusitis, which is a major feature of late-onset asthma; and
- sinus inflammation secondary to acute rhinovirus infection.

Whether the changes in the sinuses are a reflection of similar effects occurring in the lungs, or a source of mediators, or T cells that contribute to lung inflammation, is not clear.

Treatments for type I hypersensitivity

Immunotherapy is an effective treatment for hayfever and anaphylactic sensitivity to venom

Immunotherapy (or hyposensitization) with allergen extracts was introduced in 1911 by Noon and Freeman. At that time they were trying to establish immunity against pollen toxin.

Immunotherapy requires regular injections of allergen over a period of months. It is an established treatment for:

- seasonal hayfever; and
- anaphylactic sensitivity to bees, wasps, and hornets.

In addition, immunotherapy is an effective treatment for selected cases of other allergic diseases including asthma.

The dose is increased progressively, starting with between 1–10 ng and increasing up to approximately 10 μg allergen per dose.

The response to treatment includes:

- an increase in serum IgG antibodies;
- a striking decrease in the response of peripheral blood T cells to antigen *in vitro*; and
- a marked decrease in late reactions in the skin.

Over a longer period of time there is a progressive decrease in IgE antibodies in the serum (Fig. 23.21).

The change in antibodies, lymphocyte responses, and symptoms could all be secondary to changes in T cells. Given the known mechanisms of allergic inflammation, a

Effects of immunotherapy on allergic rhinitis

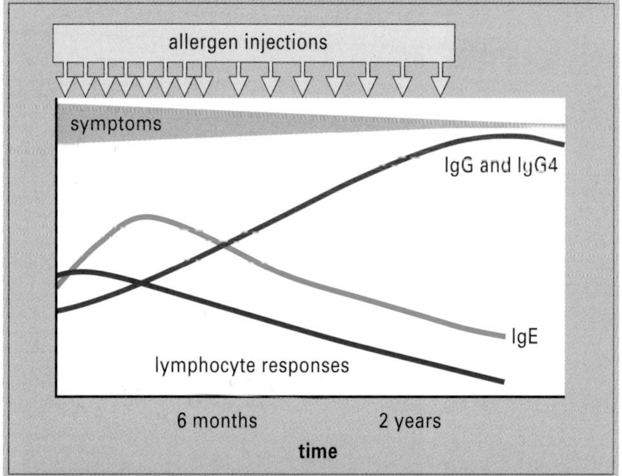

Fig. 23.21 During desensitization or immunotherapy the allergic patient receives regular subcutaneous injections of the relevant allergen. The immunological changes that occur include an initial increase in IgE antibodies followed by a gradual decline, which in pollen-allergic patients is largely due to a blunting of the seasonal increase. Antibodies of the IgG and specifically IgG4 isotype increase progressively and may reach concentrations of ten times those present before treatment. Symptoms decline, starting as early as 3 months, but generally not maximally until 2 years. Changes in T cells are less well defined, but include decreased *in-vitro* response to allergens and increased production of IL-10.

response of T cells to allergen injections could influence symptoms in several ways:

- decreased local recruitment of mast cells and basophils;
- decreased recruitment of eosinophils to the nose or lungs;
- increased IgG including IgG4 antibodies with progressive decreases in IgE – the IgG antibodies may act as blocking antibodies by binding allergen before it cross-links IgE on mast cells.

Some studies of cytokine RNA have suggested that immunotherapy produces a shift in T cells from a TH2 profile (i.e. IL-4 and IL-5) towards a profile that is more typical of TH1 (i.e. IFNγ). Although this could explain decreased help for IgE, and decreased eosinophil recruitment, this would not explain the production of IgG4. The expression of the gene for IgG4 is dependent on IL-4, and may also require the cytokine IL-10. The response to immunotherapy is therefore better seen as a modification of the TH2 response.

Modified forms of allergen-specific immunotherapy

Peptides from the primary sequence of an allergen that can stimulate T cells *in* vitro

Peptides from the primary sequence of an allergen, usually approximately 20 amino acids in length, stimulate T cells *in vitro* and *in vivo*.

In theory, peptides provide a mechanism for stimulating or desensitizing T cells without the risk of anaphylaxis, which is always present with traditional allergens.

Whether incomplete stimulation of T cells by peptides can lead to 'tolerance' or a change in the cytokine profile is not clear. Problems with peptide immunotherapy include:

- significant reactions in the lung with a fall in FEV_1; and
- the fact that multiple peptides are necessary to allow presentation of antigen in patients with different HLA types.

Modified recombinant allergens have decreased binding to IgE

Genetically modified recombinant allergens that have decreased binding to IgE can be produced. Their advantage is that the primary sequence with the T cell epitopes is preserved. Even if the molecule is extensively modified, any full-length protein has the potential to induce anaphylaxis in allergic individuals. Thus, the use of genetically modified molecules would always require precautions similar to those for traditional immunotherapy. A potential but unlikely problem is that patients would develop IgE antibodies against new epitopes.

Adjuvants can shift the immune response away from a simple TH2 response

Adjuvants 'attached' to allergen molecules have been designed to shift the immune response from TH2 towards TH1. Possible co-molecules that act like an adjuvant include:

- the cytokine IL-12; or
- immunostimulatory sequences (ISSs). ISSs are DNA sequences such as cytosine phosphoguanidine (CpG) that are common in bacterial DNA and have a profound effect on the mammalian immune system.

In mice combining an antigen with two or three molecules of CpG can induce a TH1 response or downregulate IgE responses.

Combining CpG with allergen not only influences the response, but also reduces the reactivity of the allergen with IgE.

Thus immunization with allergen and CpG may produce a greater immune response with less potential for an acute allergic reaction.

Although preliminary trials with CpG were encouraging large trials were not. It is important to remember that CpG acts through TLR9 which is on the nuclear membrane. An alternative approach is to use flagellin attached to allergen because it binds to TLR-5 which is on the cell surface.

DNA vaccines are being designed to change the immune response

The concept of immunizing with the gene for an antigen is well established (i.e. DNA vaccines). Experiments with DNA vaccines have been very successful in mice, both in inducing a TH1 response initially and in controlling an existing IgE antibody response. However, the consequences of expressing an allergen within the tissue of an allergic individual are not known. Equally, it is not clear whether inducing a TH1 response to a high dose allergen such as cat dander which is present in almost all houses would give rise to other forms of inflammatory disease.

Other forms of immune based non-specific therapy

Humanized monoclonal anti-IgE

Humanized monoclonal anti-IgE treatment can reduce sensitivity and significantly decrease the number of acute episodes of asthma per year.

Antibodies directed against the binding site for FcεRI on IgE bind to IgE in the circulation, but not when it is attached to mast cells or basophils. An antibody of this kind can therefore remove IgE from the circulation but will not induce anaphylaxis. A mouse monoclonal antibody to IgE has been progressively humanized so that the molecule can be safely injected into patients and will bind IgE with high affinity.

Treatment with anti-IgE antibodies has reduced exacerbations of asthma and the symptoms of hayfever. In addition, continued treatment that controls free IgE below 10 ng/mL leads to a progressive decrease in the number of IgE receptors on mast cells. Thus, the treatment may achieve a secondary effect, further decreasing the sensitivity of histamine-containing cells to allergen. Although there have been small studies on the role of anti-IgE in treating food allergy, atopic dermatitis, urticaria and drug allergy, this treatment remains to be established.

Recombinant soluble IL-4R can block the biological activity of IL-4

Given the central role of IL-4 in the TH2 response, it is not surprising that several efforts have been made to block its action. These include:

- a mutated IL-4 (Y124D);
- antibodies to IL-4; and
- recombinant soluble IL-4 receptor (sIL-4R). Treatment with sIL-4R has proved moderately effective in clinical trials of allergic asthma. The mechanism is that sIL-4R binds to IL-4 before it can react with the receptor on T cells or B cells, and thus blocks its biological activity. However, it is less clear which of the many actions of IL-4 is relevant to the clinical effects:
  - blocking the action of IL-4 on B cells may reduce IgE production, but this would probably require many

weeks to produce a clinical effect; because IgE plasma cells are long lived;
  - the autocrine effect of IL-4 on TH2 cells may be an essential growth factor.

The efficacy of sIL-4R provides indirect evidence for the role of T cells in allergic disease.

Humanized monoclonal anti-IL-5 decreases circulating eosinophils

Anti-IL-5 (like anti-IgE) is a humanized mouse monoclonal antibody.

Following successful studies in baboons, anti-IL-5 has been shown to decrease circulating eosinophils in patients. It is therefore assumed that binding IL-5 produced by T cells (or mast cells) can decrease the production of eosinophils in the bone marrow. However, the results do not answer whether the treatment acts on IL-5 in the circulation or on IL-5 produced by T cells (or mast cells) locally in the bone marrow and/or the respiratory tract.

In initial studies, anti-IL-5 was not effective as a treatment for asthma despite an approximately 90% decrease in circulating eosinophils.

Some new treatment approaches may not be practical

The primary treatment of allergic disease is based on:

- allergen avoidance;
- pharmacological management including disodium cromoglycate, theophyline, leukotriene antagonists, and local corticosteroids; and
- immunotherapy.

The treatment approaches using peptides, modified allergens, or allergens linked to TLR ligands such as CpG or Flagellin have the disadvantage that each allergen would have to go through clinical trials.

Although specific antagonists to other cytokines appear to be an attractive target for treatment, it is increasingly unlikely that they will be clinically successful in competition with anti-IgE, inhaled corticosteroids, and leukotriene antagonists.

CRITICAL THINKING: SEVERE ANAPHYLACTIC SHOCK (SEE P. 442 FOR EXPLANATIONS)

Sixty-two-year-old Mrs Young was stung by a bee from a hive in her back garden. Harvesting the honey had left her with several stings during the course of the summer. Several minutes after the recent sting she complained of an itching sensation in her hands, feet, and groin accompanied by cramping abdominal pain. Shortly afterwards she felt faint and acutely short of breath. Moments later she collapsed and lost consciousness. Her husband, a doctor, noticed that her breathing was rapid and wheezy and that she had swollen eyelids and lips. She was pale and had patchy erythema across her neck and arms.

On examination her apex beat could be felt, but her radial pulse was weak. Her husband immediately administered 0.5 mL of 1/1000 epinephrine (adrenaline) intramuscularly and 10 mg of chlorpheniramine (chlorphenamine) (an H_1-receptor antihistamine) intravenously with 100 mg of hydrocortisone. She regained consciousness and her respiratory rate dropped. By the following day she had recovered completely. Results of investigations at this time are shown in the table.

Investigation	Result (normal range)
hemoglobin (g/dL)	14.2 (11.5–16.0)
white cell count ($\times 10^9$/L)	7.5 (4.0–11.0)
neutrophils ($\times 10^9$/L)	4.4 (2.0–7.5)
eosinophils ($\times 10^9$/L)	0.40 (0.04–0.44)
total lymphocytes ($\times 10^9$/L)	2.4 (1.6–3.5)
platelet count ($\times 10^9$/L)	296 (150–400)
serum immunoglobulins IgG (g/L) IgM (g/L) IgA (g/L) IgE (IU/mL)	 10.2 (5.4–16.1) 0.9 (0.5–1.9) 2.1 (0.8–2.8) 320 (3–150)
RAST bee venom wasp venom	 class 4 class 0
skin prick tests	grade (0–5)
bee venom (10 µg/mL)	3+

Mrs Young had no previous history of adverse reactions to bee venom, foods, or antibiotics. In addition there was no history of asthma, allergic rhinitis, food allergy, or atopic dermatitis. A diagnosis of anaphylactic shock due to bee venom sensitivity was made based on the history and investigations, and a decision taken to commence desensitization therapy.

Mrs Young was made aware of the possible risk of the procedure and consented to it. She was injected subcutaneously with gradually increasing doses of bee venom, the procedures being performed in hospital with access to resuscitation apparatus. No further allergic reactions occurred and she was maintained on a dose of bee venom at 1-month intervals for the next 2 years. She was stung by a bee the following summer and had no adverse reaction.

1   What mechanisms are involved in anaphylaxis?

2   What are the clinical features and management of acute anaphylaxis?

3   How may such sensitivity be detected and what can be done to desensitize patients?

Further reading

Akdis CA, Blaser K. IL-10-induced anergy in peripheral T cell and reactivation by microenvironmental cytokines: two key steps in specific immunotherapy. FASEB J 1999;13:603–609.

Ali FR, Kay AB, Larche M. Airway hyperresponsiveness and bronchial mucosal inflammation in T cell peptide-induced asthmatic reactions in atopic subjects. Thorax 2007;62:750–757.

Beaven MA, Metzger H. Signal transduction by Fc receptors: the FcεRI case. Immunol Today 1993;14:222–226.

Borish L, Rosenwasser L. TH1/TH2 lymphocytes: doubt some more. J Allergy Clin Immunol 1997;99:161–164.

Chung CH, Mirakhur B, Chan E, et al. Cetuximab-induced anaphylaxis and IgE specific for galactose-alpha-1,3-galactose. N Engl J Med 2008;358:1109–1117.

Commins SP, Satinover SM, Hosen J, et al. Delayed anaphylaxis, angioedema, or urticaria after consumption of red meat in patients with IgE antibodies specific for galactose-alpha-1,3-galactose. J Allergy Clin Immunol 2009;123:426–433.

Coyle AJ, Wagner K, Bertrand C, et al. Central role of immunoglobulin (Ig) E in the induction of lung eosinophil infiltration and T helper 2 cell cytokine production: inhibition by a non-anaphylactogenic anti-IgE antibody. J Exp Med 1996;183:1303–1310.

Ege MJ, Mayer M, Normand AC, et al. Exposure to environmental microorganisms and childhood asthma. N Engl J Med 2011;364:701–709.

Galli SJ. New concepts about the mast cell. N Engl J Med 1993;328:257–265.

Geha RF. Regulation of IgE synthesis in humans. J Allergy Clin Immunol 1992;90:143–150.

Haselden BM, Kay AB, Larch M. Immunoglobulin E-independent major histocompatibility complex-restricted T cell peptide epitope-induced late asthmatic reactions. J Exp Med 1999;189:1885–1894.

Miller JS, Schwartz LB. Human mast cell proteases and mast cell heterogeneity. Curr Opin Immunol 1989;1:637–642.

Montford S, Robinson HC, Holgate ST. The bronchial epithelium as a target for inflammatory attack in asthma. Clin Exp Immunol 1992;22:511–520.

Platts-Mills TAE, Vervloet D, Thomas WR, et al. Indoor allergens and asthma: report of the Third International Workshop. J Allergy Clin Immunol 1997;100:S2–S24.

Platts-Mills TAE, Vaughan JW, Squillace S, et al. Sensitisation, asthma and a modified TH2 response in children exposed to cat allergen. Lancet 2001;357:752–756.

Prausnitz C, Kustner H. In: Gell PGH, Coombes RRA, eds. Clinical aspects of immunology, Oxford: Blackwell Scientific Publications; 1962:808–816.

Sporik R, Holgate ST, Platts-Mills TAE, Cogswell JJ. Exposure to house-dust mite allergen (Der p I) and the development of asthma in childhood. A prospective study. N Engl J Med 1990;323:502–507.

Wan H, Winton HL, Soeller C, et al. Der p1 facilitates transepithelial allergen delivery by disruption of tight junctions. J Clin Invest 1999;104:123–133.

Wark PA, Johnston SL, Bucchieri F, et al. Asthmatic bronchial epithelial cells have a deficient innate immune response to infection with rhinovirus. J Exp Med 2005;201:937–947.

Wide L, Bennich H, Johansson SGO. Diagnosis of allergy by an in-vitro test for allergen antibodies. Lancet 1967;ii:1105.

CHAPTER 24

Hypersensitivity (Type II)

SUMMARY

- **Type II hypersensitivity is mediated by antibodies binding to specific cells.** Type II hypersensitivity reactions are caused by IgG, IgA, or IgM antibodies against cell surface and extracellular matrix antigens. The antibodies damage cells and tissues by activating complement, and by binding and activating effector cells carrying Fc γ receptors.

- **Red blood cells (blood groups) must be cross-matched for transfusion.** Transfusion reactions to erythrocytes are produced by antibodies to blood group antigens, which may occur naturally or may have been induced by previous contact with incompatible tissue or blood following transplantation, transfusion, or during pregnancy.

- **Hemolytic disease of the newborn** occurs when maternal antibodies to fetal blood group antigens cross the placenta and destroy the fetal erythrocytes.

- **Type II hypersensitivity reactions may target tissues.** Damage to tissues may be produced by autoantibodies to extracellular matrix, cell surface molecules, or intracellular proteins. Examples of diseases caused by these mechanisms are myasthenia gravis, pemphigus, and Goodpasture's syndrome.

- **The role of autoantibodies in disease is not always clear.** Antibodies to intracellular components are not necessarily pathogenic, but they may be diagnostically useful.

Mechanisms of tissue damage

Type II hypersensitivity reactions are mediated by IgG and IgM antibodies binding to specific cells or components of the extracellular matrix. The damage caused is therefore restricted to the specific cells or tissues bearing the antigens. In general:

- antibodies directed against cell surface antigens are usually pathogenic;
- antibodies directed against internal antigens are usually not pathogenic.

Type II reactions therefore differ from type III reactions, which involve antibodies directed against soluble antigens in the serum, leading to the formation of circulating antigen–antibody complexes. Damage occurs when the complexes are deposited non-specifically onto tissues and/or organs (see Chapter 25).

Effector cells engage their targets using Fc and C3 receptors

In type II hypersensitivity, antibody directed against cell surface or tissue antigens interacts with the **Fc receptors (FcR)** on a variety of effector cells and can activate complement to bring about damage to the target cells (Fig. 24.1).

Once the antibody has attached itself to the surface of the cell or tissue, it can bind and activate complement component C1, with the following consequences:

- complement fragments (C3a and C5a) generated by activation of complement attract macrophages and polymorphs to the site, and also stimulate mast cells and basophils to produce chemokines that attract and activate other effector cells;
- the classical complement pathway and activation loop lead to the deposition of C3b, C3bi, and C3d on the target cell membrane;
- the classical complement pathway and lytic pathway result in the production of the C5b–9 membrane attack complex (MAC) and insertion of the complex into the target cell membrane.

Effector cells – in this case macrophages, neutrophils, eosinophils, and NK cells – bind to either:

- the complexed antibody via their Fc receptors; or
- the membrane-bound C3b, C3bi, and C3d, via their C3 receptors (CR1, CR3, CR4).

The mechanisms by which these antibodies trigger cytotoxic reactions *in vivo* have been investigated in FcR-deficient mice. Anti-red blood cell antibodies trigger erythrophagocytosis of IgG-opsonized red blood cells in an FcR-dependent manner. Fc receptor γ chain-deficient

Antibody-dependent cytotoxicity

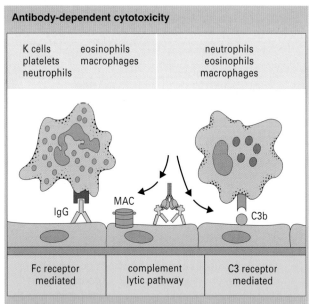

Fig. 24.1 Effector cells – K cells, platelets, neutrophils, eosinophils, and cells of the mononuclear phagocyte series – all have receptors for Fc, which they use to engage antibody bound to target tissues. Activation of complement C3 can generate complement-mediated lytic damage to target cells directly, and also allows phagocytic cells to bind to their targets via C3b, C3bi, or C3d, which also activate the cells. (MAC, membrane attack complex.)

Damage mechanisms

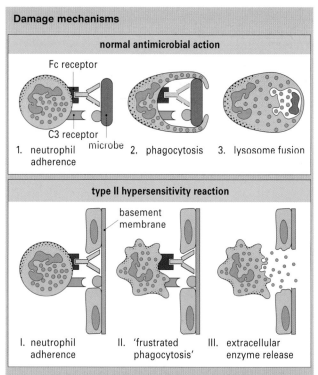

Fig. 24.2 Neutrophil-mediated damage is a reflection of normal antibacterial action. (**1**) Neutrophils engage microbes with their Fc and C3 receptors. (**2**) The microbe is then phagocytosed and destroyed as lysosomes fuse to form the phagolysosome (**3**). In type II hypersensitivity reactions, individual host cells coated with antibody may be similarly phagocytosed, but where the target is large, for example a basement membrane (**I**), the neutrophils are frustrated in their attempt at phagocytosis (**II**). They exocytose their lysosomal contents, causing damage to cells in the vicinity (**III**).

mice were protected from the pathogenic effect of these antibodies whereas complement-deficient mice were indistinguishable from wild-type animals in their ability to clear the targeted red cells.

Q. How do you interpret this observation?

A. These experiments indicate that phagocytosis of antibody-sensitized red cells depends on FcR-mediated binding to the phagocytes and is not dependent on opsonization by C3b deposited via the classical pathway.

Cells damage targets by releasing their normal immune effector molecules

The mechanisms by which neutrophils and macrophages damage target cells in type II hypersensitivity reactions reflect their normal methods of dealing with infectious pathogens (Fig. 24.2).

Normally pathogens would be internalized and then subjected to a barrage of microbicidal systems including defensins, reactive oxygen and nitrogen metabolites, hypohalites, enzymes, altered pH, and other agents that interfere with metabolism (see Chapters 7 and 14).

If the target is too large to be phagocytosed, the granule and lysosome contents are released in apposition to the sensitized target in a process referred to as **exocytosis**. Cross-linking of the Fc and C3 receptors during this process causes activation of the phagocyte with production of reactive oxygen intermediates, as well as activation of phospholipase A2 with consequent release of arachidonic acid from membrane phospholipids.

Q. What inflammatory mediators are synthesized from arachidonic acid?

A. This metabolite is the precursor of eicosanoids – prostaglandins and leukotrienes.

In some situations, such as the eosinophil reaction against schistosomes (see Chapter 15), exocytosis of granule contents is normal and beneficial. However, when the target is host tissue that has been sensitized by antibody, the result is damaging (Fig. 24.3).

Antibodies may also mediate hypersensitivity by NK cells. In this case, however, the nature of the target, and whether it can inhibit the NK cells' cytotoxic actions, are as important as the presence of the sensitizing antibody.

The resistance of a target cell to damage varies. Susceptibility depends on:

- the amount of antigen expressed on the target cell's surface; and
- the inherent ability of different target cells to sustain damage.

For example, an erythrocyte may be lysed by a single active C5 convertase site, whereas it takes many such sites to destroy most nucleated cells – their ion-pumping capacity and ability to maintain membrane integrity with anti-complementary defenses is so much greater.

Phagocytes attacking a basement membrane

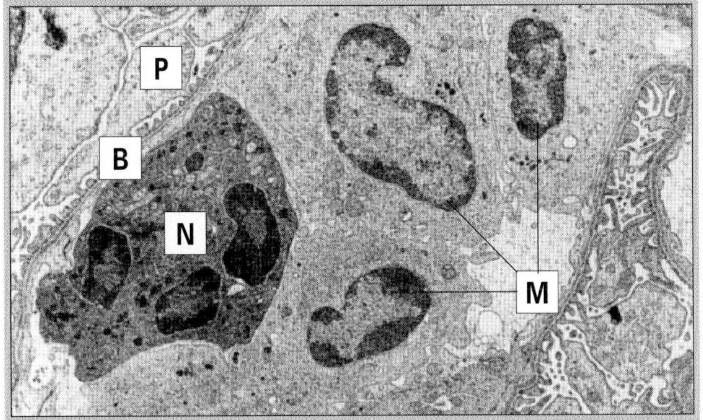

Fig. 24.3 This electron micrograph shows a neutrophil (N) and three monocytes (M) binding to the capillary basement membrane (B) in the kidney of a rabbit containing anti-basement membrane antibody. × 3500. (P, podocyte.) *(Courtesy of Professor GA Andres.)*

Q. What molecules protect the surface of nucleated cells from complement-mediated damage?
A. Decay accelerating factor (CD55) and CD59.

We now examine some instances where type II hypersensitivity reactions are thought to be of prime importance in causing target cell destruction or immunopathological damage.

Type II reactions against blood cells and platelets

Some of the most clearcut examples of type II reactions are seen in the responses to erythrocytes. Important examples are:

- incompatible blood transfusions, where the recipient becomes sensitized to antigens on the surface of the donor's erythrocytes;
- hemolytic disease of the newborn, where a pregnant woman has become sensitized to the fetal erythrocytes;
- autoimmune hemolytic anemias, where the patient becomes sensitized to his or her own erythrocytes.

Reactions to platelets can cause thrombocytopenia, and reactions to neutrophils and lymphocytes have been associated with systemic lupus erythematosus (SLE).

Transfusion reactions occur when a recipient has antibodies against donor erythrocytes

More than 20 blood group systems, generating over 200 genetic variants of erythrocyte antigens, have been identified in humans.

A blood group system consists of a gene locus that specifies an antigen on the surface of blood cells (usually, but not always, erythrocytes).

Within each system there may be two or more phenotypes. In the ABO system, for example, there are four phenotypes (A, B, AB, and O), and therefore four possible blood groups.

Five major blood group systems involved in transfusion reactions

system	gene loci	antigens	phenotype frequency (%)
ABO	1	A, B, or O	A 42 B 8 AB 3 O 47
Rhesus	2 closely linked loci: major antigen=RhD	C or c D or d E or e	RhD+ 85 RhD− 15
Kell	1	K or k	K 9 k 91
Duffy	1	Fyᵃ, Fyᵇ, or Fy	FyᵃFyᵇ 46 Fyᵃ 20 Fyᵇ 34 Fy 0.1
MN	1	M or N	MM 28 MN 50 NN 22

Fig. 24.4 Not all blood groups are equally antigenic in transfusion reactions – thus RhD evokes a stronger reaction in an incompatible recipient than the other Rhesus antigens; and Fyᵃ is stronger than Fyᵇ. Frequencies stated are for Caucasian populations – other races have different gene frequencies.

An individual with a particular blood group can recognize erythrocytes carrying allogeneic (non-self) blood group antigens, and will produce antibodies against them. However, for some blood group antigens such antibodies can also be produced 'naturally' (i.e. without previous sensitization by foreign erythrocytes).

Some blood group systems (e.g. ABO and Rhesus) are characterized by antigens that are relatively strong immunogens; such antigens are more likely to induce antibodies.

When planning a blood transfusion, it is important to ensure that donor and recipient blood types are compatible with respect to these major blood groups, otherwise transfusion reactions will occur.

Some major human blood groups are listed in Figure 24.4.

The ABO blood group system is of primary importance

The epitopes of the **ABO blood group system** occur on many cell types in addition to erythrocytes and are located on the carbohydrate units of glycoproteins. The structure of these carbohydrates, and of those determining the related Lewis blood group system, is determined by genes coding for enzymes that transfer terminal sugars to a carbohydrate backbone (Fig. 24.5).

Most individuals develop antibodies to allogeneic specificities of the ABO system without previous sensitization by foreign erythrocytes. This sensitization occurs through contact with identical epitopes, coincidentally expressed on a wide variety of microorganisms.

Antibodies to ABO antigens are therefore extremely common, making it particularly important to match donor blood to the recipient for this system. However, all people are tolerant to the O antigen, so O individuals are **universal donors** with respect to the ABO system.

The Rhesus system is a major cause of hemolytic disease of the newborn

The Rhesus system is also of great importance because it is a major cause of **hemolytic disease of the newborn (HDNB)**.

Rhesus antigens are associated with membrane proteins of 30 kDa, which are expressed at moderate levels on the erythrocyte surface. The antigens are encoded by two closely linked loci, RhD and RhCcEe, with 92% homology.

RhD is the most important clinically due to its high immunogenicity, but in RhD⁻ individuals the RhD locus is missing completely. The RhCcEe locus encodes a molecule that expresses the RhC/c and RhE/e epitopes.

ABO blood group antigens

blood group (phenotype)	genotypes	antigens	antibodies to ABO in serum
A	AA, AO	A	anti-B
B	BB, BO	B	anti-A
AB	AB	A and B	none
O	OO	H	anti-A and anti-B

Fig. 24.5 The diagram shows how the ABO blood groups are constructed. The enzyme produced by the H gene attaches a fucose residue (Fuc) to the terminal galactose (Gal) of the precursor oligosaccharide. Individuals possessing the A gene now attach N-acetylgalactosamine (NAGA) to this galactose residue, whereas those with the B gene attach another galactose, producing A and B antigens, respectively. People with both genes make some of each. The table indicates the genotypes and antigens of the ABO system. Most people naturally make antibodies to the antigens they lack. (NAG, N-acetylglucosamine.)

Cross-matching ensures that a recipient does not have antibodies against donor erythrocytes

The aim of cross-matching is to ensure that the blood of a recipient does not contain antibodies that will be able to react with and destroy transfused (donor) erythrocytes. For example:

- antibodies to ABO system antigens cause incompatible cells to agglutinate in a clearly visible reaction;
- minor blood group systems cause weaker reactions that may only be detectable by an indirect Coombs' test (see Fig. 24.9).

If the individual is transfused with whole blood, it is also necessary to check that the donor's serum does not contain antibodies against the recipient's erythrocytes. However, transfusion of whole blood is unusual – most blood donations are separated into cellular and serum fractions, to be used individually.

Transfusion reactions involve extensive destruction of donor blood cells

Transfusion of erythrocytes into a recipient who has antibodies to those cells produces an immediate reaction. The symptoms include:

- fever;
- hypotension;
- nausea and vomiting; and
- pain in the back and chest.

The severity of the reaction depends on the class and the amounts of antibodies involved:

Antibodies to ABO system antigens are usually IgM, and cause agglutination, complement activation, and intravascular hemolysis. Other blood groups induce IgG antibodies, which cause less agglutination than IgM. The IgG-sensitized cells are usually taken up by phagocytes in the liver and spleen, though severe reactions may cause erythrocyte destruction by complement activation. This can cause circulatory shock, and the released contents of the erythrocytes can produce acute tubular necrosis of the kidneys. These transfusion reactions are often seen in previously unsensitized individuals and develop over days or weeks as antibodies to the foreign cells are produced. This can result in anemia or jaundice.

> **Q. Why do antibodies to the ABO blood group that are normally present in a mother not damage the erythrocytes that are present in a fetus she is carrying when the fetus has a different blood group?**
> A. Antibodies to the ABO blood group are usually IgM, which is not transported across the placenta.

Transfusion reactions to other components of blood may also occur, but their consequences are not usually as severe as reactions to erythrocytes.

Hyperacute graft rejection is related to the transfusion reaction

Hyperacute graft rejection occurs when a graft recipient has preformed antibodies against the graft tissue. It is only seen in tissue that is revascularized directly after transplantation, in kidney grafts for example.

The most severe reactions in this type of rejection are due to the ABO group antigens expressed on kidney cells. The damage is produced by antibody and complement activation in the blood vessels, with consequent recruitment and activation of neutrophils and platelets.

Donors and recipients are now always cross-matched for ABO antigens, and this reaction has become extremely rare. Antibodies to other graft antigens (e.g. MHC molecules) induced by previous grafting can also produce this type of reaction.

HDNB is due to maternal IgG reacting against the child's erythrocytes *in utero*

Hemolytic disease of the newborn (HDNB) occurs when the mother has been sensitized to antigens on the infant's erythrocytes and makes IgG antibodies to these antigens. These antibodies cross the placenta and react with the fetal erythrocytes, causing their destruction (Figs 24.6 and 24.7). Rhesus D (RhD) is the most commonly involved antigen.

A risk of HDNB arises when a Rh⁺-sensitized Rh⁻ mother carries a second Rh⁺ infant. Sensitization of the Rh⁻ mother to the Rh⁺ erythrocytes usually occurs during the birth of the first Rh⁺ infant, when some fetal erythrocytes leak back across the placenta into the maternal circulation and are recognized by the maternal immune system. The first incompatible child is therefore usually unaffected, whereas subsequent children have an increasing risk of being affected, as the mother is resensitized with each successive pregnancy.

Reactions to other blood groups may also cause HDNB, the second most common being the Kell system K antigen. Reactions due to anti-K are much less common than reactions due to RhD because of the relatively low frequency (9%) and weaker antigenicity of the K antigen.

The risk of HDNB due to Rhesus incompatibility is known to be reduced if the father is of a different ABO group to the mother. This observation led to the idea that these Rh⁻ mothers were destroying Rh⁺ cells more rapidly because they were also ABO incompatible. Consequently, fetal Rh⁺ erythrocytes would not be available to sensitize the maternal immune system to RhD antigen.

This notion led to the development of **Rhesus prophylaxis** – preformed anti-RhD antibodies are given to Rh⁻ mothers immediately after delivery of Rh⁺ infants, with the aim of destroying fetal Rh⁺ erythrocytes before they can cause Rh⁻ sensitization. This practice has successfully reduced the incidence of HDNB due to Rhesus incompatibility (Fig. 24.8). Although the number of cases of HDNB has fallen dramatically and progressively, the proportion of cases caused by other blood groups, including Kell and the ABO system, has increased.

Autoimmune hemolytic anemias arise spontaneously or may be induced by drugs

Reactions to **blood group antigens** also occur spontaneously in the autoimmune hemolytic anemias, in which patients produce antibodies to their own erythrocytes.

Autoimmune hemolytic anemia is suspected if a patient gives a positive result on a **direct antiglobulin test** (Fig. 24.9), which identifies antibodies present on the patient's erythrocytes. These are usually antibodies directed

A child with hemolytic disease of the newborn

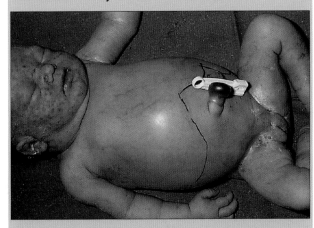

Fig. 24.7 There is considerable enlargement of the liver and spleen associated with erythrocyte destruction caused by maternal anti-erythrocyte antibody in the fetal circulation. The child had elevated bilirubin (breakdown product of hemoglobin). The facial petechial hemorrhaging was due to impaired platelet function. The most commonly involved antigen is RhD. *(Courtesy of Dr K Sloper.)*

Hemolytic disease of the newborn

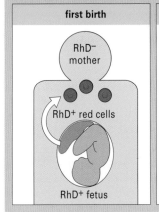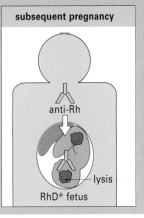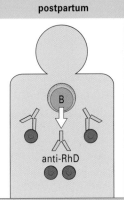

Fig. 24.6 Erythrocytes from a RhD⁺ fetus leak into the maternal circulation, usually during birth. This stimulates the production of anti-Rh antibody of the IgG class postpartum. During subsequent pregnancies, IgG antibodies are transferred across the placenta into the fetal circulation (IgM cannot cross the placenta). If the fetus is again incompatible, the antibodies cause erythrocyte destruction.

Rhesus prophylaxis

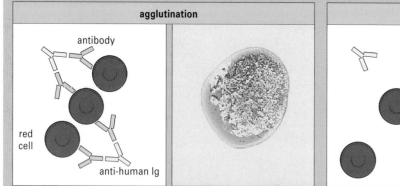

Fig. 24.8 (**1**) Without prophylaxis, Rh⁺ erythrocytes leak into the circulation of a Rh⁻ mother and sensitize her to the Rh antigen(s). (**2**) If anti-Rh antibody (anti-D) is injected immediately postpartum it eliminates the Rh⁺ erythrocytes and prevents sensitization. The incidence of deaths due to HDNB fell during the period 1950–1966 with improved patient care. The decline in the disease was accelerated by the advent of Rhesus prophylaxis in 1969.

Direct antiglobulin test

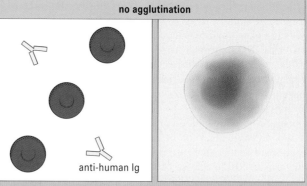

Fig. 24.9 This test, also called a Coombs' test, is used to detect antibody on a patient's erythrocytes. If antibody is present the erythrocytes can be agglutinated by anti-human immunoglobulin. If no antibody is present on the red cells, they are not agglutinated by anti-human immunoglobulin.

towards erythrocyte antigens, or immune complexes adsorbed onto the erythrocyte surface.

The direct antiglobulin test is also used to detect antibodies on red cells in mismatched transfusions, and in HDNB.

Autoimmune hemolytic anemias can be divided into three types, depending upon whether they are caused by:

- warm-reactive autoantibodies, which react with the antigen at 37 °C;
- cold-reactive autoantibodies, which can only react with antigen at below 37 °C;
- antibodies provoked by allergic reactions to drugs.

Warm-reactive autoantibodies cause accelerated clearance of erythrocytes

Warm-reactive autoantibodies are frequently found against Rhesus system antigens, including determinants of the RhC and RhE loci as well as RhD. They differ from the antibodies responsible for transfusion reactions in that they appear to react with different epitopes.

Warm-reactive autoantibodies to other blood group antigens exist, but are relatively rare.

Most of these hemolytic anemias are of unknown cause, but some are associated with other autoimmune diseases, including SLE and rheumatoid arthritis.

Q. What mechanisms could lead to the anemia associated with these autoantibodies?
A. Fc receptor-mediated erythrophagocytosis or complement-dependent lysis.

The anemia appears to be a result of accelerated clearance of the sensitized erythrocytes by spleen macrophages more often than being caused by complement-mediated lysis.

Cold-reactive autoantibodies cause erythrocyte lysis by complement fixation

Cold-reactive autoantibodies are often present in higher titers than the warm-reactive autoantibodies. The antibodies are primarily IgM and fix complement strongly. In most cases they are specific for the Ii blood group system. The I and i epitopes are expressed on the precursor polysaccharides that produce the ABO system epitopes, and are the result of incomplete glycosylation of the core polysaccharide.

The reaction of the antibody with the erythrocytes takes place in the peripheral circulation (particularly in winter), where the temperature in the capillary loops of exposed skin may fall below 30 °C. In severe cases, peripheral necrosis may occur due to aggregation and microthrombosis of small vessels caused by complement-mediated destruction in the periphery.

The severity of the anemia is therefore directly related to the complement-fixing ability of the patient's serum. (Fc-mediated removal of sensitized cells in the spleen and liver is not involved because these organs are too warm for the antibodies to bind.)

Most cold-reactive autoimmune hemolytic anemias occur in older people. Their cause is unknown, but it is notable that the autoantibodies produced are usually of very limited clonality.

Q. Why would you expect the autoimmune response to Ii antigens to be of limited clonality? There are two reasonable explanations, which are not mutually exclusive.

A. The numbers of autoreactive clones may have been curtailed by negative selection during B cell development. In addition, the antigens are carbohydrate and induce an IgM response (T independent) which has not been subject to diversification.

However, some cases may follow infection with *Mycoplasma pneumoniae*, and these are acute-onset diseases of short duration with polyclonal autoantibodies. Such cases are thought to be due to cross-reacting antigens on the bacteria and the erythrocytes, producing a bypass of normal tolerance mechanisms (see Chapter 19).

Drug-induced reactions to blood components occur in three different ways

Drugs (or their metabolites) can provoke hypersensitivity reactions against blood cells, including erythrocytes and platelets. This can occur in three different ways (Fig. 24.10).

- **The drug binds to the blood cells and antibodies are produced against the drug.** In this case it is necessary for both the drug and the antibody to be present to produce the reaction. This phenomenon was first recorded by Ackroyd, who noted thrombocytopenic purpura (destruction of platelets leading to purpuric rash) following administration of the drug sedormid. Hemolytic anemias have been reported following the administration of a wide variety of drugs, including penicillin, quinine and sulfonamides. All of these conditions are rare.
- **Drug–antibody immune complexes are adsorbed onto the erythrocyte cell membrane.** When drug–antibody immune complexes are adsorbed on to the erythrocyte cell membrane damage occurs by complement-mediated lysis.
- **The drug induces an allergic reaction.** The drug induces an allergic reaction and autoantibodies are directed against the erythrocyte antigens themselves, as occurs in 0.3% of patients given α-methyldopa. The antibodies produced are similar to those in patients with warm-reactive antibody. However, the condition remits shortly after the cessation of drug treatment.

Drug-induced reactions to blood cells

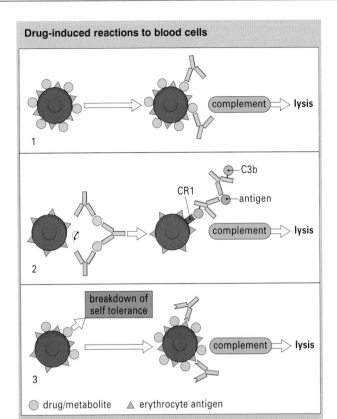

○ drug/metabolite   ▲ erythrocyte antigen

Fig. 24.10 Three ways that drug treatment can cause damage are illustrated. **(1)** The drug adsorbs to cell membranes. Antibodies to the drug bind to the cell and complement-mediated lysis occurs. **(2)** Immune complexes of drugs and antibody become adsorbed to the red cell. This could be mediated by an Fc receptor, but is more probably via the C3b receptor CR1. Damage occurs by complement-mediated lysis. **(3)** Drugs, presumably adsorbed onto cell membranes, induce a breakdown of self tolerance, possibly by stimulating T_H cells. This leads to the formation of antibodies to other blood group antigens on the cell surface. Note that in examples 1 and 2 the drug must be present for cell damage to occur, whereas in 3 the cells are destroyed whether they carry adsorbed drug or not.

Autoantibodies to platelets may cause thrombocytopenia

Autoantibodies to platelets are seen in up to 70% of cases of **idiopathic thrombocytopenic purpura (ITP)**, a disorder in which there is accelerated removal of platelets from the circulation, mediated primarily by splenic macrophages. The mechanism of removal is via the immune adherence receptors on these cells.

ITP most often develops after bacterial or viral infections, but may also be associated with autoimmune diseases including SLE. In SLE, antibodies to cardiolipin, which is present on platelets, can sometimes be detected. Autoantibodies to cardiolipin and other phospholipids can inhibit one aspect of blood clotting (**lupus anticoagulant**) and can be associated, in some cases, with venous thrombosis and recurrent abortions.

Thrombocytopenia may also be induced by drugs by similar mechanisms to those outlined in Figure 24.10.

Type II hypersensitivity reactions in tissues

A number of autoimmune conditions occur in which antibodies to tissue antigens cause immunopathological damage by activation of type II hypersensitivity mechanisms. The antigens are mostly extracellular, and may be expressed on structural proteins or on the surface of cells. The resulting diseases discussed here include Goodpasture's syndrome, pemphigus and myasthenia gravis.

It is often possible to demonstrate autoantibodies to particular cytoplasmic proteins, but it has been debated whether such antibodies could actually reach the intracellular antigens to cause damage. For this reason it had been thought that recognition of autoantigen by T cells is probably more important pathologically. More recently, a role for endocytosed, intracellular antibodies has been described in protection against viral infections, and this indicates that autoantibodies could potentially follow similar routes to target their antigens.

Antibodies against basement membranes produce nephritis in Goodpasture's syndrome

A number of patients with nephritis are found to have **antibodies to collagen type IV**, which is a major component of basement membranes. Collagen type IV undergoes alternate RNA splicing, which produces a number of variant proteins (**Goodpasture antigen**), but the antibodies appear to bind just those forms that retain the characteristic N terminus. The antibody is usually IgG and, in at least 50% of patients, it appears to fix complement.

Goodpasture's syndrome usually results in severe necrosis of the glomerulus, with fibrin deposition. The association of this type of nephritis with lung hemorrhage was originally noticed by Goodpasture (hence Goodpasture's syndrome). Although the lung symptoms do not occur in all patients, the association of lung and kidney damage is due to cross-reactive autoantigens in the basement membranes of the two tissues.

Pemphigus is caused by autoantibodies to an intercellular adhesion molecule

Pemphigus vulgaris is a serious blistering disease of the skin and mucous membranes. Patients have **autoantibodies against desmoglein-1 and desmoglein-3**, components of desmosomes, which form junctions between epidermal cells (Fig. 24.11). The antibodies disrupt cellular adhesion, leading to breakdown of the epidermis with separation of the superficial layers to form blisters.

Clinical disease profiles can be related to the specificity of the antibodies. For example:

- patients with only anti-desmoglein-3 tend to show mucosal disease;
- those with anti-desmoglein-1 and anti-desmoglein-3 have skin and mucosal involvement.

The disease profile is also partly dependent on the isotype of the antibodies produced; some patients show strong

Autoantibodies in pemphigus

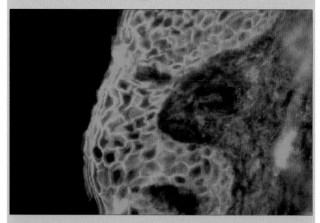

Fig. 24.11 The antibodies in pemphigus bind to components of the desmosome involved in cell adhesion. Desmoglein-1 and desmoglein-3 are most commonly involved, but other molecules, including the plakins and desmocollin, may also act as autoantigens. Immunofluorescence of human skin stained with anti-IgA. *(Courtesy of Dr R Mirakian and Mr P Collins.)*

deposition of IgA (see Fig. 24.11) whereas other have particularly high titres of IgG4. Recently, antibodies to mitochondrial components have also been implicated in the pathology, by inducing apoptosis in keratinocytes.

Pemphigus is strongly linked to a rare haplotype of HLA-DR4 (DRB1*0402), and this molecule has been shown to present a peptide of desmoglein-3, which other DR4 subtypes cannot. This is therefore a clear example of an autoimmune disease producing pathology by type II mechanisms.

In myasthenia gravis autoantibodies to acetylcholine receptors cause muscle weakness

Myasthenia gravis, a condition in which there is extreme muscular weakness, is associated with **antibodies to the acetylcholine receptors** on the surface of muscle membranes. The acetylcholine receptors are located at the motor endplate where the neuron contacts the muscle. Transmission of impulses from the nerve to the muscle takes place by the release of acetylcholine from the nerve terminal and its diffusion across the gap to the muscle fiber.

It was noticed that immunization of experimental animals with purified acetylcholine receptors produced a condition of muscular weakness that closely resembled human myasthenia. This suggested a role for antibody to the acetylcholine receptor in the human disease.

Analysis of the lesion in myasthenic muscles indicated that the disease was not due to an inability to synthesize acetylcholine, nor was there any problem in secreting it in response to a nerve impulse – the released acetylcholine was less effective at triggering depolarization of the muscle (Fig. 24.12).

Myasthenia gravis

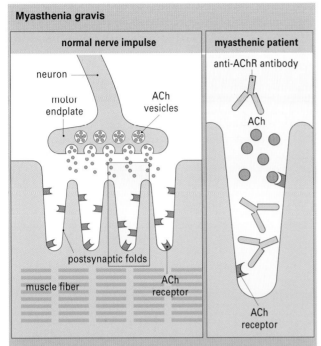

normal nerve impulse	myasthenic patient

normal nerve impulse:
neuron
motor endplate
ACh vesicles
postsynaptic folds
muscle fiber
ACh receptor

myasthenic patient:
anti-AChR antibody
ACh
ACh receptor

Fig. 24.12 Normally a nerve impulse passing down a neuron arrives at a motor endplate and causes the release of acetylcholine (ACh). This diffuses across the neuromuscular junction, binds ACh receptors (AChR) on the muscle, and causes ion channels in the muscle membrane to open, which in turn triggers muscular contraction. In myasthenia gravis, antibodies to the receptor block binding of the ACh transmitter. The effect of the released vesicle is therefore reduced, and the muscle can become very weak. Antibody blocking receptors are only one of the factors operating in the disease.

Motor endplate in myasthenia gravis

G
P
1
C
D
M
2

Fig. 24.13 (**1**) Electron micrograph showing IgG deposits (G) in discrete patches on the postsynaptic membrane (P). × 13 000. (**2**) Electron micrograph illustrating C9 (C) shows the postsynaptic region denuded of its nerve terminal – it consists of debris and degenerating folds (D). There is a strong reaction for C9 on this debris. × 9000. (M, muscle fiber.) *(Courtesy of Dr AG Engel.)*

Examination of neuromuscular endplates by immunochemical techniques has demonstrated IgG and the complement proteins, C3 and C9, on the postsynaptic folds of the muscle (Fig. 24.13).

Further evidence for a pathogenetic role for IgG in this disease was furnished by the discovery of transient muscle weakness in babies born to mothers with myasthenia gravis. This is significant because it is known that IgG can and does cross the placenta, entering the blood stream of the fetus.

IgG and complement are thought to act in two ways:

- by increasing the rate of turnover of the acetylcholine receptors; and
- by partial blocking of acetylcholine binding.

Cellular infiltration of myasthenic endplates is rarely seen, so it is assumed that damage does not involve effector cells.

Lambert–Eaton syndrome is a condition with similar symptoms to myasthenia gravis, where the muscular weakness is caused by defective release of acetylcholine from the neuron. In this case the autoantibodies are directed against components of voltage-gated calcium channels or the synaptic vesicle protein synaptogamin. The different forms of Lambert–Eaton syndrome are thought to relate to the target antigen and the class and titer of antibodies involved.

Q. Predict whether inhibitors of acetylcholinesterase will have any value in alleviating the symptoms of myasthenia gravis or Lambert–Eaton syndrome.

A. These drugs are often useful in myasthenia gravis because acetylcholine is present and an inhibitor of acetylcholinesterase will prolong its activity. They are less useful in Lambert–Eaton syndrome because acetylcholine is not released in the first place.

Autoantibodies and autoimmune disease

Although many autoantibodies react with tissue antigens, their significance in causing tissue damage and pathology *in vivo* is not always clear. For example, although autoantibodies to pancreatic islet cells can be detected *in vitro* using sera from some diabetic patients (Fig. 24.14), most of the immunopathological damage in autoimmune diabetes is thought to be caused by autoreactive T cells.

Until recently it was thought that autoantibodies against intracellular antigens would not usually cause immunopathology because they could not reach their antigen within a living cell. However, it now appears that antibodies such as anti-ribonucleoprotein (anti-RNP) and anti-DNA can reach the cell nucleus and modulate cell function – in some cases, they can induce apoptosis.

Islet cell autoantibodies

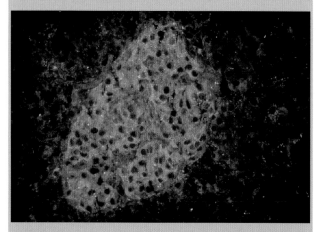

Fig. 24.14 Autoantibodies to the pancreas in diabetes mellitus may be demonstrated by immunofluorescence. The antibodies are diagnostically useful, and may contribute to the pathology. *(Courtesy of Dr B Dean.)*

Although the relative importance of antibody in causing cell damage is still debated, autoantibodies against internal antigens of cells often make excellent disease markers because they are frequently detectable before immunopathological damage occurs.

Finally, there are a group of conditions where autoantibodies actually stimulate the target cells. For example in some forms of autoimmune thyroid disease antibodies to the thyroid-stimulating hormone (TSH) receptor mimic TSH, thereby stimulating thyroid function (see Chapter 21).

CRITICAL THINKING: BLOOD GROUPS AND HEMOLYTIC DISEASE OF THE NEWBORN (SEE P. 443 FOR EXPLANATIONS)

Mrs Chareston has the blood group O, Rhesus negative, and her husband Mr Chareston is A, Rhesus positive. They have had four children, of which two have been affected by hemolytic disease of the newborn (HDNB), as follows:

- first child born 1968 – unaffected;
- second child born 1974 – mildly affected;
- third child born 1976 – seriously affected, required intrauterine blood transfusion;
- fourth child born 1980 – unaffected.

In both affected cases (second and third), the cause of the hemolytic disease was identified as antibodies to Rhesus D binding to the child's red cells. Following the second, third, and fourth deliveries, Mrs Chareston was given antibodies to the Rhesus D blood group (Rhesus prophylaxis was introduced in the UK in 1972).

1   From this information, what can you deduce about the blood group of the first child?

2   Why does HDNB usually become more serious with successive pregnancies?

3   What is the reason for giving anti-Rhesus D antibodies to the mother?

4   Why are the antibodies given postpartum and not earlier?

5   Give an explanation of why the Rhesus prophylaxis after the second delivery failed to prevent HDNB in the third child.

6   What explanation can be given to account for the fact that the fourth child is unaffected?

When the blood groups of the children are examined it is found that they are:

- first child – O, Rh$^+$;
- second child – B, Rh$^+$;
- third child – A, Rh$^+$;
- fourth child – A, Rh$^-$.

7   As Mrs Chareston has antibodies to blood group A, why was the fourth child not affected by HDNB caused by these antibodies?

8   One of these children was definitely not fathered by Mr Chareston – which child?

Further reading

Alarcón-Segovia D, Ruiz-Argüelles A, Llorente L. Broken dogma: penetration of autoantibodies into living cells. Immunol Today 1996;17:163–164.

Amagai M. Autoantibodies against desmosomal cadherins in pemphigus. J Dermatol Sci 1999;20:92–102.

Anstee DJ. Blood group active substances of the human red blood cell. Vox Sang 1990;58:1.

Black M, Mignogna MD, Scully C. Pemphigus vulgaris. Oral Dis 2005;11:119–130.

Dean FG, Wilson GR, Li M, Edgtton KL, et al. Experimental autoimmune Goodpasture's disease: a pathogenetic role for both effector cells and antibody injury. Kidney Int 2005;67:566–575.

Engelfriet CP, Reesink HW, Judd WJ, et al. Current status of immunoprophylaxis with anti-D immunoglobulin. Vox Sang 2003;85:328–337.

Lang B, Newsom-Davis J. Immunopathology of the Lambert–Eaton myasthenic syndrome. Springer Semin Immunopathol 1995;17:3–15.

Mauro I, Colin Y, Chenif-Zahar B, et al. Molecular genetic basis of the human Rhesus blood group system. Nat Genet 1993; 5:62–65.

Payne AS, Hanakawa Y, Amagai M, Stanley JR. Desmosomes and disease: pemphigus and bullous impetigo. Curr Opin Cell Biol 2004;16:536–543.

Race R, Sanger R. Blood groups in man. 6th edn. Oxford: Blackwell Scientific Publications; 1975.

Russo D, Redman C, Lee S. Association of XK and Kell blood group proteins. J Biol Chem 1998;273:13950–13956.

Schulz DR, Tozman EC. Anti-neutrophil cytoplasmic antibodies: major autoantigens, pathophysiology, and disease associations. Semin Arthritis Rheum 1995;25:143–159.

Vincent A. Antibody-mediated disorders of neuro-muscular transmission. Clin Neurophysiol Suppl 2004;57:147–158.

Yamamoto F-I, Clausen H, White T, et al. Molecular genetic basis of the histo-blood group ABO system. Nature 1990; 345:229.

CHAPTER 25

Hypersensitivity (Type III)

SUMMARY

- **Immune complexes are formed when antibody meets antigen**. They are removed by the mononuclear phagocyte system following complement activation. Persistence of antigen from chronic infection or in autoimmune disease can lead to immune complex disease.

- **Immune complexes can trigger a variety of inflammatory processes.** Fc–FcR interactions are the key mediators of inflammation. Most importantly, Fc regions within immune deposits within tissues engage Fc receptors on activated neutrophils, lymphocytes, and platelets to induce inflammation. During chronic inflammation B cells and macrophages are the predominant infiltrating cell type, and activation of endogenous cells within the organ participates in fibrosis and disease progression.

- **Experimental models demonstrate the main immune complex diseases.** Serum sickness can be induced with large injections of foreign antigen. Autoimmunity causes immune complex disease in the NZB/NZW mouse. Injection of antigen into the skin of presensitized animals produces the Arthus reaction.

- **Immune complexes are normally removed by the mononuclear phagocyte system.** Complement helps to disrupt antigen–antibody bonds and keeps immune complexes soluble. Primate erythrocytes bear a receptor for C3b and are important for transporting complement-containing immune complexes to the spleen for removal. Complement deficiencies lead to the formation of large, relatively insoluble complexes, which deposit in tissues.

- **The size of immune complexes affects their deposition.** Deposition of circulating, soluble immune complexes is limited by physical factors, such as the size and charge of the complexes. Small, positively charged complexes have the greatest propensity for deposition within vessels. Large immune complexes are rapidly removed in the liver and spleen.

- **Immune complex deposition in the tissues results in tissue damage.** Immune complexes can form both in the circulation, leading to systemic disease, and at local sites such as the lung. Charged cationic antigens have tissue-binding properties, particularly for the glomerulus, and help to localize complexes to the kidney. Factors that tend to increase blood vessel permeability enhance the deposition of immune complexes in tissues.

Immune complex diseases

Immune complexes are formed when antibody meets antigen, and generally they are removed effectively by the liver and spleen via processes involving complement, mononuclear phagocytes and erythrocytes.

Immune complexes may persist and eventually deposit in a range of tissues and organs. The complement and effector cell-mediated damage that follows is known as a type III hypersensitivity reaction or immune complex disease.

The sites of immune complex deposition are partly determined by the localization of the antigen in the tissues and partly by how circulating complexes become deposited.

Immune complex formation can result from:

- persistent infection;
- inhalation of antigenic material (Fig. 25.1);
- autoimmune disease;
- cryoglobulins.

Type II and type III hypersensitivity reactions are similar in concept and action and are not mutually exclusive. Both types of reactions may be seen in autoimmune rheumatic disorders such as systemic lupus erythematosus where autoimmune haemolytic anaemia and immune thrombocytopenic purpura may occur.

Three categories of immune complex disease

cause	antigen	site of complex deposition
persistent infection	microbial antigen	infected organ(s), kidney
autoimmunity	self antigen	kidney, joint, arteries, skin
inhaled antigen	mold, plant, or animal antigen	lung

Fig. 25.1 This table indicates the source of the antigen and the organs most frequently affected.

Immunofluorescence study of immune complexes in infectious disease

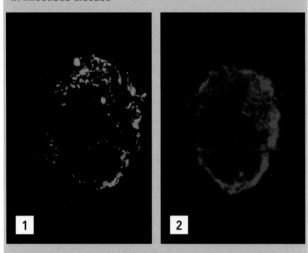

Fig. 25.2 These serial sections of the renal artery of a patient with chronic hepatitis B infection are stained with fluoresceinated anti-hepatitis B antigen (**1**) and rhodaminated anti-IgM (**2**). The presence of both antigen and antibody in the intima and media of the arterial wall indicates the deposition of complexes at this site. IgG and C3 deposits are also detectable with the same distribution. *(Courtesy of Dr A Nowoslawski.)*

Persistent infection with a weak antibody response can lead to immune complex disease

The combined effects of a low-grade persistent infection and a weak antibody response lead to chronic immune complex formation, and eventual deposition of complexes in the tissues (Fig. 25.2). Diseases with this etiology include:

- leprosy;
- malaria;
- dengue hemorrhagic fever;
- viral hepatitis; and
- staphylococcal infective endocarditis.

Immune complexes can be formed with inhaled antigens

Immune complexes may be formed at body surfaces following exposure to extrinsic antigens.

Such reactions are seen in the lungs following repeated inhalation of antigenic materials from molds, plants, or animals. This is exemplified in:

- farmer's lung, where there are circulating antibodies to actinomycete fungi (found in moldy hay); and
- pigeon fancier's lung, where there are circulating antibodies to pigeon antigens.

Both diseases are forms of **extrinsic allergic alveolitis**, and occur only after repeated exposure to the antigen. Note that the antibodies induced by these antigens are primarily IgG, rather than the IgE seen in type I hypersensitivity reactions. When antigen again enters the body by inhalation, local immune complexes are formed in the alveoli leading to inflammation and fibrosis (Fig. 25.3).

Precipitating antibodies to actinomycete antigens are found in the sera of 90% of patients with farmer's lung. However, they are also found in some people with no disease, and are absent from some patients, so it seems that other factors are also involved in the disease process, including type IV hypersensitivity reactions.

Immune complex disease occurs in autoimmune rheumatic disorders

Immune complex disease is common in autoimmune disease, where the continued production of autoantibody to a self antigen leads to prolonged immune complex formation. As the number of complexes in the blood increases, the systems responsible for the removal of complexes (mononuclear phagocyte, erythrocyte, and complement) become overloaded, and complexes are deposited in the tissues (see Fig. 25.16). Systemic lupus erythematosus (SLE) is the classic disease characterized by immune complex deposition and others include Henoch-Schönlein purpura and primary Sjögren's syndrome.

Cryoglobulins precipitate at low temperature

Cryoglobulins are immunoglobulins that precipitate reversibly at low temperature. They may be divided into three classes:

- type I consists of a single monoclonal immunoglobulin and is typically found in association with lymphoproliferatve diseases;
- type II is monoclonal IgM with rheumatoid factor activity, i.e. it binds to IgG;
- type III consists of polyclonal IgM rheumatoid factors.

Types II and III, also referred to as mixed cryoglobulins, are found in association with infectious, immunological, and neoplastic diseases. Mixed cryoglobulinemic vasculitis is a major extra-hepatic manifestation of chronic hepatitis C virus infection. Clinical features include arthralgia, cutaneous purpuric vasculitis, glomerulonephritis and peripheral neuropathy. Hepatitis C virus associated mixed cryoglobulinemia is characterized by a clonal expansion of B cells secreting IgM-RF which may be found in the liver, bone marrow and in the peripheral blood mononuclear cells of hepatitis C virus infected patients.

Immune complexes and inflammation

Immune complexes are capable of triggering a wide variety of inflammatory processes:

- they interact directly with basophils and platelets (via Fc receptors) to induce the release of vasoactive amines (Fig. 25.4);

Extrinsic allergic alveolitis

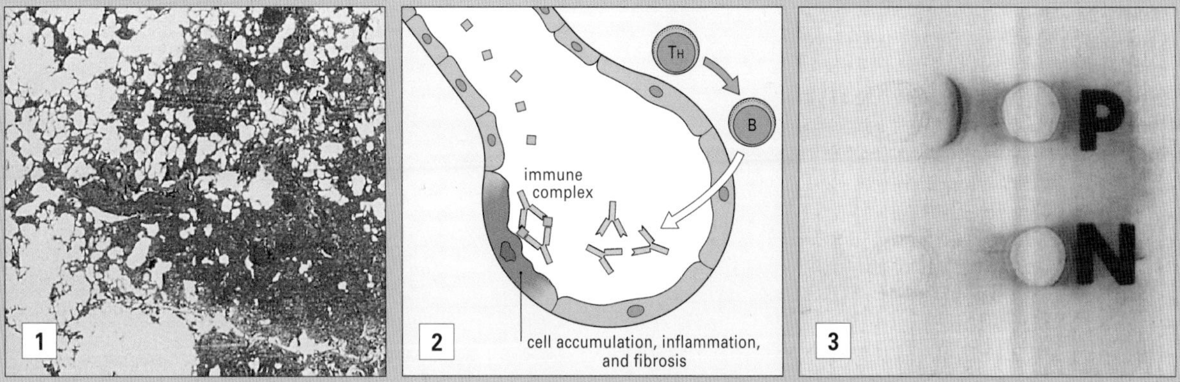

Fig. 25.3 The histological appearance of the lung in extrinsic allergic alveolitis (**1**) shows consolidated areas due to cell accumulation. When fungal antigen is inhaled into the lung of a sensitized individual, immune complexes are formed in the alveoli (**2**). Complement fixation leads to cell accumulation, inflammation, and fibrosis. Precipitin antibody (**P**) present in the serum of a patient with pigeon fancier's lung (**3**) is directed against the fungal antigen *Micropolyspora faeni*. Normal serum (**N**) lacks antibodies to this fungus.

- macrophages are stimulated to release cytokines, particularly tumor necrosis factor-α (TNFα) and interleukin-1 (IL-1), which have important roles in inflammation;
- they interact with the complement system to generate **C3a** and **C5a**, which stimulate the release of vasoactive amines (including histamine and 5-hydroxytryptamine) and chemotactic factors from mast cells and basophils; C5a is also chemotactic for basophils, eosinophils, and neutrophils.

Studies with knockout mice indicate that complement has a less proinflammatory role than previously thought, whereas cells bearing Fc receptors for IgG and IgE appear to be critical for developing inflammation, with complement having a protective effect.

The vasoactive amines released by platelets, basophils, and mast cells cause endothelial cell retraction and thus increase vascular permeability, allowing the deposition of immune complexes on the blood vessel wall (Fig. 25.5). The deposited complexes continue to generate C3a and C5a.

Platelets also aggregate on the exposed collagen of the vessel basement membrane to form microthrombi.

> **Q. Aggregation may be directly enhanced by the presence of immune complexes on the basement membrane. How can platelets recognize immune complexes?**
> A. They have an Fc receptor, FcγRIIa (see Fig. 25.4).

The aggregated platelets continue to produce vasoactive amines and to stimulate the production of C3a and C5a. Platelets are also a rich source of growth factors – these may be involved in the cellular proliferation seen in immune complex diseases such as **glomerulonephritis**.

Polymorphs are chemotactically attracted to the site by C5a. They attempt to engulf the deposited immune complexes, but are unable to do so because the complexes are bound to the vessel wall. Therefore they exocytose their lysosomal enzymes onto the site of deposition (see Fig. 25.5). If simply released into the blood or tissue fluids these lysosomal enzymes are unlikely to cause much inflammation, because they are rapidly neutralized by serum enzyme inhibitors. But if the phagocyte applies itself closely to the tissue-trapped complexes through Fc binding, then serum inhibitors are excluded and the enzymes may damage the underlying tissue.

Complement is an important mediator of immune complex disease

In many diseases, complement activation is triggered inappropriately and drives a vicious cycle, causing:

- further tissue damage;
- increased inflammation; and
- perpetuation of the disease.

This scenario is particularly evident in autoimmune diseases where immune complexes deposit in tissues and activate complement, causing damage and destruction of host cells. Examples include:

- the kidney in various autoimmune glomerular diseases; and
- the skin in autoimmune diseases where cutaneous vasculitis is a feature such as SLE, Sjögren's syndrome and Henoch–Schönlein purpura.

Staining of these tissues for complement deposits reveals the full extent of involvement. The tissues are often packed with C3 fragments and other complement proteins. Complement activation is also evident in the blood in these diseases; complement activity and the plasma concentrations of the major components C3 and C4 are reduced due to consumption in the tissues and levels of complement activation fragments are increased.

In SLE, autoantibodies are generated against cell contents including DNA, cytoplasmic proteins, and small nuclear ribonucleoproteins. The source of these autoantigens is apoptosis and failure to effectively clear apoptotic bodies has been demonstrated in SLE, resulting in the accumulation of apoptotic cell remnants. Immune complexes form when autoantibodies bind post-apoptotic debris and these deposit in capillary beds in organs such as skin, kidney, joint, and brain where they activate complement causing further tissue damage. Here complement is playing dual roles:

Immune complexes as a trigger for increasing vascular permeability

blood   tissue

endothelium

immune complexes

complement

platelets

CR1

erythrocyte

basophil

vasoactive amines

increase in endothelial permeability

liver and spleen   deposition in vessels

Fig. 25.4 Immune complexes normally bind complement and are removed to the liver and spleen after binding to CR1 on erythrocytes. In inflammation, immune complexes act on basophils and platelets (in humans) to produce vasoactive amine release. The amines released (e.g. histamine, 5-hydroxytryptamine) cause endothelial cell retraction and thus increase vascular permeability.

- the important immune complex solubilizing roles will prevent immune complex deposition until the capacity of the system is exceeded;
- beyond this threshold complexes deposit and activate complement in the tissues, causing pathology.

Patients with active SLE often have markedly decreased plasma levels of complement activity and the components C3 and C4 due to the massive and widespread activation of the system.

Autoantibodies to complement components can modulate complement activity

Autoantibodies may also develop that directly target the complement components and complexes. For example, autoantibodies against C1q are commonly found in SLE, correlating particularly with renal involvement.

Deposition of immune complexes in blood vessel walls

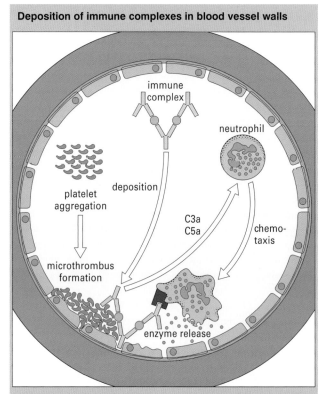

immune complex

neutrophil

platelet aggregation

deposition

C3a C5a

chemo-taxis

microthrombus formation

enzyme release

Fig. 25.5 Increased vascular permeability allows immune complexes to be deposited in the blood vessel wall. This induces platelet aggregation and complement activation. The aggregated platelets form microthrombi on the exposed collagen of the basement membrane of the endothelium. Neutrophils are attracted to the site by complement products, but cannot ingest the complexes. They therefore exocytose their lysosomal enzymes, causing further damage to the vessel wall.

Antibodies against the alternative pathway C3 convertase bind and stabilize the complex, markedly increasing its functional half-life and thus consuming C3. These autoantibodies were first identified in patients with **membranoproliferative glomerulonephritis (MPGN)** and were therefore termed **C3 nephritic factors (C3NeF)**, but they may also be found in SLE.

Immune complexes clearance by the mononuclear phagocyte system

Immune complexes are opsonized with C3b following complement activation, and removed by the mononuclear phagocyte system, particularly in the liver and spleen. Removal is mediated by the complement C3b receptor, CR1.

In primates, the bulk of CR1 in blood is found on erythrocytes. (Non-primates do not have erythrocyte CR1, and must therefore rely on platelet CR1.) There are about 700 receptors per erythrocyte, and their effectiveness is enhanced by the grouping of receptors in patches, allowing high-avidity binding to the large complexes.

CR1 readily binds immune complexes that have fixed complement, as has been shown by experiments with animals lacking complement (Fig. 25.6).

Effects of complement depletion on handling of immune complexes

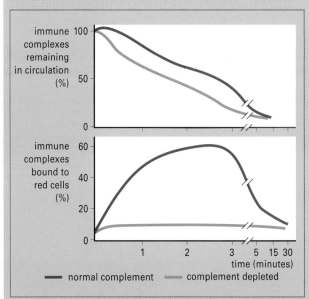

Fig. 25.6 A bolus of immune complexes was infused into the circulation of a primate. In animals with a normal complement system the complexes were bound quickly by the CR1 on erythrocytes. In animals whose complement had been depleted by treatment with cobra venom factor, the erythrocytes hardly bound immune complexes at all. Paradoxically, this results in slightly faster removal of complexes in the depleted animals, with the complexes being deposited in the tissues rather than being removed by the spleen. *(Based on data from Waxman FJ, et al. J Clin Invest 1984;74:1329–1340.)*

Clearance of immune complexes in the liver

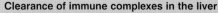
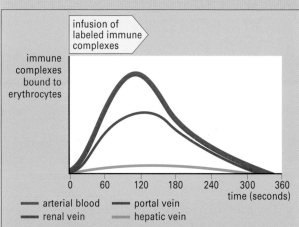

Fig. 25.7 ^{125}I-BSA/anti-BSA complexes were infused into a primate over a period of 120 seconds. Blood was sampled from renal, portal, and hepatic veins, and the level of immune complexes bound to the erythrocytes was measured by radioactive counting. The levels of complexes in the renal and portal veins were similar to that in arterial blood. However, complexes were virtually absent from hepatic venous blood throughout, indicating that complexes bound to erythrocytes are removed during a single transit through the liver. *(Based on data from Cornacoff JB, et al. J Clin Invest 1983;71:236–247.)*

In normal primates the erythrocytes provide a buffer mechanism, binding complexes that have fixed complement and effectively removing them from the plasma. In small blood vessels 'streamline flow' allows the erythrocytes to travel in the center of the vessel surrounded by the flowing plasma. Thus it is only the plasma that makes contact with the vessel wall. Only in the sinusoids of the liver and spleen, or at sites of turbulence, do the erythrocytes make contact with the lining of the vessels.

The complexes are transported to the liver and spleen, where they are removed by fixed tissue macrophages (Fig. 25.7). Most of the CR1 is also removed in the process, so in situations of continuous immune complex formation the number of active receptors falls rapidly, impairing the efficiency of immune complex handling.

In patients with SLE, for example, the number of receptors may well be halved. With fewer complement receptors the complexes are cleared rapidly to the liver, but these complexes, which arrive directly rather than on red cells, are later released into the circulation again and may then deposit in the tissues elsewhere and lead to inflammation.

Complexes can also be released from erythrocytes in the circulation by the enzymatic action of factor I.

Q. What action does factor I have in the complement system?
A. It cleaves C3b and C4b into fragments (see Fig. 4.7).

This action leaves a small fragment (C3dg) attached to the CR1 on the cell membrane. These soluble complexes are then removed by phagocytic cells, particularly those in the liver, bearing receptors for IgG Fc (Fig. 25.8).

Complement solubilization of immune complexes

It has been known since Heidelberger's work on the precipitin curve in the 1930s that complement delays precipitation of immune complexes, though this information was forgotten for a long time.

The ability to keep immune complexes soluble is a function of the classical complement pathway. The complement components reduce the number of antigen epitopes that the antibodies can bind (i.e. they reduce the valency of the antigen) by intercalating into the lattice of the complex, resulting in smaller, soluble complexes. In primates these complement-bearing complexes are readily bound by the C3b receptor (CR1) on erythrocytes.

Complement can rapidly resolubilize precipitated complexes through the alternative pathway. The solubilization appears to occur by the insertion of complement C3b and C3d fragments into the complexes.

It may be that complexes are continually being deposited in normal individuals, but are removed by solubilization. If this is the case, then the process will be inadequate in hypocomplementemic patients and lead to prolonged complex deposition.

Solubilization defects have indeed been observed in sera from patients with systemic immune complex disease, but whether the defect is primary or secondary is not known.

409

Immune complex clearance

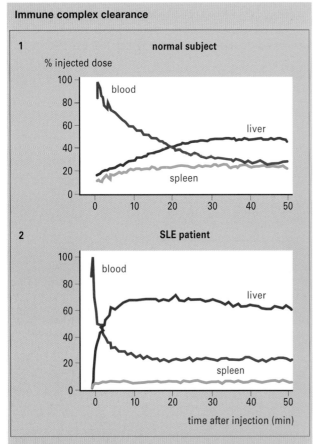

Fig. 25.8 (**1**) Immune complex clearance in a healthy normal subject. (**2**) Immune complex clearance in a patient with SLE. Radiolabeled soluble complexes were injected intravenously and immune complex localization monitored by dynamic imaging. In the normal subject complexes remained longer in the blood through binding to CR1 on red cells, followed by clearance to the liver and the spleen, where immune complexes take part in immunoregulation. In the hypocomplementemic patient with SLE there was little binding to red cells, but rapid clearance to organs such as the liver, with little localizing to the spleen, leading to impaired immunoregulation, which may be a factor in the persistence of autoimmunity.

Q. What evidence implies that defective solubilization of complexes is a primary cause of immune complex disease?

A. Genetic deficiency of classical pathway components (i.e. primary defects) are associated with SLE and some other immune complex diseases (see Figs. 4.16, 16.13, and Chapter 20).

Complement deficiency impairs clearance of complexes

In patients with low levels of classical pathway components there is poor binding of immune complexes to erythrocytes. The complement deficiency may result from:

- depletion, caused by immune complex disease; or
- a hereditary disorder, as is the case in C2 deficiency.

This might be expected to result in persistent immune complexes in the circulation, but in fact the reverse occurs, with the complexes disappearing rapidly from the circulation.

Immune complex transport and removal

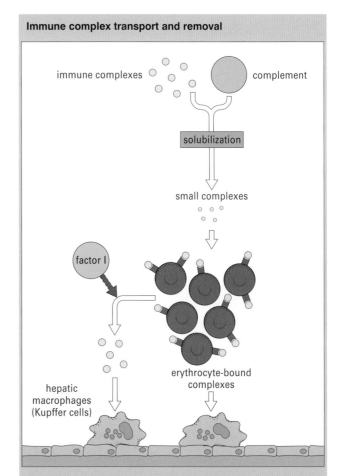

Fig. 25.9 In primates, complexes solubilized by complement are bound by CR1 on erythrocytes and transported to the liver where they are removed by hepatic macrophages. Complexes released from erythrocytes by factor I are taken up by cells (including macrophages) bearing receptors for Fc and complement.

These non-erythrocyte-bound complexes are taken up rapidly by the liver (but not the spleen) and are then released to be deposited in tissues such as skin, kidney, and muscle, where they can set up inflammatory reactions (Fig. 25.9).

Infusion of fresh plasma, containing complement, restores the clearance patterns to normal, illustrating the importance of complement in the clearance of immune complexes.

Failure to localize in the spleen not only results in immune complex disease, but may also have important implications for the development of appropriate immune responses. This is because the spleen plays a vital role in antigen processing and the induction of immune responses (see Chapter 2).

The size of immune complexes affects their deposition

In general, larger immune complexes are rapidly removed by the liver within a few minutes, whereas smaller complexes circulate for longer periods (Fig. 25.10). This is because larger complexes are:

- more effective at binding to Fc receptors and at fixing complement, so binding better to erythrocytes;
- released more slowly from the erythrocytes by the action of factor I.

Complex clearance by mononuclear phagocytes

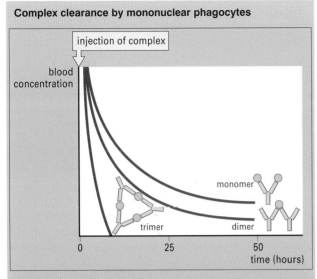

Fig. 25.10 Large immune complexes are cleared most quickly because they present an IgG–Fc lattice to mononuclear phagocyte cells with Fc receptors, permitting higher avidity binding to these cells. They also fix complement better than small complexes.

Anything that affects the size of complexes is therefore likely to influence clearance.

It has been suggested that a genetic defect that favors the production of low-affinity antibody could lead to the formation of smaller complexes, and so to immune complex disease.

Antibodies to self antigens may have low affinity and recognize only a few epitopes. This results in small complexes and long clearance times because the formation of large, cross-linked lattices is restricted.

Affinity maturation is dependent on efficient somatic mutation and selection of B cells within germinal centers following binding of antigen. This process is far more effective when B cells are stimulated by antigen or immune complexes coated with complement. Patients with complement deficiencies are particularly prone to develop immune complex disease and recent evidence indicates that another way that this is brought about is through poor targeting of antigen complexes to germinal centers, so preventing affinity maturation.

Immunoglobulin classes affect the rate of immune complex clearance

Striking differences have been observed in the clearance of complexes with different immunoglobulin classes:

- IgG complexes are bound by erythrocytes and are gradually removed from the circulation;
- IgA complexes bind poorly to erythrocytes, but disappear rapidly from the circulation, with increased deposition in the kidney, lung, and brain.

Q. Provide an explanation for the different patterns of localization of immune complexes containing IgG and those containing IgA

A. IgG-containing immune complexes activate the complement classical pathway and can bind to CR1 on erythrocytes. IgA does not activate the classical pathway, but can bind to Fcα receptors on mononuclear phagocytes (see Fig. 3.15).

Phagocyte defects allow complexes to persist

Opsonized immune complexes are normally removed by the mononuclear phagocyte system, mainly in the liver and spleen. However, when large amounts of complex are present, the mononuclear phagocyte system may become overloaded, leading to a rise in the level of circulating complex and increased deposition in the glomerulus and elsewhere.

Defective mononuclear phagocytes have been observed in human immune complex disease, but this may be the result of overload rather than a primary defect. In SLE, defects in macrophage clearance of apoptotic debris increase the exposure of intracellular constituents to the immune system. Immune complexes formed between autoantibodies and nucleic acids from apoptotic material can activate plasmacytoid dendritic cells which then produce large quantities of pro-inflammatory Type I interferons – a hallmark cytokine in SLE.

Dendritic cells can also capture immune complexes containing DNA fragments via FcγRIII receptors and TLR 9, generating TNFα production in the presence of granulocyte-macrophage colony-stimulating factor (GM-CSF). Dendritic cells can also be activated by immune complexes containing RNA fragments, which activate intracellular TLR7.

Carbohydrate on antibodies affects complex clearance

Carbohydrate groups on immunoglobulin molecules have been shown to be important for the efficient removal of immune complexes by phagocytic cells.

Abnormalities of these carbohydrates occur in immune complex diseases such as rheumatoid arthritis, thus aggravating the disease process. Oligosaccharides associated with the Fc region of IgG lack the normally terminating galactose residue, enhancing rheumatoid factor binding and mannan-binding protein has been shown to bind agalactosyl IgG and subsequently activate complement.

Immune complex deposition in tissues

Immune complexes may persist in the circulation for prolonged periods of time. However, simple persistence is not usually harmful in itself; the problems start only when complexes are deposited in the tissues.

Two questions are relevant to tissue deposition:

- Why are complexes deposited?
- Why do complexes show affinity for particular tissues in different diseases?

The most important trigger for immune complex deposition is probably an increase in vascular permeability

Animal experiments have shown that inert substances such as colloidal carbon will be deposited in vessel walls following the administration of vasoactive substances, such as histamine or serotonin. Circulating immune complexes are deposited in a similar way following the infusion of agents that cause the liberation of mast cell vasoactive amines (including histamine). Pretreatment with antihistamines blocks this effect.

Effect of a vasoactive amine antagonist on immune complex disease

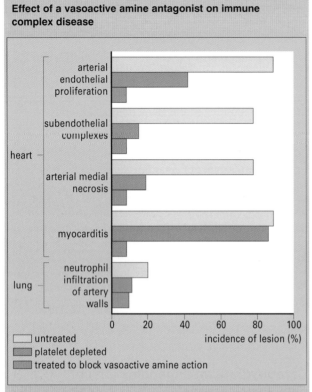

untreated
platelet depleted
treated to block vasoactive amine action

Fig. 25.11 Serum sickness was induced in rabbits with a single injection of bovine serum albumin. The animals were either untreated, platelet depleted, or treated with drugs to block vasoactive amine action. The incidence of serum sickness lesions in the heart and lung was scored. Drug treatment considerably reduced the signs of disease by lowering vascular permeability and thus minimizing immune complex deposition.

In studies of experimental immune complex disease in rabbits, long-term administration of vasoactive amine antagonists, such as chlorpheniramine and methysergide, has been shown to reduce immune complex deposition considerably (Fig. 25.11). More importantly young NZB/NZW mice which normally develop proteinuria by 9 months old, have less renal pathology, when treated with methysergide. Methysergide blocks the formation of the vasoactive amine 5-hydroxytryptamine (5-HT), and thus blocks a variety of inflammatory events (e.g. deposition of complexes, neutrophil infiltration of capillary walls, and endothelial proliferation), all of which produce the glomerular pathology.

Increases in vascular permeability can be initiated by a range of mechanisms, which vary in importance, depending on the diseases and species concerned. This variability makes interpretation of some of the animal models difficult. In general, however, complement, mast cells, basophils, and platelets must all be considered as potential producers of vasoactive amines.

Immune complex deposition is most likely where there is high blood pressure and turbulence

Many macromolecules deposit in the glomerular capillaries, where the blood pressure is approximately four times that of most other capillaries (Fig. 25.12).

Hemodynamic factors affecting complex deposition

Fig. 25.12 Factors that affect complex deposition include filtration and high blood pressure, both of which occur in the formation of ultrafiltrate in the renal glomerulus (**1**). Turbulence at curves or bifurcations of arteries (**2**) also favors deposition of immune complexes.

If the glomerular blood pressure of a rabbit is reduced by partially constricting the renal artery or by ligating the ureter, deposition is also reduced. If the glomerular blood pressure is increased by experimentally induced hypertension, immune complex deposition is enhanced as shown by the development of serum sickness. Elsewhere, the most severe lesions also occur at sites of turbulence:

• at turns or bifurcations of arteries,
• in vascular filters such as the choroid plexus and the ciliary body of the eye.

Q. Why should the site of bifurcation in an artery be more susceptible to damage than other sites?
A. This site is subject to high pressure and more erratic shear forces, which may affect the integrity of the endothelium (see Fig. 25.12). In addition blood cells and platelets are not segregated from the vessel wall by laminar flow.

Affinity of antigens for specific tissues can direct complexes to particular sites

Local high blood pressure explains the tendency for deposits to form in certain organs, but does not explain why complexes are deposited on specific organs in certain diseases. In SLE, the kidney is a particular target, whereas in rheumatoid arthritis, although circulating complexes are present, the kidney is usually spared and the joints are the principal target.

It is possible that the antigen in the complex provides the organ specificity, and a convincing model has been established to support this hypothesis. In the model, mice are given endotoxin causing cell damage and release of DNA, which then binds to healthy glomerular basement membrane. Anti-DNA is then produced by polyclonal activation of B cells, and is bound by the fixed DNA leading to local immune complex formation (Fig. 25.13). The production of rheumatoid factor (IgM anti-IgG) allows further immune complex formation to occur in situ.

Tissue binding of antigen with local immune complex formation

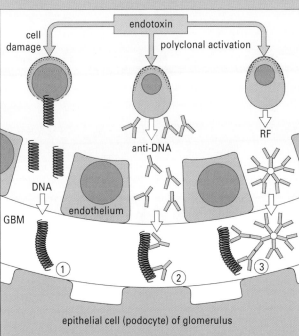

Fig. 25.13 Endotoxin injected into mice increases vascular permeability and induces cell damage and release of DNA. The DNA can then become deposited (**1**) on the collagen of the glomerular basement membrane (GBM) in the kidney. Endotoxin can also induce a polyclonal stimulation of B cells, some of which produce autoantibodies such as anti-DNA and anti-IgG – the latter are known as rheumatoid factors (RFs). Anti-DNA antibody can then bind to the deposited DNA forming a local immune complex (**2**). RFs have a low affinity for monomeric IgG, but bind with high avidity to the assembled DNA–anti-DNA complex (**3**). Thus further immune complex formation occurs in situ.

Immune complex deposition in the kidney

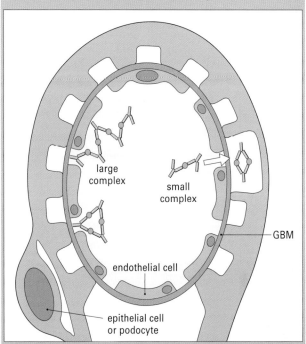

Fig. 25.14 The site of complex deposition in the kidney is dependent on the size of the complexes in the circulation. Large complexes become deposited on the glomerular basement membrane, whereas small complexes pass through the basement membrane and are seen on the epithelial side of the glomerulus.

It is possible that in other diseases antigens will be identified with affinity for particular organs.

The charge of the antigen and antibody may be important in some systems. For example, positively charged antigens and antibodies are more likely to be deposited in the negatively charged glomerular basement membrane.

The degree of glycosylation also affects the fate of complexes containing glycoprotein antigens because certain clearance mechanisms are activated by recognition of sugar molecules (e.g. mannan-binding protein).

In certain diseases the antibodies and antigens are both produced within the target organ. The extreme of this is reached in rheumatoid arthritis, where IgG anti-IgG rheumatoid factor is produced by plasma cells within the synovium; these antibodies then combine with each other (self-association), so setting up an inflammatory reaction.

The site of immune complex deposition depends partly on the size of the complex

The fact that the site of immune complex deposition depends partly on the size of the complex is exemplified in the kidney:

- small immune complexes can pass through the glomerular basement membrane, and end up on the epithelial side of the membrane;
- large complexes are unable to cross the membrane and generally accumulate between the endothelium and the basement membrane or the mesangium (Fig. 25.14).

The size of immune complexes depends on the valency of the antigen, and on the titer and affinity of the antibody.

The class of immunoglobulin in an immune complex can influence deposition

There are marked age- and sex-related variations in the class and subclass of anti-DNA antibodies seen in SLE.

Similarly, as NZB/NZW mice grow older there is a class switch, from predominantly IgM to IgG2a. This occurs earlier in females than in males and coincides with the onset of renal disease, indicating the importance of antibody class in the tissue deposition of complexes (Fig. 25.15).

Diagnosis of immune complex disease

The ideal place to look for immune complexes is in the affected organ (Figs. 25.2, 25.16).

Tissue samples may be examined by immunofluorescence for the presence of immunoglobulin and complement. The composition, pattern, and particular area of tissue affected all provide useful information on the severity and prognosis of the disease. For example:

Antibody classes in immune complex disease

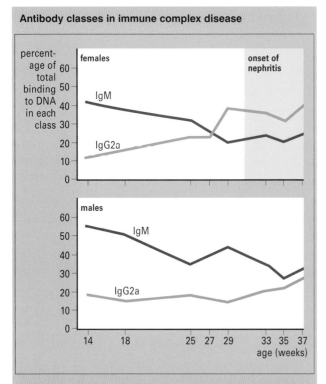

Fig. 25.15 Immune complex disease is automatic in the NZB/NZW mouse and follows a class switch during early development, from IgM to IgG2a. The graphs show the proportions of anti-DNA antibodies of the IgM and IgG2a isotypes in females and males. Both the class switch and fatal renal disease occur earlier in the female mice of this strain.

Immunofluorescence study of immune complexes in autoimmune disease

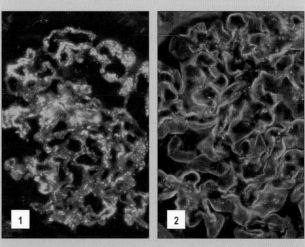

Fig. 25.16 These renal sections compare the effect of systemic lupus erythematosus (type III hypersensitivity) (**1**) and Goodpasture's syndrome (type II hypersensitivity) (**2**). In each case the antibody is detected with fluorescent anti-IgG. Complexes, formed in the blood and deposited in the kidney, form characteristic 'lumpy bumpy' deposits (**1**). The anti-basement membrane antibody in Goodpasture's syndrome forms an even layer on the glomerular basement membrane (**2**). *(Courtesy of Dr S Thiru.)*

- patients with the continuous, granular, subepithelial deposits of IgG found in membranous glomerulonephritis have a poor prognosis with prolonged heavy proteinuria;
- in contrast, those whose complexes are localized in the mesangium have a good prognosis and respond to immunosuppressive therapies.

Not all tissue-bound complexes give rise to an inflammatory response; for example, in SLE complexes are frequently found in skin biopsies from normal-looking skin, as well as from inflamed skin.

Assays for immune complexes in serum are more readily performed than in-situ immunofluorescence, although the results have to be interpreted carefully (see Method box 25.1).

CRITICAL THINKING: TYPE III SERUM SICKNESS AFTER FACTOR IX ADMINISTRATION (SEE P. 444 FOR EXPLANATIONS)

An 8-year-old boy with factor IX deficiency has had repeated episodes of bleeding into his joints and skin, despite requiring administration of factor IX. Ten days after receiving a dose, he developed fever, swelling of multiple joints, and a skin rash. On physical exam, his temperature was 39 °C, he had a diffuse maculopapular skin rash involving his torso and extremities, and both elbows and knees were red, warm, and appeared inflamed. His mother thought the appearance and distribution were very different from the typical appearance after either minor trauma or bleeding into his joints, which he had sustained on multiple previous occasions. His pediatrician ordered the following tests

(results shown in Table 25.1) and prescribed a short course of corticosteroids.

1 What immunologic mechanisms are involved in this inflammatory reaction after the boy received the factor IX?

2 Why were corticosteroids prescribed?

3 What is the likelihood that this type of reaction will develop again?

4 What measures would you take to prevent this reaction from occurring again?

Table 25.1

Variable	Result (normal range)
C3 (mg/dL)	38 (85–155)
C4 (mg/dL)	4 (12–45)
anti-nuclear antibody	Negative
hemoglobin (g/dL)	11.2
white cell count (cells/mm^3)	11 000
eosinophils (%)	1

He responds to treatment and his symptoms resolve, but 1 year later his mother notices that his face is swollen in the morning and his feet are swollen at the end of the day. Otherwise the boy feels well.

On physical exam, his blood pressure is elevated at 140/90 mmHg and his ankles are very edematous. His joints do not appear inflamed and the skin does not show either evidence of recent bleeding or inflammation. Results of tests are shown in Table 25.2.

5 What immunologic mechanisms are involved in this inflammatory reaction after the boy received the factor IX? How do they differ from the previous episode?

6 What is the likelihood that this type of reaction will develop again?

7 What measures would you take to prevent this reaction again?

Table 25.2

Variable	Result (normal range)
C3 (mg/dL)	142 (85–155)
C4 (mg/dL)	44 (12–45)
anti-nuclear antibody	Negative
hemoglobin (g/dL)	11.6
white cell count (cells/mm^3)	8600
eosinophils (%)	<1
albumin (g/dL)	2.5 (3.5–5.5)
urine protein (g/24 h)	8 (<0.2)

Further reading

Agnello V. Immune complex assays in rheumatic diseases. Hum Pathol 1983;14:343–349.

Arthus M. Injections répétées de sérum de cheval chez le lapin. C R Seances Soc Biol Fil 1903;55:817.

Birmingham DJ, Herbert LA, Cosio FG, et al. Immune complex erythrocyte complement receptor interactions in vivo during induction of glomerulonephritis in non-human primates. J Lab Clin Med 1990;116:242–252.

Boackle SA, Holer VM, Karp DR. CD21 augments antigen presentation in immune individuals. Eur J Immunol 1997;27:122–129.

Boruchov AM, Heller G, Veri MC, et al. Activating and inhibitory IgG Fc receptors on human DCs mediate opposing functions. J Clin Invest 2005;115:2914–2923.

Bruhns P, Samuelsson A, Pollard JW, Ravetch JV. Colony-stimulating factor-1-dependent macrophages are responsible for IVIG protection in antibody-induced autoimmune disease. Immunity 2003;18:573–581.

Clynes R, Maizes JS, Guinamard R, et al. Modulation of immune complex-induced inflammation in vivo by the co-ordinate expression of activation and inhibitory Fc receptors. J Exp Med 1999;189:179–185.

Cornacoff JB, Hebert LA, Smead WL, et al. Primate erythrocyte immune complex clearing mechanism. J Clin Invest 1983;71:236–247.

Czop J, Nussenzweig V. Studies on the mechanism of solubilization of immune precipitates by serum. J Exp Med 1976;143:615–630.

Davies KA, Hird V, Stewart S, et al. A study of in vivo immune complex formation and clearing in man. J Immunol 1990;144:4613–4620.

Davies KA, Peters AM, Beynon HLC, Walport MJ. Immune complex processing in patients with systemic lupus erythematosus – in vivo imaging and clearance studies. J Clin Invest 1992;90:2075–2083.

Davies KA, Chapman PT, Norsworthy PJ, et al. Clearance pathway of soluble immune complexes in the pig. Insights into the adaptive nature of antigen clearance in humans. J Immunol 1995;155:5760–5768.

Davies KA, Schifferli JA, Walport MJ. Complement deficiency and immune complex diseases. Springer Semin Immunopathol 1994;15:397–416.

Dixon FJ, Joseph D, Feldman JD, et al. Experimental glomerulonephritis: the pathogenesis of a laboratory model resembling the spectrum of human glomerulonephritis. J Exp Med 1961;113:899–919.

Dixon FJ, Vazquez JJ, Weigle WO, et al. Pathogenesis of serum sickness. Arch Pathol 1958;65:18–28.

Emlen W, Carl V, Burdick CG. Mechanism of transfer of immune complexes from red blood cell CR1 to monocytes. Clin Exp Immunol 1992;89:8–17.

Finbloom DS, Magilvary DB, Harford JB, et al. Influence of antigen on immune complex behaviour in mice. J Clin Invest 1981;68:214–224.

Fukuyama H, Nimmerjahn F, Ravetch JV. The inhibitory Fc gamma receptor modulates autoimmunity by limiting the accumulation of immunoglobulin G+ anti-DNA plasma cells. Nat Immunol 2005;6:99–106.

Heidelberger M. Quantitative chemical studies on complement or alexin. J Exp Med 1941;73:681–709.

Inman RD. Immune complexes in SLE. Clin Rheum Dis 1982;8:49–62.

Johnston A, Auda GR, Kerr MA, et al. Dissociation of primary antigen–antibody bonds is essential for complement mediated solubilization of immune complexes. Mol Immunol 1992;29:659–665.

Kijlstrea H, Van Es LA, Daha MR. The role of complement in the binding and degradation of immunoglobulin aggregates by macrophages. J Immunol 1979;123:2488–2493.

Lachmann PJ. Complement deficiency and the pathogenesis of autoimmune complex disease. Chem Immunol 1980;49:245–263.

Lucisano Valim M, Lachmann PJ. The effects of antibody isotype and antigenic epitope density on the complement-fixing activity of immune complexes: a systematic study using chimaeric anti-NIP antibodies with human Fc regions. Clin Exp Immunol 1991;84:1–8.

McGaha TL, Sorrentino B, Ravetch JV. Restoration of tolerance in lupus by targeted inhibitory receptor expression. Science 2005;307:590–593.

McKenzie SE, Taylor SM, Malladi P, et al. The role of the human Fc receptor FcγRIIA in the immune clearance of platelets: a transgene mouse model. J Immunol 1999;162:4311–4318.

Miller GW, Nussenzweig V. A new complement function: solubilization of antigen–antibody aggregates. Proc Natl Acad Sci USA 1975;72:418–422.

Muñoz LE, Lauber K, Schiller M, et al. The role of defective clearance of apoptotic cells in systemic autoimmunity. Nat Rev Rheumatol 2010;6:280–289.

Moll T, Nitschke L, Carroll M, et al. A critical role for Fc gamma RIIB in the induction of rheumatoid factors. J Immunol 2004;173:4724–4728.

Olsson M, Bruhns P, Frazier WA, et al. Platelet homeostasis is regulated by platelet expression of CD47 under normal conditions and in passive immune thrombocytopenia. Blood 2005;105:3577–3582.

Park SY, Ueda S, Ohno H, et al. Resistance of Fc receptor-deficient mice to fatal glomerulonephritis. J Clin Invest 1998;102:1229–1238.

Qiao J-H, Castellani LW, Fishbein MC, et al. Immune complex-mediated vasculitis increases coronary artery lipid accumulation in autoimmune-prone MRL mice. Arterioscler Thromb 1993;13:932–943.

Ravetch JV. Fc receptors. Curr Opin Immunol 1997;9:121–125.

Ravetch JV. A full complement of receptors in immune complex diseases. J Clin Invest 2002;110:1759–1761.

Schifferli JA, Ng YC, Peters DK. The role of complement and its receptor in the elimination of immune complexes. N Engl J Med 1986;315:488–495.

Sylvestre DL, Ravetch JV. A dominant role for mast cell Fc receptors in the Arthus reaction. Immunity 1996;5:387–390.

Takata Y, Tamura N, Fujita T. Interaction of C3 with antigen–antibody complexes in the process of solubilisation of immune precipitates. J Immunol 1984;132:2531–2537.

Terino FL, Powell MS, McKenzie IF, Hogarth PM. Recombinant soluble human FcγRII: production, characterization, and inhibition of the Arthus reaction. J Exp Med 1993;178:1617–1628.

Theofilopoulos AN, Dixon FJ. The biology and detection of immune complexes. Adv Immunol 1979;28:89–220.

Warren JS, Yabroff KR, Remick DG, et al. Tumour necrosis factor participates in the pathogenesis of acute immune complex alveolitis in the rat. J Clin Invest 1989;84:1873–1882.

Waxman FJ, Hebert LE, Cornacoff JB, et al. Complement depletion accelerates the clearance of immune complexes from the circulation of primates. J Clin Invest 1984;74:1329–1340.

Whaley K. Complement and immune complex diseases. In: Whaley K, ed. Complement in health and disease, Lancaster: MTP Press Ltd; 1987.

Williams RC. Immune complexes in clinical and experimental medicine. Massachusetts: Harvard University Press 1980.

World Health Organization Scientific Group. Technical report 606. The role of immune complexes in disease. Geneva: WHO; 1977.

CHAPTER 26

Hypersensitivity (Type IV)

SUMMARY

- **DTH reflects the presence of antigen-specific T cell-mediated inflammation.**

- **There are three variants of type IV hypersensitivity reaction** – contact, tuberculin, and granulomatous.

- **Contact hypersensitivity occurs at the site of contact with an allergen.** Sensitization occurs when skin dendritic cells internalize and process epicutaneously applied hapten and migrate to the draining lymph nodes where they activate antigen-specific T cells. On re-exposure to antigen, cytokines produced by skin cells (e.g. keratinocytes, Langerhans' cells), recruit antigen-specific, and also non-specific T cells, and macrophages.

- **Tuberculin-type hypersensitivity is induced by CD4 T cell responses to soluble antigens from a** variety of organisms. It is useful as a diagnostic test to detect infection with a number of infectious agents.

- **Granulomatous hypersensitivity is clinically the most important form of type IV hypersensitivity.** Persistence of antigen leads to chronic T cell activation, differentiation of macrophages into epithelioid cells, and their fusion to form giant cells. This granulomatous reaction results in tissue pathology. Granuloma formation is driven by T cell activation of macrophages, and is dependent on TNF. Inhibition of TNF leads to breakdown in granulomas.

- **Many chronic diseases manifest type IV granulomatous hypersensitivity.** These include tuberculosis, leprosy, schistosomiasis, sarcoidosis, and Crohn's disease.

Delayed hypersensitivity

Delayed-type hypersensitivity (DTH) is a T cell-mediated inflammatory response in which the stimulation of antigen-specific effector T cells leads to macrophage activation and localized inflammation and edema within tissues. This effector T cell response is essential for the control of intracellular and other pathogens. If the response is excessive, however, it can damage host tissues.

The T cell response may be directed against exogenous agents, such as microbial antigens and sensitizing chemicals, or against self-antigens. Typically T cells are sensitized to the foreign antigen during infection with the pathogen or by absorption of a contact sensitizing agent across the skin.

Q. Where in the body are T cells sensitized and how?
A. Typically, T cells are sensitized in the T cell areas of secondary lymphoid tissues by dendritic cells, which carry infectious or sensitizing agents from the peripheral sites.

Subsequent exposure of the sensitized individual to the exogenous antigen, either injected intradermally or applied to the epidermis, results in the recruitment of antigen-specific T cells to the site and the development of a local inflammatory response over 24–72 hours.

If the foreign antigen persists in the tissues, chronic activation of T cells and macrophages may lead to granuloma formation and tissue damage.

If the antigen is an organ-specific self antigen, autoreactive T cells may produce localized cellular inflammation and autoimmune disease, such as type I diabetes mellitus.

According to the Coombs and Gell classification, type IV or DTH reactions take more than 12 hours to develop and involve cell-mediated immune reactions rather than antibody responses to antigens. Some other hypersensitivity reactions may straddle this definition because they have:

- a rapid antibody-mediated phase;
- a later cell-mediated phase.

For example, the late-phase IgE-mediated reaction may peak 12–24 hours after contact with allergen, and TH2 cells and eosinophils contribute to the inflammation as well as IgE (see Chapter 23).

In contrast to other forms of hypersensitivity, type IV hypersensitivity is transferred from one animal to another by T cells, particularly CD4 TH1 cells in mice, rather than by serum. Therefore DTH can develop in antibody-deficient humans, but is lost as CD4 T cells fall in HIV infection and AIDS.

Delayed hypersensitivity reactions

type	reaction time	clinical appearance	histology	antigen
contact	48–72 hours	eczema	lymphocytes, later macrophages; edema of epidermis	epidermal (e.g. antigen, nickel, rubber, poison ivy)
tuberculin	48–72 hours	local induration	lymphocytes, monocytes, macrophages	intradermal (e.g. tuberculin)
granuloma	21–28 days	hardening (e.g. skin of lung)	macrophages, epithelioid cells, giant cells, fibrosis	persistent antigen or antibody complexes or non-immunoglobulin stimuli (e.g. talc)

Fig. 26.1 The characteristics of type IV reactions comparing contact, tuberculin, and granulomatous reactions.

Type IV hypersensitivity reflects the presence of antigen-specific CD4 T cells and is associated with protective immunity against intracellular and other pathogens. However, there is not a complete correlation between type IV hypersensitivity and protective immunity, and progressive infections can develop despite the presence of strong DTH reactivity.

There are three variants of type IV hypersensitivity reaction

Three variants of type IV hypersensitivity reaction are recognized (Fig. 26.1):

- **contact hypersensitivity** and **tuberculin-type hypersensitivity** both occur within 72 hours of re-exposure to antigen;
- **granulomatous hypersensitivity** reactions develop over a period of 21–28 days – the granulomas are formed by the aggregation of macrophages and lymphocytes and may persist for weeks – this is the most important type of type IV hypersensitivity response for producing clinical consequences.

These three types of DTH were originally distinguished according to the reaction they produced when antigen was applied directly to the skin (epicutaneously) or injected intradermally. The degree of the response is usually assessed in animals by measuring thickening of the skin. This local response is accompanied by evidence of T cell activation systemically, such as antigen-specific T cell proliferation and cytokine synthesis, such as interferon-γ (IFNγ).

> **Q. What causes the skin to become thickened during a chronic immune response?**
> A. The migration of lymphocytes and macrophages into the dermis, the proliferation of cells in the dermis in response to cytokines, and the deposition of new extracellular matrix components can all contribute to skin thickening.

Contact hypersensitivity

Contact hypersensitivity is characterized by an eczematous skin reaction at the site of contact with an allergen (Fig. 26.2). Sensitizing agents for humans include metal ions, such as nickel and chromium, many industrial chemicals including those in rubber and leather and natural products present in dyes, drugs, fragrances and plants, such as pentadecacatechol, the sensitizing chemical in poison ivy.

Clinical and patch test appearances of contact hypersensitivity

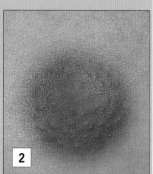
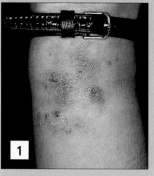

Fig. 26.2 (1) The eczematous area at the wrist is due to sensitivity to nickel in the watch-strap buckle. (2) The suspected allergy may be confirmed by applying potential allergens, in the relevant concentrations and vehicles, to the patient's upper back (patch testing). A positive reaction causes a localized area of eczema at the site of the offending allergen 2–4 days after application.

This is distinct from the non-immune-mediated inflammatory response to irritants.

Sensitizing agents behave as **haptens**. Haptens are:

- low molecular weight chemicals (< 1 kDa) that are not immunogenic by themselves
- lipophilic and penetrate the epidermis and dermis where they bind covalently to cysteine or lysine residues in self proteins to form new antigenic determinants.
- metal ions, which chelate with self-peptides in the groove of MHC class II.

Some contact allergens are modified by detoxifying enzymes encountered in the skin to form highly reactive metabolites that bind to self-proteins.

Potent haptens, such as dinitrochlorobenzene (DNCB), sensitize nearly all individuals and are used in animal models of allergic contact dermatitis.

A contact hypersensitivity reaction has two stages – sensitization and elicitation

Dendritic cells and keratinocytes have key roles in the sensitization phase

Antigen presenting cells (APC) in the skin include **Langerhans' cell** (LCs), located in the suprabasal epidermis, and dermal dendritic cells (dDCs). Contact hypersensitivity is

Langerhans' cells

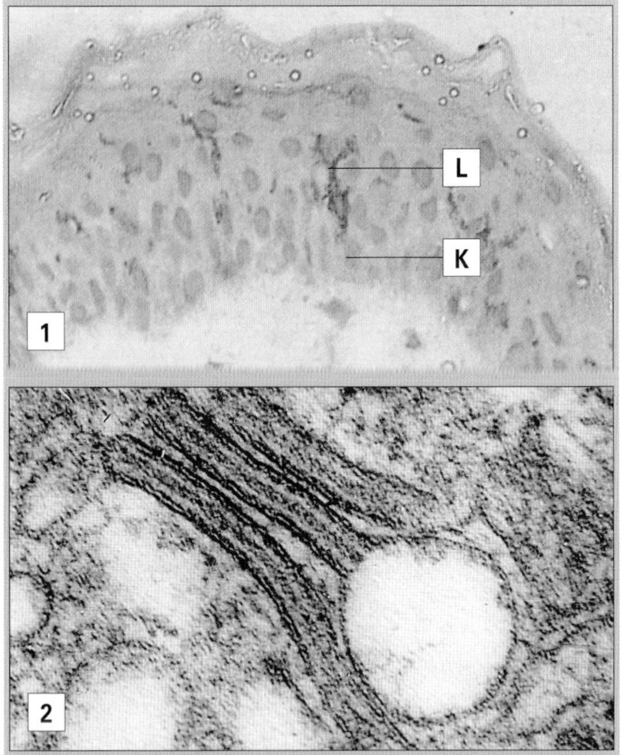

Fig. 26.3 **(1)** These dendritic cells constitute 3% of all cells in the epidermis. They express a variety of surface markers, including Langerin and CD1. Here they have been identified in normal skin using an anti-CD1 monoclonal antibody (counterstained with Mayer's hemalum). (L, Langerhans' cell; K, keratinocyte.) × 312. **(2)** Electron micrograph of a Langerhans' cell showing the characteristic 'Birbeck granule'. This organelle is a platelike structure derived from cell membranes, often with a bleb-like extension at one end. × 132 000.

primarily an epidermal reaction, and epidermal LCs were considered to be the APC responsible for initiating contact sensitivity (Fig. 26.3). More recent studies have established that dDCs are essential for stimulating hapten-specific T cells.

Langerhans' cells (see Chapter 2) are specialized DCs which extend dendritic processes throughout the epidermis, allowing them to sample environmental antigens. LCs express MHC class II, CD1 and the C-type lectin, **langerin** (CD207), which is responsible for the development of **Birbeck granules**, the cell membrane-derived organelle characteristic of LCs (see Fig. 26.3). The majority of dermal DCs are Langerin⁻, but there is a small population of Langerin⁺ dDCs, which are distinct from LCs, but also migrate rapidly to draining lymph nodes on exposure to sensitizers and activate hapten-specific CD8⁺ T cells. Both LCs and dDCs take up hapten-modified proteins by micropinocytosis but they also absorb lipid-soluble haptens, which modify cytoplasmic proteins. Under the influence of IL-1 and TNF secreted by keratinocytes and other cells, these DCs undergo maturation and increase expression of MHC and co-stimulatory molecules. Both LCs and dDCs are inactivated by ultraviolet B, which can therefore prevent or alleviate the effects of contact hypersensitivity.

Keratinocytes produce cytokines important to the contact hypersensitivity response

Keratinocytes provide the structural integrity of the epidermis and have a central role in epidermal immunology. Keratinocytes can be activated by a number of stimuli, including sensitizing agents and irritants. They may express MHC class II molecules and intercellular adhesion molecule-1 (ICAM-1) in the cell membrane.

Activated keratinocytes produce a wide range of cytokines, including:

- TNF, IL-1, and granulocyte–macrophage colony stimulating factor (GM–CSF), which activate LCs and dDCs;
- IL-3 which activates LCs and co-stimulates T cell proliferative responses, recruits mast cells, and induces secretion of immunosuppressive cytokines, such as IL-10 and transforming growth factor-β (TGFβ). These dampen the immune response and may induce clonal anergy or immunological unresponsiveness in TH1 cells.

Sensitization stimulates a population of memory T cells

Sensitization takes 10–14 days in humans. Hapten-bearing LCs and dDCs bearing modified proteins migrate as veiled cells through the afferent lymphatics to the paracortical areas of regional lymph nodes, where they activate CD4⁺ and CD8⁺ T cells.

MHC class I-restricted CD8⁺ T cells are important in contact hypersensitivity responses in humans and mice and are the major effector cells for many allergens. For example, lipid-soluble urushiol from poison ivy enters the cytoplasm of APCs and haptened cytoplasmic proteins are processed through the MHC class I pathway, leading to the activation of allergen-specific CD8⁺ T cells. Hapten-specific CD4 T cells are also activated hapten–peptide conjugates in association with MHC class II molecules and become effector/memory CD4⁺ T cells, which contribute to the skin inflammation, or regulatory CD4⁺ T cells (Fig. 26.4).

Activated T cells change the pattern of adhesion molecules on their surface by downregulating the chemokine receptor, CCR7, and CD62L.

> **Q. What effect will loss of CCR7 and CD62L have on T cell function?**
> **A.** CD62L promotes adhesion of lymphocytes to high endothelial venules and CCR7 allows the cells to respond to CCL21 expressed in secondary lymphoid tissues (see Fig. 6.15). Hence cells lacking these receptors will lose their propensity to traffic into lymph tissues.

The expression of leukocyte functional antigen-1 (LFA-1), very late antigen-4 (VLA-4), and the chemokine receptors CXCR3 and CCR5 is increased. As a result the activated/memory T cells remain within the circulation rather than trafficking through lymphoid tissue, and are able to bind to adhesion molecules on the endothelium of inflamed tissues.

Elicitation involves recruitment of CD4⁺ and CD8⁺ lymphocytes and monocytes

The application of a contact allergen leads to:

- rapid expression of proinflammatory cytokines; and
- recruitment of effector T cells and monocytes to the site (Fig. 26.5).

Sensitization phase of contact hypersensitivity

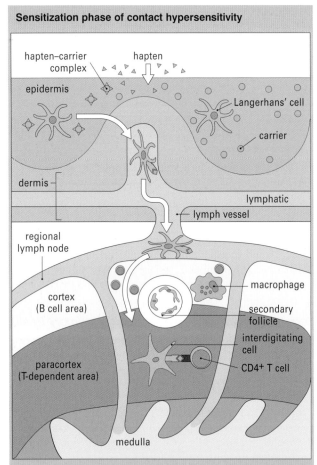

Fig. 26.4 The hapten forms a hapten–carrier complex in the epidermis or within cytoplasm. Langerhans' cells and dermal Dendritic cells internalize the antigen, undergo maturation, and migrate via afferent lymphatics to the paracortical area of the regional lymph node where peptide–MHC molecule complexes on the surface of the Langerhans' cell can also be directly haptenated. As interdigitating cells, they present antigen to CD4$^+$ and CD8$^+$ T cells.

There is induction of mRNA for TNF, IL-1β, and GM–CSF in Langerhans' cells within 30 minutes of exposure to allergen, and increased transcription of mRNA for IL-1α, macrophage inflammatory protein-2 (CXCL2), and interferon-induced protein-10 (CXCL10) by keratinocytes.

TNF and IL-1 are potent inducers of endothelial cell adhesion molecules, including:

- E-selectin and vascular cell adhesion molecule-1 (VCAM-1) within 2 hours; and
- ICAM-1 within 8 hours (Fig. 26.6).

VCAM-1 and ICAM-1 are the receptors for VLA-4 and LFA-1, respectively, on the surface of effector/memory T cells and contribute to their recruitment across the endothelium. These locally released cytokines and chemokines also produce a gradient signal for the movement of mononuclear cells towards the dermoepidermal junction and epidermis.

The earliest histological change, seen after 4–8 hours, is the appearance of mononuclear cells around blood vessels.

Macrophages and lymphocytes invade the dermis and epidermis, peaking at 48–72 hours (Fig. 26.7).

The recruitment of memory T cells is antigen non-specific, with less than 1% of infiltrating lymphocytes bearing hapten-specific αβ T cell receptors. However, the hapten-specific T cells are stimulated by dermal DCs expressing hapten–peptide complexes to expand and to increase the expression of adhesion molecules. This leads to the retention of hapten-specific T cells at the inflamed site.

Infiltrating lymphocytes include CD4$^+$ TH1-like T cells secreting IFNγ, and up to 50% CD8$^+$ T cells. CD8$^+$ T cells are essential for inducing experimental allergic sensitivity through their direct cytolytic effect on keratinocytes and the release of IFNγ.

Effector αβ T cells are essential for experimental contact sensitivity in mice, but NK T cells and γδ T cells also contribute to the induction and elicitation of this response.

Interestingly, hapten-specific IgM antibodies from B-1 cells are also important during the elicitation phase in mice by activating complement and recruiting T cells to the challenge site.

Experiments in gene-targeted mice show that selectins, ICAM-1, and the integrins, LFA-1 and VLA-4, are all required for the elicitation of contact and delayed hypersensitivity.

Suppression of the inflammatory reaction is mediated by multiple mechanisms

The reaction to cutaneous application of sensitizer wanes after 48–72 hours. This is due to the removal of antigenic stimulus following degradation of the hapten–conjugate and a variety of inhibitory mechanisms (see Fig. 26.6) including:

- keratinocytes, dermal mast cells and macrophages secrete the anti-inflammatory cytokines, IL-10 and TGFβ, and the prostaglandin PGE, which inhibit T cell proliferation, cytokine production and inflammation;
- FoxP3$^+$ CD4$^+$ regulatory T cells and IL-10 secreting TH1 cells directly inhibit activation of effector T cells;
- external factors, such as UV light, also may inhibit the expression of contact sensitivity.

Tuberculin-type hypersensitivity

Tuberculin-type hypersensitivity was originally described by Koch. He observed that if patients with tuberculosis were injected subcutaneously with a tuberculin culture filtrate (antigens derived from the causative agent, *Mycobacterium tuberculosis*) they reacted with fever and generalized sickness. An area of hardening and swelling developed at the site of injection.

Soluble antigens from other organisms, including *Mycobacterium leprae* and *Leishmania tropica*, induce similar Tuberculin-type hypersensitivity reactions in sensitized people. The skin reaction is frequently used to test for T cell-mediated responses to the organisms following previous exposure (Fig. 26.8).

This form of hypersensitivity may also be induced by T cell responses to non-microbial antigens, such as beryllium and zirconium.

Elicitation phase of contact hypersensitivity

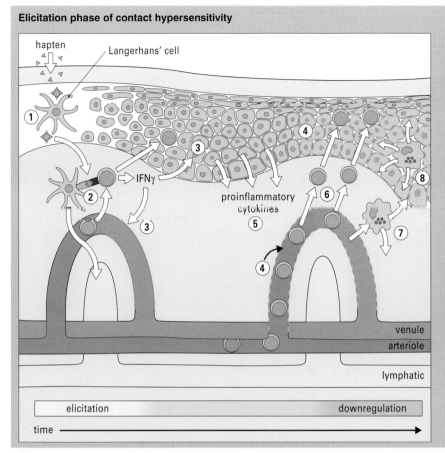

Fig. 26.5 Langerhans' cells carrying the hapten–carrier complex (**1**) move from the epidermis to the dermis, where they present the hapten–carrier complex to memory CD4$^+$ and CD8$^+$ T cells (**2**). Activated CD4$^+$ and CD8$^+$ T cells release IFNγ, which induces expression of ICAM-1 (**3**) and, later, MHC class II molecules (**4**) on the surface of keratinocytes and on endothelial cells of dermal capillaries, and activates keratinocytes, which release proinflammatory cytokines such as IL-1, IL-6, and GM–CSF (**5**). Hapten specific CD8$^+$ T cells induce apoptosis of keratinocytes expressing haptenated self-peptides (6). Non-antigen-specific T cells are attracted to the site by cytokines (**7**) and may bind to keratinocytes via ICAM-1 and MHC class II molecules. Activated macrophages are also attracted to the skin, but this occurs later. Thereafter the reaction starts to downregulate. This suppression is driven by eicosanoids such as prostaglandin E2 (PGE2), produced by activated keratinocytes and macrophages, and the inhibitory cytokines, IL-10 and TGFβ (**8**).

The tuberculin skin test reaction involves monocytes and lymphocytes

The tuberculin skin test is an example of the recall response to soluble antigen previously encountered during infection. Dendritic cells infected with *M. tuberculosis* in the lung undergo maturation and migrate to the draining mediastinal lymph nodes where they activate CD4$^+$ and CD8$^+$ T cells.

Q. How can dendritic cells activate CD8$^+$ T cells?
A. This involves the process of cross-presentation (see Chapter 8).

Following intradermal tuberculin challenge in a previously infected individual, mycobacteria-specific memory T cells are recruited and activated by dermal DCs to secrete IFNγ, which activates macrophages to produce TNFα and IL-1. These proinflammatory cytokines and chemokines from T cells and macrophages act on endothelial cells in dermal blood vessels to induce the sequential expression of the adhesion molecules E-selectin, ICAM-1, and VCAM-1. These molecules bind receptors on leukocytes and recruit them to the site of the reaction.

The initial influx at 4 hours is of neutrophils, but this is replaced at 12 hours by monocytes and T cells. The infiltrate, which extends outwards and disrupts the collagen bundles of the dermis, increases to a peak at 48 hours. CD4$^+$ T cells outnumber CD8$^+$ cells by about 2:1. A few CD4$^+$ cells infiltrate the epidermis between 24–48 hours.

Monocytes constitute 80–90% of the total cellular infiltrate. Both infiltrating lymphocytes and macrophages express MHC class II molecules, and this increases the efficiency of activated macrophages as APCs. CD1$^+$ DCs also are present at 24–48 hours. Overlying keratinocytes express HLA-DR molecules 48–96 hours after the appearance of the lymphocytic infiltrate. These events are summarized in Figure 26.9.

Q. What is the function of CD1?
A. It can present pathogen-derived glycolipid antigens to T cells (see Fig. 5.w3).

The circulation of immune cells to and from the regional lymph nodes is thought to be similar to that for contact hypersensitivity. The tuberculin lesion normally resolves within 5–7 days, but if there is persistence of antigen in the tissues it may develop into a granulomatous reaction.

Tuberculin-like DTH reactions are used practically in two ways

First, reaction to soluble antigens from a pathogen demonstrates past infection with that pathogen. Thus, tuberculin reactivity confirms past or latent infection with *M. tuberculosis*, but not necessarily active disease. However, subjects with latent tuberculosis infection have an increased lifelong risk of 7–10% for the reactivation of active tuberculosis.

Second, DTH responses to frequently encountered microbes are a general measure of cell-mediated immunity. This can be tested with intradermal injection of single antigens from common pathogens or vaccine antigens, such as *Candida albicans* or tetanus toxoid. Loss of recall responses

Cytokines, prostaglandins, and cellular interactions in contact hypersensitivity

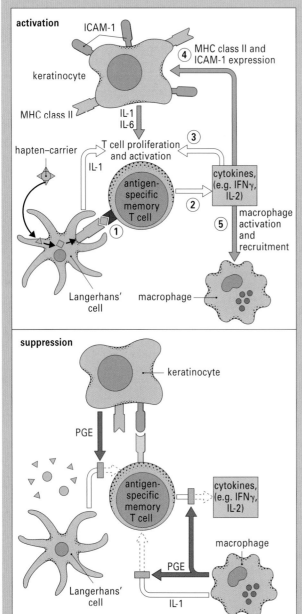

Fig. 26.6 Cytokines and prostaglandins are central to the complex interactions between Langerhans' cells, CD8⁺ and CD4⁺ T cells, keratinocytes, macrophages, and endothelial cells in contact hypersensitivity. The act of antigen presentation (**1**) causes the release of a cascade of cytokines (**2**). This cascade initially results in the activation and proliferation of CD4⁺ T cells (**3**), the induction of expression of ICAM-1 and MHC class II molecules on keratinocytes and endothelial cells (**4**), and the attraction of further T cells and macrophages to the skin (**3, 5**). Subsequently, influx of FoxP3⁺ CD25⁺ CD4⁺ regulatory T cells inhibits T cell activation and function by direct CTLA4-mediated effects and secretion of IL-10 and TGFβ. IL-10 is also released by keratinocytes and mast cells, while keratinocytes and macrophages produce PGE, which inhibits IL-1 and IL-2 production. The combined effects of enzymatic and cellular degradation of the hapten–carrier complex, regulatory CD4⁺ T cells and suppressive cytokines and PGE released by skin cells lead to downregulation of the reaction.

Histological appearance of the lesion in contact hypersensitivity

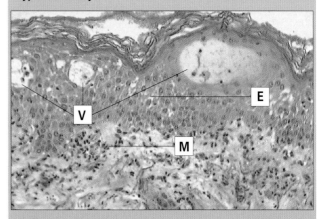

Fig. 26.7 Mononuclear cells (M) infiltrate both dermis and epidermis. The epidermis is pushed outwards and microvesicles (V) form within it due to edema (E). H&E stain. × 130.

Clinical and histological appearances of tuberculin-type sensitivity

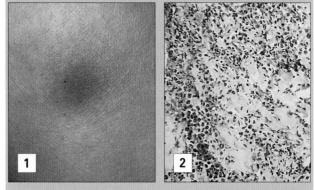

Fig. 26.8 The response to an injection of leprosy bacillus into a sensitized individual is known as the Fernandez reaction. The reaction is characterized by an area of firm red swelling of the skin and is maximal 48–72 hours after challenge (**1**). Histologically (**2**), there is a dense dermal infiltrate of leukocytes. H&E stain. × 80.

to specific antigens occurs in a wide range of diseases and infections, including HIV infection, which impair T cell function, and during therapy with corticosteroids or immunosuppressive agents.

Granulomatous hypersensitivity

Granulomatous hypersensitivity is clinically the most important form of type IV hypersensitivity, as it is responsible for the immunopathology in many diseases that involve T cell-mediated immunity. It usually results from the persistence within macrophages of:

- intracellular microorganisms, which are able to resist macrophage killing; or
- other particles that the cell is unable to destroy.

Tuberculin-type hypersensitivity

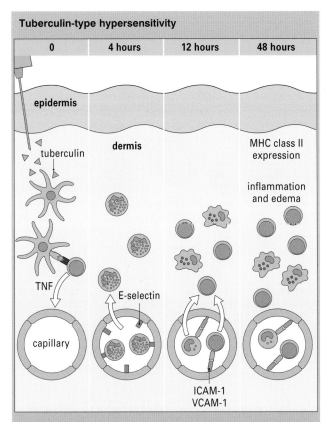

Fig. 26.9 This diagram illustrates cellular movements following intradermal injection of tuberculin. Within 1–2 hours there is expression of E-selectin on capillary endothelium leading to a brief influx of neutrophil leukocytes. By 12 hours ICAM-1 and VCAM-1 on endothelium bind the integrins LFA-1 and VLA-4 on monocytes and lymphocytes, leading to accumulation of both cell types in the dermis. This peaks at 48 hours and is followed by expression of the MHC class II molecules on keratinocytes. There is no edema of the epidermis.

This leads to chronic stimulation of T cells and the release of cytokines. The process results in the formation of **epithelioid cell granulomas** with a central collection of epithelioid cells and macrophages surrounded by lymphocytes.

The histological appearance of the granuloma reaction is quite different from that of the tuberculin-type reaction, although both types of reaction are caused by T cells sensitized to similar microbial antigens, for example those of *M. tuberculosis* and *M. leprae*.

Granulomas occur with chronic infections associated with predominantly TH1-like T cell responses, such as tuberculosis, leprosy, and leishmaniasis, and with TH2-like T cells, as in schistosomiasis.

Immune-mediated granuloma formation also occurs in the absence of infection, as in the sensitivity reactions to zirconium and beryllium, and in sarcoidosis and Crohn's disease where the antigens are unknown.

Foreign body granuloma formation occurs in response to talc, silica, and a variety of other particulate agents, when macrophages are unable to digest the inorganic matter. These non-immunological granulomas may be distinguished by the absence of lymphocytes in the lesion.

Epithelioid cells and giant cells are typical of granulomatous hypersensitivity

Epithelioid cells are large and flattened with increased endoplasmic reticulum (Fig. 26.10). They:

- are derived from activated macrophages under the chronic stimulation of cytokines;
- continue to secrete TNF and thus potentiate continuing inflammation.

Giant cells are formed when epithelioid cells fuse to form multinucleate giant cells (Fig. 26.11), sometimes referred to as **Langhans' giant cells** (not to be confused with the Langerhans' cell discussed earlier). Giant cells have several nuclei at the periphery of the cell. There is little endoplasmic reticulum, and the mitochondria and lysosomes appear

Electron micrograph of an epithelioid cell

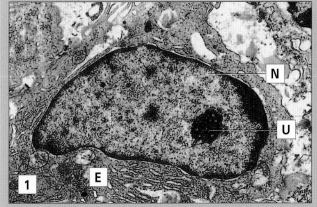
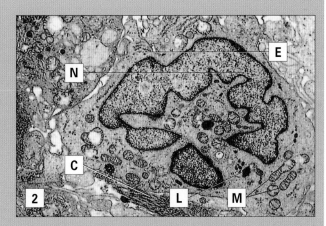

Fig. 26.10 The epithelioid cell is the characteristic cell of granulomatous hypersensitivity. Compare the extent of the endoplasmic reticulum (E) in the epithelioid cell (**1**, × 4800) with that of a tissue macrophage (**2**, × 4800). (C, collagen; L, lysosome; M, mitochondria; N, nucleus; U, nucleolus) *(Courtesy of MJ Spencer.)*

Clinical and histological appearances of the Mitsuda reaction in leprosy seen at 28 days

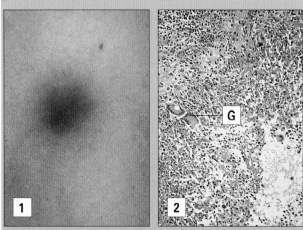

Fig. 26.11 (**1**) The resultant skin swelling (which may be ulcerated) is much harder and better defined than at 48 hours. (**2**) Histology shows a typical epithelioid cell granuloma (H&E stain. × 60). Giant cells (G) are visible in the center of the lesion, which is surrounded by a cuff of lymphocytes. This response is more akin to the pathological granulomatous processes in delayed hypersensitivity diseases than the self-resolving tuberculin-type reaction. The reaction is due to the continued presence of mycobacterial antigen.

Transformed lymphocytes

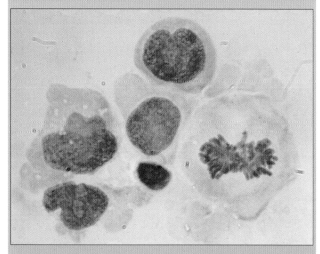

Fig. 26.12 Following stimulation with appropriate antigen, T cells undergo lymphoblastoid transformation before cell division. Blast cells with expanded nuclei and cytoplasm (as well as one lymphocyte in the metaphase of cell division) are shown. The resulting cell division can be measured by the uptake of tritiated thymidine.

to be undergoing degeneration. The giant cell may therefore be a terminal differentiation stage of the monocyte/macrophage line.

A granuloma contains epithelioid cells, macrophages, and lymphocytes

An immunological granuloma typically has a core of epithelioid cells and macrophages, sometimes with giant cells. In some diseases, such as tuberculosis, this central area may have a zone of necrosis, with complete destruction of all cellular architecture.

The macrophage/epithelioid core is surrounded by a cuff of lymphocytes, and there may also be considerable fibrosis (deposition of collagen fibers) caused by proliferation of fibroblasts and increased collagen synthesis. An example of a granulomatous reaction is the delayed **Mitsuda reaction** to dead *M. leprae* (see Fig. 26.11).

The three types of delayed hypersensitivity are summarized in Figure 26.1.

Cellular reactions in type IV hypersensitivity

T cells bearing αβ TCRs are essential

Experiments with gene knockout mice have confirmed that T cells bearing αβ TCRs rather than γδ TCRs are essential for initiating delayed hypersensitivity reactions in response to infection with intracellular bacteria.

Sensitized αβ T cells, stimulated with the appropriate antigen and APCs, undergo lymphoblastoid transformation before cell division (Fig. 26.12). This forms the basis of the lymphocyte stimulation test as a measure of T cell

function. Lymphocyte stimulation is accompanied by DNA synthesis and this can be measured by assaying the uptake of radiolabeled thymidine, a nucleoside required for DNA synthesis. Lymphocytes from a patient are stimulated in culture with the suspect antigen to determine whether it induces proliferation. It is important to stress that this is a test for T cell memory only, and does not necessarily imply the presence of protective immunity.

Following activation by APCs, T cells release a number of proinflammatory cytokines, which attract and activate macrophages. These include IFNγ, lymphotoxin-α, IL-3, and GM–CSF. The presence of memory T cells can be detected by antigen-specific IFNγ release assays.

Q. How can IFNγ cause the attraction of macrophages to an inflammatory site?
A. It causes the production of chemokines, including CCL2, CCL5, and CXCL10, and induces adhesion molecules ICAM-1 and VCAM-1 on the endothelium (see Chapter 6).

This TH1-like pattern of cytokines is enhanced by activation of the naive T cells in the presence of IL-12 which is released by dendritic cells on exposure to bacterial products. IL-12 suppresses the cytokine response of TH2 cells.

IFNγ is required for granuloma formation in humans

The role of individual cytokines can be analyzed in gene knockout mice deficient for a single cytokine. For example, IFNγ gene knockout mice are unable to activate macrophages and control infection with *M. tuberculosis* (Fig. 26.13).

The absolute requirement of IFNγ for granuloma formation in humans is illustrated by the syndrome of Mendelian susceptibility to mycobacterial disease. Subjects deficient in

The importance of IFNγ in the activation of macrophages

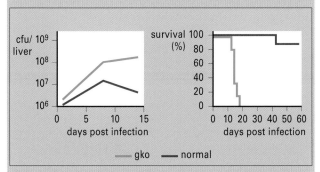

Fig. 26.13 Mice deficient in IFNγ (gene knockout [gko] mice), infected with a sublethal dose of *M. tuberculosis*, are unable to activate macrophages in response to infection with an intracellular bacterium. Macrophages initially accumulate at the site of infection, but do not form typical granulomas. Uncontrolled infection (graph, left) causes widespread tissue necrosis and death (graph, right). (cfu, colony forming units of infectious agent in the liver.)

the IFNγ receptor have markedly increased susceptibility to environmental mycobacteria and the vaccine strain, BCG, and fail to develop granulomas.

TNF and lymphotoxin-α are essential for granuloma formation during mycobacterial infections

TNF and the related cytokine, lymphotoxin-α, are both essential for the formation of granulomas during mycobacterial infections (Fig. 26.14), and act in part through the regulation of chemokine production.

Both macrophage- and T cell-derived TNF contribute to this process, but within granulomas activated macrophages become the major source of TNF, driving the differentiation of macrophages into epithelioid cells and the fusion of epithelioid cells to form giant cells (Figs 26.14 and 26.15). The maintenance of granulomas is also dependent on TNF. Consequently, inhibition of TNF activity suppresses the granulomatous inflammation in Crohn's disease and sarcoidosis.

Granulomatous reactions in chronic diseases

There are many chronic human diseases that manifest type IV hypersensitivity. Most are due to infectious agents, such as mycobacteria, protozoa, and fungi, although in other granulomatous diseases such as sarcoidosis and Crohn's disease no infectious agent has been established.

A common feature of these infections is that the pathogen causes a persistent, chronic, antigenic stimulus. Activation of macrophages by lymphocytes limits the infection, but continuing stimulation leads to tissue damage through the release of macrophage products including reactive oxygen intermediates and hydrolases.

Although delayed hypersensitivity is a measure of T cell activation, the infection is not always controlled, with the result that protective immunity and delayed hypersensitivity do not necessarily coincide. Therefore some subjects

Macrophage differentiation

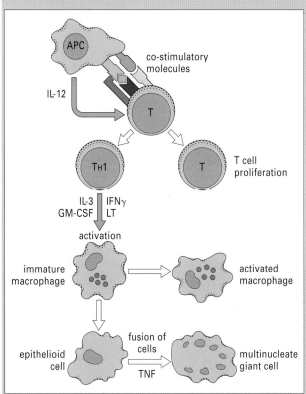

Fig. 26.14 Bacterial products stimulate macrophages to secrete IL-12. Activation of T cells in the presence of IL-12 leads to the release of IFNγ and other cytokines, lymphotoxin (LT), IL-3, and GM–CSF. These cytokines activate macrophages to kill intracellular parasites. Failure to eradicate the antigenic stimulus causes persistent cytokine release and promotes differentiation of macrophages into epithelioid cells, which secrete large amounts of TNFα. Some fuse to form multinucleate giant cells.

The importance of TNF in the formation of granulomas

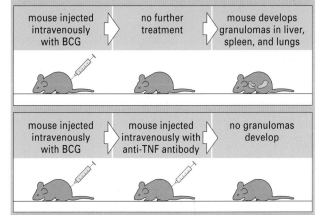

Fig. 26.15 TNF is essential for the development of epithelioid cell granulomas. If BCG-injected mice are injected with anti-TNFα antibodies, they do not develop granulomas.

showing delayed hypersensitivity may not be protected against disease in the future.

The immune response in leprosy varies greatly between individuals

Leprosy is a chronic granulomatous disease of skin and nerves caused by infection with *M. leprae*. It is divided clinically into three main types – tuberculoid, borderline, and lepromatous:

- in tuberculoid leprosy, the skin may have a few well-defined hypopigmented patches, which show an intense lymphocytic and epithelioid cell infiltrate and no microorganisms;
- by contrast, the polar reaction of lepromatous leprosy shows multiple confluent skin lesions characterized by numerous bacilli, 'foamy' macrophages, and a paucity of lymphocytes;
- borderline leprosy has characteristics of both tuberculoid and lepromatous leprosy (Fig. 26.16).

In leprosy, protective immunity is usually associated with cell-mediated immunity, but this declines across the leprosy spectrum towards the lepromatous pole with an increase in mycobacteria and rise in non-protective anti-*M. leprae* antibodies.

The borderline leprosy reaction is a dramatic example of delayed hypersensitivity. Borderline reactions occur either spontaneously or following drug treatment. In these reactions, hypopigmented skin lesions containing *M. leprae* become swollen and inflamed (Fig. 26.17) because the patient is now able to mount a T cell response to the mycobacteria resulting in a delayed-type hypersensitivity reaction. The histological appearance shows a more tuberculoid pattern with an infiltrate of IFNγ-secreting lymphocytes. The process may occur in peripheral nerves, where Schwann cells contain *M. leprae*; this is the most important cause of nerve destruction in this disease. The lesion in borderline leprosy is typical of granulomatous hypersensitivity (see Fig. 26.17).

In patients with a tuberculoid-type reaction, T cell sensitization may be assessed *in vitro* by lymphocyte proliferation or the release of IFNγ following stimulation with *M. leprae* antigens.

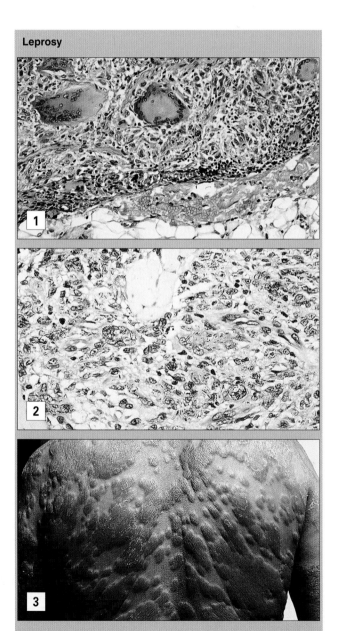

Leprosy

Fig. 26.17 (1) A borderline leprosy reaction. This small nerve is almost completely replaced by the granulomatous infiltrate. (2) Lepromatous leprosy. Large numbers of bacilli are present. (3) Borderline lepromatous leprosy. There are gross infiltrated erythematous plaques with well-defined borders. *((2) Courtesy of Dr Phillip McKee. (3) Courtesy of Dr S Lucas.)*

The immunological spectrum of leprosy

| tuberculoid | borderline | lepromatous |

cell-mediated immunity

antibody response

M. leprae in tissues

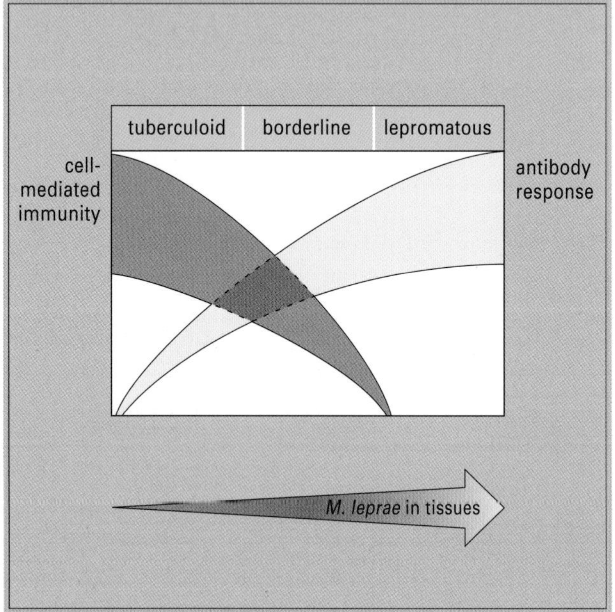

Fig. 26.16 The clinical spectrum of leprosy ranges from tuberculoid disease with few lesions and bacteria to lepromatous leprosy, with multiple lesions and uncontrolled bacterial proliferation. This range reflects host immunity as measured by specific cellular and antibody responses to *M. leprae*, and the tissue expression of cytokines.

Granulomatous reactions are necessary to control tuberculosis

In tuberculosis, the granuloma provides the microenvironment in which lymphocytes stimulate macrophages to kill the intracellular *M. tuberculosis*. The formation and maintenance of granulomas are essential to control the infection.

In most (>90%) subjects with latent tuberculosis infection, the mycobacteria remain dormant within small granulomas in the lung. There is, however, a balance between the effects of activated macrophages:

- controlling the bacterial growth; and
- causing tissue damage in infected organs. In those who progress to clinical tuberculosis, granulomatous reactions erode airways leading to cavitation in the lung and spread of bacteria. The reactions are frequently accompanied by extensive fibrosis and the lesions are visible in the chest radiographs of affected patients (Fig. 26.w1).

Q. What factors might affect the balance that controls a latent infection with tuberculosis?
A. Immunosuppression by drugs or infection (e.g. AIDS) (see Chapter 17) can allow reactivation of infection with tuberculosis.

The histological appearance of the lesion is typical of a granulomatous reaction, with central caseous (cheesy) necrosis (Fig. 26.18). This is surrounded by an area of epithelioid cells with a few giant cells. Mononuclear cell infiltration occurs around the edge.

Granulomas surround the parasite ova in schistosomiasis

In schistosomiasis, which is caused by parasitic trematode worms (schistosomes), the host becomes sensitized to the eggs of the worms, leading to a typical granulomatous reaction in the parasitized tissue mediated essentially by TH2 cells (Fig. 26.19; see also Chapter 15). In this case the cytokines IL-5 and IL-13 are responsible for the recruitment of eosinophils and the formation of the granulomas around the ova. When the eggs have been deposited in the liver, the subsequent IL-13-dependent fibrosis causes hepatic scarring and portal hypertension.

The cause of sarcoidosis is unknown

Sarcoidosis is a chronic disease of unknown etiology in which activated macrophages and non-caseating granuloma accumulate in many tissues, frequently accompanied by fibrosis (Fig. 26.20). The disease particularly affects lymphoid tissue and the lungs, as well as bone, nervous tissue, and skin. Enlarged lymph nodes may be detected in chest radiographs of affected patients (Fig. 26.w2). No infectious agent has been isolated, though mycobacteria have been implicated because of the similarities in the pathology.

One of the paradoxes of clinical immunology is that this disease is usually associated with depression of delayed hypersensitivity both *in vivo* and *in vitro*. Patients with sarcoidosis are anergic on testing with tuberculin; however, when cortisone is injected with tuberculin antigen the skin

Histological appearance of the liver in schistosomiasis

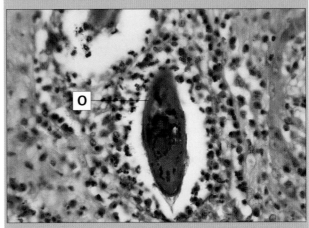

Fig. 26.19 The epithelioid cell granuloma surrounds the schistosome ovum (O) and eosinophils are prominent. H&E stain. × 300. *(Courtesy of Dr Phillip McKee.)*

Histological appearance of a tuberculous section of lung

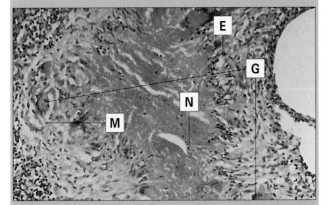

Fig. 26.18 This shows an epithelioid cell granuloma (E) with giant cells (G). Mononuclear cell infiltration can be seen (M). There is also marked caseation and necrosis (N) within the granuloma. H&E stain. × 75.

Histological appearance of sarcoidosis in a lymph node biopsy

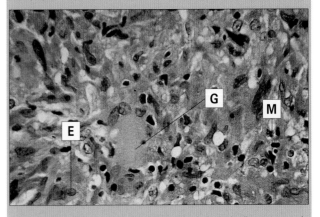

Fig. 26.20 The granuloma of sarcoidosis is typically composed of epithelioid cells (E) and multinucleate giant cells (G), but without caseous necrosis. There is only a sparse mononuclear cell infiltrate (M) evident at the periphery of the granuloma. H&E stain. × 240.

tests are positive, suggesting that cortisone-sensitive T inhibitory cells are responsible for the anergy.

Q. What effect does cortisone normally have on an immune response, and why does its effect here appear paradoxical?
A. Cortisone would normally suppress delayed hypersensitivity, principally by its actions on macrophages.

Patients may present acutely with fever and malaise, though in the longer term those with pulmonary involvement develop shortness of breath caused by lung fibrosis. The diagnosis is often suggested by the clinical pattern and radiographic changes and confirmed by tissue biopsy. Angiotensin converting enzyme (ACE) and serum calcium levels are sometimes elevated because activated macrophages are a source of both ACE and 1,25-dihydroxy-cholecalciferol (the active metabolite of vitamin D_3).

The cause of Crohn's disease is unknown

Crohn's disease is a chronic inflammatory disease of the ileum and colon, in which lymphocytes and macrophages accumulate in all layers of the bowel. The granulomatous reaction and fibrosis cause stricture of the bowel and penetrating fistulas into other organs (see Fig. 7.17). Although the antigens initiating this granulomatous reaction are unknown, there appears to be defect in inflammasome-mediated intracellular signaling responses to bacterial products in Crohn's disease. This may result an excessive T cell-driven immune response to microbial antigens in genetically predisposed individuals.

Infiltrating T cell show a restricted T cell receptor repertoire and the cytokine profile of pro-inflammatory TH17 cells, driven by IL-23, as well as TH1 T cells. These are responsible for macrophage activation and the release of inflammatory cytokines, such as IL-17, IL-21, IL-22, and TNF, reactive oxygen metabolites, and nitric oxide. These initiate and maintain the transmural intestinal inflammation.

Inhibition of TNF activity with antibody or soluble TNF receptor reduces inflammation in patients with Crohn's disease, but this therapy may be associated with reactivation of tuberculosis in subjects with latent tuberculosis infection and with other granulomatous infectious diseases.

CRITICAL THINKING: A HYPERSENSITIVITY TYPE IV REACTION (SEE P. 444 FOR EXPLANATIONS)

An 8-year-old boy with recent weight loss and mild fever is found to have an enlarged lymph node on the right side of the neck. He has no cough and his chest radiograph is normal. Surgical biopsy of the lymph node reveals a granulomatous infiltrate with no evident acid-fast bacilli. The result of microbiological culture for *Mycobacterium tuberculosis* is awaited. Intradermal skin testing with tuberculin causes swelling and erythema of 20 mm in diameter after 48 hours.

1 What cell types make up the granulomas in the lymph node and what cytokines are involved in their formation?

2 What is the pathology at the site of the skin testing and how does it differ from that in the lymph node?

3 What type of lymphocyte is responsible for the skin test reactivity?

4 What other conditions cause granulomas in lymph nodes and how are they diagnosed?

5 When the family members are tested, the boy's 5-year-old brother is found to have a positive tuberculin reaction (18 mm at 48 hours), but he is well with a normal chest radiograph. What does this result indicate about his immune responses and what is its significance?

Further reading

Ananworanich J, Shearer WT. Delayed-type hypersensitivity skin testing. In: Manual of Clinical Laboratory Immunology, 6th edn. Washington: ASM Press; 2002:212–219.

Askenase PW. Yes T cells, but three different T cells ($\alpha\beta$, $\gamma\delta$ and NK T cells) and also B-1 cells mediate contact sensitivity. Clin Exp Immunol 2001;125:345–350.

Baughman RP, Lower EE, du Bois RM. Sarcoidosis. Lancet 2003;361:1111–1118.

Bean AGD, Roach DR, Briscoe H, et al. Structural deficiencies in granuloma formation in tumor necrosis factor gene-targeted mice underlie the heightened susceptibility to aerosol *Mycobacterium tuberculosis* infection which is not compensated for by lymphotoxin. J Immunol 1999;162:3504–3511.

Brand S. Crohn's disease: TH1, TH17 or both? The change of a paradigm: new immunological and genetic insights implicate TH17 cells in the pathogenesis of Crohn's disease. Gut 2009;58:1152–1167.

Britton WJ, Lockwood DN. Leprosy. Lancet 2004;363:1209–1219.

Casanova J-L, Abel L. Genetic dissection of immunity to mycobacteria: the human model. Annu Rev Immunol 2002;40:581–620.

Cavani A, De Luca A. Allergic contact dermatitis: novel mechanisms and therapeutic perspectives. Curr Drug Metabol 2010;11:228–233.

Cho JH. The genetics and immunopathogenesis of inflammatory bowel disease. Nat Rev Immunol 2008;8:458–466.

Cooper AM. Cell-mediated immune responses in tuberculosis. Ann Rev Immunol 2009;27:393–422.

Daniel H, Present MD, Rutgeerts P, et al. Infliximab for the treatment of fistulas in patients with Crohn's disease. N Engl J Med 1999;18:1398–1405.

Flynn JL, Chan J, Triebold KJ, et al. An essential role for interferon-γ in resistance to *Mycobacterium tuberculosis* infection. J Exp Med 1993;178:2249–2254.

Hagge DA, Saunders BM, Ebenezer GJ, et al. Lymphotoxin-alpha and TNF have essential but independent roles in the evolution of the granulomatous response in experimental leprosy. Am J Pathol 2009;174:1379–1389.

Igyarto BZ, Kaplan DH. The evolving function of Langerhans cells in adaptive skin immunity. Immunol Cell Biol 2010;88:361–365.

Kalish RS, Wood JA, LaPorte A. Processing of urushiol (poison ivy) hapten by both endogenous and exogenous pathways for presentation to T cells in vitro. J Clin Invest 1994;93:2039–2047.

Kaplan DH. In vivo function of Langerhans cells and dermal dendritic cells. Trends Immunol 2010;27:446–451.

Kindler V, Sappino A-P, Gran GE, et al. The inducing role of tumour necrosis factor in the development of bactericidal granulomas during BCG infection. Cell 1989;56:731–740.

Klimas N. Delayed hypersensitivity skin testing. In: Manual of clinical laboratory immunology, 5th edn. Washington: ASM Press; 1997:276–280.

Martin SF, Esser PR, Schmucker S, et al. T-cell recognition of chemicals, protein allergens and drugs: towards the development of in vitro assays. Cell Mol Life Sci 2010;67:4171–4184.

Roach DR, Briscoe H, Saunders B, et al. Secreted lymphotoxin-alpha is essential for the control of intracellular bacterial infection. J Exp Med 2001;193:239–246.

Roach DR, Bean AGD, Demangel C, et al. Tumor necrosis factor regulates chemokine induction essential for cell recruitment, granuloma formation and clearance of mycobacterial infection. J Immunol 2002;168:4620–4628.

Salgame P. Host innate and TH1 responses and the bacterial factors that contain *Mycobacterium tuberculosis* infection. Curr Opin Immunol 2005;17:374–380.

Saunders BM, Britton WJ. Life and death in the granuloma: immunopathology of tuberculosis. Immunol Cell Biol 2007;85:103–111.

Vocanson M, Hennino A, Rozieres A, et al. Effector and regulatory mechanisms in allergic contact dermatitis. Allergy 2009;64:1699–1714.

Von Andrian UH, Mackay CR. T cell function and migration: two sides of the same coin. N Engl J Med 2000;343:1020–1034.

Wallis RS, Broder MS, Wong JY, et al. Granulomatous infectious disease associated with tumor necrosis factor. Clin Infect Dis 2004;38:1261–1265.

Wynn TA, Thompson RW, Cheever AW, Mentink Kano MM. Immunopathogenesis of schistosomiasis. Immunol Rev 2004;201:156–167.

Yamamura M, Uyemura K, Deans RJ, et al. Defining protective immune responses to pathogens: cytokine profiles in leprosy lesions. Science 1991;254:277–279.

Websites

http://www.who.int/lep/disease/disease.htm–a home page describing leprosy infection.

Critical thinking: Explanations

1. Specificity and memory in vaccination

1.1 The immunological 'memory' induced by vaccination does not depend just on the antibodies. Memory is due to long-lived memory lymphocytes, which persist in the lymphoid tissues for many years. They will be reactivated if the individual encounters the toxin or the vaccine on a later occasion.

1.2 The tetanus toxoid is a stable molecule – it does not change or mutate, so antibodies and lymphocytes that recognize it continue to be effective. By contrast, influenza A mutates every year. Last year's antibodies are marginally effective or ineffective against this year's virus. Researchers must identify newly emerging virus strains and prepare vaccine from those strains they think will produce new epidemics. Often they get it right, but not always.

1.3 Recommendations are based on practicality. It is impossible to prepare sufficient vaccine each year to immunize everyone against influenza. There is not enough time to do it and not enough laboratory resources available. So the highest risk groups are targeted – health workers because they will likely be in contact with the disease and old people because the disease can lead to serious complications.

Discussion point

If we could immunize every person in the world against influenza A in 1 year, do you think that this would lead to total eradication of the disease?

2. Development of the immune system

2.1 The total numbers of blood lymphocytes are drastically reduced, with T cells being virtually absent and B cells significantly reduced – B cells require T cells to complete their own development. The lymph nodes are much reduced in size, and this particularly affects the paracortex (T cell areas). Compare this with DiGeorge syndrome. The animals have a reduced ability to fight infections, but this is selective, affecting

particularly some viruses and parasites – possibly because there is still good NK cell activity and macrophage-mediated antibacterial defenses.

2.2 Adult thymectomy has very little effect on the individual's ability to fight infection. By adulthood, there is a large pool of peripheral T cells that may to some extent self renew. The thymus progressively involutes and becomes less important as a site of T cell development in the adult.

2.3 Because the lymphocyte precursors fail to make productive rearrangements of their antigen receptor genes, they die by apoptosis during development. This leads to a profound immune deficiency of all lymphocytes, which is analogous to severe combined immunodeficiency (SCID) in humans.

2.4 Interleukin-7 is required for lymphocyte development in primary lymphoid organs. There is a profound reduction in thymocytes and peripheral lymphocytes and a total absence of $\gamma\delta$ T cells.

2.5 The $\alpha_4\beta_7$-integrin is required for binding of cells to adhesion molecules on the high endothelial venule (HEV) of gut-associated lymphoid tissue (GALT), so this knockout results in drastically reduced lymphocyte numbers in these tissues.

3. The specificity of antibodies

3.1 In the presence of the antibodies, mutated variants of the virus are selected that do not bind those antibodies. By detecting which of the virus proteins are mutated, one can infer that these are the proteins that normally would bind to the antibody. Neutralizing antibodies against viruses are generally directed against proteins in the capsid of the virus, particularly against the proteins that the virus uses to attach to the surface of its target cell. Antibodies cannot gain access to the inside of the virus, so neutralizing antibodies do not bind the core protein VP4.

3.2 The antibody VP1-a binds to an epitope that includes two closely spaced residues (91 and 95). This is a 'continuous epitope' and is located on a single external loop of polypeptide. By contrast, the epitope recognized by VP1-b is located in at least two distinct areas of the polypeptide chain (83–85 and 138–139). This is a 'discontinuous epitope': examination of the VP1 antigen shows that these residues are located on two adjacent areas of β-pleated sheet.

3.3 A mutation of residue 138 does not affect the epitope recognized by antibody VP1-a, so it continues to bind with high affinity to the antigen. This confirms that the epitopes recognized by VP1-a and VP1-b are physically separate. The mutant with Gly at position 95 still binds the VP1-a antibody weakly. Glycine is a smaller amino acid than aspartate, which is present in the wild type, hence the antibody can still bind to the epitope, although the 'fit' is less good, so the affinity of binding is lower. By contrast, lysine (Lys) is a larger residue than aspartate. It protrudes further out into the antibody's binding site and completely disrupts the antigen–antibody bond.

4. Complement deficiency

4.1 Deficiencies of components of the classical or alternative pathways, particularly of C3, produce a reduced ability to opsonize bacteria, resulting in impaired phagocytosis by macrophages and neutrophils. Patients suffer from repeated bacterial infections from Gram-positive bacteria (e.g. staphylococci, streptococci). These children are unable to clear bacterial infections because their phagocytes do not take up bacteria efficiently. Deficiencies in the lytic pathway components (C5–C9) can render patients more susceptible to neisserial infections because the lytic pathway can damage the outer membrane of Gram-negative bacteria such as *Neisseria* spp.

4.2 There is a clear deficiency in C3 and components of the alternative pathway. Components of the classical pathway are on the lower end of normal. At first this looks surprising, because the initial assay for lytic complement required the activity of the classical and lytic pathways. Nevertheless, both the bacterial infections and the lack of total hemolytic complement can be explained by the very low levels of C3. Note that the genes for C3, fB, and fI are not genetically linked, so we cannot explain this apparent multiple deficiency of alternative pathway components by some multiple gene deletion. The explanation lies in the alternative pathway amplification loop. Because the children lack fI, they cannot break down the alternative pathway C3 convertase C3bBb. Therefore C3 is continuously activated and binds fB. All the fB is consumed, as is most of the free C3. The genetic deficiency of fI therefore leads to secondary deficiencies in the components of the alternative pathway and this then affects C3 and the function of the classical and lytic pathways.

4.3 The children have a homozygous fI deficiency – both copies of the gene are missing. Replacing fI, either by an infusion of normal serum or by providing pure fI, restores all other components to normal levels, and allows the children to clear bacterial infections.

Antibiotic prophylaxis will help prevent bacterial infections.

Discussion point

What problem might occur if you inject a protein such as fI into an individual who lacks it due to a genetic deficiency?

5. Somatic hypermutation

5.1 There are at least three theories why TCRs do not undergo somatic hypermutation.

1. T cells control most antibody responses – they therefore represent an important mechanism for maintaining self tolerance. According to this view, the immune system can afford to let immunoglobulin genes undergo somatic hypermutation because (non-mutating) T cells retain control.
2. TCRs must retain the ability to recognize self (MHC), and therefore cannot be allowed to undergo somatic hypermutation.
3. The main purpose of somatic hypermutation of antibodies is to give a more robust secondary response.

In the case of T cells, as opposed to antibodies, it is possible to increase the efficacy/avidity of the memory T cell by affecting TCR density, presence of co-stimulatory/inhibitory molecules, or other aspects of the wiring of T cell signaling. Mutating the receptor is therefore simply not necessary because it is potentially dangerous as well. According to this theory, it is best avoided.

5.2 This is an example of genetic restriction in antigen presentation. The SM/J T cells are primed with antigen on MHC molecules of the SM/J haplotype and will only respond to this combination of antigen–MHC. They do not recognize the same antigen presented by other MHC molecules. Because MHC molecules are co-dominantly expressed, the H-2v MHC molecules are present on the APCs from the F1 animal and so they too stimulate the T cells.

5.3 The minimum peptide needed to activate the T cells appears to be 80–94, which is 15 residues long and therefore corresponds well to the expected size of antigen peptides that can fit into the MHC class II binding site. This peptide is included within peptide 80–102, which also stimulates strongly. Peptides 84–98 and 73–88 lack the N and C terminals of the antigenic peptide, respectively, and therefore lack some of the anchor residues needed to hold them in the MHC peptide-binding groove.

5.4 This is called a superagonist or a strong agonist peptide. Typically such a peptide will have a stronger binding affinity for the MHC molecule and/or the TCR.

6. The role of adhesion molecules in T cell migration

6.1 IL-1 induces the expression of a number of adhesion molecules, including ICAM-1 and VCAM-1, both of which can potentially mediate leukocyte migration by their interaction with the integrins LFA-1 and VLA-4, respectively.

6.2 Because it takes several hours to increase migration, and ICAM-1 and VCAM-1 appear to be involved in the process, one can infer that their expression is increased as a result of protein synthesis (which takes several hours) rather than by a relatively rapid release from intracellular stores.

6.3 Antibodies to ICAM-1/LFA-1 reduce migration of cells across unstimulated endothelium. Therefore, this pair of adhesion molecules is required for migration across resting endothelium.

6.4 Antibodies to both ICAM-1/LFA-1 and VCAM-1/VLA-4 reduce migration across IL-1-activated cells, therefore both pairs of adhesion molecules control this event. In practice it is known that ICAM-1 is present on unstimulated brain endothelium and is increased by IL-1, whereas VCAM-1 is virtually absent from unstimulated brain endothelium, but may be synthesized following stimulation with inflammatory cytokines.

7. The role of macrophages in toxic shock syndrome

7.1 TNFα, IL-1, IL-6, IL-10.

7.2 Lack of activity, ruffling of fur, respiratory distress, possibly leading to death within 24 hours.

7.3 BCG activates macrophages via infection of APCs and induction of IFNγ by NK and CD4+ T cells, which primes macrophages. LPS delivers stimulus via LPS binding protein, CD4, Toll-like receptors, and NFκB activation, to enhance proinflammatory cytokine release. TNFα and IL-1, especially, act locally and systemically on vascular endothelium, neutrophils, and central nervous centers, causing hypotension and circulatory collapse.

7.4 CD14 knockout mice are extremely resistant to septic shock. Scavenger receptor A knockout mice are more susceptible to septic shock. IFNγ knockout mice are relatively resistant to septic shock.

7.5 CD14 is central to the LPS recognition and signaling pathway. SR-A clears LPS from the circulation to protect the host. IFNγ is needed to prime macrophages.

7.6 Evaluate the kinetics of pro- and anti-inflammatory cytokine production to establish the endogenous regulation of macrophage activation. Use blocking antibodies for TNFα and other cytokines, and receptor knockout mice to establish the roles of each. Evaluate cytokine production by peritoneal macrophages taken from BCG-primed mice after LPS challenge *in vitro*.

7.7 Septic shock is a major complication of Gram-negative (e.g. *Neisseria meningitidis*) infection. Therapeutic approaches include circulatory support, antibiotics, and possibly combinations of cytokine and receptor antagonists (blocking antibodies, inhibitors of TNFα cleavage, soluble receptors).

Relevant references

Haworth R, Platt N, Keshav S, et al. The macrophage scavenger receptor type A (SR-A) is expressed by activated macrophages and protects the host against lethal endotoxic shock. J Exp Med 1997;186:1431–1439.

Haziot A, Ferrero E, Kontgen F, et al. Resistance to endotoxin shock and reduced dissemination of Gram-negative bacteria in CD14 deficient mice. Immunity 1996;4:407–414.

7.8 Use blocking antibodies for phagocytic receptors (e.g. vitronectin receptors) or cells from knockout mice, if available.

7.9 Ligation and cross-linking of phagocytic receptors by apoptotic cells induce signaling pathways resulting in suppression of inflammatory and antimicrobial responses.

7.10 Use antibodies and antagonists to receptors to study candidate inhibitory responses such as production of prostaglandin E₂ and TGFβ.

7.11 Pathogens can exploit and induce the downregulation of inflammation by apoptotic cells to evade killing by host cells. This may be counteracted by the use of drugs to prevent inhibitory pathways, even *in vivo*.

Relevant references

Stein M, Keshav S, Harris N, Gordon S. IL-4 potently enhances murine macrophage MR activity; a marker of alternative immunologic macrophage activation. J Exp Med 1992;176:287–292.

Freire-de-Lima CG, Nascimento DO, Soares MBP, et al. Uptake of apoptotic cells drives the growth of a pathogenic trypanosome in macrophages. Nature 2000;403:199–203.

7.12 Macrophage activation involves a complex pattern of altered gene expression, covering a spectrum of activities and not just polar opposites between activation (TH1, IFNγ) and deactivation (TH2, IL-10). IL-4 and IL-13, TH2 cytokines, use common receptor chains to induce an alternative pathway of macrophage activation involved in humoral immunity and possibly repair (enhanced APC function via MHC class II expression and MRs, as well as other effects on B cell production of antibody). IFNγ and IL-10 regulate cellular immune effector functions.

7.13 Broaden the range of macrophage markers examined, ultimately by DNA gene chip analysis, and look for consistency and reproducibility of similar patterns of altered gene expression by the cytokines above. Analyze macrophage functions in mice with knockouts of cytokines or their receptors.

7.14 Find model antigens (e.g. parasites) that induce TH2 responses *in vivo*, and establish whether these are recognized by APC receptors that enhance IL-4/IL-13 or inhibit IFNγ production by appropriate cells.

8. Antigen processing and presentation

8.1 Macrophages express both MHC class I and class II molecules, and can therefore present antigen to either of the clones. Fibroblasts do not generally express MHC class II molecules and one would not expect them to stimulate the MHC class II-restricted clone.

8.2 Live flu virus infects the macrophages and flu virus polypeptides are synthesized in the cytoplasm of the cell, so the viral antigens are presented by the internal (MHC class I) pathway as well as the external (MHC class II) pathway. Inactivated virus is taken up by the macrophage, processed and presented via the class II pathway only – because there is no viral protein synthesis there is no presentation via the MHC class I pathway.

8.3 Emetine blocks protein synthesis, so no protein fragments are fed into the MHC class I pathway by the proteasomes. Chloroquine prevents phagosome/lysosome fusion so endocytosed virus cannot be broken down into peptides. Consequently no peptides are available for the MHC class II pathway.

8.4 The MHC class I-restricted T cells express CD8 and the MHC class II-restricted cells express CD4 because CD8 and CD4 are co-receptors for MHC class I and class II molecules, respectively.

9. Development of the antibody response

9.1 In a developing immune response to a TD antigen, B cells will switch from IgM production to IgG. Because the antigen is continuously present as a depot, by day 14 the response has the characteristics of a secondary response – IgG antibody titers are climbing rapidly.

9.2 Perhaps the two mice have already been infected by mouse hepatitis virus. By day 5 they are already making a secondary IgG response. This could be a problem in the colony, though usually all animals housed together would become infected. If these mice have been naturally infected it would be through the gut (unlike the vaccine) and one would therefore expect a stronger IgA response.

9.3 IgA-producing clones tend to be located in the mucosa-associated lymphoid tissues (see Chapter 2) and it is not surprising that no IgA-producing clones were generated from the spleen.

9.4 IgG-producing clones at day 14 are likely to be of higher affinity than IgM producers.

10. Mechanisms of cytotoxicity

10.1 CTLs and NK cells effect cytotoxicity by inducing apoptosis in their targets. In this assay, targets with fragmented DNA are assumed to be undergoing apoptosis. Note that there is always a low level of DNA fragmentation in the controls that contain no effector cells.

10.2 Tumor line 1 is susceptible to killing by CTLs but less so to killing by NK cells. Tumor line 1S is susceptible to killing by NK cells, but resistant to killing by CTLs. These observations are consistent with tumor line 1 expressing MHC class I molecules, which are recognized as foreign by CTLs, while tumor line 1S is MHC class I negative, and thus a target for NK cells.

10.3 NK cells do effect some killing of tumor line 1, even though it expresses MHC class I. Therefore, the NK cells must be recognizing the tumor cells via activating receptors. Tumor cells often express surface proteins that can activate NK cells via NKG2D, so this is a likely candidate. You could test this hypothesis by blocking the interaction of NKG2D with its cellular ligands

either using a blocking antibody or soluble NKG2D ligands.

10.4 Blocking interactions with MHC class I prevents CTL killing of tumor line 1 because it is no longer able to recognize the target cell class I molecules as foreign. In this condition, however, NK cell killing of tumor line 1 actually increases. This is likely to be because NK cells are now able to recognize the antibody-coated target cells via their Fc receptor, CD16. Note that the addition of anti-class I has no effect on the MHC class I negative tumor line 1S.

11. Regulation of the immune response

11.1 Over excessive immune activation is harmful to the host. An incorrect or excessive immune response can lead to autoimmunity or allergy. Anergy, cell death, and suppression by cytokines and regulatory cells are three ways of inducing tolerance and preventing this.

11.2 Antibody regulates the immune system through a number of feedback mechanisms. Antibodies can form immune complexes with antigen; these can lead to expansion or suppression of immune responses. Passive IgM can enhance an immune response whereas passive IgG suppresses the response through antibody blocking or receptor cross-linking. In addition, some immunoglobulins are idiotypic and they have an immunogenic sequence within them. During an immune response antibodies can be generated against this idiotypic sequence leading to downregulation of the response.

11.3 Transfer of regulatory T cells into mice with autoimmunity can cause a reduction in the disease, however it is not known how this would affect other immune responses if the system was used in the treatment of human autoimmunity. It is possible that there could be a decreased immune response to viral and bacterial infections leading to an increase in these diseases.

12. Immune reactions in the gut

Oysters are a food item that is normally tolerated by the body. Eating an infected shellfish causes the antigens in the food to be presented in association with components of the pathogen that can activate PAMP receptors, induce co-stimulatory molecules, and break tolerance. Additionally bacterial toxins may damage the gut epithelium again, enhancing antigen presentation and allowing antigens to access the gut-associated lymphoid tissues more readily. Once tolerance is broken the TH2-type response, which is characteristic of the gut, will lead to production of antigen-specific IgE antibodies. Consequently, eating another oyster, even a good one, will lead to an allergic reaction to antigen in the food.

13. Virus–immune system interactions

13.1 The non-neutralizing antibodies may have mediated protection by activating complement to mediate virolysis, virion opsonization for uptake and destruction by macrophages, or destruction of virus-infected cells expressing glycoprotein D on their surface. They may also have mediated protection by mobilizing Fc receptor-expressing effector cells to combat the infection, promoting virion uptake by macrophages or targeting macrophages or NK cells to lyse virus-infected cells and produce soluble antiviral factors.

13.2 Whether the protective capacity of the non-neutralizing antibodies was dependent on the presence of their Fc region could be evaluated by testing the capacity of the $F(ab')_2$ portion of the antibody to mediate protection. Although the antibodies were not able to neutralize virus *in vitro* alone, whether they were capable of doing so in the presence of complement, macrophages or NK cells could be assessed. The roles played by complement, macrophages and NK cells in antibody-mediated virus neutralization *in vivo* could also be explored by depleting mice of complement or these innate subsets just prior to antibody administration and determining whether or not the antibodies were still able to mediate protection in their absence.

13.3 CD8$^+$ T cells mediate effector activity against virus-infected cells, i.e. they are unable to block the acquisition of infection altogether. If there were sufficient vaccine-induced effector-memory CD8$^+$ T cells present at the mucosal sites where HIV infection is typically initiated these cells may be able to extinguish the infection before the virus disseminates to establish a widespread systemic infection and generate a pool of latently-infected cells (which cannot be detected by the host immune system). However if moderate numbers of resting memory CD8$^+$ T cells were present in a vaccinated individual at the time of infection, the time taken for these cells to be reactivated and expand following HIV exposure permit virus amplification and dissemination to establish a systemic infection that the T cells are then unable to eliminate.

13.4 No. Although epitopes derived from all of the HIV proteins can be presented on infected cells and target these cells for T cell recognition, T cells recognizing epitopes in proteins that are present in cells early after the cell becomes infected are likely to be able to control virus replication most effectively, as these T cells will have a longer window of opportunity to detect and lyse the infected cell before new virus particles start to be produced from it. Epitopes derived from structural proteins that are present in virions in sufficient quantities for the protein introduced into the cytoplasm as infection occurs to be processed and presented (e.g. the HIV Gag protein) will be displayed on an infected cell most rapidly, followed by epitopes derived from proteins that are synthesized in infected cells relatively early in the viral lifecycle (e.g. the HIV Nef protein).

13.5 One way in which this could be achieved is by designing vaccines to induce T cell responses to epitopes in the most invariant regions of the virus, where any amino acid changes introduced to confer escape from T cell recognition are likely to have a high cost to viral fitness. It would also be helpful for vaccines to stimulate strong T cell responses to a large number of different viral epitopes so that the virus will need to acquire multiple mutations to escape from the entire vaccine-induced response.

14. Immunoendocrine interactions in the response to infection

14.1 The immune system cannot be understood in isolation from the rest of mammalian physiology. One of the many effects of stress is increased production of adrenocorticotropic hormone (ACTH) from the pituitary. This in turn drives increased production of cortisol by the adrenal. The proof is that, in the animal models mentioned, the stressor can be replaced by mimicking the stress-induced levels of cortisol (or the rodent equivalent, corticosterone) with implanted slow-release cortisol pellets. The cortisol downregulates cell-mediated immunity to tuberculosis.

14.2 These observations provide clues as to why increased cortisol levels can lead to reduced immunity to tuberculosis. Raised cortisol levels cause APCs to release more IL-10 and less IL-12, so newly recruited T cells tend to develop a TH2 cytokine profile. Moreover, cortisol actually synergizes with some functions of TH2 cytokines, and enhances the ability of IL-4 to drive IgE production. It is interesting that BCG vaccination does not lead to protective immunity if the BCG is given to animals bearing cortisol pellets that mimic stress levels of cortisol. Cortisol also reduces the antimycobacterial functions of macrophages.

These points emphasize the need for a physiological approach to the understanding of infection. A narrowly immunological approach has solved some infections, but global emergencies such as tuberculosis, HIV infection and septic shock may require integrated physiological thinking as well as pure immunology.

15. Immunity to protozoa and helminths

15.1 Protozoa replicate within the host, so there is usually a balance between the effectiveness of the immune response and the virulence of the parasite. With certain parasites the infections may be short-lived and may kill the host, but this may not be a disadvantage to the parasite if it has already been transmitted to a new host. A good example is falciparum malaria, which is potentially fatal, particularly in children in endemic areas who have not developed any immunity, but are likely to have been bitten during the course of the infection by mosquitos, which will ensure further transmission. Helminths, by contrast, do not replicate within the host and are generally long-lived chronic infections. Transmission is by the release of eggs and larvae from an adult parasite, which may be excreted or be taken up by a vector.

15.2 By adopting an intracellular mode of existence parasites may be able to 'hide' from the immune response. A good example is falciparum malaria, which lives in mature red blood cells. Because this cell type has no nucleus it cannot express MHC class I molecules on its surface, so the parasite is invisible to $CD8^+$ cytotoxic T cells. Other parasites live in nucleated cells, which will express class I MHC molecules, but experiments have shown this to be downregulated in cells infected with some parasites. *T. gondii* avoids being killed by the macrophage by inhibiting the fusion of the lysosome with the phagosome; *T. cruzi* escapes from the phagosome into the cytoplasm of the cell; and *Leishmania* spp. can resist the low pH of the phagolysosomes and are resistant to lysosomal enzymes.

15.3 Extracellular parasites can adopt a number of ways of avoiding immune attack. Parasites may 'disguise' themselves, for example by undergoing antigenic variation (African trypanosomes) or by adsorbing host molecules or undergoing molecular mimicry of the host (schistosomes). Parasites may 'hide' from the host immune response by becoming cysts (*Entamoeba* spp.) or by living in an immunoprivileged location (*Toxoplasma* in brain). They may 'resist' attack by having a physical barrier (helminths) or by producing enzymes that resist the oxidative burst or disable antibodies. Many parasites are able to 'modulate' the host immune response to their advantage.

16. Hyper-IgM immunodeficiency

16.1 This child presented with bacterial pneumonia, a history of recurrent respiratory tract infections, lymphadenopathy and abnormal immunoglobulin levels, with increased IgM and low IgG and IgA. These features are consistent with a hyper-IgM phenotype. The normal number and distribution of T and B lymphocytes rules out both SCID and congenital agammaglobulinemia. CD40L deficiency is inherited as an X-linked trait, and is characterized by severe infections (including opportunistic infections) and neutropenia. The patient was a female child, and she did not present with opportunistic infections or neutropenia. This makes the diagnosis of CD40L very unlikely.

16.2 The association of hyper-IgM phenotype and recurrent lymphadenopathy is typical of AID deficiency, which is inherited as an autosomal trait, affecting both males and females. This is the most likely diagnosis in this patient.

16.3 Antibodies formed to tetanus toxoid immunization are of the IgG class. Because this child is incapable of undergoing isotype switching, she cannot make IgG antibodies. However, antibodies to the blood group substances are predominantly of the IgM isotype, which this child can synthesize.

16.4 The child should be given intravenous immunoglobulins (IVIG), at regular intervals (every 3–4 weeks) to protect her against bacterial infections. As this child is incapable of making IgG, she will need IVIG for life. She may benefit also from prophylactic antibiotics, along with IVIG administration. This treatmemt should

result in a significant reduction of infectious episodes. However, AID deficiency also carries an increased risk of autoimmune manifestations.

17. Secondary immunodeficiency

17.1 Approximately 95% of HIV-positive individuals seroconvert within 3 months of infection. ELISAs for antibodies to gp41, an HIV surface glycoprotein, and p24, a core protein, are the most widely used to detect HIV infection. Confirmation is obtained by Western blot analysis to decrease the rate of false-positive results. The Centers for Disease Control and Prevention recommends that the blot should be positive for two of the p24, gp41, and gp120/160 markers (gp160 is the precursor form of gp41 and gp120, the envelope protein). ELISAs for p24 antigen can also be used, though the false-negative rate is higher. The PCR is a technique for amplifying specific sequences of DNA or RNA to produce quantities that are readily detectable. The test in the context of HIV is highly sensitive and specific, but is more costly than ELISA techniques.

17.2 The mother's serological state should be tested by ELISA and confirmed by Western blot if positive. Around 20–30% of infants born to HIV-positive mothers are infected with the virus. Transmission can occur *in utero* or very rarely by breastfeeding. Diagnosis presents a problem because maternal IgG specific for HIV antigens crosses the placenta and can be detected in the infant even if the infant has not become infected. The presence of HIV-specific antibodies of IgA and IgM classes in the infant should imply infection because they do not cross the placenta. Current tests lack sensitivity and remain in development. The method most widely used in the UK and USA is the PCR, which demonstrates the virus directly. Below the age of 1 month the PCR may be negative in infected children. It has been shown that, in many children, HIV is sequestered into regional lymph nodes at this age. After establishing infection at these sites a viremia follows.

17.3 The figure shows the change in a variety of indices of HIV infection over time. Acute seroconversion causes an infectious mononucleosis-like illness in up to 50% of those infected with HIV. Common symptoms are fever, lymphadenopathy, pharyngitis, rashes, and myalgia. At this point there is a drop in the CD4 (and also CD8) lymphocyte count and a rise in plasma viremia and p24 antigen concentration. Antibodies to HIV surface glycoproteins gp120 and gp41 are produced from approximately 6 weeks after infection and are initially of the IgM class. IgG antibodies of the same specificities follow the IgM response and persist during the latent phase. Viremia and p24 antigenemia are generally low during this period. Disease progression is heralded by a declining CD4 lymphocyte count and a rise in plasma viremia. Clinically, CD4 counts have become a widely used index of progression. Plasma viremia is the most accurate measure of disease progression, and is becoming a more commonly used method.

A typical course of HIV infection

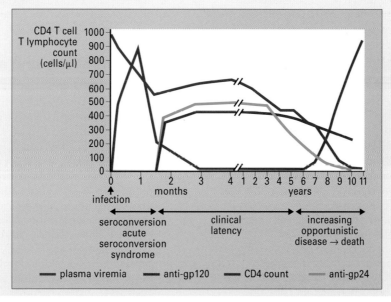

18. Vaccination

18.1 Successful attenuation results in an organism still capable of generating an immune response against the wild-type virulent organism, but no longer capable of causing disease. This is a delicate balance to achieve. In some instances (e.g. hepatitis B and C viruses) the organisms cannot be cultured, so attenuation by repeated *in-vitro* passage is impossible.

18.2 There is no reason to believe that a vaccine cannot improve on nature. Many organisms express gene products that interfere with immune responses. Removal of these from the vaccine may allow protective responses to be generated.

18.3 Although smallpox was eliminated because there was no animal reservoir or carrier state, this is also the case for some other microorganisms and it should be possible to eliminate them. For other organisms, elimination will be difficult and maintenance of herd immunity will remain important.

18.4 Vaccines are unlikely ever to replace antibiotics completely. Microorganisms evolve very rapidly and vaccine production against complex organisms, such as mycobacteria, has proved very difficult. In addition, immunodeficient individuals and the elderly remain at risk even after vaccination.

18.5 BCG clearly has multiple effects. Specific immune responses to BCG antigens can be detected, but cell wall and other components of the bacterium have potent immunomodulatory effects. The efficacy of BCG as a vaccine has been suggested to depend on cross-reactions of BCG with environmental mycobacteria as well as *Mycobacterium tuberculosis* itself.

18.6 Strong immune responses may cause tissue damage in individuals with parasites already present. However, a vaccine that prevented establishment of infection would be unlikely to be damaging.

18.7 Antigens that induce T cell immunity may be useful vaccine antigens. Molecules that contribute to virulence, such as toxins, may be the best targets for vaccines. Because the genomes of many pathogens have been or are being sequenced, searching homologous gene products may identify potential targets.

19. Immunological tolerance

19.1 **Clonal deletion:** Immature B cells that recognize antigen in the bone marrow can undergo clonal deletion. T cells start rearranging their antigen receptors in the thymus where they undergo the processes of positive and negative selection. T cells that do not receive survival signals during positive selection and T cells that recognize self antigens with high affinity will undergo apoptosis.

Receptor editing: This is a B-cell specific tolerance mechanism. Immature B cells that recognize antigen in the bone marrow get a second chance: they can continue V(D)J recombination to assemble another, non self reactive antigen receptor. Only if that fails will they undergo apoptosis. T lymphocytes assemble one receptor that cannot be changed during development.

Anergy: describes the inability of a lymphocyte to respond to antigenic stimulation. This was first described for B cells but also occurs in T cells. The molecular mechanisms for anergy may differ between the two lymphocyte populations.

Lack of T-cell help: B cells need T cell help to switch from IgM to other isotypes. Therefore, robust tolerance in the T-cell compartment will also help to ensure B cell tolerance. T cells depend on co-stimulatory signals from antigen presenting cells. This could be viewed as somewhat similar to the B cells' dependance on T cell help.

19.2 Mutations in AIRE have been identified as the cause of the APECED (**a**utoimmune **p**olyendocrinopathy-candidiasis-**e**ctodermal **d**ystrophy) syndrome and mice that lack AIRE have a similar phenotype. AIRE has been shown to direct the ectopic expression of otherwise strictly tissue restricted antigens by medullary thymic epithelial cells (mTECs) in the thymus.

19.3 T cells which have rearranged their TCR in the thymus need to receive survival signals (cytokines) from cortical thymic APC. In order to receive these signals the TCR must be able to recognize self MHC. Only T cells that express TCRs capable of recognizing self-MHC will receive survival signals, the other T cells will undergo apoptosis. T cells recognize only antigen that is complexed with self MHC. Therefore, a T cell that cannot recognize self-MHC would be useless. B cells in contrast can recognize antigen without the help of antigen presenting cells. Therefore, B cells do not need to be selected for self-MHC recognition.

19.4 Dendritic cells in the thymus contribute to thymic selection of the T cell repertoire. Outside the thymus dendritic cells are important antigen presenting cells for T cells, in particular for naive T cells. Dendritic cells are located in many organs and constantly take up antigen, both self and non-self. Only if the dendritic cells recognize danger signals (PAMPs), via their pattern recognition receptors (PRRs, e.g. TLRs), will they undergo certain maturation steps, including the upregulation of co-stimulatory ligands for T cells, which transform them into powerful antigen presenting cells. To become activated effector cells T cells need to recognize antigen and receive co-stimulatory signals. If a DC presents only antigen but does not provide co-stimulatory signals the corresponding T cell will become anergic or undergo apoptosis. Self-antigens usually do not provide danger signals for the DC. Therefore, the DC will not provide co-stimulatory signals for the T cells and the T cells recognizing self antigen presented by a non-activated DC will become anergic or apoptotic rather than activated.

19.5 These pathogens do not present danger signals to the antigen presenting cells in the tissue. Consequently, the APC do not take up the pathogen and deliver it to the T cell zones in the draining lymph nodes. Therefore, an adaptive immune response against such pathogens is not primed.

19.6 Immunological ignorance describes a state in which fully functional T cells are kept away from the antigen which they recognize *in vivo*. Anergy describes a state in which lymphocytes do not respond with effector functions upon recognizing antigen. If the TCR transgenic T cells were ignorant *in vivo*, they would still respond to antigen *in vitro*, e.g. they would proliferate and produce cytokines. These effector functions can be assayed *in vitro*. If the TCR transgenic T cells were anergic they would proliferate very little and fail to produce IL-2 in response to antigen presentation *in vitro*.

19.7 This is still an open question. The two most likely explanations are (i) the effector cells have become

resistant to regulation by Tregs, or (ii) the Tregs lack the relevant effector functions necessary to prevent the effector cells from causing damage.

20. Autoimmunity and autoimmune disease

20.1 It is thought that free DNA filtered in the kidney fixes to the glomerular basement membrane and can then bind anti-DNA antibodies, which then form an immune complex in situ. Complement is then fixed, resulting in local damage.

20.2 This is a vexed question. Although DNA–anti-DNA complexes are found in tissues, efforts to find these complexes in the serum have failed. In addition, immunizing lupus-prone animals with DNA does not produce clinical lupus. However, introduction of transgenes encoding anti-ds DNA in mice can produce lupus.

20.3 A possible explanation is that the mononuclear–phagocyte system becomes saturated and is therefore unable to clear the soluble complexes, which are thought to be most likely pathogenic. It is also possible that the reduction in the complement receptors on red cells (complement receptor-1, CR1) might also predispose to poor clearance of complexes.

20.4 Over 95% of patients with SLE have ANA as the major autoantibody. Antibodies to extractable nuclear antigens are also seen, but much less frequently. Anti-dsDNA antibodies are the most specific to SLE because anti-single-stranded antibodies are found in a variety of other situations, such as other autoimmune disease, a variety of infections, and inflammatory conditions.

21. Kidney transplantation

21.1 There is a great shortage of donor organs. The supply of cadaveric organs depends on the deaths of healthy individuals and the willingness of their relatives to allow donation. In addition, the available organs are given to recipients with the best HLA tissue match. At random there is less than a 1 in 20 000 chance of finding a perfect match. In the case of kidney transplantation the blood group antigens must be taken into account. Mrs X is blood group B, which is uncommon (<10%), and will therefore have antibodies to tissues from blood group A donors. Blood group A is the most common blood group (about 45% of individuals).

21.2 Mrs X is HLA identical to her brother Fred and shares one HLA haplotype with her brother Gary. There is a 1 in 4 chance of siblings inheriting the same mendelian characteristics from their parents.

21.3 Like Mrs X and her brother Fred, Bert and Edna are HLA identical to each other. Of the five children of Mrs X, four have Mr X as their biological father. However, it is clear that Dave was fathered by a man other than Mr X! This is not uncommon. Approximately 5–10% of children may be like Dave!

21.4 HLA identical: Fred; HLA haplotype match: Anne, Bert, Chas, Dave, Gary; complete HLA mismatch: Mr X.

21.5 If only HLA matching is considered, Fred would be the best donor because there would be no HLA mismatch between the donor and recipient.

21.6 Mrs X is blood group B, and therefore has antibodies to blood group A, thus excluding Mr X, Anne, Bert, Edna, and Fred. Only Chas, Dave, and Gary would be suitable. Because Mrs X is Rhesus positive (has antigen D) she will not have anti-Rh antibodies, so typing for this blood group can be ignored in this instance.

21.7 Chas is first choice. He is HLA haplotype matched, he is ABO compatible, and is a young man. In general, younger kidneys last for longer than older kidneys, and younger people respond better to surgery. Gary might be considered. He too is haplotype identical and ABO compatible. In fact, in terms of his ABO blood group, being blood group O he is the 'universal donor', having no A or B blood group antigens on his tissues. However, he is older and therefore not an ideal donor. Dave is like his brother Chas, HLA haplotype identical and ABO compatible with his mother. However, he is only 15 years of age and minors are generally excluded from this kind of surgery.

21.8 The organ from Chas suffered hyperacute rejection. This is mediated by preformed antibodies in the recipient binding to antigens in the graft. The antibodies fix complement and initiate the process of graft thrombosis. Platelet aggregation in the blood vessels blocks blood flow and the graft dies from lack of oxygen (ischemia).

21.9 The main stimuli for antibodies that cause hyperacute rejection are rejection of a previous graft, blood transfusions, and multiple pregnancies by the same partner. Mrs X has had four children by the same father, Mr X, and is likely to have become sensitized towards class I HLA antigens that Mr X has but Mrs X does not possess. In this case antibodies to either HLA-A3 or HLA-B7 could have been responsible for the hyperacute rejection.

21.10 Cross-match tests are used to detect anti-donor antibodies before transplantation. These tests are becoming more and more sensitive, but occasionally an antibody in low titer may go undetected. It appears that the cross-match test used at the time of the transplantation failed to detect an antibody to a HLA class I antigen. Fortunately this seldom happens today and hyperacute rejection is now very rare.

21.11 There were three family members who were originally suitable for donation, Chas, Dave, and Gary. The kidney from Chas was transplanted and rejected by Mrs X. Gary is now 60 and is less attractive as a donor. In any case he shares the HLA-B14 antigen with Mr X, which, because Mrs X is sensitized to Mr X, may be a target for hyperacute rejection. The possibility that Mrs X has an antibody to HLA-B14 would have to be investigated very carefully! Dave has by now reached the age of majority and could be considered as a donor. He is HLA haplotype identical to his mother, and is ABO compatible. Furthermore, because he has a different father, Dave is less likely to express antigens that might be the target of hyperacute rejection. It seems that Dave would be the most suitable donor. You might like to consider the emotional pressure this puts on Dave, given the seriousness of his mother's condition and how his family are likely to react if he wants to change his mind about donation.

21.12 Triple immunosuppression is standard in most transplant centers. It consists of corticosteroids plus either ciclosporin or tacrolimus and either azathioprine or mycophenolate. Some centers add other agents such as anti-lymphocyte serum or a monoclonal antibody to T cells (OKT3).

21.13 About one-third of all transplant recipients suffer an episode of acute rejection in the first few weeks. This is mainly a cell-mediated immune response.

21.14 The anti-rejection therapy often used is to give three large doses of corticosteroid on three consecutive days (totaling 2–3 g of corticosteroid). This causes apoptosis (programmed cell death) of activated lymphocytes and stops the rejection episode very effectively. Other anti-rejection therapies are used, such as OKT3 anti-T cell monoclonal antibody.

21.15 Because of the immunosuppression, patients are more prone to infection. The immunosuppressive drugs used can be toxic, so a dose reduction or a change in medication may be required. In addition, transplant patients on high doses of immunosuppression may develop a post-transplant lymphoproliferative disorder caused by Epstein–Barr virus infection. Reduction of the dose usually helps. In the longer term transplant patients have a higher risk of cancer because of depressed immune surveillance.

21.16 Mrs X finally lost her kidney transplant to chronic rejection. This may involve both immunological and non-immunological damage. The damage initiates a repair process involving the production of growth factors in the graft. None of the drugs in current use controls this process very well, so although the doctors change drugs and doses it is very difficult to control chronic rejection.

22. Immunity to cancers

22.1 When animals are immunized prophylactically, an adaptive immune response to the tumors is generated. When the same animal is challenged with live cancer cells later, the pre-existing immune response is amplified rapidly and can eliminate the tumor challenge. In contrast, when a naive animal is challenged, the tumor has generally already grown to a considerable size by the time an immune response to it is generated. At the same time, this developing immune response is compromised by a number of immune downregulatory mechanisms (immunosuppressive cytokines, $CD4^+$ suppressor T cells, etc.) that get activated in a host with a growing tumor. Thus, even as the tumor keeps growing, the immune response to it is compromised, and the host succumbs to the tumor.

22.2 The immunity elicited by HSP preparations does not derive from the HSP molecules per se, but from the antigenic peptides chaperoned by them. The HSPs isolated from tumors are associated with antigenic tumor-specific peptides in addition to the normal non-immunogenic peptides. In contrast, HSPs isolated from normal tissues are associated with only the non-immunogenic, normal peptides. This difference accounts for the lack of immunogenicity of normal tissue-derived HSPs and immunogenicity of tumor-derived HSPs.

22.3 Tumor antigens have been defined by a number of methods, such as by their ability to elicit tumor rejection in animal models or by recognition by T cells or antibodies in animals or in patients with cancer. Altogether, tumor antigens may be classified into the following classes:
- differentiation antigens;
- cancer testes antigens;
- unique mutated antigens;
- common mutated antigens (including oncogene-encoded antigens);
- viral antigens; and
- heat-shock proteins (which act as carriers of all of the above categories of antigen).

22.4 Concomitant immunity is defined as the presence in a host of an anti-tumor immune response that is able to successfully eradicate a tumor at one site in the concomitant presence of another tumor, which is apparently unresponsive to it. This phenomenon is a dramatic demonstration of the two opposing forces in cancer immunity – the immune response to a growing cancer, and the subversion of that response.

22.5 Several observations can be cited in support of down-regulation of immune response in the tumor-bearing state, as follows:

- The phenomenon of concomitant immunity is clear evidence in this regard. Tumor-reactive and tumor-protective T cells can be isolated early during tumor growth. At a later stage, one can show the presence of immune-suppressive T cells in the same animal. The CD4$^+$CD25$^+$ regulatory T cells have also been shown to play a downregulatory influence on the anti-cancer immune response.
- The phenomenon that the same animal can reject a skin allograft while not rejecting a tumor expressing the same allo-MHC shows that there are local factors that make the tumor apparently resistant to the existing systemic anti-tumor immune response.
- The extensive murine and emerging clinical data that blocking of the CTLA-4 molecule (which transmits an inhibitory signal to activated T cells) leads to tumor regression or other forms of protection from tumor growth suggest strongly that the anti-tumor immune response in a cancer-bearing host is downregulated.

23. Severe anaphylactic shock

23.1 Traditionally, the term anaphylaxis has been used to describe a systemic clinical syndrome caused by IgE-mediated degranulation of mast cells and basophils.

Susceptible individuals exposed to a sensitizing antigen produce specific IgE antibodies, which bind to high-affinity IgE receptors (FcεRI) found on mast cells and basophils. The receptor binds the Fc portion of the antibody, leaving the Fab binding sites available to interact with antigen. The avidity of this Fc binding reaction is high and therefore the dissociation of IgE from the receptors is slow, with a long half-life. On subsequent exposure, the antigen is bound by the IgE-receptor complexes, which causes receptor-mediated activation of the cells with release of preformed and de-novo synthesized mediators. Degranulation is rapid and completed within 30 minutes. These mediators, released on a large scale, are responsible for the clinical manifestations of anaphylaxis. The IgE-mediated mechanism of mast cell degranulation has been implicated in the pathogenesis of anaphylaxis triggered by a variety of agents. These include antibiotics (e.g. penicillins, cephalosporins), foods (e.g. milk, nuts, shellfish), foreign proteins (e.g. insulin, bee venom, latex), and pharmacological agents (e.g. streptokinase, vaccines). Patients who have anaphylaxis may or may not have a history of atopy. Natural exposure to common allergens such as pollen or dust mites is only very rarely a cause of anaphylaxis. However, when patients who also have asthma develop anaphylaxis due to venom, penicillin, or food antigens, the reactions are more dangerous because they can include rapid onset of bronchospasm.

Mast cell degranulation can occur by IgE-independent pathways. In these cases prior exposure is not a prerequisite because specific IgE antibodies are not involved. Three putative mechanisms of anaphylactoid reactions are given below.

- Blood, blood products, and immunoglobulins can cause an anaphylactoid reaction. The suggested mechanism is the formation of immune complexes with subsequent complement activation and production of C3a and C5a. Both of these complement components (anaphylatoxins) are capable of degranulating mast cells directly. In addition, both components increase vasopermeability and may induce hypotension.
- Certain therapeutic and diagnostic agents such as opiates, muscle relaxants, and contrast media are also capable of directly causing mast cell degranulation and anaphylaxis.
- 5–10% of asthmatic subjects produce a reaction to non-steroidal anti-inflammatory drugs (NSAIDs), such as aspirin or indometacin. Symptoms commonly include bronchospasm, rhinorrhea, and, rarely, vascular collapse. The ability of these agents to cause anaphylaxis appears to correlate with their effectiveness in inhibiting prostaglandin synthesis. The mechanism of this sensitivity is unknown, but increased leukotriene production occurs, which suggests that triggering of mast cells is part of the reaction.

23.2 There is a great variation in the timing and nature of anaphylactic symptoms. The onset is usually within seconds or minutes of exposure, though delays of an hour have been reported. The following are common presentations, which may occur singly or in combination:

- cutaneous – erythema, pruritus of hands, feet, and abdomen, urticaria, angioedema;
- respiratory – laryngeal edema causing hoarseness, which may progress to asphyxia, bronchoconstriction causing wheezing, rhinorrhea;
- cardiovascular – hypotension, arrhythmias, tachycardia, vascular collapse;
- gastrointestinal – cramping abdominal pain, nausea, vomiting, diarrhea.

The majority of cases of anaphylactic reaction are not fatal. It has been estimated that 1–2% of courses of penicillin therapy are complicated by systemic reactions, but only 10% of these are serious. In the USA some 400–800 people die annually from penicillin anaphylaxis, with a similar figure for contrast media – 70% of deaths result from respiratory complications (laryngeal edema and/or bronchospasm) with 25% resulting from cardiovascular dysfunction. Prompt treatment of anaphylaxis is essential because death may occur rapidly. The patient is placed in the recovery position, oxygen is given by mask, and 0.5–1.0 mL epinephrine 1:1000 w/v is injected intramuscularly. This has the effect of raising the blood pressure, relaxing bronchial smooth muscle, and preventing further mediator release. Intravenous antihistamines (e.g. 10 mg chlorpheniramine) can be useful because histamine can cause vasodilation, cardiac arrhythmias, and bronchospasm. Corticosteroids (e.g. 100 mg hydrocortisone) intravenously may help to reduce any late-phase response.

23.3 The first step is to obtain a thorough history of previous adverse reactions. The timing and nature of such reactions should be noted. Skin prick testing with insect venom is a fast and sensitive method of detecting anti-venom IgE. Radioallergosorbent tests can detect venom-specific IgE, but are positive in only 80% of those with significant reactions to venom skin prick tests. Immunotherapy is best reserved for those with life-threatening systemic reactions to insect venom. The patient is given increasing subcutaneous dosages and then a monthly maintenance dose of 100 µg. The clinical protection rate is in the order of 98% for both adults and children.

24. Blood groups and hemolytic disease of the newborn

24.1 Because Mrs Chareston has clearly becomed sensitized to Rhesus D, it is most likely that her first child is RhD⁺. The alternative explanation, that she has become sensitized by a blood transfusion, is highly unlikely, because of the routine matching of this blood group when carrying out transfusions.

24.2 HDNB usually becomes more serious with successive pregnancies because the mother has become sensitized to the fetal red cells and successive sensitizations produce progressively stronger responses in the mother, and more serious disease in susceptible children.

24.3 Anti-Rhesus D antibodies are given to the mother to clear the fetal RhD⁺ erythrocytes before they have a chance to sensitize the mother's immune system.

24.4 If the antibodies are given pre-partum, they would cross the placenta and produce or exacerbate HDNB in the fetus.

24.5 Rhesus prophylaxis is not always successful, but in this case there was no treatment after the first pregnancy and Mrs Chareston was already sensitized to RhD. Preventing further responses in an individual who is already sensitized is less likely to succeed because of the nature of secondary immune responses – less antigen is required to trigger the response.

24.6 The most likely explanation is that the child is Rh⁻. Indeed this turns out to be the case. A Rh⁻ child must have received a Rh⁻ gene from both parents. Assuming that Mr Chareston is the father of the fourth child, we can say that his genotype is RhD⁺/RhD⁻ (heterozygote), and that the child received RhD⁻ genes from both parents.

24.7 Antigens of the ABO blood group are carbohydrates and tend to induce IgM antibodies, which do not undergo affinity maturation or class switching (see Chapter 8). IgM does not cross the placenta (see Chapter 3) and so does not produce HDNB.

24.8 The second child was definitely not fathered by Mr Chareston because ABO blood groups are co-dominantly expressed. For a child to have the blood group B, one or both parents must have blood group B. As neither Mr or Mrs Chareston has this blood group, the B gene must have come from someone else.

25. Type III serum sickness after factor IX administration

25.1 This is a classic example of serum sickness induced by a 'foreign protein' factor IX because the boy does not produce it.

25.2 Corticosteroids were prescribed to decrease inflammation and for immunosuppression.

25.3 The likelihood that this type of reaction will develop again is relatively high because a memory response will be produced; T cells and plasma cells will respond more rapidly during re-exposure to the same foreign antigen (i.e. factor IX).

25.4 Short courses of corticosteroids with/without transient immunosuppression.

25.5 In this case, the clinical presentation is associated with an apparent non-inflammatory process (inferred because there is only proteinuria and inflammation has not reduced the glomerular filtration rate). Although the precise pathogenesis is uncertain, it is thought that the administered factor IX gets modified (becomes more positively charged) in the circulation. Because of its charge, it becomes trapped during normal filtration between the negatively charged glomerular basement membrane and glomerular epithelial cells, where it serves as a 'planted antigen' for circulating anti-factor IX antibodies. The Fc regions of local or 'in-situ' formed immune complexes activate the classical complement system, whereby C5b–9 causes sublytic injury to the epithelial cells, leading to their detachment. Because these cells normally participate in maintaining the glomerular integrity and limiting protein filtration, this pathologic process causes loss of large amounts of protein in the urine. Inflammation is not observed because FcR engagement on circulating inflammatory cells is prevented by the intact basement membrane. Pathologically there is epithelial cell 'effacement' from the basement membrane, but a conspicuous absence of inflammation. By contrast, in acute serum sickness, when immune deposits form between the endothelium and the basement membrane (or on the basement membrane), the deposited IgG engages FcR on circulating cells, and inflammation (with cellular infiltration) is the predominant feature.

25.6 The likelihood that this type reaction will develop again is relatively high because a memory response will be produced; T cells and plasma cells will respond more rapidly during re-exposure to the same foreign antigen (i.e. factor IX).

25.7 Immunosuppression until the proteinuria resolves to treat the present episode. Because the probability of immunologic recall is high, transient immunosuppression with each factor IX therapy is indicated to reduce the production of antibodies to factor IX.

26. A hypersensitivity type IV reaction

26.1 Granulomas are composed of lymphocytes, macrophages, and epithelioid cells. The latter develop from macrophages following chronic antigenic stimulation and may fuse to form multinucleate giant cells, typical of granulomas. Cytokines involved in this process include T cell-derived IFNγ and TNF, both for the activation of macrophages and for the organization of the granuloma.

26.2 Histological examination at the site of a DTH reaction reveals edema of the dermis with an infiltrate of monocytes and lymphocytes. This resolves over 1–2 weeks. Granulomas do not form at the sites of DTH reactions if soluble antigen, such as tuberculin, is used. By contrast, in the lymph node a chronic granulomatous response develops as the mycobacteria survive within macrophages, leading to persistent stimulation of T cells and chronic inflammation.

26.3 CD4 T lymphocytes are the major cells responsible for the recognition of soluble recall antigens and the stimulation of DTH reactions.

26.4 Other infections, such as cat scratch fever due to *Bartonella henselae*, histoplasmosis, and tularemia, may cause granulomas in lymph nodes. These are diagnosed by the clinical pattern and microbial cultures. Sarcoidosis causes non-caseating granulomas and is diagnosed by clinical features, histology, and the absence of an infectious cause. Granulomas may also develop in response to foreign bodies, such as talc and silica, or exposure to beryllium.

26.5 The brother's DTH reaction is evidence of a strong T cell response to soluble antigens from *M. tuberculosis*. This indicates that he has been infected with *M. tuberculosis*, but does not mean that he has active tuberculosis disease at present. Normally he would have investigations to exclude active tuberculosis, and if this is not present he would be considered for chemoprophylaxis to eradicate the infection and prevent progression to disease in later life.

Glossary

Acquired immune deficiency syndrome (AIDS). A progressive immune deficiency caused by infection of CD4 T cells with the human retrovirus HIV.

Activation-induced cytidine deaminase (AID). An enzyme expressed in activated B cells that causes somatic mutation in the immunoglobulin gene locus.

Acute phase proteins. Serum proteins whose levels increase during infection or inflammatory reactions.

ADCC (antibody-dependent cell-mediated cytotoxicity). A cytotoxic reaction in which Fc receptor-bearing killer cells recognize target cells via specific antibodies.

Adhesion molecules. Cell surface molecules involved in the binding of cells to extracellular matrix or to neighboring cells, where the principal function is adhesion rather than cell activation (e.g. integrins and selectins).

Adjuvant. A substance that non-specifically enhances the immune response to an antigen.

AFCs (antibody-forming cells). Functionally equivalent to plasma cells.

Affinity. A measure of the binding strength between an antigenic determinant (epitope) and an antibody-combining site.

Affinity maturation. The increase in average antibody affinity frequently seen during a secondary immune response.

AIRE. A transcription factor that promotes expression of multiple tissue genes within the thymus, and is hence involved in T cell education.

Allelic exclusion. This occurs when the use of a gene from the maternal or paternal chromosome prevents the use of the other. It is seen with antibody and T cell receptor genes.

Allergen. An agent (e.g. pollen, dust, animal dander) that causes IgE-mediated hypersensitivity reactions.

Allergy. Originally defined as altered reactivity on second contact with antigen; now usually refers to a type I hypersensitivity reaction.

Allotype. The protein of an allele that may be detectable as an antigen by another member of the same species.

Alternative pathway. The activation pathways of the complement system involving C3 and factors B, D, P, H, and I, which interact in the vicinity of an activator surface to form an alternative pathway C3 convertase.

Amplification loop. The alternative complement activation pathway that acts as a positive feedback loop when C3 is split in the presence of an activator surface.

Anaphylatoxins. Complement peptides (C3a and C5a) that cause mast cell degranulation and smooth muscle contraction.

Anaphylaxis. An antigen-specific immune reaction mediated primarily by IgE that results in vasodilation and constriction of smooth muscle, including those of the bronchus, and may result in death.

Anergy. Failure to make an immune response following stimulation with a potential antigen.

Antagonist peptides. Analogs of antigenic peptides that bind to MHC molecules and prevent stimulation of specific clones of T cells.

Antibody. A molecule produced by animals in response to antigen that has the particular property of combining specifically with the antigen that induced its formation.

Antigen. A molecule that reacts with preformed antibody and the specific receptors on T and B cells.

Antigen receptors. The lymphocyte receptors for antigens including the T cell receptor (TCR) and surface immunoglobulin on B cells, which acts as the B cell's antigen receptor (BCR).

Antigen presentation. The process by which certain cells in the body (antigen-presenting cells) express antigen on their cell surface in a form recognizable by lymphocytes.

Antigen processing. The conversion of an antigen into a form in which it can be recognized by lymphocytes.

Antigenic determinants. See 'epitopes'.

Antigenic peptides. Peptide fragments of proteins that bind to MHC molecules and induce T cell activation.

Antiviral proteins. Proteins whose synthesis is induced by interferons. They become activated if the cell is infected by virus and limit viral replication.

APCs (antigen-presenting cells). A variety of cell types that carry antigen in a form that can stimulate lymphocytes.

Apoptosis. Programmed cell death that involves nuclear fragmentation and condensation of cytoplasm, plasma membranes, and organelles into apoptotic bodies.

Arthus reaction. Inflammation seen in the skin some hours following injection of antigen. It is a manifestation of a type III hypersensitivity reaction.

Atopy. The clinical manifestation of type I hypersensitivity reactions, including eczema, asthma, rhinitis, and food allergy.

Autocrine. This refers to the ability of a cytokine to act on the cell that produced it.

Autoimmunity. Immune recognition and reaction against the individual's own tissue.

Avidity. The functional combining strength of an antibody with its antigen, which is related to both the affinity of the reaction between the epitopes and paratopes, and the valencies of the antibody and antigen.

β_2-Microglobulin. A polypeptide that constitutes part of some membrane proteins including the class I MHC molecules.

B7–1 (CD80), B7–2 (CD86). Two molecules that are present on antigen-presenting cells. They ligate CD28 on T cells and act as powerful co-stimulatory signals.

B cells. Lymphocytes that develop in the bone marrow in adults and produce antibody. They can be subdivided into two groups, B1 and B2. B1 cells use minimally mutated receptors, which are close to the germline immunoglobulin sequences, whereas B2 cells are the major responding population in conventional immune responses to protein antigens.

B cell co-receptor complex. A group of cell surface molecules consisting of complement receptor type 2 (CD21), CD81, and CD19, which act as a co-stimulatory receptor on mature B cells.

B cell receptor complex (BCR). B cell surface immunoglobulin and its associated signaling molecules, CD79a and CD79b.

Basophil. A population of polymorphonuclear leukocytes that stain with basic dyes and have important roles in the control of inflammation.

BCG (bacille Calmette–Guérin). An attenuated strain of *Mycobacterium tuberculosis* used as a vaccine, an adjuvant, or a biological response modifier in different circumstances.

Bcl-2. A molecule expressed transiently on activated B cells that have been rescued from apoptosis.

Biozzi mice. Lines of mice bidirectionally bred to produce low or high antibody responses to a variety of antigens (originally sheep erythrocytes).

Blood groups. Sets of allelically variable molecules expressed on red cells and sometimes other tissues that may be the target of transfusion reactions.

Bradykinin. A vasoactive nonapeptide that is the most important mediator generated by the kinin system.

Bursa of Fabricius. A lymphoepithelial organ that is the site of B cell maturation and is found at the junction of the hindgut and cloaca in birds.

Bystander lysis. Complement-mediated lysis of cells in the immediate vicinity of a complement activation site that are not themselves responsible for the activation.

C domains. The constant domains of antibody and the T cell receptor. These domains do not contribute to the antigen-binding site and show relatively little variability between receptor molecules.

C genes. The gene segments that encode the constant portion of the immunoglobulin heavy and light chains and the α, β, γ, and δ chains of the T cell antigen receptor.

c-Kit (CD117). A receptor for stem cell factor, which is required for the early development of leukocytes.

C1–C9. The components of the complement classical and lytic pathways, which are responsible for mediating inflammatory reactions, opsonization of particles, and lysis of cell membranes.

C3 convertases. The enzyme complexes C3b, Bb, and C4b2a that cleave complement C3.

Capping. A process by which cell surface molecules are caused to aggregate (usually using antibody) on the cell membrane.

Carrier. An immunogenic molecule or part of a molecule that is recognized by T cells in an antibody response.

Caspases. A group of enzymes that are particularly involved in the transduction of signals for apoptosis.

Cathelicidins. A group of cytotoxic peptides produced by granulocytes.

CD markers. Cell surface molecules of leukocytes and platelets that are distinguishable with monoclonal antibodies and may be used to differentiate different cell populations.

CDRs (complementarity determining regions). The sections of an antibody or T cell receptor V region responsible for antigen or antigen–MHC molecule binding.

Cell adhesion molecules (CAMs). A group of proteins of the immunoglobulin supergene family involved in intercellular adhesion, including ICAM-1, ICAM-2, ICAM-3, vascular cell adhesion molecule-1 (VCAM-1), mucosal addressin cell adhesion molecule-1 (MAd-CAM-1), and platelet endothelial cell adhesion molecule (PECAM).

Central tolerance. Tolerance of T cells or B cells induced during their development in the thymus or bone marrow.

Chemokines. A large group of cytokines falling into four families, of which the main families are the CC and the CXC group. Chemokines are designated as ligands belonging to a particular family (e.g. CCL2). Many chemokines have older descriptive names, for example CCL2 is macrophage chemotactic protein-1 (MCP-1). They act on G protein-linked, seven-transmembrane pass receptors and have a variety of chemotactic and cell-activating properties.

Chemokinesis. Increased random migratory activity of cells.

Chemotaxis. Increased directional migration of cells, particularly in response to concentration gradients of certain chemotactic factors.

Ciclosporin. A T cell suppressive drug that is particularly useful in suppression of graft rejection.

Class I/II/III MHC molecules. Three major classes of molecule are coded within the MHC. Class I molecules have one MHC-encoded peptide complexed with β_2-microglobulin, class II molecules have two MHC-encoded peptides which are non-covalently associated, and class III molecules are other molecules including complement components.

Class I/II restriction. The observation that immunologically active cells will cooperate effectively only when they share MHC haplotypes at either the class I or class II loci.

Class switching. The process by which an individual B cell can link immunoglobulin heavy chain C genes to its recombined V gene to produce a different class of antibody with the same specificity. This process is also reflected in the overall class switch seen during the maturation of an immune response.

Classical pathway. The pathway by which antigen–antibody complexes can activate the complement system, involving components C1, C2, and C4, and generating a classical pathway C3 convertase.

Clonal selection. The fundamental basis of lymphocyte activation in which antigen selectively causes activation, division, and differentiation only in those cells that express receptors with which it can combine.

CMI (cell-mediated immunity). A term used to refer to immune reactions that are mediated by cells rather than by antibody or other humoral factors.

Collectins. A group of large polymeric proteins, including conglutinin and mannan-binding lectin (MBL), that can opsonize microbial pathogens.

Complement. A group of serum proteins involved in control of inflammation, activation of phagocytes, and lytic attack on cell membranes. The system can be activated by interaction with the antibodies of the immune system (classical pathway).

Complement control protein (CCP) domains (also called short consensus repeats). A domain structure found in many proteins of the complement classical and alternative pathways and in some complement receptors and control proteins.

Complement receptors (CR1–CR4 and C1qR). A set of four cell surface receptors for fragments of complement C3. CR1 and CR2 have numerous complement control protein (CCP) domains, and CR3 and CR4 are integrins. C1qR binds C1q.

ConA (concanavalin A). A mitogen for T cells.

Congenic. Animals that are genetically constructed to differ at one particular locus.

Conjugate. A reagent that is formed by covalently coupling two molecules together, such as fluorescein coupled to an immunoglobulin molecule.

Constant regions. The relatively invariant parts of immunoglobulin heavy and light chains, and the α, β, γ, and δ chains of the T cell receptor.

Contact hypersensitivity. A delayed inflammatory reaction on the skin seen in type IV hypersensitivity.

Co-stimulation. The signals required for the activation of a lymphocyte, in addition to the antigen-specific signal delivered via their antigen receptors. CD28 is an important co-stimulatory molecule for T cells and CD40 for B cells.

Cross-reaction. The sharing of antigenic determinants by two different antigens.

CSFs (colony stimulating factors). A group of cytokines that control the differentiation of hematopoietic stem cells.

CTLA-4 (CD152). A downregulatory signaling molecule of T cells that competes with CD28 for ligation by B7 on antigen-presenting cells.

Cytokines. A generic term for soluble molecules that mediate interactions between cells.

Cytotoxic T cells (Tc). Cells that can kill virally infected targets expressing antigenic peptides presented by MHC class I molecules.

D genes. Sets of gene segments lying between the V and J genes in the immunoglobulin heavy chain genes, and in the T cell receptor β and δ chain genes, which are recombined with V and J genes during ontogeny.

DAMPs. Damage associated molecular patterns are signatures associated with damaged or apoptotic cells.

Decay accelerating factor (DAF). A cell surface molecule on mammalian cells that limits activation and deposition of complement C3b.

Defensins. A group of small antibacterial proteins produced by neutrophils.

Degranulation. Exocytosis of granules from cells such as mast cells and basophils.

Dendritic cells. A set of cells present in tissues that capture antigens and migrate to the lymph nodes and spleen, where they are particularly active in presenting the processed antigen to T cells. Dendritic cells can be derived from either the lymphoid or mononuclear phagocyte lineages.

DM molecules. Molecules related to MHC class II molecules that are required for loading antigenic peptides onto class II molecules.

Domain. A region of a peptide having a coherent tertiary structure. Both immunoglobulins and MHC class I and II molecules have immunoglobulin supergene family domains.

DTH (delayed-type hypersensitivity). This term includes the delayed skin reactions associated with type IV hypersensitivity.

Education of T cells. The process by which developing thymocytes are selected for those that recognize peptides on self MHC molecules, but not for those that recognize self antigenic peptides.

Effector cells. A functional concept, which in context means those lymphocytes or phagocytes that produce an end effect.

Eicosanoids. Products of arachidonic acid metabolism including prostaglandins, leukotrienes, and thromboxanes.

Endocytosis. Internalization of material by a cell by phagocytosis or pinocytosis.

Endothelium. Cells lining blood vessels and lymphatics.

Endotoxin. Lipolysaccharide produced by Gram-negative bacteria that activates B cells and macrophages.

Enhancement. Prolongation of graft survival by treatment with antibodies directed towards the graft alloantigens.

Eosinophils. A population of polymorphonuclear granulocytes that stain with acidic dyes and are particularly involved in reactions against parasitic worms and in some hypersensitivity reactions.

Epithelioid cells. A population of activated mononuclear phagocytes present in granulomatous reactions.

Epitopes. The parts of an antigen that contact the antigen-binding sites of an antibody or the T cell receptor.

Epstein–Barr virus (EBV). Causal agent of Burkitt's lymphoma and infectious mononucleosis that has the ability to transform human B cells into stable cell lines.

Fab. The part of an antibody molecule that contains the antigen-combining site consisting of a light chain and part of the heavy chain; it is produced by enzymatic digestion.

Factors B, P, D, H, and I. Components of the alternative complement pathway.

Fas (CD95). A molecule expressed on a variety of cells that acts as a target for ligation by Fas ligand (FasL) on the surface of cytotoxic lymphocytes.

Fc. The portion of an antibody that is responsible for binding to antibody receptors on cells and the C1q component of complement.

Fc receptors. Surface molecules on a variety of cells that bind to the Fc regions of immunoglobulins. They are antibody class specific and isotype selective.

Ficolins. A group of opsonins that recognize carbohydrate PAMPs.

Flow cytometry. Analysis of cell populations in suspension according to each individual cell's expression of selected surface markers.

Fluorescence-activated cell sorter (FACS). A machine that analyzes cells by flow cytometry and then allows them to be sorted into different populations and collected separately.

Follicular dendritic cells (FDCs). Antigen-presenting cells in the B cell areas of lymphoid tissues that retain stores of antigen.

Formyl-methionyl peptides. Prokaryotes initiate protein synthesis with f-Met. Peptides such as f-Met-Leu-Phe are highly chemotactic for mononuclear phagocytes and neutrophils.

Foxp3. A transcription factor required for differentiation of regulatory T cells.

Framework segments. Sections of antibody V regions that lie between the hypervariable regions.

Freund's adjuvant. An emulsion of aqueous antigen in oil. Complete Freund's adjuvant contains killed *Mycobacterium tuberculosis*, whereas incomplete Freund's adjuvant does not.

Frustrated phagocytosis. A term to describe the events that occur when a phagocyte attempts to internalize an antigen or antigenic particle, but is unable to do so (e.g. because of its size).

γδ T cells. The minor subset of T cells that express the γδ form of the T cell receptor.

GALT (gut-associated lymphoid tissue). The accumulation of lymphoid tissue associated with the gastrointestinal tract.

Genetic association. The condition where particular genotypes are associated with other phenomena, such as particular diseases.

Genetic restriction. The term used to describe the observation that lymphocytes and antigen-presenting cells cooperate most effectively when they share particular MHC haplotypes.

Genome. The total genetic material contained within the cell.

Genotype. The genetic material inherited from parents; not all of it is necessarily expressed in the individual.

Germinal centers. Areas of secondary lymphoid tissue in which B cell differentiation and antibody class switching occur.

Germline. The genetic material that is passed down through the gametes before it is modified by somatic recombination or maturation.

Giant cells. Large multinucleated cells sometimes seen in granulomatous reactions and thought to result from the fusion of macrophages.

GPI (glycosylphosphatidylinositol)-linkage. A way in which proteins become attached to the outer leaflet of the phospholipid bilayer that forms the plasma membrane.

Granulocytes. Neutrophils, eosinophils, and basophils.

Granulomatous reactions. Chronic inflammatory reactions (often a manifestation of type IV hypersensitivity) caused by a failure to clear antigen.

Granzymes. Granule-associated enzymes of Tc cells and large granular lymphocytes.

GVHD (graft-versus-host disease). A condition caused by allogeneic donor lymphocytes reacting against host tissue in an immunologically compromised recipient.

H-2. The mouse major histocompatibility complex.

Hemagglutination. Clumping of erythrocytes caused by antibody. This forms the basis of a number of immunoassays and blood group typing.

Haplotype. A set of genetic determinants located on a single chromosome.

Hapten. A small molecule that can act as an epitope, but is incapable by itself of eliciting an antibody response.

Helper T cells (TH). A functional subclass of T cells that can help to generate cytotoxic T cells (Tc) and cooperate with B cells in the production of antibody responses. TH cells recognize antigen in association with MHC class II molecules.

Heterologous. Refers to interspecies antigenic differences.

HEV (high endothelial venule). An area of venule from which lymphocytes migrate into lymph nodes, Peyer's patches and other encapsulated secondary lymphoid tissues.

Hinge. The portion of an immunoglobulin heavy chain between the Fc and Fab regions that permits flexibility within the molecule and allows the two combining sites to operate independently. The hinge region is usually encoded by a separate exon.

Histamine. A major vasoactive amine released from mast cell and basophil granules.

Histocompatibility. The ability to accept grafts between individuals.

HIV (human immunodeficiency virus). The causative agent of acquired immune deficiency syndrome (AIDS).

HLA. The human major histocompatibility complex.

Homologous restriction factors. Complement components that restrict the action of the membrane attack complex on cells of the host.

Humoral. Pertaining to the extracellular fluids, including the serum and lymph.

Hybridoma. Cell line created in vitro by fusing two different cell types, usually lymphocytes, one of which is a tumor cell.

5-Hydroxytryptamine (serotonin). A vasoactive amine present in platelets and a major mediator of inflammation in rodents.

Hypersensitivity. An inordinately strong immune response that causes more damage than the antigen or pathogen that induced the response.

Hypervariable region. The most variable areas of the V domains of immunoglobulin and T cell receptor chains. These regions are clustered at the distal portion of the V domain and contribute to the antigen-binding site.

ICAM-1 (CD54), ICAM-2 (CD102), and ICAM-3 (CD50) (intercellular adhesion molecules). Cell surface molecules found on a variety of leukocytes and non-hematogenous cells that interact with leukocyte functional antigen-1 (LFA-1).

Iccosomes. Immune complexes in the form of small inclusion bodies found in follicular dendritic cells.

Idiotope. A single antigenic determinant on an antibody V region.

Idiotype. The antigenic characteristic of the V region of an antibody.

IELs (intraepithelial lymphocytes). A population of lymphocytes defined according to location in which γδ T cells are strongly represented.

Immune complex. The product of an antigen–antibody reaction that may also contain components of the complement system.

Immune response (Ir) genes. Genes that affect the level of immune responses. MHC class II genes are very important in controlling responses to specific antigens.

Immunoblotting (western blotting). A technique for identifying and characterizing proteins using antibodies.

Immunofluorescence. A technique used to identify particular antigens microscopically in tissues or on cells by the binding of a fluorescent antibody conjugate.

Immunogenic. Having the ability to evoke B cell- and/or T cell-mediated immune reactions.

Immunoglobulins. The serum antibodies, including IgG, IgM, IgA, IgE, and IgD.

Immunoglobulin supergene family (IgSF). Molecules that have domains homologous to those seen in immunoglobulins, including MHC class I and II molecules, the T cell receptor, CD2, CD3, CD4, CD8, ICAMs, VCAM, and some of the Fc receptors.

Immunological synapse. The closely apposed region of plasma membrane in the interaction between T cells and antigen-presenting cells, centered on interacting TCRs and MHC–peptide complexes.

Induced fit. A description of the way in which an antigen can alter the normal tertiary structure of the binding site on a receptor following binding, by displacing amino acids.

Inducible nitric oxide synthase (iNOS). An enzyme induced by inflammatory cytokines in macrophages that catalyzes the synthesis of nitric oxide (NO).

Inflammasome. A multi-protein complex that assembles within a cell in response to PAMPS, and which can activate caspase-1. The exact composition depends on the initiating stimulus.

Inflammation. A series of reactions that bring cells and molecules of the immune system to sites of infection or damage. This appears as an increase in blood supply, increased vascular permeability, and increased transendothelial migration of leukocytes.

Integrins. A large family of cell surface adhesion molecules, some of which interact with cell adhesion molecules (CAMs), others with complement fragments, and others with components of the extracellular matrix.

Interferons (IFNs). A group of molecules involved in signaling between cells of the immune system and in protection against viral infections.

Interleukins (IL-1–IL-35). A group of molecules involved in signaling between cells of the immune system and the tissues.

Isotype. Refers to genetic variation within a family of proteins or peptides such that every member of the species will have each isotype of the family represented in its genome (e.g. immunoglobulin classes).

ITAMs (immunoreceptor tyrosine activation motifs) and ITIMs (immunoreceptor tyrosine inhibitory motifs). These are target sequences for phosphorylation by kinases involved in cell activation or inhibition.

JAKs (Janus kinases). A group of enzymes with two catalytic domains. They activate by cross-phosphorylation and are particularly involved in signaling from type I and II cytokine receptors.

J chain. A monomorphic polypeptide present in polymeric IgA and IgM, and essential to their formation.

J genes. Sets of gene segments in the immunoglobulin heavy and light chain genes and in the genes for the chains of the T cell receptor, which are recombined during lymphocyte ontogeny and contribute toward the genes for variable domains.

K cells. A group of lymphocytes that are able to destroy their target by antibody-dependent cell-mediated cytotoxicity.

κ (kappa) chains. One of the immunoglobulin light chain isotypes.

Karyotype. The chromosomal constitution of a cell that may vary between individuals of a single species depending on the presence or absence of particular sex chromosomes or on the incidence of translocations between sections of different chromosomes.

Killer immunoglobulin-like receptors (KIRs). Receptors on NK cells that belong to the Ig superfamily, having either two or three extracellular domains. They may either inhibit or activate cytotoxicity, depending on their intracellular domains.

Kinins. A group of vasoactive mediators produced following tissue injury.

Knockout. An animal whose endogenous gene for a particular protein has been deleted or mutated to be non-functional.

Kupffer cells. Phagocytic cells that line the liver sinusoids.

λ (lambda) chains. One of the immunoglobulin light chain isotypes.

Langerhans' cells. Antigen-presenting cells of the skin that emigrate to local lymph nodes to become dendritic cells; they are very active in presenting antigen to T cells.

Large granular lymphocytes (LGLs). A group of morphologically defined lymphocytes containing the majority of K cell and NK cell activity. They have both lymphocyte and monocyte/macrophage markers.

Lectin pathway. A pathway of complement activation initiated by mannan-binding lectin (MBL) that intersects the classical pathway.

Leukotrienes. A collection of metabolites of arachidonic acid that have powerful pharmacological effects.

LFAs (leukocyte functional antigens). A group of three molecules that mediate intercellular adhesion between leukocytes and other cells in an antigen non-specific fashion. LFA-1 is CD11a/CD18, LFA-2 is CD2, and LFA-3 is CD58.

Ligand. A linking (or binding) molecule.

Line. A collection of cells produced by continuous growth of a particular cell culture in vitro. Such a cell line will usually contain a number of individual clones.

Linkage. The condition where two genes are both present in close proximity on a single chromosome and are usually inherited together.

Linkage disequilibrium. A condition where two genes are found together in a population at a greater frequency than that predicted simply by the product of their individual gene frequencies.

LPS (lipopolysaccharide). A product of some Gram-negative bacterial cell walls that can act as a B cell mitogen.

Ly antigens. A group of cell surface markers found on murine T cells that relate to the differentiation of T cell subpopulations. Many are now assigned to the CD system.

Lymphokines. A generic term for molecules other than antibodies that are involved in signaling between cells of the immune system and are produced by lymphocytes (cf. interleukins).

Lymphokine activated killer cells (LAKs). Cytotoxic cells generated ex vivo by stimulation with interleukin-2 (IL-2) and possibly other cytokines.

Lymphotoxins. A group of cytokines, related to tumor necrosis factors, that act on TNF receptors and mediate inflammatory reactions and leukocyte activation.

Lysosomes. Intracellular vesicles containing stored enzymes, adhesion molecules, or toxic molecules depending on the cell type.

Lysozyme. An enzyme secreted by mononuclear phagocytes that hydrolyzes bonds present in bacterial cell walls.

Lytic pathway. The complement pathway effected by components C5–C9 that is responsible for lysis of sensitized cell plasma membranes.

MALT (mucosa-associated lymphoid tissue). Generic term for lymphoid tissue associated with the gastrointestinal tract, bronchial tree, and other mucosas.

Mannose receptor (MR). A lectin-like receptor found on mononuclear phagocytes.

MAMPs. Microbe-associated molecular patterns are molecular signatures that originate from bacteria, parasites and fungi and which are recognized by the innate immune system.

MAP kinases. A group of intracellular enzymes involved in signaling cascades that lead to the activation of transcription factors.

Marginal zone. An area surrounding the splenic white pulp that separates the lymphoid areas from the surrounding red pulp.

Mast cells. Cells found distributed near blood vessels in most tissues. These cells are full of granules containing inflammatory mediators.

Matrix metalloproteases. A group of zinc-containing degradative enzymes that can break down components of the extracellular matrix (e.g. collagenase).

MCPs (macrophage chemotactic proteins). The old name for a group of chemokines.

Membrane attack complex (MAC). The assembled terminal complement components C5b–C9 of the lytic pathway that becomes inserted into cell membranes.

Memory cells. Long-lived lymphocytes that have already been primed with their antigen, but have not undergone terminal differentiation into effector cells. They react more readily than naive lymphocytes when restimulated with the same antigen.

MHC (major histocompatibility complex). A genetic region found in all mammals, the products of which are primarily responsible for the rapid rejection of grafts between individuals and function in signaling between lymphocytes and cells expressing antigen.

MHC restriction. A characteristic of many immune reactions in which cells cooperate most effectively with other cells that share a MHC haplotype.

Microglia. Mononuclear phagocytes resident in the brain and spinal cord. Microglial precursors colonize the human central nervous system early in gestation.

MIF (migration inhibition factor). A group of peptides produced by lymphocytes that are capable of inhibiting macrophage migration.

MIIC compartment. An endosomal compartment where MHC class II molecules are loaded with antigenic peptides.

MIPs (macrophage inflammatory proteins). The old name for a group of chemokines.

Mitogens. Substances that cause cells, particularly lymphocytes, to undergo cell division.

MLR/MLC (mixed lymphocyte reaction/mixed lymphocyte culture). Assay system for T cell recognition of allogeneic cells in which response is measured by proliferation in the presence of the stimulating cells.

Mononuclear phagocyte system. The lineage of fixed and mobile long-lived phagocytic cells including blood monocytes and tissue macrophages.

Myeloid cells. The lineages of bone marrow-derived phagocytes, including neutrophils, eosinophils, and monocytes.

Myeloma. A lymphoma produced from cells of the B cell lineage that can invade bone.

N regions. Gene segments present in recombined antigen receptor genes that are not present in the germline DNA.

Neoplasm. A synonym for cancerous tissue.

Neutrophils. Polymorphonuclear granulocytes, which form the major population of blood leukocytes.

NF-κB. A transcription factor that is widely used by different leukocyte populations to signal activation – sometimes called the master-switch of the immune system.

NK (natural killer) cells. A group of lymphocytes that have the intrinsic ability to recognize and destroy some virally infected cells and some tumor cells.

Nod-like receptors (NLRs) Nucleotide oligomerization domain-like receptors are pattern recognition receptors that sense intracytoplasmic pathogens

Nucleotide oligomerization domains (NODs). Domains in intracellular receptors for pathogen-associated molecular patterns.

Nude mouse. A genetically athymic mouse that lacks a transcription factor, which is also required for hair production.

Opsonization. A process by which phagocytosis is facilitated by the deposition of opsonins (e.g. antibody and C3b) on the antigen.

PAF (platelet activating factor). A factor released by basophils that causes platelets to aggregate.

PALS (periarteriolar lymphatic sheath). The accumulations of lymphoid tissue constituting the white pulp of the spleen.

Paneth cells. Cells present in the crypts of the small intestine that secrete antimicrobial peptides.

Paracrine. The action of a cytokine on a cell distinct from the cell that produced it.

Passenger cells. Donor leukocytes present in a tissue graft that may sensitize the recipient to the graft.

Patch test. Application of antigen to skin on a patch to test for type IV hypersensitivity reactions.

Pathogen. An organism that causes disease.

Pathogen-associated molecular patterns (PAMPs). Biological macromolecules produced by microbial pathogens that are recognized by receptors on mononuclear phagocytes and some opsonins in serum and tissue fluids.

PC (phosphorylcholine). A commonly used hapten that is also found on the surface of a number of microorganisms.

Pentraxins. A group of acute-phase pentameric molecules present in serum that recognize PAMPs and opsonize bacteria for phagocytosis.

Perforin. A granule-associated molecule of cytotoxic cells, homologous to complement C9. It can form pores on the membrane of a target cell.

Peyer's patches. Collections of lymphoid cells in the wall of the gut that form a secondary lymphoid tissue.

PFC (plaque forming cell). An antibody-producing cell detected in vitro by its ability to lyze antigen-sensitized erythrocytes in the presence of complement.

PHA (phytohemagglutin). A mitogen for T cells.

Phagocytosis. The process by which cells engulf material and enclose it within a vacuole (phagosome) in the cytoplasm.

Phenotype. The expressed characteristics of an individual (cf. genotype).

Plasma cell. An antibody-producing B cell that has reached the end of its differentiation pathway.

Plasmin system. One of the plasma enzyme systems that generates the fibrinolytic enzyme, plasmin, and also contributes to inflammation and tissue remodeling.

Pokeweed mitogen. A mitogen for B and T cells.

Polymorphs. A common acronym for polymorphonuclear leukocytes, including basophils, neutrophils, and eosinophils.

Prick test. Introduction of minute quantities of antigen into the skin to test for type I hypersensitivity.

Primary lymphoid tissues. Lymphoid organs in which lymphocytes complete their initial maturation steps; they include the fetal liver, adult bone marrow, and thymus, and bursa of Fabricius in birds.

Primary response. The immune response (cellular or humoral) following an initial encounter with a particular antigen.

Prime. To induce an initial sensitization to antigen.

Privileged tissues/sites. In the context of transplantation these are tissues that induce weak immune responses or sites of the body that are partly shielded from graft rejection reactions.

Prostaglandins. Pharmacologically active derivatives of arachidonic acid. Different prostaglandins are capable of modulating cell mobility and immune responses.

Proteasomes. Organelles that degrade cellular proteins tagged for breakdown by ubiquitination.

Protein A and protein G. Components of the cell wall of some strains of staphylococci that bind to Fc of most IgG isotypes.

PRRs (pattern recognition receptors) are groups of molecules that can detect PAMP, for example the Toll-like receptors and the collectins.

Pseudoalleles. Tandem variants of a gene: they do not occupy a homologous position on the chromosome (e.g. C4).

Pseudogenes. Genes that have homologous structures to other genes, but are incapable of being expressed (e.g. *Jk3* in the mouse).

Pyrogen. A microbial product or chemokine that induces fever (e.g. LPS, IL-1).

Radioimmunoassay (RIA). A number of different sensitive techniques for measuring antigen or antibody titers using radiolabeled reagents.

RAG-1 and RAG-2. Recombination activating genes required for recombination of V, D, and J gene segments during generation of functional antigen receptor genes.

Rapamycin. A bacterial product, used as an immunosuppressive agent in transplantation.

Receptor. A cell surface molecule that binds specifically to particular extracellular molecules.

Receptor editing. A process by which immunoglobulin genes can undergo a secondary recombination event, in order to rescue B cells that are producing non-functional or autoreactive antibodies.

Recombination. A process by which genetic information is rearranged during meiosis. This process also occurs during the somatic rearrangements of DNA, which occur in the formation of genes encoding antibody molecules and T cell antigen receptors.

Relative risk. A number that expresses how much more likely (>1) or less likely (<1) an individual is to develop a particular disease if they possess a particular genotype.

Respiratory burst. Increase in oxidative metabolism of phagocytes following uptake of opsonized particles.

Reticuloendothelial system. A diffuse system of phagocytic cells derived from the bone marrow stem cells that are associated with the connective tissue framework of the liver, spleen, lymph nodes, and other serous cavities. An old-fashioned term that is rarely used – mononuclear phagocyte system is the preferred term.

RLRs (rig-like receptors). A group of intracellular helicases that can detect dsRNA and act as sensors of viral infection.

ROIs/RNIs (reactive oxygen intermediates/reactive nitrogen intermediates). Bactericidal metabolites produced by phagocytic cells, including hydrogen peroxide, hypohalites, and nitric oxide.

Scavenger receptors. A group of receptors that recognize cell debris and are involved in the phagocytosis of apoptotic cells and some pathogens.

SCID (severe combined immunodeficiency). A group of genetic conditions leading to major deficiencies or absence of both B cells and T cells.

Secondary response. The immune response that follows a second or subsequent encounter with a particular antigen.

Secretory component. A polypeptide produced by cells of some secretory epithelia that is involved in transporting secreted polymeric IgA across the cell and protecting it from digestion in the gastrointestinal tract.

Selectins. Three adhesion molecules (P-selectin (CD62P), E-selectin (CD62E), and L-selectin (CD62L)) involved in slowing leukocytes during their transit through venules.

Serotonin. 5-Hydroxytryptamine.

SLE (systemic lupus erythematosus). An autoimmune disease (non-organ specific) of humans usually involving anti-nuclear antibodies.

Somatic mutation. A process occurring during B cell maturation and affecting the antibody gene region that permits refinement of antibody specificity.

Spleen. A major secondary lymphoid organ in the peritoneal cavity next to the stomach.

STATs. A group of proteins that form components of transcription factors following activation by kinases.

Stem cell factor (SCF). Also called steel factor. A cytokine required for the earliest stages of leukocyte development in bone marrow.

Superantigens. Antigens that stimulate clones of T cells with different antigen specificity but using the same TCR V genes.

Suppressor (Ts) cells. Functionally defined populations of T cells that reduce the immune responses of other T cells or B cells, or switch the response into a different pathway to that under investigation. See also 'Tregs'.

Surface plasmon resonance. A biophysical phenomenon that can be used to measure the association and binding constants of proteins in solution interacting with bound ligands.

Synergism. Cooperative interaction.

Syngeneic. Strains of animals produced by repeated inbreeding so that each pair of autosomes within an individual is identical.

T cells. Lymphocytes that differentiate primarily in the thymus and are central to the control and development of immune responses. The principal subgroups are cytotoxic T cells (Tc) and T helper cells (TH0, TH1, TH2, and TH17).

Tregs (regulatory T cells). A functionally defined group of T cells which control (especially) autoimmune reactions, and inflammation in the gut and skin.

TAP transporters. A group of molecules that transport proteins and peptides between intracellular compartments.

TCR (T cell receptor). The T cell antigen receptor consisting of either an αβ dimer (TCR-2) or a γδ dimer (TCR-1) associated with the CD3 molecular complex.

T-dependent/T-independent antigens. T-dependent antigens require immune recognition by both T and B cells to produce an immune response. T-independent antigens can directly stimulate B cells to produce specific antibody.

TGFs (transforming growth factors). A group of cytokines identified by their ability to promote fibroblast growth; they are also generally immunosuppressive.

Thoracic duct. Drains efferent lymph into the venous system.

Thromboxanes. Products of arachidonic acid metabolism, some of which are involved in inflammation.

Thymus. A primary lymphoid organ in the thoracic cavity over the heart.

Tissue inhibitors of matrix metalloproteases (TIMPs). A group of proteins released by cells in tissues, that limit the activity of matrix metalloproteases.

Tissue typing. Determination of an individual's allotypic variants of MHC molecules.

TNF (tumor necrosis factor). A cytokine released by activated macrophages that is structurally related to lymphotoxin released by activated T cells.

Tolerance. A state of specific immunological unresponsiveness.

Toll-like receptors (TLRs). A group of receptors, mostly located on the plasma membrane, that recognize PAMPs and transduce signals for inflammation.

Tonsils. Paired lymphoid organs in the throat that form part of the mucosa-associated lymphoid tissue (MALT).

Transformation. Morphological changes in a lymphocyte associated with the onset of division. Also used to denote the change to the autonomously dividing state of a cancer cell.

Transgenic animal. An animal in which one or more new genes have been incorporated. These are often placed under specific promoters so that they are expressed only in particular tissues for limited periods.

Tumor necrosis factors (TNFs). A group of proinflammatory cytokines encoded within the MHC.

V domains. The N terminal domains of antibody heavy and light chains and the α, β, γ, and δ chains of the T cell receptor that become recombined with appropriate sets of D and J genes during lymphocyte ontogeny.

Vaccination. A general term for immunization against infectious disease, originally derived from immunization against smallpox, which uses the vaccinia virus.

Vasoactive amines. Products such as histamine and 5-hydroxytryptamine (serotonin) released by basophils, mast cells, and platelets that act on the endothelium and smooth muscle of the local vasculature.

Veiled cells. Cells of the dendritic cell lineage as seen in afferent lymph. They may be derived from Langerhans' cells or other dendritic cell types.

VLA-1–VLA-6 (very late antigens). The set of integrins that share a common β1 chain (CD29).

Waldeyer's ring. The secondary lymphoid tissues of the nasopharynx that includes the tonsils and adenoids.

Western blotting. A technique for identifying and characterizing proteins using antibodies. Synonymous with immunoblotting.

White pulp. The lymphoid component of spleen consisting of periarteriolar sheaths of lymphocytes and antigen-presenting cells.

Xenogeneic. Refers to interspecies antigenic differences.

Index

Note: Page numbers followed by *b* indicate boxes, *f* indicate figures and *t* indicate tables.

A